W9-BLM-093

PERCUTANEOUS

BALLOON VALVULOPLASTY

AND

RELATED TECHNIQUES

PERCUTANEOUS
BALLOON VALVULOPLASTY
AND
RELATED TECHNIQUES

EDITORS

THOMAS M. BASHORE, M.D.
Associate Professor of Medicine
Director, Cardiac Catheterization Laboratories
Duke University Medical Center
Durham, North Carolina

CHARLES J. DAVIDSON, M.D.
Assistant Professor of Medicine
Associate Director
Cardiac Catheterization Laboratories
Duke University Medical Center
Durham, North Carolina

WILLIAMS & WILKINS
BALTIMORE · HONG KONG · LONDON · MUNICH
PHILADELPHIA · SAN FRANCISCO · SYDNEY · TOKYO

Editor: Jonathan W. Pine, Jr.
Associate Editor: Linda Napora
Copy Editor: Martha Wolf
Designer: Dan Pfisterer
Illustration Planner: Ray Lowman
Production Coordinator: Adèle Boyd-Lanham

Copyright © 1991
Williams & Wilkins
428 East Preston Street
Baltimore, Maryland 21202, USA

All rights reserved. This book is protected by copyright. No part of this book may be reproduced in any form or by any means, including photocopying, or utilized by any information storage and retrieval system without written permission from the copyright owner.

Accurate indications, adverse reactions, and dosage schedules for drugs are provided in this book, but it is possible that they may change. The reader is urged to review the package information data of the manufacturers of the medications mentioned.

Printed in the United States of America

Library of Congress Cataloging-in-Publication Data

Percutaneous balloon valvuloplasty and related techniques / editors, Thomas M. Bashore,
    Charles J. Davidson.
        p.   cm.
    Includes index.
    ISBN 0-683-00345-3
    1. Percutaneous balloon valvuloplasty.   2. Percutaneous balloon valvotomy.
3. Aortic valve stenosis—Surgery.   4. Mitral stenosis—Surgery.   I. Bashore,
Thomas M.   II. Davidson, Charles J.
    [DNLM: 1. Aortic Valve Stenosis—therapy.   2. Balloon Dilatation.   3. Heart
Valve Disease—therapy.   4. Mitral Valve Stenosis—therapy.   5. Congenital Heart
Disease—therapy.   WG 265 P429]
RD598.35.P37P47   1991
617.4′12059—dc20
DNLM/DLC
for Library of Congress   90-13140
                                                                                      CIP

91 92 93 94 95
1 2 3 4 5 6 7 8 9 10

Preface

The renowned physician Austin Flint once commented that in regard to valvular heart lesions, "the anatomic changes which the valves and orifices have undergone are irremediable, and therefore, do not claim any special medical treatment. The existing lesions must remain. The damage which they have occasioned cannot be repaired. Medication employed for that object will be worse than useless . . . Truth and justice to the physician himself, as well as good faith toward the patient, require that fact should be candidly stated." (Quoted from Flint A: *A Practical Treatice on the Diagnoses, Pathology and Treatment of Diseases of the Heart.* Philadelphia: Blanchard and Lea, 1859, pp 217 and 229.)

We have come a long way since the days of Austin Flint's bleak assessment of the therapy of valvular heart disease. Not only have there been tremendous advances in the surgical therapy of valvular heart disease, there is now growing excitement regarding the role catheter therapy might play. *Percutaneous Balloon Valvuloplasty and Related Techniques* is an effort to put a current perspective on the catheter treatment of both valvular and congenital heart disease.

Section I includes a general discussion of the indications for balloon valvuloplasty, the pathology involved in aortic and mitral stenosis, and the vagaries in the hemodynamic assessment of stenotic valve lesions. The next two sections are an overview of the aortic (Section II) and mitral (Section III) valvuloplasty/valvotomy procedures. Within each section, the clinical evaluation and the indications for *any* therapy in these patients are outlined in a separate chapter. There is discussion of the use of noninvasive techniques in the evaluation of these lesions followed by the details regarding the actual balloon procedure, the complications that have been reported, and both the acute and the follow-up results that can be expected using current technology. Finally, a cardiovascular surgical perspective is presented for balance. Section IV is devoted to reviewing the catheter treatment of children and neonates suffering from a wide variety of congenital heart disease syndromes. A cardiovascular surgical perspective is again provided. Each chapter has been written by a known authority in the field. Not only are summary data provided, but the opinions of each of these experts are expressed openly and candidly.

The advances in catheter techniques described herein represent the dawn of a new era in valvular and congenital heart disease therapy. Though the entire field is in its infancy, it is becoming increasingly clear that there are a variety of valvular and congenital lesions that can be repaired without splitting the sternum. This is a natural evolution for cardiovascular medicine regarding the therapy for these disorders. Austin Flint would have been impressed.

THOMAS M. BASHORE
CHARLES J. DAVIDSON

Contributors

THOMAS M. BASHORE, M.D.
Associate Professor of Medicine
Director, Cardiac Catheterization Laboratories
Duke University Medical Center
Durham, North Carolina

PETER C. BLOCK, M.D.
Director, Cardiac Catheterization Laboratories
Massachusetts General Hospital
Associate Professor of Medicine
Harvard Medical School
Boston, Massachusetts

RAOUL BONAN, M.D.
Assistant Professor of Medicine
University of Montreal Faculty of Medicine
Director, Cardiac Catheterization Laboratory
Montreal Heart Institute
Montreal, Quebec, Canada

HARISIOS BOUDOULAS, M.D.
Professor of Medicine
Division of Cardiology
The Ohio State University
College of Medicine
Columbus, Ohio

CHARLES J. DAVIDSON, M.D.
Assistant Professor of Medicine
Associate Director
Cardiac Catheterization Laboratories
Duke University Medical Center
Durham, North Carolina

JOHN FAHEY, M.D.
Assistant Professor of Pediatrics
Yale University School of Medicine
New Haven, Connecticut

FRANK L. HANLEY, M.D.
Assistant Professor of Surgery
Harvard Medical School

Associate in Surgery
The Children's Hospital
Boston, Massachusetts

WILLIAM E. HELLENBRAND, M.D.
Associate Professor of Pediatrics and Diagnostic
    Imaging
Yale University School of Medicine
Director, Pediatric Cardiac Catheterization
    Laboratory at Yale-New Haven Hospital
New Haven, Connecticut

PAUL J. HENDRY, M.D.
Assistant Professor
Department of Surgery
University of Ottawa Heart Institute
Ottawa, Ontario, Canada

RONALD J. KANTER, M.D.
Assistant Professor
Pediatric Cardiology
Duke University Medical Center
Durham, North Carolina

DAVID KASS, M.D.
Assistant Professor of Medicine
Division of Cardiology
The Johns Hopkins University School of Medicine
Baltimore, Maryland

THIERRY LEFÈVRE
Centre Chirurgical Henri Hartman
UCVI
Neuilly sur Seine, France

JAMES E. LOWE, M.D.
Associate Professor of Surgery and Pathology
Director, Surgical Electrophysiology Service
Duke University Medical Center
Durham, North Carolina

CHARLES McKAY, M.D.
Associate Professor
Department of Cardiology
University of Iowa College of Medicine
Iowa City, Iowa

CATHERINE M. OTTO, M.D.
Assistant Professor of Medicine
University of Washington School of Medicine
Seattle, Washington

IGOR F. PALACIOS, M.D.
Director, Interventional Cardiology
Cardiac Catheterization Laboratories
Massachusetts General Hospital
Associate Professor of Medicine
Harvard Medical School
Boston, Massachusetts

STANTON B. PERRY, M.D.
Division of Pediatric Cardiology
The Children's Hospital
Boston, Massachusetts

P. SYAMASUNDAR RAO, M.D.
Professor of Pediatrics
Head, Division of Pediatric Cardiology
University of Wisconsin Medical School
University of Wisconsin Children's Hospital
Madison, Wisconsin

ROBERT D. SAFIAN, M.D.
Assistant Professor of Medicine
Harvard Medical School
Associate Director, Interventional
   Cardiology
Beth Israel Hospital
Boston, Massachusetts

ANTONIO SERRA, M.D.
Servei de Cardiologia
Hospital Clinic i Provincial
Barcelona, Spain

KHALID SHEIKH, M.D.
Assistant Professor of Medicine
Duke University Medical Center
Durham, North Carolina

ELIZABETH A. SPARKS, R.N.
Coordinator of James W. Overstreet Research
   and Teaching Laboratory
Ohio State University
Columbus, Ohio

E. MURAT TUZCU, M.D.
Cardiac Catheterization Laboratories
Massachusetts General Hospital
Instructor in Medicine
Harvard Medical School
Boston, Massachusetts

ROSS M. UNGERLEIDER, M.D.
Assistant Professor, General and Thoracic Surgery
Chief, Pediatric Cardiac Surgery
Duke University Medical Center
Durham, North Carolina

JAMES W. VanTASSEL, M.D.
Nasser, Smith, Pinkerton, Cardiology, Inc.
The Indiana Heart Institute
Cardiovascular Pathology Registry
St. Vincent Hospital
Indianapolis, Indiana

PETER VAN TRIGT, M.D.
Assistant Professor, General and Thoracic Surgery
Duke University Medical Center
Durham, North Carolina

BRUCE F. WALLER, M.D.
Nasser, Smith, Pinkerton, Cardiology, Inc.
The Indiana Heart Institute
Cardiovascular Pathology Registry
St. Vincent Hospital
Indianapolis, Indiana

ROBERT A. WAUGH, M.D.
Associate Professor of Medicine
Duke University Medical Center
Durham, North Carolina

CHARLES F. WOOLEY, M.D.
Professor of Medicine
Division of Cardiology
The Ohio State University College of Medicine
Columbus, Ohio

Contents

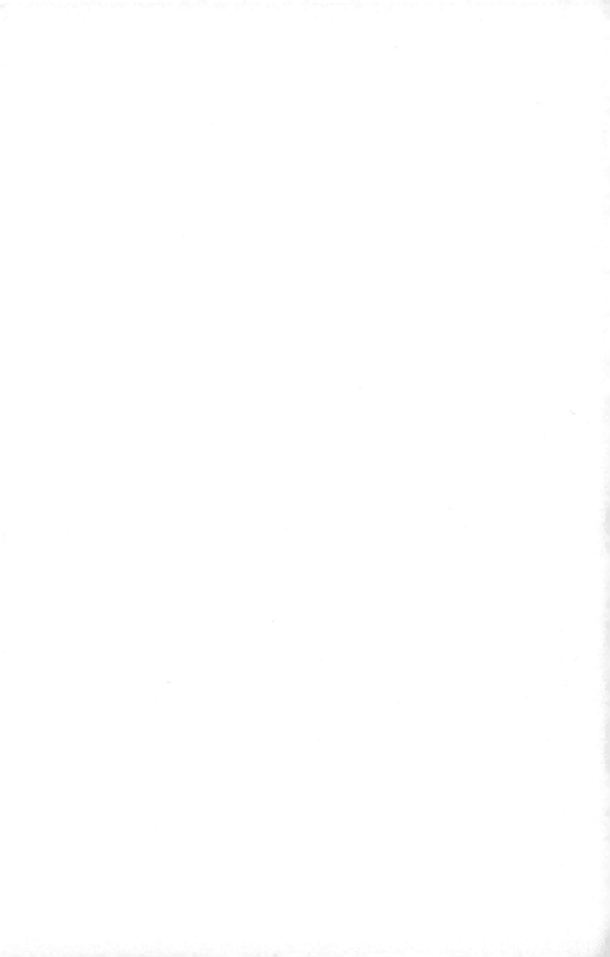

SECTION I.

INTRODUCTION

1

Current Indications for Percutaneous Valvuloplasty and Valvotomy Procedures in the Adult

CHARLES J. DAVIDSON and THOMAS M. BASHORE

The emergence of catheter-based balloon dilation of adult valvular stenoses has been undertaken with both enthusiasm and caution. Since these procedures represent a relatively new modality as a therapeutic alternative to medical or surgical therapy, only data on short-term and intermediate-term outcome are available, with long-term results yet to be defined. Thus, the current indications for percutaneous balloon valvuloplasty outlined in this chapter must be tempered by the realization that 5- and 10-year follow-up are yet to be reported.

However, based on the differing types of valvular stenoses and the emerging knowledge regarding mechanisms of successful balloon dilation, certain indications are now evident. A general overview of potential indications for stenotic aortic, mitral, tricuspid, pulmonic, and bioprosthetic valves will be discussed. More specific data regarding each of these procedures as well as other catheter-based interventions are provided in the chapters dealing with each subject individually.

PERCUTANEOUS BALLOON AORTIC VALVULOPLASTY

The initial enthusiasm and hope for widespread application of percutaneous balloon aortic valvuloplasty (BAV) have been tempered by evidence for early restenosis and early return of clinical symptoms in many patients. Thus, the clearest indications for BAV of critical aortic stenosis are limited in adults to those particular situations in which the surgical risk for aortic valve replacement is considered high or the procedure is meant to be temporizing measure prior to eventual aortic valve replacement. The procedure still can be beneficial in certain subsets and does provide a therapeutic option for many patients that had none prior to the emergence of BAV as an alternative.

When evaluating a potential candidate for BAV, awareness of the surgical risk is essential. A variable perception of the risk often exists between the cardiologist and the surgeon. Therefore, consultation with a cardiac surgeon is highly desirable prior to attempting any catheter intervention, but particularly prior to aortic valvuloplasty. Surgical risk has been addressed in a number of studies describing the characteristics that are most predictive of morbidity and mortality following cardiac surgery.[1–5] The most consistent factors that predict early mortality include advanced age (i.e., >70 years), the need for emergent surgery, and the presence of depressed preoperative left ventricular function. Although aortic valve replacement combined with coronary artery bypass grafting has a higher operative mortality, the independent negative predictive value of the combined operations has yet to be demonstrated in a large series.[3]

Indications for percutaneous balloon aortic valvuloplasty can be classified into two broad categories. The first are those patients with symptomatic, calcific aortic stenosis (AS) (generally degenerative), and the second are those with symptomatic, noncalcific aortic stenosis (generally bicuspid). Table 1.1 summarizes these current indications. In most situations, a determined aortic valve area of ≤ 0.8 cm^2 should be present prior to considering the procedure.

Table 1.1.
Indications for Percutaneous Balloon
Aortic Valvuloplasty

I. Symptomatic severe *calcific* aortic stenosis with ≤ 2 +
   aortic regurgitation
   A. High risk for aortic valve replacement
      1. Advanced physiologic age
      2. Presence of associated serious comorbid dis-
         ease that may limit longevity or functional
         improvement
      3. Apparent severely depressed LV function
         (valvuloplasty as a diagnostic intervention)
   B. Need for temporizing or "bridge" procedure in
      patients with serious, but potentially reversible,
      cardiac disease
      1. Cardiogenic shock or severe CHF
      2. Recent myocardial infarction
      3. As a "bailout" during acute decompensation
II. Symptomatic *noncalcific* aortic stenosis with ≤ 2 +
    aortic regurgitation
    A. High risk for aortic valve replacement
       1. Associated serious comorbid disease present
       2. Apparent severely depressed LV function
    B. As a "bridge" procedure
       1. During pregnancy
       2. As a "bailout" during acute decompensation
    C. As possible primary therapy
       1. Pediatric or neonatal AS
       2. Rheumatic AS

Patients with calcific AS can be subdivided into
those patients at high risk for aortic valve replacement and into those in whom the procedure is
meant to provide interim relief only. High-risk
patients are those physiologically 80 years or older
in whom symptomatic improvement is the primary
and only goal.[6-8] Since survival may not be altered
by BAV, especially at this age, but short-term
functional status is usually improved, this procedure appears to be well suited to physiologically
elderly patients with severely symptomatic aortic
stenosis. However, these patients should not be
considered a uniform group, and in many cases,
aortic valve replacement can be performed at only
slight additional risk even in octogenarians. Patients with serious comorbid disease such as
malignancy, renal or hepatic failure, severe COPD,
or altered mental or neurologic status are generally
considered poor surgical candidates and may
derive benefit from BAV by improving their
cardiac functional class.

The role of BAV as a temporizing or palliative
procedure has now been detailed in a number of
small series and case reports[9-15] and represents a
second subset of patients in whom BAV can be
applied successfully. Patients with AS who require
noncardiac surgery are at a known increased risk
for cardiac complications that include myocardial
infarction, hemorrhage, infection, and congestive
heart failure.[16,17] Urgent noncardiac surgery and
elective noncardiac surgery can be successfully
performed in these patients soon after balloon
aortic valvuloplasty. The acute hemodynamic
improvement achieved with BAV may reduce the
risk of general anesthesia and the overall cardiac
complications from major noncardiac surgery or
noncardiac procedures.[11-13] Associated carcino-
mas (e.g., lung, colon, prostate, rectum) are the
most commonly described comorbid diseases in
which BAV has been used to improve hemodynamics prior to resection. Hip fractures and
abdominal aortic aneurysm are other commonly
associated problems that occur with some frequency in patients with severe senile calcific
aortic stenosis; BAV may help reduce surgical
risk in this subset as well. Controlled studies will
be necessary to determine whether BAV does
indeed lessen preoperative morbidity and mortality for most noncardiac surgery or procedures.
The studies to date have demonstrated an apparent improved surgical risk based only on historical controls. With the use of modern anesthesia,
the need for BAV prior to noncardiac surgery
may be less important than in years past.

The treatment of patients presenting with
cardiogenic shock secondary to AS may be a special
case in which BAV is uniquely suited to stabilize
hemodynamics prior to elective surgery.[15] These
patients are at particularly high risk for open heart
surgery and acutely often respond favorably following the procedure.

It is well documented that the hemodynamic
and symptomatic improvement observed following aortic valvuloplasty may be transient. However, in some patients, significant short-term
recovery of left ventricular (LV) function does
occur. Should improvement in LV function and
overall cardiovascular hemodynamics occur following BAV, then aortic valve replacement may be
undertaken at a lower risk. Thus, BAV can be
utilized as a planned "bridge" to eventual aortic
valve replacement. Alternatively, BAV may provide a "diagnostic intervention" to determine
whether LV function will improve by diminishing
the afterload mismatch that occurs in patients with
severe AS. The degree of LV functional improvement that can be expected is likely dependent on

the quality of the success of the valvuloplasty procedure and the inherent pathology of the aortic valve itself.

Critical AS during pregnancy presents an especially difficult management problem for both the mother and fetus. Fortunately, the association is uncommonly seen. Since cardiac output must be increased despite fixed outflow obstruction during pregnancy, AS may result in sudden death or intractable heart failure. Aortic valve replacement during pregnancy carries a 1.5% maternal mortality and a 9.5% fetal mortality.[18] Furthermore, warfarin therapy is usually considered risky due to bleeding and potential teratogenicity. A recent report describes a patient with congestive failure, angina, and syncope in whom BAV was performed at 19 weeks' gestation. Aortic valvuloplasty was successfully performed, and a normal vaginal delivery occurred at 40 weeks.[14] While severe AS in women of childbearing age is unusual, it does point out the value of using percutaneous balloon procedures for palliation until aortic valve replacement can be entertained.

The value of BAV in the neonatal and pediatric patient is still under investigation. Although early results in some series are promising, there remains the question of whether the risk:benefit ratio warrants its widespread application. The procedure and details regarding those risks and benefits are covered elsewhere in this volume, but generally a wait-and-see attitude has developed in this setting.

Diagnostic cardiac catheterization in patients with severe AS can produce hemodynamic deterioration due to ischemia or fluid overload. Balloon aortic valvuloplasty has been advocated as a "bailout" during diagnostic catheterization when resuscitation from acute hemodynamic decompensation is necessary.[9,10] Aortic valve replacement may then be contemplated following stabilization of the hemodynamics.

Combined balloon aortic and mitral valvuloplasty has recently been reported in 10 patients with rheumatic stenoses of both valves.[19] The procedures were initially successful in 9, and persistent clinical improvement was noted at 8 months in all patients. As opposed to that observed with calcific AS, the pathology of rheumatic AS routinely includes commissural fusion and thus may lend itself particularly well to valvuloplasty. Thus, despite the lack of long-term follow-up currently available, BAV may emerge a valid alternative for patients with rheumatic AS in

whom associated aortic regurgitation has not developed.

Repeat balloon aortic valvuloplasty for symptomatic restenosis generally provides hemodynamic changes similar to the initial procedure.[20] However, the clinical outcome is much poorer than that after the initial procedure and appears closely related to underlying LV function.[20] The excessively high cardiac death rate (8 of 17 within 2 months) noted after repeat BAV suggests that repeat procedure cannot be advocated as a procedure to improve survival, although short-term symptomatic and functional status may improve in the minority of patients.

Severe aortic regurgitation is generally considered a contraindication to balloon valvuloplasty. However, this is not due to a worsening of aortic regurgitation. Serial quantitative and qualitative determinations of the degree of aortic regurgitation induced by balloon aortic valvuloplasty provide evidence that significant increases in aortic regurgitation severity are unusual.[21] When mild or moderate regurgitation is present, a quantitative and qualitative decrease in the severity of regurgitation has also been observed following hemodynamically successful valvuloplasty, but this is uncommon.[21] The hemodynamic load from aortic regurgitation must be assumed to remain relatively unchanged in the vast majority of patients.

PERCUTANEOUS BALLOON MITRAL VALVOTOMY

As opposed to balloon aortic valvuloplasty, balloon mitral valvotomy (BMV) has resulted in excellent short- and long-term improvement in both hemodynamics and cardiovascular symptoms.[22–25] A mitral valve area of ≤ 1.7 cm^2 is usually required before one can be assured that symptoms are related to mitral stenosis. The favorable outcome from BMV appears to be primarily due to the rheumatic etiology of mitral stenosis, with commissural fusion predominating as opposed to the "weighted down" cusps seen in calcific AS. The mechanism of successful balloon dilation is due to commissural splitting that results in a sustained increase in mitral valve area.[25–27] In patients with significant submitral scar or valvular calcification, the results are much poorer. Similar observations have been known for years in regard to either surgical closed or open mitral commissurotomy. Overall, the same patients who are candidates for surgical commissurotomy appear to benefit from

BMV. Although long-term follow-up still is unavailable following BMV, it is anticipated that the long-term results are similar to those seen with the surgical approach.

Table 1.2 outlines those patients in whom BMV appears to be most effective. Based on the data presently available, the anatomy and pathologic features of the mitral valve as determined by echocardiography and fluoroscopy are the most important factors determining outcome of BMV.[27–30] Patients with pliable noncalcified leaflets and without subvalvular disease have achieved the best short- and intermediate-term results. An echocardiographic scoring system developed at the Massachusetts General Hospital[28,29] has proven to be quite useful in defining those patients likely to benefit from mitral valvotomy. Leaflet rigidity, leaflet thickening, leaflet calcification, and subvalvular thickening are each scored from 0 to 4+ (least to most). A high score (>8) indicates more severe disease and is an independent predictor of restenosis. Other factors, especially an elderly age or the presence of mitral regurgitation or atrial fibrillation, also reduce the chance for success. Thus, the presence of leaflet rigidity, thickening, calcium, and subvalvular disease is predictive of a poorer immediate result and earlier restenosis.[27–30] Mitral stenosis due to annular calcification and calcium invasion of the mitral valve, as seen in many elderly patients, usually responds poorly to balloon valvotomy techniques.

Other exclusionary criteria include the presence of significant or symptomatic coronary artery disease requiring surgery or the detection of a left atrial thrombus by either surface or transesoph-ageal echocardiography. Since surface echocardiography is limited in its ability to detect small thrombi or left atrial in the appendage,[31] it is highly desirable that a transesophageal echocardiogram be obtained prior to attempted BMV in all patients. Although a left atrial thrombus is generally considered an absolute contraindication to balloon valvotomy, resolution of thrombus has been noted after prolonged warfarin therapy.[32] As a consequence, in our institution warfarin is recommended in all patients for a minimum of 4 weeks before the valvotomy procedure. Since thrombi can form on the ulcerated valve as well as in the left atrium, 4 weeks of anticoagulation is advised regardless of whether the patient is in sinus rhythm or in atrial fibrillation. As with aortic stenosis, the presence of more than mild ($\geq 2+$) mitral insufficiency precludes performance of BMV. In addition, excessive thickening of the interatrial septum may hinder passing of the balloon catheter into the left atrium during the procedure.[33] This feature should be added to the list of echocardiographic descriptors considered when assessing patients for this procedure.

Patients with recurrent mitral stenosis after surgical commissurotomy represent a special subgroup of patients. Once again, valvular and leaflet morphology appear to be the predominant factors identifying patient outcome,[34] and these patients are good candidates for percutaneous mitral valvotomy if the valve apparatus is favorable. A discussion of neonatal and pediatric balloon mitral valvotomy can be found in Chapters 16 and 17. The value of the procedure in nonrheumatic or mitral prosthetic valve stenosis has yet to be demonstrated.

Table 1.2.
Indications for Percutaneous Balloon Mitral Valvotomy

Symptomatic rheumatic mitral stenosis with $\leq 2+$ mitral regurgitation
A. Favorable echocardiographic descriptors
   1. Commissural fusion with pliable leaflets
   2. Insignificant fusion of submitral apparatus
   3. Minimal valvular calcification
   4. $\leq 2+$ mitral regurgitation
   5. Interatrial septal thickness ≤ 1.5 cm
   6. No evidence for left atrial thrombus or recent embolus
B. Favorable angiographic descriptors
   1. Pliable mitral valve motion
   2. $\leq 2+$ mitral regurgitation
   3. Minimal valvular calcification

BALLOON PULMONIC VALVULOPLASTY

Surgical pulmonary valvotomy has previously been the treatment of choice when patients present with moderate to severe pulmonic valvular obstruction with or without symptoms.[35–37] Moderate pulmonic stenosis is usually considered present when the transvalvular gradient is 50–79 mm Hg, and severe stenosis when > 80 mm Hg. Balloon pulmonic valvuloplasty achieves a similar immediate and sustained reduction in transvalvular gradient and an improvement in patient symptomatology.[35–38] Therefore, the recommendations for percutaneous balloon pulmonic valvuloplasty are the same as those for the surgical procedure (Table

Table 1.3.
Indications for Percutaneous Pulmonic Balloon Valvuloplasty

1. Symptomatic pulmonary valvular stenosis
2. Asymptomatic, severe pulmonary valvular stenosis (> 80 mm Hg gradient).
3. No evidence for the following:
   a. Severe pulmonic valvular regurgitation
   b. Significant subpulmonic stenosis
   c. Severe pulmonary annular hypoplasia

1.3). Since mild pulmonic stenosis (< 50 mm Hg gradient) generally is not progressive and tends to be well tolerated, balloon valvuloplasty is generally not recommended or required in these patients.

Balloon pulmonic valvuloplasty should be considered the treatment of choice for both primary valvular pulmonic stenosis and restenosis after previous surgical valvotomy even if some pulmonic valve dysplasia exists.[39–41]

The pathology of pulmonic stenosis plays a key role in the success of the procedure. Dysplastic valves may require more aggressive dilation with larger balloons to achieve an adequate result. Hypertrophic subpulmonic stenosis may also contribute to the gradient, and there are reports of severe subpulmonic stenosis occurring after pulmonic valvuloplasty.[42] This can be so severe at times that a "suicide ventricle" results. This subpulmonic obstruction may be reduced by pretreatment with beta-blockers. The presence of severe pulmonic insufficiency rarely accompanies pulmonic stenosis and when present may be difficult to detect due to high right ventricular diastolic pressures and low pulmonary artery diastolic pressures. Severe pulmonic insufficiency and markedly dysplasic pulmonary valves or significant pulmonary annular hypoplasia precludes successful pulmonic valvuloplasty.

PERCUTANEOUS BALLOON TRICUSPID VALVOTOMY

Since the etiology of tricuspid stenosis is usually due to rheumatic heart disease, commissural fusion is often the predominant mechanism of stenosis. Balloon valvotomy has been described in several case reports to represent an alternative therapy for the treatment of tricuspid stenosis.[43–45] Surgical commissurotomy has not always been effective in this setting due to resultant tricuspid regurgitation. This may also limit the widespread application of percutaneous balloon valvotomy.

Balloon dilation of the tricuspid valve produces commissural separation in a similar manner as mitral valvotomy.[43] Marked reduction in the transvalvular gradient and improved symptoms have also been described. However, no long-term follow-up or any large series of patients exist at this time in the literature. Thus, definitive recommendations cannot be made.

Based on the existing experience with balloon mitral valvotomy, the anatomic substrate may be similar. The patient with primary commissural fusion and without significant tricuspid regurgitation, valvular calcification, or subvalvular apparatus scarring is likely the ideal candidate. The tricuspid valvular apparatus differs considerably from the mitral apparatus (particularly in regard to chordal attachments to the ventricular endomyocardium as well as to papillary muscles). This difference may result in a higher likelihood of tricuspid regurgitation, especially if the right ventricle is dilated.

PERCUTANEOUS BALLOON BIOPROSTHESIS VALVULOPLASTY

Balloon dilation of bioprosthetic valves has been advocated for stenosis of porcine prosthesis in extracardiac conduits.[46,47] Transvalvular gradients have been reduced by 50%, without necessarily producing a "valveless" conduit. Some investigators have recommended balloon dilation to allow deferral of conduit replacement, thereby, permitting insertion of a larger conduit at a later date when the child is older.

Balloon dilation has also been reported for stenotic bioprostheses in both the mitral and tricuspid position[48–51] with successful reduction of the transvalvular gradient by approximately 50%. However, early restenosis appears to occur in some.[48]

Although acute valvular insufficiency does not invariably occur following dilation of bioprosthetic valves, results have been variable. McKay et al. have reported unpredictable results of balloon dilation of stenotic prosthetic aortic valves.[52] Degenerative porcine valves usually display a primary calcific degenerative process involving the cusps. Commissural fusion does not generally contribute to the etiology of the obstruction. Thus, the mechanism of prosthetic valve stenosis is a primary limitation to its applicability. We have attempted balloon dilation of autopsied specimens with destructive results. Balloon dilation of tricuspid, aortic, and mitral bioprosthesis should be reserved for the critically ill patient as a last resort, and only when surgical therapy is not a viable option.

REFERENCES

1. Craven JM, Weintraub WS, Jones EL, Guyton RA, Hatcher CR. Predictors of mortality, complications, and length of stay in aortic valve replacement for aortic stenosis. *Circulation 78* (Suppl I):I85–I90, 1988.
2. Edmunds LH, Stephenson LW, Edne RN, Ratcliffe MB. Open-heart surgery in octogenarians. *N Eng J Med 319*:131–136, 1988.
3. Magovern JA, Pennocle JL, Campbell DB, Pae WE, Bartholomew M, Pierce WS, Waldhausen JA. Aortic valve replacement and combined aortic valve replacement and coronary artery bypass grafting: Predicting high risk groups. *J Am Coll Cardiol 9*:38–43, 1987.
4. O'Toole JD, Geiser EA, Reddy PS, Curtiss EI, Landfair RM. Effect of preoperative ejection fraction on survival and hemodynamic improvement following aortic valve replacement. *Circulation 58*: 1175–1184, 1978.
5. Carabello BA, Green LH, Grossman W, Cohn LH, Koster JK, Collins JJ. Hemodynamic determinants of prognosis of aortic valve replacement in critical aortic stenosis and advanced congestive heart failure. *Circulation 62*:42–48, 1980.
6. Brady ST, Davis CA, Kussmaul WG, Laskey WK, Hirshfeld JW, Herrmann HC. Percutaneous aortic balloon valvuloplasty in octogenarians: Morbidity and mortality. *Annals Int Med 110*:761–766, 1989.
7. Letac B, Cribier A, Koning R, Lefebvre E. Aortic stenosis in elderly patients aged 80 or older: Treatment by percutaneous balloon valvuloplasty in a series of 92 cases. *Circulation 80*:1514–1520, 1989.
8. Cheitlin MD. Severe aortic stenosis in the sick octogenarian: A clear indication for balloon valvuloplasty as the initial procedure. *Circulation 80*: 1906–1908, 1989.
9. Losordo DW, Ramaswamy K, Rosenfeld K, Isner JM. Use of emergency balloon dilation to reverse acute hemodynamic decompensation developing during diagnostic catheterization for aortic stenosis (bailout valvuloplasty). *Am J Cardiol 63*:388–389, 1989.
10. Friedman HZ, Cragg DR, O'Neill WW. Cardiac resuscitation using emergency aortic balloon valvuloplasty. *Am J Cardiol 63*:387–388, 1989.
11. Levine MJ, Berman AD, Safian RD, Diver DJ, McKay RG. Palliation of valvular aortic stenosis by balloon valvuloplasty as preoperative preparation of noncardiac surgery. *Am J Cardiol 62*:1309–1310, 1988.

12. Hayes SN, Holmes DR, Nishimura RA, Reeder GS. Palliative percutaneous aortic balloon valvuloplasty before noncardiac operations and invasive diagnostic procedures. *Mayo Clin Proc 64*:753–757, 1989.
13. Roth RB, Palacios IF, Block PC. Percutaneous aortic balloon valvuloplasty: Its role in the management of patients with aortic stenosis requiring major noncardiac surgery. *J Am Coll Cardiol 13*:1039–1041, 1989.
14. Angel JL, Chapman C, Kruppel RA, Morales WJ, Sims CJ. Percutaneous balloon aortic valvuloplasty in pregnancy. *Obstetrics & Gynecology 72*:438–440, 1988.
15. Desnoyers MR, Salem DN, Rosenfeld K, Mackey W, O'Donnell T, Isner JM. Treatment of cardiogenic shock by emergency aortic balloon valvuloplasty. *Annals Int Med 108*:833–835, 1988.
16. Goldman L, Caldera DL, Southwich FS, Nussbaum SR, Murray B, O'Malley TA, Goroll AH, Caplan DH, Nolan J, Buke DS, Krogstad D, Carabello B, Slater EE. Cardiac risk factors and complications in non-cardiac surgery. *Medicine 57*:357–370, 1978.
17. Goldman L. Cardiac risks and complications of noncardiac surgery. *Annals Int Med 98*:504–513, 1983.
18. Bernal JM, Miralles PJ. Cardiac surgery with cardiopulmonary bypass during pregnancy. *Obstet Gynecol Surv 41*:1–6, 1986.
19. Medina A, Bethencourt A, Coello I, et al. Combined percutaneous mitral and aortic balloon valvuloplasty. *Am J Cardiol 64*:620–624, 1989.
20. Davidson CJ, Harrison JK, Leithe ME, Kisslo KB, Bashore TM. Left ventricular performance and clinical outcome after repeat balloon aortic valvuloplasty. *Annals Int Med 113*:250–252, 1990.
21. Davidson, CJ, Skelton TN, Kisslo KB, Burgess RE, Bashore TM. Quantification of aortic regurgitation after balloon aortic valvuloplasty using videodensitometric analysis of digital subtraction aortography. *Am J Cardiol 63*:585–588, 1989.
22. Lock JE, Khalilullah M, Shrivastava S, Bahl V, Keane JF. Percutaneous catheter commissurotomy in rheumatic mitral stenosis. *N Eng J Med 313*: 1515–1518, 1985.
23. Al Zaibag M, Ribeiro PA, Al Kassab S, Al Fagih MR. Percutaneous balloon mitral valvotomy for rheumatic mitral valve stenosis. *Lancet 1*:757–761, 1986.
24. Palacios I, Block PC, Brandi S, Blanco P, Casal H, Pulido JI, Munoz S, D'Empaire G, Ortega MA, Jacobs M, Vlahakes G. Percutaneous balloon valvotomy for patients with severe mitral stenosis. *Circulation 75*:778–784, 1987.
25. Reid CL, McKay CR, Chandraranta PAN, Kawanishi DT, Rahimtoola SH. Mechanisms of increase in mitral valve area and influence of anatomic features in double-balloon, catheter balloon valvuloplasty in adults with rheumatic mitral stenosis: A Doppler

and two-dimensional echocardiographic study. *Circulation 76*:628–636, 1987.

26. McKay RA, Lock JE, Safian RD, et al. Balloon dilatation of mitral stenosis in adult patients in postmortem and percutaneous mitral valvuloplasty studies. *J Am Coll Cardiol 9*:723–731, 1987.

27. Block PC, Palacios IF, Jacobs ML, Fallon MT. Mechanism of percutaneous balloon valvotomy. *Am J Cardiol 59*:178–179, 1987.

28. Palacios IF, Block PC, Wilkins GT, Weyman AE. Follow-up of patients undergoing percutaneous mitral balloon valvotomy: Analysis of factors determining restenosis. *Circulation 79*:573–579, 1989.

29. Wilkins GT, Weyman AE, Abscal VM, Block PC, Palacios CF. Percutaneous mitral valvotomy: An analysis of echocardiographic variables related to outcome and the mechanism of dilatation. *Brit Heart J 60*:299–308, 1988.

30. Nobuyoshi M, Hamasaki N, Kimura T, Nosaka H, Yokoi H, Yasumoto H, Horiuchi H, Nakashima H, Shindo T, Mori T, Miyamoto AT, Inoue K. Indications, complications, and short-term clinical outcome of percutaneous transvenous mitral commissurotomy. *Circulation 80*:782–792, 1989.

31. Shrestha NK, Moreno FL, Narciso FV, Torres L, Calleja HB. Two-dimensional echocardiographic diagnosis of left atrial thrombus in rheumatic heart disease. A clinicopathologic study. *Circulation 67*:341–347, 1983.

32. Hung JS, Lin FC, Chiang CW. Successful percutaneous transvenous catheter balloon mitral commissurotomy after warfarin therapy and resolution of left atrial thrombus. *Am J Cardiol 64*:126–128, 1989.

33. Sheikh KH, Davidson CJ, Skelton TN, Kisslo K, Bashore TM. Interatrial septal thickening preventing percutaneous mitral valve balloon valvuloplasty. *Am Heart J 177*:206–210, 1989.

34. Rediker DE, Block PC, Abascal VM, Palacios IF. Mitral balloon valvuloplasty for mitral restenosis after surgical commissurotomy. *J Am Coll Cardiol 11*:252–256, 1988.

35. Nadas AS. Pulmonary stenosis: Indications for surgery in children and adults. *N Eng J Med 287*:1196–1197, 1972.

36. Nugent EW, Freedom RM, Nora JJ, Ellison RC, Rowe RD, Nadas AS. Clinical course of pulmonic stenosis. *Circulation 56*:I38–I47, 1977.

37. Kan JS, White RI, Mitchell SE, Gardner TJ. Percutaneous balloon valvuloplasty: A new method for treating congenital pulmonary valve stenosis. *N Eng J Med 307*:540–543, 1982.

38. Rao PS, Fawzy ME, Solymar L, Mardini MK. Long-term results of balloon pulmonary valvuloplasty of valvular pulmonic stenosis. *Am Heart J 115*:1291–1296, 1988.

39. Rao PS. Balloon pulmonary valvuloplasty: A review. *Clin Cardiol 12*:55–94, 1989.

40. Tynan M, Baker EJ, Bohmer J, Jones ODH, Reidy JF, Joseph MC, Ottenkamp J. Percutaneous balloon pulmonary valvuloplasty. *Brit Heart J 53*:520–524, 1985.

41. Miller GAH. Balloon valvuloplasty and angioplasty in congenital heart disease. *Brit Heart J 54*:285–289, 1986.

42. Ben-Shacher G, Cohen MH, Sivakoff MC, Portman MA, Riemenschneider TA, Van Heeckeren DW. Development of infundibular obstruction after percutaneous pulmonary balloon valvuloplasty. *J Am Coll Cardiol 5*:754–756, 1985.

43. Bourdillon PD, Hookman LD, Morris SN, Waller BF. Percutaneous balloon valvuloplasty for tricuspid stenosis: Hemodynamic and pathologic findings. *Am Heart J 117*:492–495, 1989.

44. Goldenberg IF, Pederson W, Olson J, Madison JD, Mooney MR, Gobel FL. Percutaneous double balloon valvuloplasty for severe tricuspid stenosis. *Am Heart J 118*:417–419, 1989.

45. Khalilullah M, Tyagi S, Yadav BS, Jain P, Choudhry A, Lochan R. Double-balloon valvuloplasty for tricuspid stenosis. *Am Heart J 114*:1232–1233, 1987.

46. Waldman JD, Schoen FJ, Kirkpatrick SE, Mathewson JW, George L, Lamberti JJ. Balloon dilatation of porcine bioprosthetic valves in the pulmonary position. *Circulation 76*:109–114, 1987.

47. Lloyd TR, Marvin WJ, Mahoney LT, Lauer RM. Balloon dilation valvuloplasty of bioprosthetic valves in extracardiac conduits. *Am Heart J 114*:268–274, 1987.

48. Fernandez JJ, Desando J, Leff RA, Ord M, Sabbagh AH. Percutaneous balloon valvuloplasty of a stenosed mitral bioprosthesis. *Cathet Cardiovasc Diagn 19*: 39–41, 1990.

49. DeFelice CA, Mullins CE, Kumpuris AG, Raizner AE. Percutaneous balloon valvuloplasty of a porcine xenograft bioprosthesis in the mitral position: Late hemodynamic observation. *J Interven Cardiol 2*:103–107, 1989.

50. Feit F, Stecy PJ, Nachamie MS. Percutaneous balloon valvuloplasty for stenosis of a porcine bioprosthesis in the tricuspid valve position. *Am J Cardiol 58*:363–364, 1986.

51. McKay CR, Waller BF, Hong R, Rubin N, Reid CL, Rahimtoola SH. Problems encountered with catheter balloon valvuloplasty of bioprosthetic aortic valves. *Am Heart J 115*:463–465, 1988.

52. Calvo OL, Sobrino N, Gamallo C, et al. Balloon percutaneous valvuloplasty for stenotic bioprosthetic valves in the mitral position. *Am J Cardiol 60*:736–737, 1987.

2

Anatomic Basis For and Morphologic Changes Produced By Catheter Balloon Valvuloplasty

BRUCE F. WALLER, JAMES W. VanTASSEL, and CHARLES McKAY

During the last several years, catheter balloon valvuloplasty has been used as a nonsurgical treatment of stenotic mitral, aortic, tricuspid, and pulmonic valves. The technique has been used successfully in children and adults. This chapter will review the anatomic basis for successful balloon valvuloplasty procedures and describe various morphologic changes observed following in vitro and in vivo dilation of various human stenotic cardiac valves.

EXAMINATION OF THE DILATED STENOTIC CARDIAC VALVE

As more and more catheter balloon valvuloplasty procedures are performed, pathologists will be called upon to examine operatively excised or necropsy valves previously subjected to balloon dilation. It behooves the cardiac surgeon to remove these valves intact if at all possible, and it behooves the pathologist to evaluate the valves intact without destroying the specimen by taking histologic sections. The valves should be photographed from top and bottom surfaces and radiographed for calcific deposits. Valves examined early (< 30 days) after valvuloplasty procedures should have documentation regarding various injuries produced: splitting of commissures, cracking of leaflets or cusps, fracture of chordae tendineae, and annular damage. Necropsy specimens should be cut leaving the cardiac valve(s) intact. Initial short axis views of the cardiac valves provide an excellent overall assessment of the stenotic valve following dilation. Further examination may require opening the valve circumference in a "flow of blood" method.

ANATOMIC BASIS FOR SUCCESSFUL BALLOON VALVULOPLASTY OR VALVOTOMY

Morphologic changes of stenotic cardiac valves include[1-3] fibrous thickening of cusps (semilunar valves) or leaflets (atrioventricular valves); fusion of commissures; calcific deposits within cusps, sinuses of Valsalva, or leaflets; fibrous thickening and fusion of chordae tendineae; or abnormal development of valve structure (absent or reduced number of commissures, cusps, leaflets, or chordae). Based on the pattern and distribution of these changes, specific etiologies for valve stenoses can be established. Determination of specific etiology for valve stenoses will result in improved initial success, reduced complication rate, and a better long-term success in catheter balloon valvuloplasty procedures.

Mitral Valve

The etiology of mitral valve stenosis in the Western world is nearly exclusively secondary to previous acute rheumatic fever ("rheumatic heart disease"). The terms "mitral stenosis" and "rheumatic heart disease" are used interchangeably. Morphologic changes associated with "rheumatic mitral stenosis" include fusion of one or both commissures, diffuse fibrosis of the anterior and posterior leaflets, and occasionally thickening and fusion of chordae tendineae (Figs. 2.1, 2.2). Fusion of mitral valve commissures is the most common basis for mitral valve stenosis but occasionally a secondary level ("subvalvular level") of stenosis is created by extensive fusion of chordae tendineae.

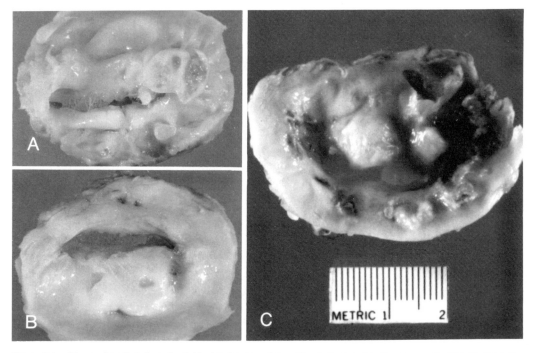

Figure 2.1.   Rheumatic mitral stenosis. **A,** Ventricular view of stenotic mitral valve showing narrowed orifice. **B,** Atrial view of mitral valve showing diffuse fibrosis of leaflets and fusion of commissures. **C,** Atrial view of stenotic mitral valve showing calcific deposits (nodules).

In the latter situation simply splitting of commissures may not result in significant reduction in gradient between left atrium and left ventricle. Calcific deposits can be associated with fused commissures and fibrotic leaflets (Fig. 2.3). The more severe the degree of calcific deposits, the greater the stenosis across the mitral valve. Furthermore, the more heavily calcified mitral valves are less likely to be successfully dilated (surgical commissurotomy or catheter balloon valvuloplasty). Calcific deposits generally increase with advancing age of the patient or in association with chronic renal failure, renal dialysis, or hypercalcemic states. Other rarer causes of mitral valve stenosis include active infective endocarditis, congenital abnormalities (developmental lack of commissures, chordae tendineae, or papillary muscles, or the reduction in the number and size of mitral leaflets, anulus, or chordae), and calcified mitral anulus. Mitral valve stenosis secondary to acute or active endocarditis results from a large vegetation obstructing the orifice of the mitral valve. This condition is obviously not a suitable etiology for catheter balloon valvotomy. Certain congenital abnormalities of the mitral valve such as fusion or absence of commissures may be amenable to balloon dilation. Mitral valves with congenitally shortened or absent chordae tendineae or with chordae tendineae totally inserted into a single papillary muscle (single papillary muscle syndrome, parachute mitral valve) are not suitable stenotic mitral valves for balloon dilation. Mitral valve annular calcium represents a degenerative disease in which the anulus fibrosa behind the posterior mitral valve leaflet becomes calcified. In rare instances of massive annular calcium, an element of mitral valve orifice obstruction can result. In this instance, the mitral leaflets and chordae are focally fibrotic, but the commissures are not fused. Mitral valve stenosis secondary to mitral annular calcium does not appear amenable to balloon dilation procedures.

Thus, rheumatic mitral stenosis with fused commissures is virtually the only etiology of mitral stenosis suitable for successful dilation with catheter balloon valvotomy procedures.

Aortic Valve

The etiology of aortic valve stenosis consists of three major conditions: congenital abnormalities, and rheumatic and degenerative changes (Fig. 2.4).

Congenitally malformed aortic valves are primarily of two types: unicuspid and bicuspid (Fig. 2.5–2.8). In the congenitally unicuspid aortic

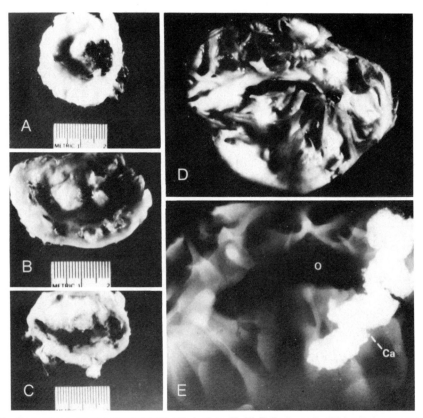

Figure 2.2.   Series of operatively excised stenotic mitral valves. (**A–D**). **E,** Radiograph of Valve D showing calcific deposits (Ca) in commissure. O = orifice.

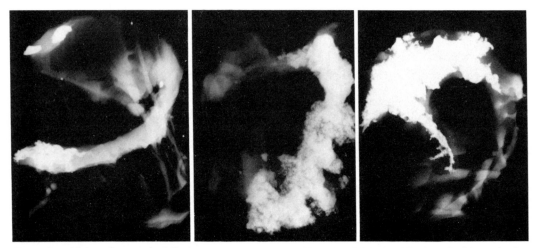

Figure 2.3.   Various degrees of calcific deposits in stenotic mitral valves. *Left,* Minimal calcific deposits (ideal valve for balloon dilation). *Middle and Right,* Heavy calcific deposits (not a valve for balloon dilation).

STENOTIC AORTIC VALVES OF VARIOUS ETIOLOGIES

Morphologic Definitions

1. **Congenital**
   a) **unicuspid** (unicommissural):
   Single "wrap-around" cusp with one commissure producing an "exclamation point" type orifice.

   b) **bicuspid**:
   Two generally equal sized cusps with false commissure (raphe) in one cusp generally unassociated with commissural fusion.

2. **Rheumatic**
   a) Three cuspid

   b) Commissural fusion of 2 and usually 3 commisures

   c) Associated with stenotic mitral valve

3. **Degenerative ("Old age", "Wear and tear")**
   a) Three-cuspid
   b) Absent commissural fusion
   c) Mounds of calcium in sinuses of Valsalva
   d) Normal mitral valve leaflets

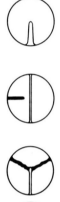

Figure 2.4.   Diagram showing various etiologies of stenotic aortic valves.

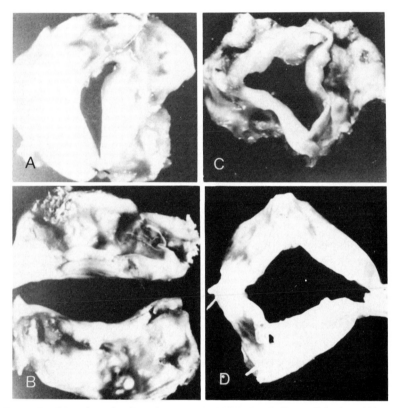

Figure 2.5. Composite of stenotic aortic valves showing various etiologies: **A,** Congenital unicuspid (unicommissural); **B,** Congenital bicuspid; **C,** Rheumatic; **D,** Congenital quadricuspid.

valve, there is a single "wrap-around cusp" with one commissure (unicommissural). The valve orifice appears as an "exclamation point." Unicuspid aortic valves are inherently stenotic at birth and generally cause symptoms early in life. Occasionally, the unicuspid aortic valve is present in young adults. Of isolated aortic stenosis in patients aged 15 to 65 years, about 10% of the aortic valves will be unicommissural unicuspid.[4] The single aortic valve cusp is diffusely fibrotic and generally heavily calcified early in adult life. The single commissure is not fused. Without fusion, this valve would be difficult to dilate with the hope of achieving short-or long-term success. Two-dimensional echocardiographic differentiation of the unicuspid valve from a bicuspid valve with fusion of one or two commissures is difficult if not impossible.

The congenitally bicuspid aortic valve consists of two nearly equal-sized cusps generally unassociated with commissural fusion (Figs. 2.5–2.8). The cusps are densely fibrotic and contain calcific deposits in early to mid adulthood. In about half of the bicuspid valves, a false commissure (false raphe) is found in one of the two cusps. Of patients with isolated aortic stenosis aged 15 to 65 years, about 60% of the valves will be congenitally bicuspid.[4] Two-dimensional echocardiography is a useful tool in establishing this etiology of aortic stenosis except in the instances of severely calcified valves. In the latter case, little structural information can be obtained by the use of the echocardiogram.

Rheumatic aortic stenosis is characterized by a three-cuspid aortic valve with fusion of one to three commissures and densely fibrotic cusps (Fig. 2.9). This diagnosis is established only in the presence of a diseased (almost exclusively stenotic) mitral valve. In the classic rheumatic aortic valve stenosis, all three commissures are fused, producing a triangular, central orifice. Calcific deposits are also commonly present. As with the mitral valve with fusion of commissures, the rheumatic aortic valve is ideally suitable for catheter balloon valvuloplasty. The

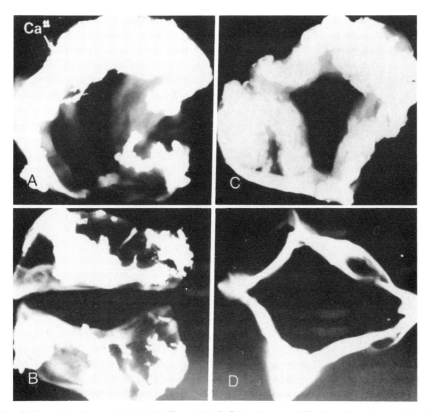

Figure 2.6. Radiographs of valves illustrated in Figure 2.5. **A–C** have heavy calcific deposits and are not ideally suited for balloon dilation. **D,** Absent calcific deposits but associated regurgitation precludes this valve for effective balloon dilation.

BICUSPID AORTIC VALVES

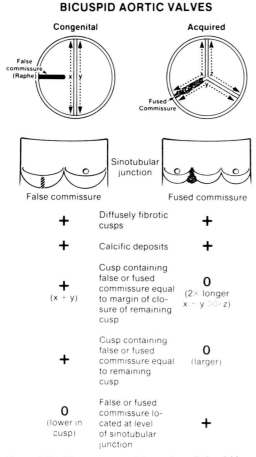

Figure 2.7. Diagram summarizing various distinguishing features of the congenitally bicuspid aortic valve from the acquired (rheumatic) bicuspid aortic valve.

degree of calcific deposits would be a limiting factor in the early and late success of the dilation.

Degenerative aortic stenosis is characterized by a three-cusp aortic valve without commissural fusion and mounds of calcific deposits in the sinuses of Valsalva (Fig. 2.9). The mitral valve leaflets are normal. This condition is most common in patients over the age of 65 years. In patients with isolated aortic valve stenosis who are over 65 years of age, 90% of the valves are degenerative in etiology.

Rarely, active infective endocarditis or homogeneous type II hyperlipoproteinemia produces aortic valve stenosis.[5] In the former condition, valvuloplasty is not indicated. In the latter condition, accelerated atherosclerotic disease of the ascending aorta thickens the aortic valve cusps, and

depending on the presence of fusion of commissures, this valve may be suitable for dilation.[5]

Tricuspid Valve

The etiology of tricuspid valve stenosis consists of the following conditions: rheumatic, carcinoid, congenital abnormalities, and active infective endocarditis. Rheumatic tricuspid valve stenosis is not an isolated condition. The mitral valve is also stenotic in rheumatic tricuspid stenosis. Pathologic charges of the rheumatic stenotic tricuspid valve are similar to that described previously with the mitral valve including commissural fusion and leaflet fibrosis (Fig. 2.10). Fibrosis and/or fusion of the chordae tendineae of the tricuspid valve in rheumatic disease is less frequent than with the mitral valve. Leaflet calcific deposits are very uncommon in rheumatic tricuspid valve stenosis. Like the mitral valve, this condition should be ideally suited to successful catheter balloon valvotomy procedures. Carcinoid heart disease may be a cause of tricuspid valve stenosis and in the instance of isolated tricuspid valve stenosis, carcinoid heart disease is the most likely diagnosis. In contrast to rheumatic disease, carcinoid involves the valve by coating the leaflets and chordae with a fibrotic carcinoid plaque. These plaques thicken the leaflets and chordae tendineae without disturbing the underlying valve structure. Commissural fusion is not a specific consequence of the carcinoid plaque. Catheter balloon valvotomy may have a limited role in the nonsurgical management of carcinoid-induced tricuspid valve stenosis.

Congenital tricuspid valve stenosis results from abnormalities of the leaflets (absent or decreased number), chordae tendineae (absent, reduced, or shortened), and papillary muscles (reduced number) similar to conditions described under the mitral valve pathology. Large vegetations from active infective endocarditis obstructing the orifice to the tricuspid valve are not treatable with balloon dilation.

Pulmonic Valve

The etiology of pulmonic valve stenosis consists of congenital abnormalities, active infective endocarditis, and carcinoid and rheumatic disorders. The most frequent etiology for pulmonic valve stenosis is congenital. Congenital pulmonic stenosis consists of several forms: domed-shaped three-cusp pulmonic valve ("volcano-shaped orifice") (Fig. 2.11), dysplastic three-cusp (mucopolysaccharide increase), and the bicuspid pul-

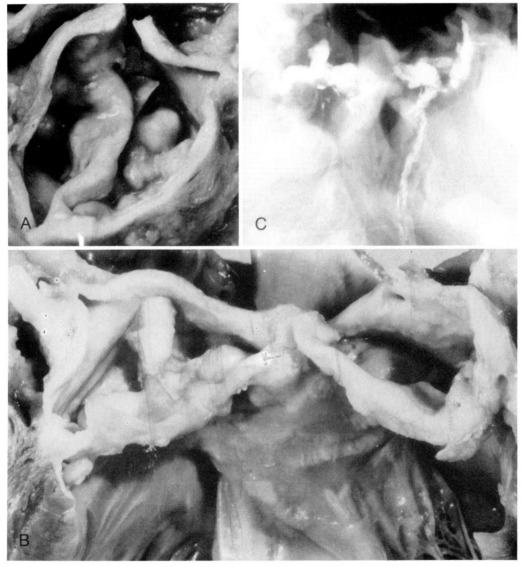

Figure 2.8.   Composite showing a severely stenotic congenitally bicuspid aortic valve. **A,** Aortic view. **B,** Opened view showing false raphe. **C,** Radiograph shows heavy calcific deposits.

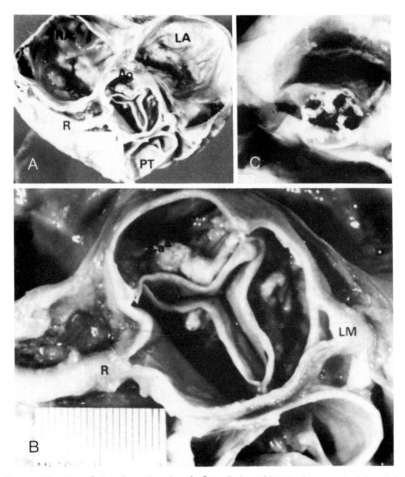

Figure 2.9.   Degenerative type of stenotic aortic valve. **A,** Overall view of heart—Ao = aorta, LA = left atrium, PT = pulmonary trunk, R = right coronary artery, RA = right atrium. **B,** Close-up of aortic valve seen in **A.** LM = left main. **C,** Radiograph shows mounds of calcium in the sinuses of Valsalva.

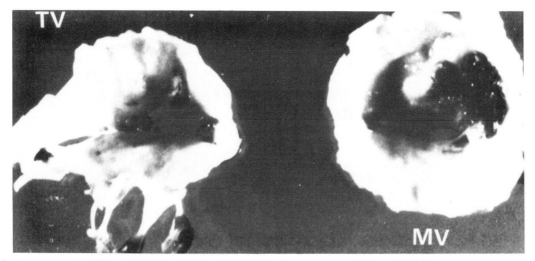

Figure 2.10. Stenotic tricuspid (TV) and mitral (MV) valves of rheumatic etiology.

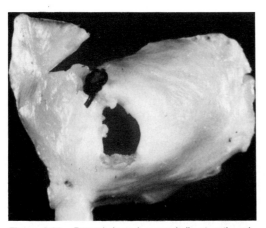

Figure 2.11. Domed-shaped congenitally stenotic pulmonic valve.

monic valve. The domed-shape valve is amenable to balloon valvuloplasty, but without truly identifiable commissures, leaflet tearing is the probable mechanism. In the dysplastic pulmonic valve, no commissural fusion is present, so stretching of the cusps and/or pulmonary trunk at sites of nonfused commissures is a likely mechanism. The most frequent cause of acquired pulmonic valve stenosis is carcinoid followed by rheumatic disease.[1,6,7] As with carcinoid involvement of the tricuspid valve, carcinoid plaques thicken the pulmonic valve cusps. Commissures are not a preferential site for the carcinoid plaque.

MECHANISMS OF CATHETER BALLOON VALVULOPLASTY OR VALVOTOMY AS OBSERVED IN HUMAN VALVES DILATED IN VITRO OR DURING LIFE (IN VIVO) AND EXAMINED AFTER REMOVAL

Mitral Balloon Valvotomy

The mechanism for catheter balloon valvotomy of stenotic mitral valves was initially described as "splitting of fused commissures." To test this theory, we performed an extensive in vitro dilation experiment using fresh and formalin-preserved operatively excised and necropsy stenotic mitral valves. A split-image video-recording system provided detailed and simultaneous views of both surfaces of the valve during the dilation experiments. Slow-motion playback of the dilation recordings provided information on the location(s) and timing of various injuries produced by the valvotomy experiments. Single and double balloons were employed and the size of the balloon(s) determined using standard clinical parameters of orifice diameter and balloon cross-sectional area. The mitral valves were examined before and after each dilation procedure to record various injury patterns. Each valve was radiographed for the presence and location of calcific deposits.

Twelve stenotic mitral valves were studied from patients aged 44–73 years (Table 2.1). Catheterization data during life (10 patients) indicated the

Table 2.1.
Incremental Changes Following Single and Double Catheter Balloon Valvotomy of 12 Stenotic Mitral Valves

1. Number of valves examined	12
a) operatively excised = 10	
b) intact necropsy = 2	
2. Ages of patients	44–73 yrs (54)
Gender (M:F)	(1:11)
3. Catheterization data during life	
(10 pts)	
a) range and mean MV end-	10–29
diastolic gradients (mm Hg)	(15.2)
b) MV orifice area (cm²)	0.4–0.9 (0.7)
4. Number of MV with previous	3
clinical commissurotomy	
procedures 10–24 years	
before MV excision	
5. Number of MV with double	5 (1)
catheter balloon dilations	
(or overdilation)	

Table 2.2.
Incremental Changes Following Single and Double Catheter Balloon Valvotomy of 12 Stenotic Mitral Valves

Mitral Valves with Previous Surgical Commissurotomy Sites	#1	#2	#3
1. Years from previous commissurotomy to MV excision	21	20	17.9
2. Morphologic evidence of healed previous commissurotomy	+	+	+
3. Calcific deposits at commissurotomy site (0–4+)	2+	3+	0–½+
4. Commissural cracks after catheter balloon valvotomy	0	0	+
5. Leaflet cracks adjacent to commissurotomy site	(7mm, AML)	(3mm, AML)	0

AML = anterior mitral leaflet

mean end-diastolic gradients ranged from 10 to 29 mm Hg (average 15.2). Calculated mitral valve areas ranged from 0.4 to 0.9 cm² (average 0.7). Three mitral valves had previous surgical commissurotomy procedures 9 to 21 years before valve excision (Table 2.2). Of the 12 valves, 7 had single balloon dilation and the remaining 5 had single followed by double balloon dilation (Tables 2.3, 2.4). One valve was specifically overdilated in order to define possible areas of dissection. Morphologic findings of the dilation study are summarized in Tables 2.3 and 2.4 and Figures 2.12–2.21. Of the 7 valves (12 fused commissures) dilated with a single balloon, 14 of 14 commissures were split (superficial splitting [defined as split length ≤ 2 mm] in 9 and deep splitting [defined as split length ≥ 2 mm] in 5). No leaflet cracking, anulus splitting, or left atrial wall tears were observed after single balloon dilation. Of the 5 stenotic mitral valves initially dilated with a single balloon followed by double balloon dilation, 9 of 10 commissures were split after one balloon (5 superficial, 4 deep) and 10 of 10 commissures were split after two balloons (10 of 10 deep). After double balloon dilation, 3 of the 5 leaflets had injury (cracking), but the mitral anulus and left atrial walls were intact. Overdilation of one stenotic mitral valve with oversized balloons was associated with anulus splitting and left atrial wall tears in addition to severe leaflet cracking.

Incremental increases in mitral valve internal orifice diameters following single and double balloon valvuloplasty are shown in Figures 2.18 and 2.19 and Table 2.4. Diameters increased 1 to 6 mm (average 3.5 mm) after single balloon dilation, and increased an additional 2 to 9 mm (average 4.0 mm) after the use of two balloons. The use of two balloons resulted in an increase in the internal mitral valve diameter of 3 to 15 mm (average 7.5 mm).

Mitral valve orifice areas pre- and post-balloon dilation were measured using a jeweler's ring sizer pushed gently into the orifice to accommodate the largest fit. The increase in mitral valve orifice areas ranged from 3 to 65% (average 35%) (Figs. 2.20, 2.21, Table 2.5). Five valves initially dilated with single balloons resulted in increased orifice areas of 1 to 124% (average 42%), which increased further after double balloon inflation (an additional 12 to 125%, average 38%).

Thus, single balloon valvotomy resulted in increased orifice diameters and cross-sectional areas. These changes increased further with double balloon dilation.

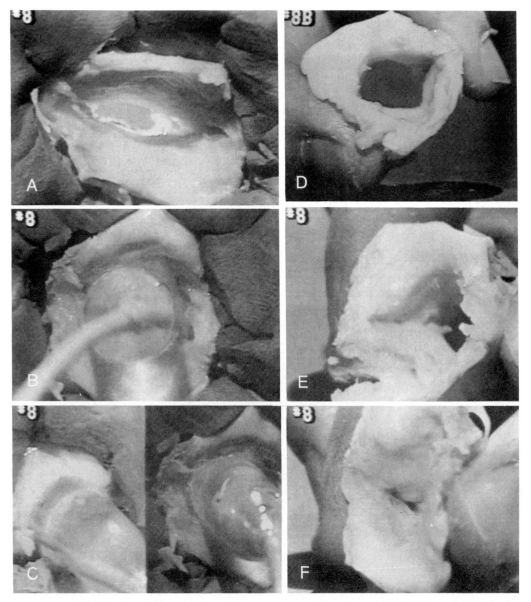

Figure 2.12.   Panel of catheter balloon valvotomy views dilating a stenotic mitral valve (left-sided frames). Following the single balloon dilation, a lateral commisural crack improves mobility of the fibrotic leaflets (right-sided frames).

Table 2.3.
Incremental Changes Following Single and Double Catheter Balloon Valvotomy of 12 Stenotic Mitral Valves

Morphologic Finding	Single (1) Balloon (B) Dilation	Double (2) Balloon (B) Dilation		Over Dilation
		1B	2B	
1. Number MV	7	5		1
2. Number of fused MV commissures (2/MV)	14	10		2
3. Commissurial splitting ("cracking")	14/14 (100%)	9/10		2/2
a) Superficial splits (≤ 2)	9/14 (67%)	5/10^a	0/10	
b) Deep splits (> 2)	5/14 (33%)	4/10	10/10	
4. Leaflet cracking	0	3/5 MV		—
5. Anulus splitting	0	0		—
6. Left atrial wall tear	0	0		—

^{a}Commissure had no crack after 1B but had deep crack after 2B CBV.

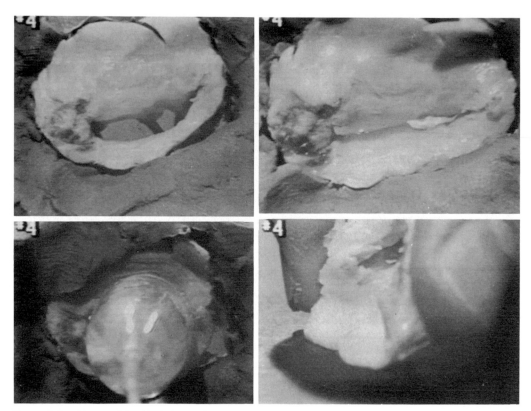

Figure 2.13. Frames of in vitro balloon dilation of stenotic mitral valve with a single balloon. Following dilation a commissural crack is present (lower right).

Table 2.4.
Incremental Changes Following Single and Double Catheter Balloon Valvotomy of 12 Stenotic Mitral Valves

Number of Catheter Balloons	Average Increase in MV Diameter (mm) Following 1 and 2 Catheter Balloon Dilation (CBD)	
	Internal (orifice)	External (anulus)
1. Single balloon only (N = 7)		
1. Baseline → 1 CBD	0–6 (3)	0–6 (2.2)
2. Single balloon followed by double balloon (N = 5)		
1. Baseline → 1 CBD	1–6 (3.5)	0–4 (1.5)
2. Baseline → 2 CBD	3–15 (7.5)	2–5 (3.3)
(Difference between 1 and 2)	(2–9 [4.0])	1–3 (1.8)

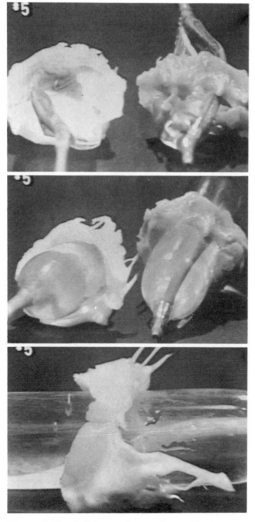

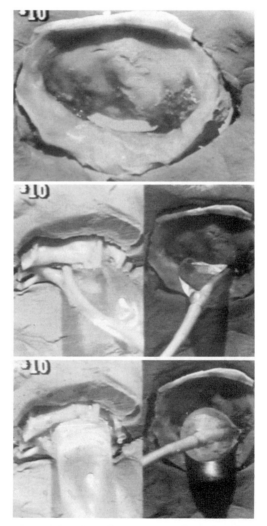

Figure 2.14. Split-image frames from video-recording showing the effects of balloon dilation on a stenotic mitral valve. Lower, Close-up shows split of previously fused commissure.

Figure 2.15. Panels from video-recording system showing placement of dilating balloon across the mitral valve and inflation of the balloon filling the orifice of the stenotic mitral valve.

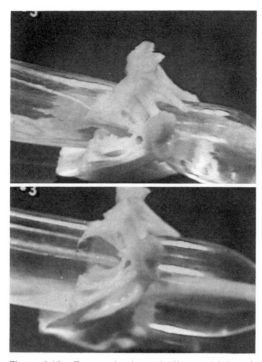

Figure 2.16. Frames showing waist-like constriction of the dilating balloon from the narrowed mitral orifice. With maximal inflation (lower), the waist constriction is gone and the fused commissure is split.

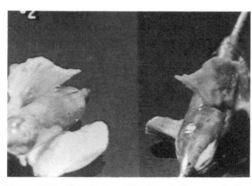

Figure 2.17. Overdilation with a large balloon cracks the commissure and splits through to the annular area.

The relationship between commissural cracking and the presence and amount of calcific deposits is summarized in Table 2.6. Radiographic calcific deposits indicated two valves without calcium (0), six valves with 1 + calcium, six valves with 2 + , six valves with 3 + , and three valves with 4 + calcium. Superficial commissural splitting occurred in three (12%) of valves with 0–2 +/4 + calcium and nine (39%) of valves with 3–4 +/4 + calcium. In contrast, of 11 commissures with deep cracking, all

MORPHOLOGIC CHANGES IN STENOTIC CARDIAC VALVES FOLLOWING CATHETER BALLOON VALVOTOMY

Stenotic Mitral Valves

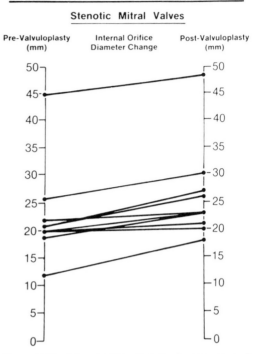

Figure 2.18. Internal orifice diameter changes pre- and post-valvuloplasty.

MORPHOLOGIC CHANGES IN STENOTIC MITRAL VALVES FOLLOWING SINGLE AND DOUBLE CATHETER BALLOON VALVOTOMY

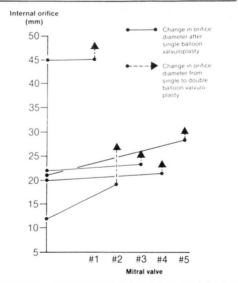

Figure 2.19. Improvement in internal diameters following single then double balloon dilation.

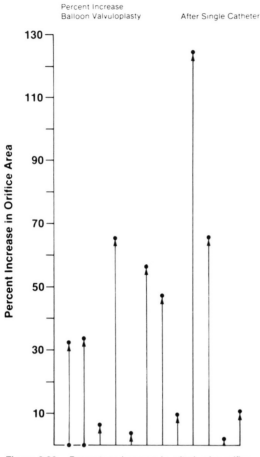

Figure 2.20.   Percentage increase in mitral valve orifice area after balloon dilation with a single balloon.

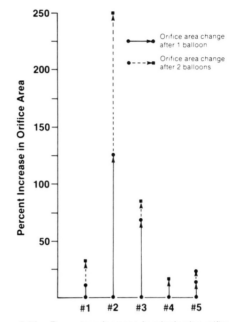

Figure 2.21.   Percentage increase in mitral valve orifice area after single and double catheter balloon valvotomy.

healed surgical commissurotomy sites was observed in the remaining two valves.

SUMMARY OF MITRAL VALVE STUDIES

1. Catheter balloon valvotomy dilates stenotic mitral valves by commissural splitting and leaflet cracking.
2. Catheter balloon valvotomy using single balloons resulted in superficial commissural cracks (67%) without leaflet cracking. Catheter balloon valvotomy using double balloons resulted in deeper commissural cracks or splitting of remaining intact commissures after a single balloon as well as deeper leaflet cracking. (Fig. 2.22).
3. Mitral valve orifice diameter and area increased after single and double balloon dilation, but the major effect of dilation was improved mobility of previously fixed leaflets.
4. Deeper cracks occurred in areas of absent or minimal calcific deposits.
5. Overdilation with oversized balloons resulted in splitting of the mitral anulus and tearing of the left atrial wall.

11 occurred in valves with absent to mild calcific deposits (0–2 + /4 +). No valve with 3–4 + /4 + calcium had deep commissural splitting (i.e., heavier calcium was associated with superficial injury and lighter or absent calcium was associated with deeper splits).

Of three stenotic valves dilated in which at least one previous surgical commissurotomy had been performed, results of balloon valvotomy are summarized in Table 2.2. The interval from previous commissurotomy to valve excision ranged from 12 to 21 years. One specimen (valve # 3, Table 2.2) had a second surgical commissurotomy procedure nine years prior to valve excision. Commissural cracking or splitting after balloon dilation was observed in only one valve. Leaflet cracking adjacent to previous

Table 2.5.
Incremental Changes Following Single and Double Catheter Balloon Valvotomy of 12 Stenotic Mitral Valves

	Baseline Area	Increase in MV Orifice Cross-Sectional Area (mm²) following 1 and 2 Catheter Balloon Dilation (CBD)	
		1 CBD (%)	2 CBD (%)
1. Single balloon dilation only (N = 7)			
1.	314	415 (32)	—
2.	530	706 (33)	—
3.	415	440 (6)	—
4.	346	572 (65)	—
5.	320	330 (3)	—
6.	340	530 (56)	—
7.	283	415 (47)	—
		Avg: 35	
2. Single balloon dilation followed by double balloon dilation (N = 5)			
1.	380	415 (9)	490 (18)
2.	113	254 (124)	572 (125)
3.	346	572 (65)	660 (15)
4.	1590	1610 (1)	1808 (12)
5.		346 (10)	415 (20)
		Avg: 42	Avg: 38

Table 2.6.
Incremental Changes Following Single and Double Catheter Balloon Valvotomy of 12 Stenotic Mitral Valves

Relationship of Commissural Cracks and Calcium

Commissurial Crack (23 Commissures)	Degree of Commissural Calcific Deposits (0–4+)				
	0	1+	2+	3+	4+
1. Superficial (≤2 mm long) (12)	0	1	2	6	3
		3 (12%)		9 (39%)	
2. Deep (>2 mm long) (11)	2	5	4	0	0
		11 (49%)		0	

Aortic Balloon Valvuloplasty

To evaluate the mechanism(s) of catheter balloon valvuloplasty in stenotic aortic valves, a similar video-recording study as described under the mitral valve was performed on 21 necropsy or operatively excised aortic valves (Table 2.7). Of the 21 valves dilated, 20 were intact necropsy stenotic aortic valves and 1 was an operatively excised unicuspid aortic valve. Ages of the patients ranged from 38 to 84 (average 63), and 15 of the 21 patients were men. Nine patients had previous cardiac catheterization, which disclosed 75 to 108 mm Hg peak systolic gradients (valve areas 0.4 to 0.6 cm²). The etiology of the aortic valve stenosis was congenital in nine (unicommissural unicuspid = 1, bicuspid = 8), rheumatic in four, and degenerative in eight. Morphologic evidence of balloon valvuloplasty based on etiologic subgroup is summarized in Table 2.7. Splitting of fused commissures was the mechanism in rheumatic aortic valves (Fig. 2.23); cracking calcific nodules and cusps or commissural stretching were the most common morphologic changes of dilation in congenitally bicuspid and degenerative aortic valves (Figs. 2.24–2.30). Combining etiologies into nonrheumatic (17 valves) and rheumatic (4 valves) disclosed that none of the nonrheumatic valves had commissural splitting, but all 17 had calcific nodule cracks, aortic wall stretching, and/or cuspal tears as mechanisms of valvuloplasty (Figs. 2.24–2.30). In contrast all four rheumatic valves had splitting of previously fused commissures with calcific nodule cracking as mechanisms of dilation (Fig. 2.23).

MORPHOLOGIC EFFECTS ON FUSED COMMISSURES, FIBROTIC LEAFLETS AND ORIFICE SIZE FOLLOWING SINGLE AND DOUBLE BALLOON VALVULOPLASTY OF STENOTIC MITRAL VALVES

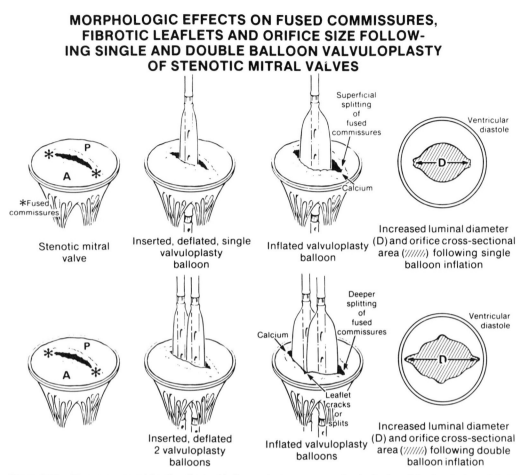

Figure 2.22.   Diagram summarizing the effects of balloon valvotomy on stenotic mitral valves following single and double balloons.

Table 2.7.
Catheter Balloon Valvuloplasty of Stenotic Aortic Valves of Various Etiologies

| | Morphologic Evidence of Balloon Valvuloplasty | | | |
| | Congenital | | | |
Morphologic Lesion	Bicuspid (N = 8)	Unicuspid (N = 1)	Rheumatic (N = 4)	Degenerative (N = 8)
1. Splitting or cracking of fused commissures	0	0	4	0
2. Calcific nodule cracks	8[a]	1	3	8[a]
3. Cuspal tears (fractures)	4	1	1	2
4. Aortic wall expansion (stretching) at commissural sites.	8[b]	1	0	8

[a]Superficial in 5 bicuspid and 7 degenerative
[b]Minimal in 3

MORPHOLOGIC EFFECTS OF PROGRESSIVE (SINGLE, DOUBLE, OVERDILATION) BALLOON VALVULOPLASTY OF STENOTIC MITRAL VALVES

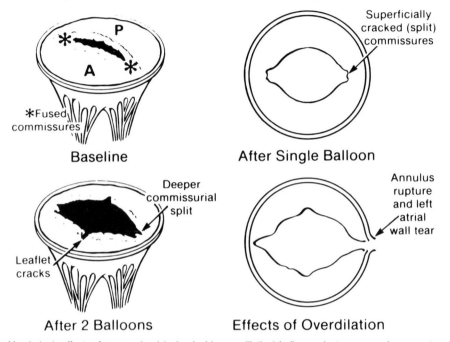

Figure 2.23. Morphologic effects of progressive (single, double, overdilation) balloon valvotomy procedures on stenotic mitral valves. A = anterior leaflet, P = posterior leaflet.

Dilation of stenotic aortic valves with one or two catheter balloons resulted in incremental morphologic changes (Table 2.8). The use of two balloons generally increased morphologic injury in all three etiology subgroups (congenital, rheumatic, degenerative): additional commissural splitting, more cuspal tears, and increased aortic wall expansion (stretching). Overdilation of three aortic necropsy valves was specifically undertaken in order to assess possible injury patterns (Figs. 2.31, 2.32). Of the three valves dilated with oversized balloons, three had aortic wall dissection, two of three had aortic wall rupture, and in one instance, avulsion of the left main coronary artery occurred (Fig. 2.31). Potential embolic complications were documented in one stenotic aortic unicuspid valve in which fracture and dislodgement of multiple pieces of calcified valve occurred during dilation (using an appropriately sized balloon).

Table 2.8.
Morphologic Changes in Stenotic Aortic Valves Following Catheter Balloon Valvuloplasty

| | Etiology of Aortic Stenosis | | |
	Bicuspid	Rheumatic	Degenerative
	One Balloon Dilation		
1. Commissural splits	−	+	−
2. Cuspal tears	+	+	+[a]
3. Aortic wall expansion at commissural sites	+	0	+
	Two Balloon Dilation		
1. Commissural splits	−	+ +	−
2. Cuspal tears	+ +	+ +	+
3. Aortic wall expansion at commissural sites	+ +	+	+ +

[a]Mounds of sinus calcium cracked

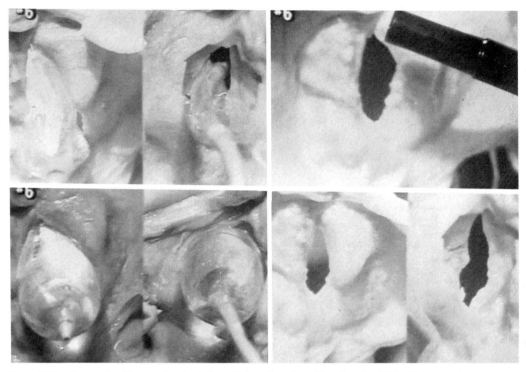

Figure 2.24. Composite of frames showing balloon dilation of a unicuspid aortic valve. Minimal injury results (pen, upper right). Small cusp crack is seen in lower right.

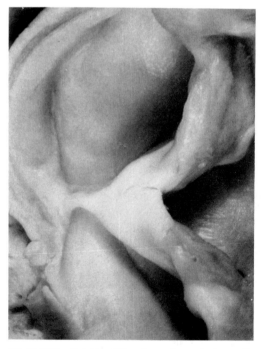

Figure 2.25. Cracking of fused commissure in rheumatic aortic valve stenosis.

SUMMARY OF IN VITRO AORTIC VALVE STENOSIS STUDIES

1. Catheter balloon valvuloplasty dilates stenotic aortic valves by various mechanisms depending in part on etiology of the aortic stenosis (Fig. 2.33).
2. Aortic stenoses without commissural fusion (i.e., congenital bicuspid, degenerative) are dilated primarily by aortic wall expansion at nonfused commissure sites and by fracture of cusps or sinus calcium.
3. Aortic stenoses with commissural fusion (i.e., rheumatic) are dilated by commissural splitting and cuspal cracking.
4. Double balloon dilation produces deeper cuspal cracks and further stretches the aortic wall.
5. Overdilation may result in aortic wall dissection and/or rupture and coronary artery ostial injury.

Aortic Balloon Valvuloplasty During Life (In Vivo) with Subsequent Tissue Examination

Twenty-three patients with aortic valve stenosis underwent catheter balloon valvuloplasty during life with subsequent surgical removal of the aortic valve within 30 days of the procedure. Of the 23 valves examined, morphologic changes are summarized in Table 2.9 and Figure 2.34. Stenotic aortic

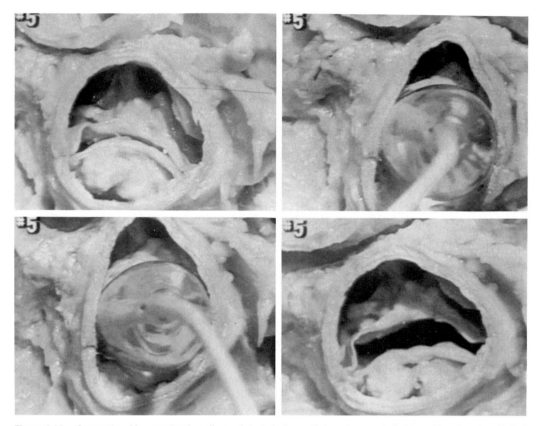

Figure 2.26.   Composite of frames showing effects of single balloon dilation of congenitally bicuspid aortic valve. Orifical stretching and stretching of aortic wall at nonfused commissural sites are seen in lower right.

valves were classified by etiology: congenital (unicuspid, bicuspid), rheumatic, and degenerative. Of the two unicuspid (unicommissural) aortic valves dilated during life, minimal injury was observed morphologically and "wrinkled" portions of the aortic wall at the single commissure site suggested that aortic wall stretching was the mechanism of dilation. Of the eight congenitally bicuspid aortic valves dilated, five had superficial calcific nodule cracking, which did little to improve flexibility or mobility of the cusps. Four of the eight valves probably had aortic wall stretching at nonfused commissural sites as the mechanism of acute valvuloplasty. Of two rheumatic aortic valves (with commissural fusion), four of four fused commissures were split, markedly improving the mobility of the valve cusps. Of 11 degenerative aortic valves (no commissural fusion), 8 had wrinkled or folded cuspal margins or aortic walls at commissural sites, indicating that balloon stretching of the valve and/or aortic wall had occurred.

Ten of the 11 valves had superficial sinus calcific nodule cracking also present, but that did little to improve the mobility of the aortic valve. Table 2.9 summarizes various morphologic changes occurring in the various etiologic subgroups.

Thus, tissue examination of stenotic aortic valves dilated during life (in vivo) and examined morphologically within 30 days of dilation confirms the previously described in vitro mechanisms of dilation based on stenosis etiology.

Clinical Recognition of Morphologic Type of Aortic Stenosis

Inasmuch as the mechanism and clinical success of aortic valvuloplasty depends in part on stenosis etiology, efforts should be directed at clinically recognizing these etiologies prior to valvuloplasty. Strategies for clinical prediction of correct etiology are summarized in Figures 2.35 and 2.36. Three items are useful in this clinical assessment: number

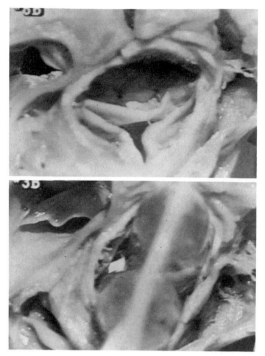

Figure 2.28. Double balloon dilation of a three-cuspid degenerative aortic valve. Stretching of aortic walls at nonfused commissural sites appears to be the mechanism of dilation.

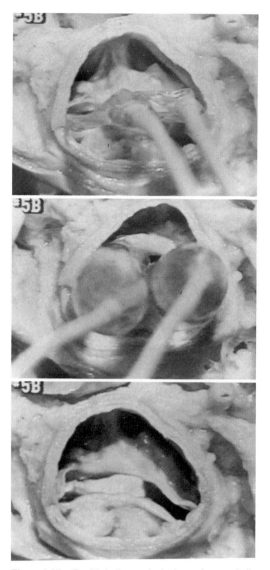

Figure 2.27. Double balloon valvuloplasty of congenitally bicuspid valve further stretches the orifice and aortic valves at nonfused commissural sites.

of aortic valve cusps seen on 2-D echocardiogram, age of the patient, and morphologic status of the mitral valve (i.e., isolated aortic stenosis or morphologically abnormal mitral valve as well). If the aortic valve stenosis is isolated (mitral valve is anatomically normal), the age of the patient is useful in predicting the aortic valve morphology: if the age is > 15 years but < 65 years, 60% of the valves are congenitally bicuspid; if the patient is > 65 years, 90% of the aortic stenoses are degenerative and 10% are congenitally bicuspid. A

more detailed flow diagram for the various possibilities is seen in Figure 2.36.

Tricuspid Valve Balloon Valvotomy

In the previously described video-dilation experiments, a few rheumatic stenotic tricuspid valves were dilated. Because of the larger internal orifice diameters compared to stenotic mitral valves of the same etiology, initial attempts to dilate using single 20 mm and/or two smaller balloons (15 mm + 18 mm) were unsuccessful in cracking commissures, and little if any orifice enlargement occurred. Subsequently, two 20 mm balloons were used, which resulted in splitting of commissures with or without adjacent leaflet injury (Fig. 2.37). Thus, balloon dilation of rheumatic tricuspid valve stenosis is similar to that previously described in stenotic rheumatic mitral valves: commissural splitting and leaflet cracking. The major difference between the two valvuloplasty techniques involves the use of larger balloons for the tricuspid valve. A second major difference between dilation of the mitral and stenotic tricuspid rheumatic valves is the lack of, or very mild, calcific deposits in the

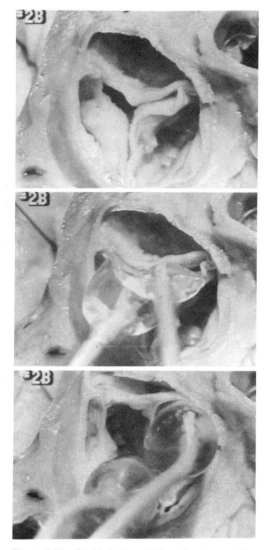

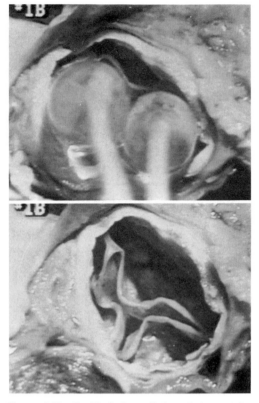

Figure 2.30. Double balloon dilation of degenerative three-cuspid aortic valve results in cusps margin wrinkling and stretching of aortic walls. No major cuspal injury is evident.

Figure 2.29. Double balloon dilation of a degenerative aortic valve shows widening of nonfused commissural spaces (bottom).

tricuspid valve stenosis. This finding will enhance the commissural splitting effect of the dilation process.

Based on these in vitro findings, we recently reported percutaneous balloon valvotomy for tricuspid stenosis in a 35-year-old woman with rheumatic heart disease. Following clinically successful balloon dilation, progressive regurgitation over the next six months led to excision of these valves. The operatively excised tricuspid valve (Fig. 2.37) showed that two of the three fused commissures had been torn. This observation confirmed

our in vitro studies, indicating the mechanisms of rheumatic tricuspid valvuloplasty were commissural splitting and/or leaflet tearing.

Pulmonic Valve Balloon Valvuloplasty

As with the preceding three cardiac valves, the mechanism(s) and clinical results of pulmonic valvuloplasty are directly related to the cause of the pulmonic stenosis. All congenital forms of pulmonic valve stenosis have thickened cusps with (bicuspid, tricuspid) or without (domed, unicuspid, bicuspid, dysplastic) commissural fusion. Tearing of pulmonic valve cusps seems to be the major mechanism of dilation without commissural fusion, whereas splitting of fused commissures with or without cuspal injury appears to be the mechanism of dilation of those congenital disorders with commissural fusion. Stretching of cusps, anulus, pulmonary truck, or combinations of factors are important mechanisms in dilation of dysplastic or unicuspid pulmonic valves. Catheter balloon valvuloplasty is likely to be more successful for acquired pulmonic valve stenosis (rheumatic or carcinoid) than for congenital stenosis because commissural fusion is the major cause of the valve dysfunction in the acquired types. Minor calcific deposits, a useful feature in dilation of left-sided stenotic valves, are rarely found in stenotic pulmonic valves.

Restenosis Following Catheter Balloon Valvuloplasty

Restenosis following catheter balloon valvuloplasty is the subject of much clinical investigation. Based on in vitro morphologic observations of valvuloplasty mechanism of dilation, mechanisms of restenosis are summarized as follows:

Mitral Valve:
1. Fibrous fusion of previously split or cracked commissures (late occurrence)
2. Fibrous healing of calcific nodule cracks

Aortic Valve:
1. Restenosis of dilated congenitally bicuspid and degenerative aortic stenoses likely results from recoil of overstretched aortic valve walls at nonfused commissural sites (early occurrence—days, weeks)

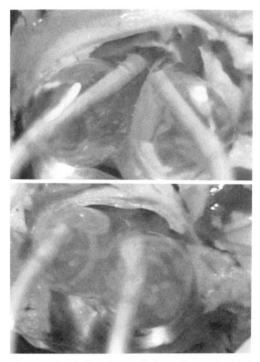

Figure 2.31. Deliberate overdilation with oversized balloons results in tearing of aortic wall (aortic dissection) and avulsion of the left main coronary artery (upper).

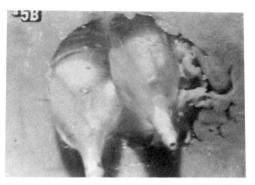

Figure 2.32. The use of two dilating balloons fully inflated causes compression (stenosis) of the normal mitral valve during dilation of a stenotic aortic valve. This reduces inflow across the mitral valve and contributes to decreased cardiac output during balloon inflation.

Table 2.9.
Catheter Balloon Valvuloplasty of Stenotic Aortic Valves of Various Etiologies

| | Balloon Valvuloplasty during Life with Subsequent Tissue Examination | | | |
| | Congenital | | | |
Morphologic Lesion	Unicuspid (N = 2)	Bicuspid (N = 8)	Rheumatic (N = 2)	Degenerative (N = 11)
1. Cuspal tear	0	1	1	1
2. Superficial calcific nodule tear	0	5	2	10
3. Fused commissures split	—	1/1[a]	4/4	1/2[a]
4. Raphe crack	—	0	—	—
5. Stretching[b]	2	4	0	8

[a]Minor fusion
[b]Wrinkled, folded cuspal margins or aortic wall at commissure sites, absent morphologic changes with increased clinical valve area.

MECHANISM(S) OF DILATION AND RESTENOSIS IN CATHETER BALLOON VALVULOPLASTY OF STENOTIC AORTIC VALVES

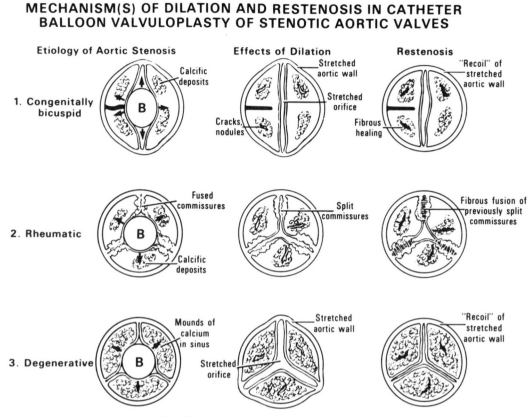

Figure 2.33. Drawing summarizing the effects of dilation with the three major types of aortic valve stenosis. The diagram also indicates the mechanism of restenosis for each type of stenotic aortic valve.

CATHETER BALLOON VALVULOPLASTY OF STENOTIC AORTIC VALVES OF VARIOUS ETIOLOGIES

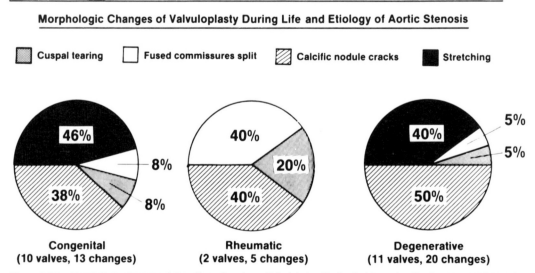

Figure 2.34. Morphologic changes of stenotic aortic valves dilated during life (in vivo) based on the three types of stenotic aortic valves.

CATHETER BALLOON VALVULOPLASTY OF STENOTIC AORTIC VALVES OF VARIOUS ETIOLOGIES

Strategies for Clinical Prediction of Aortic Valve Stenosis Etiology

1. Two-dimensional **echocardiographic view** (short axis)

2. If **isolated** aortic stenosis, **age of patient** is helpful in predicting valve morphology:

16-65 years	> 65 years
60% congenitally bicuspid	90% degenerative

3. **Status of mitral valve**: if stenotic etiology of aortic stenosis is likely rheumatic.

4. Combinations of #1 -3.

Figure 2.35.   Strategies for clinical prediction of aortic valve stenosis etiology before balloon valvuloplasty.

CATHETER BALLOON VALVULOPLASTY OF STENOTIC AORTIC VALVES OF VARIOUS ETIOLOGIES

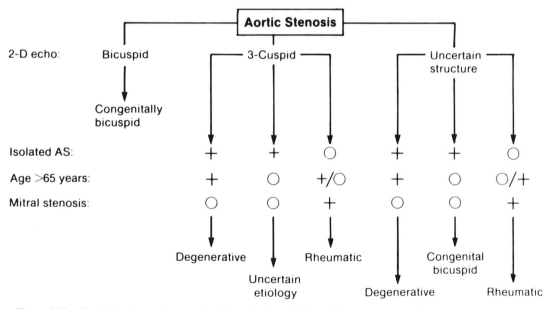

Figure 2.36.   Detailed scheme of strategy for determination of etiology of aortic stenosis. AS = aortic stenosis. + = present, 0 = absent.

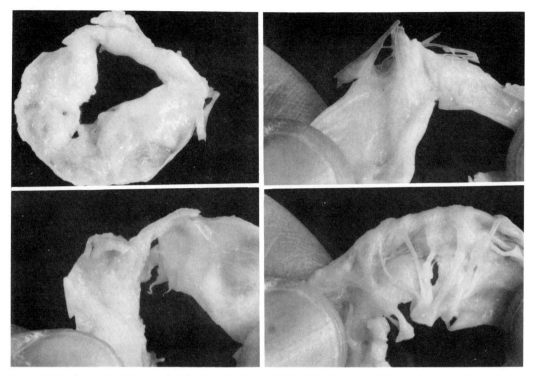

Figure 2.37. Composite of frames showing stenotic rheumatic tricuspid valve excised six months after clinical catheter balloon valvotomy. Slit commissures are seen in the upper left and bottom frames.

2. Restenosis of dilated rheumatic aortic valves results from fibrous refusion of previously split commissures (late occurrence—weeks, months, years)
3. Fibrous fusion of cracked calcific nodules

Tricuspid Valve:
1. Fibrous fusion of split commissures

Pulmonic Valve:
1. Fibrous fusion of split commissures (rheumatic and occasionally bicuspid valves) (late occurrence)
2. Elastic recoil of stretched nonfused commissural sites and/or anulus (early occurrence).

SUMMARY

This chapter has provided morphologic information in the various etiologies producing mitral, aortic, tricuspid, and pulmonic valve stenoses. Clinical recognition of conditions associated with commissural fusion will result in an increased likelihood of prolonged valvuloplasty success. In contrast, conditions (congenital or acquired) associated with no commissural fusion are likely to be associated with a limited initial balloon valvuloplasty success and an increased chance for early restenosis.

REFERENCES

1. Waller BF. Morphologic aspects of valvular heart disease. Part I. *Current Problems in Cardiology IX(7)*: 1–66, 1984.
2. Waller BF. Morphologic aspects of valvular heart disease. Part II. *Current Problems in Cardiology IX(8)*: 1–62, 1984.
3. Waller BF (ed). Pathology of the heart and great vessels. *Contemporary Issues in Surgical Pathology.* Volume 12. New York, Churchill Livingstone, Inc., 1988.
4. Roberts WC. The structural basis of abnormal cardiac function: A look at coronary, hypertensive, valvular, idiopathic, myocardial and pericardial heart disease. In: *Clinical Cardiovascular Physiology.* ed by JJ Levine, New York, Grune & Stratton, 1976.
5. Roberts WC, Ferrans VJ, Levy RI, Fredrickson DS. Cardiovascular pathology in hyperlipoproteinemia: Anatomic observations in 42 necropsy patients with normal or abnormal lipoprotein patterns. *Am J Cardiol 31*:557, 1973.
7. Waller BF. The operatively-excised pulmonic valve— A forgotten entity. *Mayo Clinic Proceedings 64*:1452–1454, 1989.
6. Bourdillon PDV, Hookman LD, Morris SN, Waller BF. Percutaneous balloon valvuloplasty for tricuspid stenosis: Hemodynamic and pathologic findings. *Am Heart J 117*:492–495, 1989.

3

Hemodynamic Assessment of Valvular Stenosis

DAVID A. KASS

The precision required of physiologic measurements in clinical medicine has been closely linked to the sophistication and nature of available therapeutic options. Thus, prior to the advent of valve replacement surgery for stenosis, accurate estimation of the severity of obstruction was of limited utility. Advances in the design of artificial valves[1] and techniques of left heart catheterization created both the need and methods for hemodynamic assessment of valve stenosis. Over the next 30 years, cardiac catheterization and valve area estimation were routinely performed in order to assess the therapeutic need for valve replacement. Yet, while measurement of valve stenosis formed an important component of preoperative evaluation, it was rarely the decisive factor. Indeed, a prominent 1981 study[2] suggested that routine invasive assessment of valve stenosis was not necessary. This argument was put forth prior to development of echo-Doppler cardiography for non-invasive quantitation of stenoses. However, the recent development of non-surgical approaches to valve stenoses reemphasizes the need for precise hemodynamic assessment of valvular disease. Beyond answering the threshold question of a given patient's suitability for therapy, these measurements are often critical for evaluating procedure outcome and efficacy.

In their 1951 paper,[3] the Gorlins first presented what has become the most widely accepted approach for assessing valvular stenosis. Using a simplified version of the Bernoulli equation, they described a relationship between mean pressure gradient, flow, and stenotic orifice area. This marked a departure from the use of Poiseuille's resistance formula to assess stenosis.[4] The Gorlins argued that rather than being primarily due to viscous losses, pressure gradients across a stenotic valve arose principally from rapid changes in flow velocity and thus reflected conversion of potential to kinetic energy. In an editorial written nearly 36 years later, Gorlin noted that "in our original presentation we pointed out that blood is a nonlinear, non-Newtonian fluid, which traverses cardiac valves in an intermittent, pulsatile, rather than steady flow. Considering that the equations were derived from systems of steady flow through fixed orifices, the surprise was that the equations worked at all!" He continues, "The problem is that while flow in and through the orifice must follow the immutable laws of physics, we cannot define all the variables that enter into the final flow equation."[5]

In light of the complexity of the underlying physics, it comes as no surprise that the Gorlin equation has been repeatedly investigated with mixed results. This chapter will review several of these studies, examine the theoretical basis for the Gorlin formula and other approaches, identify some pitfalls in pressure measurements, and present evidence supporting determination of the functional consequences of valve stenosis as well as the in vivo estimates of anatomic severity.

FLUID MECHANICS OF VALVE STENOSIS

Until the 1950s, the principal model used to explain ventricular outflow was a resistive one, using Poiseuille's relation for steady laminar flow and thus requiring that ventricular pressure exceed aortic pressure throughout systolic ejection. Improvement in the quality of pressure measurements revealed that transvalvular pressure gradients actually reversed early in systole, and this was attributed to inertial effects of flow deceleration.[6] In vitro studies by Bellhouse and Bellhouse[7,8] also demonstrated early systolic closure of aortic and mitral valves, and in addition they provided evidence for an important influence of vortex formation within the sinuses. Using a model with normal and stenotic pig valves, they found that intrasinus pressure due to vortex formation exceeded central luminal pressure, and during flow deceleration this created a gradient for valve closure. While reverse flow was normally minimal due to early valve closure, obstructing the sinuses led to sudden valve closure at end-systole and a fivefold increase in regurgitant flow (25% of stroke volume). Vortex formation was not observed with aortic stenosis, and in addition to lower deceleration rates, this contributed to late stenotic valve closure.

Despite the complexity of flow through a stenotic valve, several simplified models have been proposed. In general, these models are based on the concept of conservation of momentum embodied in the Bernoulli equation. Use of this expression requires making several assumptions: (1) blood is a Newtonian fluid, (2) cross-sectional area is circular, and (3) there are no spatial variations in pressure or velocity across a plane normal to the direction of flow (i.e., that pressure and flow are scalar rather than vector parameters). Accepting these assumptions, then for fluid with velocity (v) and pressure (p) passing through an orifice (A_2), the instantaneous pressure change over a small distance (ds) is[9] (Fig. 3.1):

$$(\delta p / \delta s) = \rho(\delta v / \delta t) + \rho v(\delta v / \delta s) + \rho \tau(v)/d \quad (1)$$

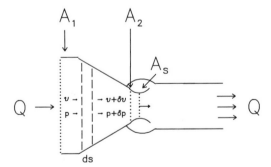

Figure 3.1. Schematic diagram of narrowing orifice. Flow (Q) enters a tube of cross-sectional area (A_1), with velocity (v) and pressure (p). Change in the velocity (δv) and pressure (δp) over a small distance (ds) are calculated in Equation 1 in text. The tube tapers to area A_2, although the effective stenotic area (A_s) just downstream of the actual orifice (vena contracta) is slightly smaller. Assuming incompressible fluid and noncompliant wall of the tube, the identical flow (Q) exits at the downstream (right-hand) end.

where ρ is fluid density, d the orifice diameter, and $\tau(v)$ viscous shear stress along the wall. Integration of Equation 1 over distance ds reveals the pressure drop (ΔP) is equal to:

$$\Delta P = \rho \int \frac{\delta v}{\delta t} \cdot ds + \text{½} \rho(v_2{}^2 - v_1{}^2) + R(v). \quad (2)$$

The first term (1) describes pressure change due to *local flow acceleration* (dv/dt) and is positive during early outflow, becoming negative during flow deceleration. The second term (2) is called *convective acceleration* and is related to the increase in velocity due to tapering of the orifice area. The last term (3) ($R(v)$) reflects *resistive influences*.

Several investigators have presented theoretical calculations and arguments as to why the resistive component can be ignored. Clark[9] estimated the ratio of resistive to convective acceleration terms in normal man to be about 0.03, indicating a minimal influence of the resistive component. Others[10] have attempted to calculate the viscous surface boundary layer of the outflow tract (or mitral inflow), yielding similarly low values for resistive losses. Finally, it has been noted that with increasing stenosis and thus greater turbulence, the ratio of inertial to viscous forces (Reynold's number) increases, making the resistive term less significant.[11] Thus in virtually all simplifying models, the third term of Equation 2 is neglected.

Calculations have also been made regarding the relative ratio of the first two terms. The ratio of local to convective acceleration is referred to as the Strouhal number and has been estimated to be nearly 1.0 in normal man.[10] However, with aortic stenosis, this number decreases markedly (to 0.01), since rates of flow change are much less in comparison to the velocity effects due to the narrowing orifice. This is consistent with delay in pressure gradient reversal.

An expression for mean pressure gradient can be derived from Equation 2 by integration over time of the cardiac cycle. This eliminates the local acceleration term (term 1) since average acceleration over the cardiac cycle is zero (i.e., for mean flow, $dv/dt = 0$). Neglecting the resistance term, this leaves only the convective acceleration term. In order to express the result in terms of volume flow (milliliters/sec) rather than flow velocity, the continuity equation is used. This simply states that flow in equals flow out (assuming fluid incompressibility and nondistensibility of the conduit). Since flow = velocity · cross-sectional area, we can write:

$$Q = v_1 \cdot A_1 = v_2 \cdot A_2 \qquad (3)$$

The effective orifice area (A_s) (Fig. 3.1) is somewhat smaller than the actual orifice (A_2) due to further narrowing of the flow stream distal to the stenosis. This is termed the vena contracta (Fig. 3.2). Thus, A_s can be written as:

$$A_s = \alpha A_2 \qquad (4)$$

with α typically equal to 0.75.[10] Combining Equations 2, 3, and 4, we obtain:

$$\Delta P = \rho Q^2/2(\alpha A_2)^2 \cdot (1 - (\alpha A_2/A_1)^2 \qquad (5)$$

Assuming valve area A_2 is much smaller than the area of the proximal chamber (A_2), then the second term can be ignored, and we are left with:

$$\Delta P = \rho Q^2/2(\alpha A_2)^2 \qquad (6)$$

Using the density of blood $\rho = 1.05$ gm/cm^3, and $\alpha = 0.75$, and converting dynes/cm^2 to conventional pressure units (mm Hg), Equation 6 becomes the familiar Gorlin equation:

$$A_2 = \frac{Q}{50.4 \, Ce} \, \frac{}{\sqrt{\Delta P}} \qquad (7)$$

The difference between the constant in Equation 7 and the usual Gorlin constant (44.3) lies in use of a hydrostatic column for manometric pressure measurement in the Gorlin derivation[3] and, therefore, incorporation of the gravitational

acceleration constant ($g = 980$ cm/sec^2). However, as shown, the formula does not critically depend on the incorporation of g.[12]

Equation 2 can also be simplified in terms of flow velocity. Assuming steady flow (i.e., $dv/dt = 0$), and no resistive term, Equation 2 becomes:

$$\Delta P = \tfrac{1}{2}\rho(v_2^2 - v_1^2). \qquad (8)$$

If $v_2 \gg v_1$ for flow through a stenosis, then after substitution for ρ and conversion of units, we get:

$$\Delta P \approx 4v^2 \qquad (9)$$

the familiar modified Bernoulli equation routinely used for Doppler pressure gradient estimation.

The essential assumptions used to derive the Gorlin expression (Eq. 7) or modified Bernoulli equation (Eq. 9) are similar (steady flow, no inertial effects, no viscous influences, and uniform spatial velocity and pressure distribution). Thus, it is not surprising that estimates of ΔP derived from both equations tend to agree.[13] The extent to which either estimate approximates physical reality is another matter, as many of these assumptions are clearly oversimplifications. For example, it has been suggested that viscous terms may well become appreciable with reductions in valve area.[5,10] Increasing downstream turbulence generates viscous losses as the jet undergoes flow separation creating marked regional differences in flow velocity. With jet reexpansion, frictional boundary layers form as fluid with the highest kinetic energy interacts with neighboring fluid, converting translational motion into thermal motion (thus viscous loss). High-speed images of transvalvular flow demonstrated that with increasing stenosis severity, the exiting jet becomes more unevenly distributed and displays eccentric flow velocity profiles.[14]

While simplified models are clearly useful, one should maintain some skepticism and empiricism regarding their application. It is probably best not to become overly fixated on a specific model framework, accepting that the extent to which reality may deviate from steady flow models under varying conditions remains unclear. Furthermore, even if a "best formula" could be agreed on, limitations in the techniques used to obtain the critical hemodynamic measurements may overshadow the theory. Thus, a desire for improved accuracy of stenosis assessment will also require that greater attention be paid to the determinations of flow and pressures.[5,15]

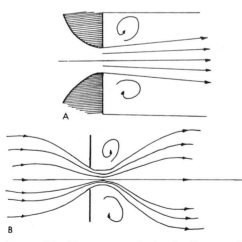

Figure 3.2. The vena contracta. **A,** Flow passing smoothly through an orifice begins to expand immediately distal to the orifice. **B,** Flow that passes more abruptly through an orifice narrows slightly further distal to the orifice (vena contracta). Reprinted with permission from American College of Cardiology.[11]

PITFALLS OF INVASIVE
PRESSURE MEASUREMENTS

Among the predictions of Equation 2 is that pressure gradients due to convective acceleration (term 2) will be observed in the presence of geometric tapering of the outflow tract. This applies at both valvular and subvalvular levels. Under normal physiologic conditions, subvalvular gradients are minimal, however, they increase significantly with aortic stenosis.[16,17] In a study of 11 aortic stenosis patients, Bird et al.[16] demonstrated significant pressure gradients between the mid-chamber and subvalvular regions of the left ventricle (Fig. 3.3). The mean transvalvular gradient was 58 ± 23 mm Hg in these patients, and the average subvalvular gradient was 41 ± 17 mm Hg. The two gradients were highly correlated ($\Delta P_{subvalve} = 0.73 \times \Delta P_{valve} - 1.9, r = 0.96$); thus, patients with high transvalvular gradients also had the highest subvalvular gradient. The authors explained the presence of significant subvalvular gradients on increased tapering of the

outflow tract due to doming of the stenotic aortic valve.[16,17]

The presence of intrachamber pressure gradients has important implications for invasive hemodynamic assessment during valvuloplasty, suggesting that pressures be reproducibly obtained at mid-chamber level. Furthermore, since reduction of afterload resistance increases the velocity of ventricular ejection, it will also increase convective acceleration and, thus, subvalvular pressure gradients. Valvuloplasty also reduces net afterload resistance (see subsequently) and thus will increase ejection velocity. This additionally emphasizes the importance of obtaining left ventricular (LV) pressures at similar mid-chamber positions to avoid under (or over) estimation of gradient change with valvuloplasty.

Another phenomenon that underlies the importance of precise manometer placement is pressure recovery downstream from the stenotic orifice. For a perfectly smooth gradually tapering stenosis at flow rates of 3.5 liters/min or more, nearly 60% of the pressure drop measured at the stenosis will be recovered within 1–2 cm distal to the valve[18]

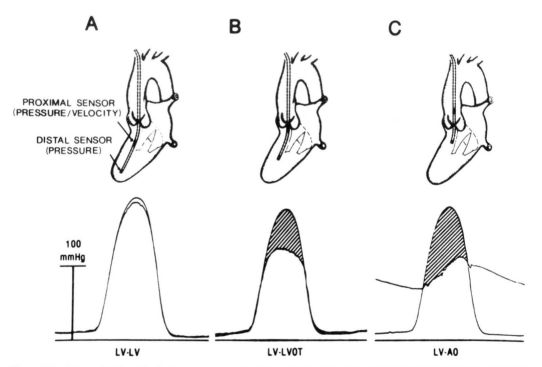

Figure 3.3.   Intraventricular subvalvular pressure gradients in a patient with aortic stenosis. The position of the proximal and distal micromanometer are shown in the upper panels, with simultaneous aortic and ventricular pressure tracings in the corresponding lower ones. With both sensors at and below mid-chamber level, there is little intrachamber pressure gradient (**A**). When the catheter is withdrawn such that the proximal sensor is subvalvular, a significant intrachamber pressure gradient is observed (**B**). Further withdrawal of the proximal sensor into the aorta demonstrates the transvalvular gradient (**C**). Reprinted with permission from *American Journal of Physiology.*[17]

(Table 3.1). This occurs as flow reexpands to the lateral wall, and kinetic energy is converted back to potential energy. Pressure recovery is much less when the stenosis is more abrupt (10%) and is even less with an eccentric stenosis (7%).

The phenomena of pressure recovery can produce Doppler gradients that appear to overestimate invasively obtained data. Rather than stemming from Doppler overestimation, this results from invasive measurement underestimation due to downstream pressure recovery. To limit the influence of varying flow rates, turbulence, and valve geometries on downstream pressure recovery, invasive aortic pressures should ideally be obtained as close to the valve as possible. Both subvalvular gradients and pressure recovery phenomena highlight the increased importance of obtaining pressures at similar locations before and after a procedure such as valvuloplasty.

THE GORLIN EQUATION: AN EMPIRICAL VIEW

As noted previously, the Gorlin formula[3] was derived using the Torricelli equation, a uniform field, steady flow, and nonresistive simplification of the Bernoulli equation. In their original paper, the Gorlins verified their formula by using a steady fixed orifice in vitro preparation and by comparing catheterization-derived measures of mitral valve area to data obtained at surgery or autopsy. Valve area was estimated using pulmonary capillary wedge pressure (for left atrial pressure) and by assuming a fixed LV mean diastolic pressure of 5 mm Hg (left heart catheterization had not yet been instituted). Data obtained before and after exercise revealed a significant increase in pulmonary capillary wedge pressure (PCWP) out of proportion to the change in estimated transmitral flow. While limited, these data supported the notion that pressure change varied by (Flow)[2]. This idea received subsequent theoretical support by Rodrigo[19] by a derivation similar to that provided previously (Eqs. 2–7).

Subsequent papers proposed modifications to the Gorlin formula. Hakki et al.[20] suggested a simplified ratio of Cardiac Output / $\sqrt{\Delta P}$. This formula "worked" due to the near constancy of the product of heart rate times systolic ejection period, and the fact that (HR · SEP · 44.5) ≈ 1000. Subsequent refinement of the Hakki formula was proposed by Angel et al.,[21] incorporating an adjustment for heart rate to reduce variability of the (HR · SEP · 44.5) product.

These studies attempted to simplify the Gorlin formula but treated the original equation as a "gold standard." Several other studies, however, critically examined the predictions of the Gorlin equation. In one study of 20 aortic stenosis patients, Bache et al.[22] found a significant disparity between valve area estimated before versus after supine bicycle exercise. Thus while cardiac output rose from 5.4 to 8.5 liters/min, and heart rate from 79 to 112 beats per minute (BPM), the valve gradient rose

Table 3.1.
Downstream pressure recovery in an in vitro model. The absolute pressure recovery, as well as the percentage of the maximal pressure gradient recovered, is shown for several valve areas from three different valve geometries. Maximal pressure recovery was observed with a gradually tapering stenosis with a narrow orifice and high downstream flows. Reprinted with permission from the American College of Cardiology.[18]

Model	Orifice Area (cm²)	Pressure Recovery (mm Hg)	Maximal Gradient (%)
Eccentric stenosis & gradual	0.25	68	60
pretaper	0.5	27	31
	0.8	22	22
Discrete eccentric stenosis	0.5	6	7
	1.1	11	10
	1.5	14	18
Discrete central stenosis	0.5	14	10
	1.1	8	7
	1.5	10	14

from 59 to 74 mm Hg, yielding an estimated area change from 0.76 ± 0.07 to 0.88 ± 0.08 cm^2. Plotting the percentage change in $\sqrt{\Delta P}$ versus %Δ in flow, the data all fell well below the line of identity (Fig. 3.4). Either the effective valve area increased with exercise or the Gorlin "constant" was not constant.

This latter idea was pursued in an in vitro and patient study of Cannon et al.[23] These experimenters used a pulsatile flow system (filled with water + glycerin + washed fixed red cells) and porcine valves with or without a 0.5-cm fixed orifice ring just distal to the valve. The valve area was determined by planimetered video images and was found to be nearly constant despite flow variation from 150 to 500 milliliters/sec. The Gorlin formula consistently overestimated valve area, and the extent of this overestimation increased as flow across the valve increased. This occurred despite the fact that true area was virtually constant. To examine this behavior, the authors plotted the Gorlin constant ($k = Q/\sqrt{\Delta P} \cdot A$) as a function of flow or pressure gradient. The authors found that k varied directly with $\sqrt{\Delta P}$ (Fig. 3.5). Setting $k = \beta\sqrt{\Delta P}$, then the Gorlin expression became:

$$A = Q/k\sqrt{\Delta P} = Q/\beta\sqrt{\Delta P} \cdot \sqrt{\Delta P} = Q/\beta P \quad (8)$$

For isolated valves in vitro, the new constant (β) averaged 1.92 ± 0.15, while in patients with porcine valve protheses, the average value of β was 80.3. In this study, use of the modified formula (Eq. 8) significantly improved correlations between known valve area and the estimates based on pressure-flow data.

Although actual changes in valve area with varying flow rates could not explain the in vitro results in Cannon's study, it remained a possible contributor in vivo. Stewart et al.[24] used a right heart bypass preparation to vary flow in anesthetized dogs and obtained echocardiographic valve area estimates along with Doppler flow velocity profiles in normal aortic, pulmonic, and mitral valves. Valve area significantly increased with higher flow rates for both aortic and mitral valves, although the change was much greater for the latter. For the group, increasing flow from 1 to 4 liters/min yielded a 63% increase in mitral valve area and a 15% increase in aortic valve area ($p < .05$ for both). Recent in vitro studies using native stenosed aortic valves in a pulsatile flow model[25] have reported similar increases in valve area (from 0.46 to 0.76 cm^2) when flow is raised from 1.5 to 5.0 liters/min.

With a renewed desire for more accurate valvular area estimates brought on by valvuloplasty, the issue of whether or not the Gorlin constant is a constant, whether valve area is constant, or whether neither is constant becomes

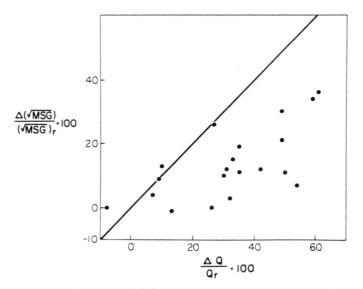

Figure 3.4. Percentage change in systolic flow ($\Delta Q/Q_r \times 100$) versus percentage change in the square root of the mean transvalvular pressure gradient in patients with aortic stenosis before and after leg exercise. Assuming valve area and the Gorlin constant as fixed values, the data should fall on the line of identity. However, the observed data fall below this line, indicating either a change in actual valve area with exercise, a change in the Gorlin constant, or both. Reproduced with permission from *Circulation*.[22]

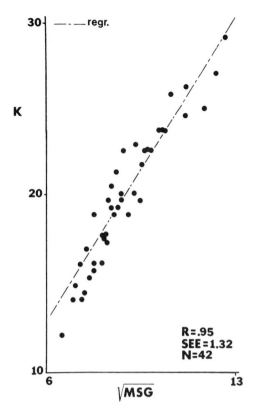

Figure 3.5. Gorlin constant *k* plotted against the square root of the mean systolic pressure gradient over a wide range of flow rates in an in vitro model of valve stenosis. Rather than a flat line, the data display a significant correlation of the constant with $\sqrt{MSG}$. Reproduced with permission from *Circulation*.[23]

increasingly relevant. These questions are difficult to answer since neither is theoretically so, and thus "constancy" must be defined empirically. This means examining many different physiologic conditions in the human model using a "gold standard" for comparison measurements, and such studies are difficult to perform. One approach is to use more functional descriptions of valvular stenosis, rather than purely relying on estimates of anatomic severity.

VALVULAR RESISTANCE

As noted previously, the relation between flow and the square root of pressure gradient makes sense if we assume a one-dimensional pressure-flow vector field, nonviscous losses, constant orifice area with a circular shape, and steady state flow. If in fact energy is required to open the valve (particularly stenotic ones) making viscous loss significant, and if an eccentric flow field and downstream turbu-

lence increase these viscous losses, and if the valve is somewhat elastic and undergoes changes in area with varying flow velocity, then whether or not the ratio of Flow: $\sqrt{\Delta P}$ is stable under varying conditions becomes unpredictable.

An alternative to area, as suggested by Equation 8 and the data of Cannon and Richards, is mean valvular resistance, which surprisingly turns out to be reasonably stable under varying flow conditions. Valvular resistance was virtually abandoned after the 1950s, yet it has several attractive features. It is easily defined (R = mean pressure gradient/mean systolic flow), displays less variability than valve area over a range of flow conditions,[26] and most importantly, provides a meaningful measure of the ventricular load posed by the stenotic valve. Since it is increased load that leads to clinical symptoms, and reductions in load following valvuloplasty or valve replacement that presumably relate to clinical improvement, why not use resistance to assess procedure efficacy?

Valvular resistance was recently reexamined by Ford.[26] Using data from several previously reported studies in which flow was varied in vitro or via hemodynamic interventions in man, he found that calculated aortic valve area by the Gorlin formula displayed much greater variability for the same valve under varying conditions than valvular resistance (Table 3.2). While area varied by 16 to as much as 210%, resistance change in the same valve was between 4 and 8%. Ford argued that despite the prevailing nonlinear theory emphasizing local and convective acceleration terms, which predicted the ratio of pressure:flow would not be constant, the empirical data suggested otherwise. Valvular resistance can be easily related to estimated valve area, since if area (A) = $Q/(k\sqrt{\Delta P})$, and $R = \Delta P/Q$, then:

$$A^2 = Q/k^2R. \qquad (9)$$

For a given range of transvalvular flows, R is inversely proportional to the square of the valve area. This relation is shown in Figure 3.6, using data from 32 patients undergoing aortic valvuloplasty.[27] Each patient contributes two data points, one before and one after valvuloplasty. The mean flow rate (Q) for the data was 186.3 ± 6.8 milliliters/sec, and using this as a constant in Equation 10, with k = 44.3 (from the Gorlin formula), area can be expressed in the form: $A = \sqrt{\kappa/R}$, with $\kappa = Q/k^2$, converted to units of dynes/cm². This model equation is also shown in Figure 3.6 by the solid line.

Valvular resistive load on the ventricle can also

Table 3.2.
Comparison of percentage change in estimated valve areas versus valve resistance from five prior studies. Data compiled and reproduced with permission from Ford.[26]

| | | | Change in Calculated Valve Area and Resistance with Changes in Flow | | | |
| | | | Change (%) | | | |
Reference	Number of valves	Kind of intervention	Systolic flow	Pressure gradient	Valve area	Valve resistance
Cannon et al.[a]	1	Controlled flow	76	69	35	−4
Ubago et al.	40	Early vs. late diastole	253	199	210	−8
Bache et al.	20	Exercise	30	25	16	−4
Casale et al.[b]	10	Dobutamine	36	27	21	−7
McCriskin et al.[b]	12	Isoproterenol	48	38	27	−7

[a]Study is of a single valve in vitro whose area was set with a nondistensible snare to 1.75 cm[2].
[b]These data are from tables in abstracts. Resistances could not be calculated separately for each patient, but ratio of mean value was calculated from mean values of pressure gradient and area.

Figure 3.6. Relation between mean aortic valve resistance and estimated valve area in 23 patients before and after aortic valvuloplasty. The two parameters follow an expected (solid line) nonlinear relation in the form: $y = \sqrt{k/x}$.

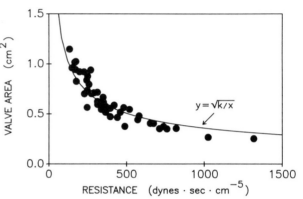

be determined from pressure-volume relations. Sunagawa et al.[28] proposed an approach to quantifying ventricular afterload resistance in the pressure-volume plane using the ratio of the chamber end-systolic pressure to stroke volume, (Pes:SV) which he termed effective arterial elastance (Ea). Increasing the steady state stroke volume ejected into the vasculature resulted in a linear rise in end-systolic vascular pressure. Ea lumps resistive, capacitative, and conduit vascular properties into a single parameter, treating the arterial system as an "effective" elastic chamber. Ea, by having units of elastance, can be coupled to the end-systolic pressure-volume relation to predict pump performance variables such as stroke work or stroke volume.[27] Under most circumstances, Ea is principally determined by the total resistance and heart rate:

$$Ea \approx R_{total} \cdot HR \quad (10)$$

Since Ea (or R_{total}) represents the total afterload resistance imposed on the ventricle, it combines both peripheral vascular and aortic valvular com-

ponents. By determining the peripheral vascular resistance and subtracting this from the total resistance ($R_{total} - R_{periph} \approx Ea/HR - R_{periph}$) the effective valvular load on the ventricle can be assessed.

We recently utilized this approach in a study of 23 patients undergoing aortic valvuloplasty.[27] Using pressure-volume loops derived by micromanometry and digitized contrast ventriculograms, the ratio of Pes:SV was determined and converted to R_{total} by Equation 10. Peripheral vascular resistance (mean arterial pressure/CO) was then subtracted from R_{total} to yield the resistance load from the aortic valve (R_{valve}) (Table 3.3). Figure 3.7 displays a typical example of steady state pressure-volume loops before (solid line) and after (dashed line) valvuloplasty. The Ea_{total} (Pes:SV) is graphically displayed for each loop by the line connecting the end-systolic pressure-volume point with the point at (EDV,0). Aortic valvuloplasty resulted in a reduction in Ea_{total} (or R_{total}), although the magnitude of change as shown in both this example and for the whole patient group

Table 3.3.
Influence of aortic valvuloplasty on total effective arterial elastance (Ea), total afterload resistance (R_{total} = Ea/HR), peripheral vascular resistance (R_{periph}), and valvular resistance (R_{valve}). Routine hemodynamic data are also provided. While the procedure yields a near 45% increase in estimated valve area, hemodynamic assessments based on a resistive model suggest far more modest reductions in net ventricular loading.

	Pre	Post	p
Ea_{total} (mm Hg/milliliter)	3.8	3.3	< .05
R_{total} (mm Hg/liter/min)	48.6	41.9	< .05
R_{periph}	20.7	20.8	NS
R_{valve}	27.4	21.2	< .01
Pes (mm Hg)	203.5	178.7	< .001
CO (liters/min)	4.4	4.6	NS
ΔP (mm Hg)	65.6	40.9	< .0001
Valve area (cm^2)	0.52	0.74	< .0001

Pes = end-systolic pressure, CO = cardiac output, ΔP = mean transaortic valvular pressure gradient.

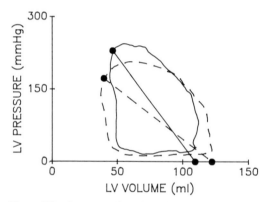

Figure 3.7. Pressure-volume loops from a patient before (solid line) and after (dashed line) aortic valvuloplasty. The points at end-systole (upper left of each loop) and end-diastolic volume (at $P = 0$) are connected to display Ea, the effective arterial elastance (Ea = Pes/SV), as a measure of ventricular afterload. Valvuloplasty reduced Ea shown by the lowering of this slope.

was modest ($-11.7 \pm 3.6\%$ ($p < .001$)). Subtraction of the peripheral vascular component revealed the average valvular resistance fell by only $- 18.7 \pm 4.5\%$ ($p < .001$). Aortic valvular stenosis contributed $55.7 \pm 1.3\%$ to the total effective afterload resistance (R_T) at baseline and still represented $49.9 \pm 1.7\%$ of the total load after valvuloplasty ($p < .01$). Thus while area estimates indicated a substantial increase postvalvuloplasty ($+42\%$, from 0.52 to 0.74, $p < .0001$), resistance calculations, which were more directly related to the ventricular pump loading and thus performance, suggested much more modest improvement.

R_{valve} also correlated with aortic valve area, in much the same way as mean valve resistance (Eq. 9 and Fig. 3.6). In fact, the two resistance measurements correlate well with each other ($R_{valve} = 2.4 \cdot R + 12.2, r = 0.8, p < .001$). The nonunity slope stems from the use of systolic ejection period for R ($\Delta P/Q$) versus cardiac cycle length for R_{valve} [(Pes-mABP)/CO].

FUNCTION VERSUS ANATOMY

An advantage of functional over anatomic assessment of valvular stenosis is that the results can be more easily related to pump function at rest and under conditions of stress. An example from the valvuloplasty study[27] derives from analysis of changes in cardiac output. Net output for the entire patient group did not change after valvuloplasty (4.4 liters/min − pre, and 4.6 − post, $p = $ NS); however, this was often due to offsetting influences of altered valvular versus peripheral vascular loading. Eleven of the 23 patients displayed less than a 9% overall change in R_{total} (mean $\%\Delta R_{total} = +2.9 \pm 3.2\%$), and in these patients, CO fell by 8% after valvuloplasty. In the majority (73%) of these patients, peripheral resistance significantly increased by 20.4%, masking the simultaneous 18% reduction in R_{valve}. In the other 12 patients, both peripheral and valvular resistances fell, yielding a greater net load reduction and significant increase in cardiac output. While the functional analysis clearly separated these two patient groups, estimated change in valve area did not but rather was similar between them.

Another example of the strength of functional over anatomic representations is presented by Ford.[26] Ventricular power (PW = rate of work change) across the valve is:

$$PW_v = Q \cdot \Delta P = Q^2 \cdot R = (CO^2 \cdot R_v)/SEF, \quad (11)$$

where SEF = systolic ejection period/RR interval, and power related to peripheral resistance is:

$$PW_{periph} = CO^2 \cdot R_{periph} \quad (12)$$

Ford showed that total power ($PW_{periph} + PW_{valve}$) normalized to rest conditions was equal to:

$$(Q' + rQ'^2)/(1 + r) \quad (13)$$

where Q' is the ratio of CO:$CO_{resting}$, and r is the ratio of R_{valve}:($R_{periph,resting} \cdot SEF$). Using Equation 13 (Fig. 3.8), a patient with a resting r ratio of 1.0 (typical of patients with aortic stenosis) would require nearly 3–6 times as much ventricular power to achieve the same degree of enhanced cardiac output as a patient without stenosis. Thus, the functional significance of doubling rest resistive load ($R_{periph} + R_{valve}$) is magnified under conditions of increased work demand. This is less directly appreciated from anatomic area measurements.

MITRAL VALVE STENOSIS

Most of the preceding discussion regarding the Gorlin formula, simplified hydraulic equations, and valvular resistance hold equally for aortic and mitral valves. The basic assumptions used to derive the Gorlin equation as well as the "modified Bernoulli" equation for Doppler gradient assessment are similar and thus predictions are internally consistent. Doppler indices have also been described for direct estimation of mitral valve area by utilization of the pressure half-time; however, this approach has recently been brought under question.

Pressure half-time, or the time for 50% fall in transvalvular pressure gradient, has been related to mitral valve area by the expression:

$$\text{Mitral Valve Area (MVA)} = 220/T_{1/2} \quad (14)$$

Thomas et al.[11,29] have recently presented both a theoretical model and in vitro and in vivo data suggesting that $T_{1/2}$ is related to factors other than just mitral valve area. During valvuloplasty, for example, these other factors become very influential, rendering Equation 14 invalid. Using a steady flow analysis similar to that presented in Equations 5–9, Thomas added consideration of left atrial and ventricular compliances and derived an analytic expression describing atrioventricular pressure difference during diastole as a function of valve area, the initial pressure gradient (ΔP_o), combined atrial (C_a) and ventricular (C_v) linear compliances ($C_n = C_a C_v /[C_a + C_v]$), and time ($t$):

$$\Delta P(t) = [\sqrt{\Delta P_o} - (25.2\alpha \cdot \text{AREA}/C_n)t]^2 \quad (15)$$

Solving Equation 15 for $T_{1/2}$ one obtains:

$$T_{1/2} = 11.6C_n\sqrt{\Delta P_o} / (\alpha\text{AREA}) \quad (16)$$

Figure 3.8. Model prediction of the influence of valvular stenosis on the incremental ventricular power required to increase cardiac output. The value (r) is the ratio of valvular:peripheral resistance (W_T:$W_{T.rest}$), the power output normalized to rest, and (CO/CO_{rest} = Q) the cardiac output normalized to rest. See text for details. Reproduced with permission from *Circulation Research*.[26]

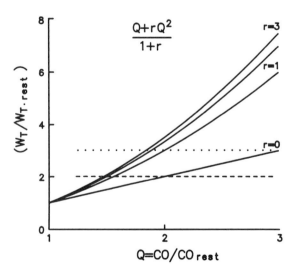

Thomas et al.[29] compared the $T_{1/2}$ predicted by the simplified formula (Eq. 14) versus the more complex formula (Eq. 16) in an in vitro model and in patients before and after mitral valvuloplasty. They reported poor correlations with the simplified model, particularly after valvuloplasty, but much better predictions using Equation 16. The source of the discrepancy was related to substantial increases in atrial compliance and a reduction in ΔP_{o} following valvuloplasty. These changes were consistent with improved emptying of the atrium and filling of the ventricle after the procedure.

There is an important lesson from this study regarding applications of models tested under rest conditions to data obtained after a procedure such as valvuloplasty. Normally $\sqrt{\Delta P_{o}}$ and C_{n} are inversely related, since for a given nonlinear passive PV relation of an atrium (or ventricle), as the pressure gradient rises, the atrium operates at higher volumes and thus lower compliance. Equation 16 reverts to Equation 14, with $T_{1/2}$ largely determined by valve area. However, valvuloplasty produces marked changes in loading, with marked sudden reductions in atrial volume and pressure; thus, the other factors incorporated in Equation 16 must be considered. One could make a similar argument concerning aortic valve calculations before and after valvuloplasty. While discrepancies between the true and idealized flow patterns and valve geometry may serve reasonably well for baseline valve area approximations, abrupt and likely highly irregular changes in valve geometry and flows with valvuloplasty may violate the simple assumptions yielding questionable results. This again highlights the benefits of combining functional and anatomic assessments in procedures such as this.

SUMMARY

While there can be no question that invasive and noninvasive estimates of in vivo valvular area will continue to play a major role in assessment of valvular heart disease, the often marked changes in loading and valve geometry produced by valvuloplasty and related techniques are forcing a reappraisal of this approach. The Gorlin formula and other formulas have their supporters and detractors, but generally there is increasing recognition that "area" estimates can change with altered physiologic conditions. The real question regards the goal of hemodynamic assessment, which is to estimate the severity of stenosis or changes in its severity following interventional procedures. In this light, a determination of functional severity, whether assessed by means of valvular resistance, altered chamber loading and compliances, or pressure half-time, can often provide valuable information regarding the outcome and efficacy of valvuloplasty. The value of these data will likely be further enhanced by examining responses both at rest and under stress. As our interventional techniques evolve, it is hoped that a broader view of hemodynamic assessment will be adapted to make full use of the available measurements.

REFERENCES

1. Effler DB, Favaloro R, Groves LK. Heart valve replacement: Clinical experience. *Ann Thorac Surg* 1:5–25, 1965.
2. St. John Sutton MG, St. John Sutton M, Oldershaw P, Sacchetti R, Paneth M, Lennox SC, Gibson RV, Gibson DG. Valve replacement without preoperative cardiac catheterization. *N Eng J Med* 305:1233–1238, 1981.
3. Gorlin R, Gorlin SG. Hydraulic formula for calculation of the area of the stenotic mitral valve, other cardiac valves, and central circulatory shunts. I. *Am Heart J* 41:1–29, 1951.
4. Dow JW, Levine HD, Elkin M, Haynes FW, Hellems HK, Whittenberger JW, Ferris BG, Goodale WT, Harvey WP, Eppinger EC, Dexter L. Studies of congenital heart disease IV. Uncomplicated pulmonic stenosis. *Circulation* 1:267–287, 1950.
5. Gorlin R. Calculations of cardiac stenosis: Restoring an old concept for advanced applications. (Editorial) *J Am Coll Cardiol* 10:920–922, 1987.
6. Spencer MP, Geiss FC. Dynamics of ventricular ejection. *Circ Res* 10:274–279, 1962.
7. Bellhouse B, Bellhouse F. Fluid mechanics of model normal and stenosed aortic valves. *Circ Res* 25:693–704, 1969.
8. Bellhouse BJ. The fluid mechanics of heart valves. In *Cardiovascular fluid dynamics*, ed by DH Bergel, New York, Academic Press, 1972.
9. Clark C. Relation between pressure difference across the aortic valve and left ventricular outflow. *Cardiovascular Research* 12:276–287, 1978.
10. Thomas JD, Weyman AE. Fluid dynamics of mitral valve flow: Description with in vitro validation. *J Am Coll Cardiol* 13:221–233, 1989.
11. Yoganathan AP, Cape EG, Sung, H-W, Williams FP, Jimoh A. Review of hydrodynamic principles for the cardiologist: Applications to the study of blood flow and jets by imaging techniques. *J Am Coll Cardiol* 12:1344–1353, 1988.
12. Gorlin WB, Gorlin R. A generalized formulation of the Gorlin formula for calculating the area of the stenotic mitral valve and other stenotic cardiac valves. *J Am Coll Cardiol* 15:246–247, 1990.

13. Wilkins GT, Gillam LD, Kritzer GL, Levine RA, Palacios IF, Weyman AE. Validation of continuous-wave Doppler echocardiographic measurements of mitral and tricuspid prosthetic valve gradients: A simultaneous Doppler-catheter study. *Circulation* 74:786–795, 1986.

14. Yoganathan AP. Fluid mechanics. *Eur Heart J* 9:13–17, 1988.

15. Carabello BA. Advances in the hemodynamic assessment of stenotic cardiac valves. *J Am Coll Cardiol 10*: 912–919, 1987.

16. Bird JJ, Murgo JP, Pasipoularides A. Fluid dynamics of aortic stenosis: Subvalvular gradients without subvalvular obstruction. *Circulation 66*:835–840, 1982.

17. Pasipoularides A, Murgo JP, Bird JJ, Craig WE. Fluid dynamics of aortic stenosis: Mechanisms for the presence of subvalvular pressure gradients. *Am J Physiol 246*:H542–H550, 1984.

18. Levine RA, Jimoh A, Cape EG, McMillan S, Yoganathan AP, Weyman AE. Pressure recovery distal to a stenosis: Potential cause of gradient "overestimation" by Doppler echocardiography. *J Am Coll Cardiol 13*:706–715, 1989.

19. Rodrigo FA. Estimation of valve area and "valvular resistance": A critical study of the physical basis of the methods employed. *Am Heart J 45:* 1–12, 1953.

20. Hakki A-H, Iskandrian AS, Bemis C, Kimbiris D, Mintz GS, Segal B, Brice C. A simplified valve formula for the calculation of stenotic cardiac valve areas. *Circulation 63*:1050–1055, 1981.

21. Angel J., Soler-Soler J, Anivarro I, Domingo E. Hemodynamic evaluation of stenotic cardiac values: II. Modification of the simplified valve formula for mitral and aortic valve area calculation. *Cath Cardiovasc Diag 11*:127–138, 1985.

22. Bache RJ, Wang Y, Jorgensen CR. Hemodynamic effects of exercise in isolated valvular aortic stenosis. *Circulation 44*:1003–1013, 1971.

23. Cannon SR, Richards KL, Crawford M. Hydraulic estimation of stenotic orifice area: A correction of the Gorlin formula. *Circulation 71*:1170–1178, 1985.

24. Stewart WJ, Jiang L, Mich R, Pandian N, Guerrero JL, Weyman AE. Variable effects of changes in flow rate through the aortic, pulmonary and mitral valves on valve area and flow velocity: Impact on quantitative Doppler flow calculations. *J Am Coll Cardiol 6*: 653–662, 1985.

25. Richards KL, Cannon SR, Lujan MS, Grewe K, Jian W-H. Anatomical valve area varies with pressure gradient and flow rate in severe aortic stenosis. *Circulation* (Suppl:II) *78*:II–209, 1988.

26. Ford LE, Feldman T, Chiu C, Carroll JD. Hemodynamic resistance as a measure of functional impairment in aortic valvular stenosis. *Circ Res 66*:1–7, 1990.

27. Kass DA, Davidson CJ, Skelton TN, Bashore TM. Altered LV afterload due to aortic valve: An alternative to valve area estimation for assessing valvuloplasty outcome. (Abstr) *Circulation 78*(II): II–528, 1988.

28. Sunagawa K, Sagawa K, Maughan WLM. Ventricular interaction with the vascular system in terms of pressure-volume relationships. In *Ventricular/Vascular Coupling*, ed. by FCP Yin, New York, Springer-Verlag, 1987, pp. 210–239.

29. Thomas JD, Wilkins GT, Choong CYP, Abascal VM, Palacois IF, Block PC, Weyman AE. Inaccuracy of mitral pressure half-time immediately after percutaneous mitral valvotomy: Dependence on transmitral gradient and left atrial and ventricular compliance. *Circulation 78*:980–993, 1988.

SECTION II.

AORTIC VALVULOPLASTY

4

Clinical Evaluation of Valvular Aortic Stenosis

ROBERT A. WAUGH

As noted in Chapter 2, the etiologies of valvular aortic stenosis are variable but most commonly include congenital leaflet deformities, rheumatic inflammation with commissural fusion, and fibrosis/calcification. The latter may occur in isolation or in combination when superimposed on a congenital or rheumatic process. Only very rarely does an infiltrative (e.g., hypercholesterolemia), infectious (e.g., fungal endocarditis), or other inflammatory process (e.g., rheumatoid arthritis) cause significant aortic stenosis.

With the decline in rheumatic fever, an increase in average longevity, and more accurate clinical and pathologic diagnosis, there has been a decline in the frequency of rheumatic aortic valve disease and an increase in degenerative aortic valve disease. In reported series, congenital and degenerative processes are now the most common etiology of pure aortic stenosis. With these changes have come alterations in the frequency of various clinical findings in the disease and, probably, in its natural history. (It should be noted parenthetically that, for comparison purposes, there is no carefully defined concurrent group of "control patients" with both aortic stenosis and no intervention.)[1]

Notwithstanding these changes and problems with defining the true natural history, these processes usually result in predictable syndromes, and the clinical evaluation of patients is typically straightforward. Thus, the history, physical examination, and laboratory evaluation combine to produce a clear and uncomplicated picture of the primary valvular problem as well as its severity. This evaluative process has been helped immeasurably by the advent of more accurate and reliable noninvasive instrumentation including echocardiography and, more recently, Doppler cardiography. The application of these technologies, however, involves significant expense, and their use still requires clinical judgment. The latter is helped immeasurably by confidence in one's bedside skills and the ability to interpret accurately cheaper and simpler laboratory tests.

This chapter will deal with the clinical evaluation of patients with known or suspected aortic valve disease beginning with the history and proceeding through the physical examination and the use of the laboratory, including the electrocardiogram and the chest roentgenogram. Chapter 5 deals separately with echo-Doppler cardiography.

CLINICAL HISTORY

The classic symptoms of valvular aortic stenosis are exertional angina, congestive heart failure, and syncope/sudden death. The following discussion will center first on angina and syncope/sudden death, two symptoms related to the severity of the valvular gradient that can occur independent of left ventricular dysfunction. This will be followed by a discussion of left ventricular heart failure, a symptom also related to the severity of the stenosis, and one that is frequently (but not invariably) superimposed on a prior history of angina or syncope. A brief discussion of a variety of additional, less common historical clues to the diagnosis then ends this section.

Chest Pain

The reported frequency of chest pain with aortic stenosis is somewhat variable but is very common with an incidence of $> 50\%$.[2-4] It is the presenting symptom in about one out of three adults.[4] In infants and young children, extracting a typical anginal history is more difficult, and its exact incidence in this subgroup remains conjectural.

The chest pain is typical of angina with a substernal location, vague localization, visceral character (aching, squeezing, burning, tight, or vice-like), and a relation to physical exertion or emotional stress. It is such a mimic of the angina of coronary atherosclerosis that it is frequently impossible, by history, to discriminate aortic stenosis alone from aortic stenosis plus coronary artery disease (CAD) or even angina due to CAD alone. A duration of angina exceeding five years, however, does favor associated CAD as the longevity of patients with angina due to aortic stenosis alone is typically more short-lived. Rest pain also favors associated CAD.[5] Nitroglycerin (TNG) relieves the pain irrespective of associated coronary artery disease, and this is not a helpful differential point. Syncope after sublingual TNG, however, hints at significant underlying aortic stenosis.

Syncope/Sudden Death

Syncope is another clue to the diagnosis of aortic stenosis; although in any population of patients with syncope, aortic stenosis is an infrequent cause of this common symptom. On the other hand, in any series of patients with aortic stenosis, syncope is common.[2-4] In Lombard and Selzer's series, it was the initial complaint in 15% and increased in frequency with chronicity of the condition.[4] The history suggests the diagnosis of aortic stenosis particularly when syncope occurs in association with angina or congestive heart failure. When syncope is a presenting complaint, however, it suggests the diagnosis only indirectly when there is an associated history of a heart murmur or when symptoms suggestive of another etiology (e.g., a vasovagal reaction, arrhythmia, or postural hypotension) are lacking. An occurrence during or following exertion is suggestive but not invariable. Some patients may experience presyncopal spells or "gray outs" either alone or mixed in with bouts of syncope. They note a dimming in their vision (hence the descriptive term) and feel as if they are about to faint but do not. Again, these episodes are more common during or immediately following exertion.

In a few patients syncope may be related to a fixed cardiac output (in turn related to the severity of the stenosis) such that with exercise and arteriolar vasodilation, the blood pressure drops with cerebral hypoperfusion and loss of consciousness. Arrhythmias are an even less frequent inciting event although they probably are the reason some syncope turns into sudden death. Most frequently

the stimulation of cardiac baroceptors (in turn related to the gradient and left ventricular transmural pressure) leads to inappropriate arteriolar and venous dilation with a fall in arterial pressure and cardiac output and ensuing syncope.[6,7]

While sudden death may occur as an initial symptom in adults, it is more frequent in children, where it is also more commonly related to exertion. This latter relationship should result in prohibition of vigorous or competitive athletics in these patients. Sudden death in adults is less frequent and only rarely occurs as the first manifestation of the disease.

Congestive Heart Failure

The frequency of the third classic symptom of aortic stenosis, congestive heart failure, also varies in different series but is common in all and becomes more frequent with increasing age and disease severity.[2-4] In general, it is a later symptom superimposed on angina or syncope. In Lombard and Selzer's series of adults, it was a presenting complaint in over one-third of patients.[4] Initially the dyspnea is mild, primarily exertional, and reflective of the stiffening of the left ventricle that is, in turn, related to hypertrophy. That is, any elevation in left ventricular end diastolic pressure, left atrial pressure, and pulmonary venous pressure may reflect diastolic dysfunction. With progression and corresponding systolic and diastolic dysfunction, orthopnea, paroxysmal nocturnal dyspnea, and nocturia appear.

The appearance of right heart failure (i.e., peripheral edema and symptoms of abdominal visceral congestion) in patients < 60 years of age is unusual and, when it does occur, should suggest associated mitral valve disease. In the elderly, concomitant coronary artery disease and/or preexistent hypertension contribute to left ventricular dysfunction with more frequent left- and right-sided congestive heart failure.

Just as with angina, the symptoms of congestive heart failure are typical of those due to any etiology. The ancillary features of the clinical syndrome are sometimes helpful, however, in suggesting aortic stenosis. For example, aortic stenosis is a well-recognized cause of heart failure in the acyanotic newborn or infant, where it invariably reflects a severe gradient and either an acommissural or a unicommissural valve. Coarctation is another cause of heart failure in infancy and has a well-documented association with congenital aortic valve disease. It may even "mask" associated aortic stenosis, and the former always demands a careful evaluation for the latter. Once past infancy, angina and syncope are the more common initial complaints, but congestive heart failure may develop subsequently in the clinical course in these patients as well. In fact, heart failure developing after angina or syncope with nothing to suggest a more common etiology (e.g., myocardial infarction with heart failure or arrhythmias) should suggest aortic stenosis.

History of Heart Murmur

When a heart murmur dates from birth or very early in childhood, particularly with no history of cyanosis, the possibility of outflow tract obstruction (and it may be either left- or right-sided) should be entertained. A murmur first noted at an older age (e.g., the child's first preschool physical examination) may reflect a valvular problem but a left to right shunt is also a possibility.

Heart murmurs due to normal flow (innocent or physiologic murmurs), however, are extremely common in children and young adults, and a history of a heart murmur may be a "red herring." A consistently detected murmur from one examination to the next, however, suggests underlying heart disease. Associated warnings to avoid exercise, ineligibility for sports, rejection from the service/employment, the denial of life insurance, and/or the administration of antibiotics for endocarditis prophylaxis are additional clues to a "pathologic" murmur. In none of these instances, however, can the history identify the specific valve or the hemodynamic derangement (shunt, stenosis, or regurgitation).

Other Symptoms

Since pure aortic stenosis is rarely, if ever, due to a rheumatic process, a history of rheumatic fever is helpful only in explaining a mixed aortic valve lesion with associated significant aortic regurgitation or in occasioning a diligent search for associated mitral valve disease.

Arrhythmias are not part of the typical picture of aortic stenosis particularly in patients < 60 years of age. In older patients with a more chronic course, associated hypertensive/coronary artery disease and/or left ventricular dysfunction, palpitations due to supraventricular and ventricular ectopy, and atrial fibrillation are more frequent.

Embolic events are also not part of the clinical picture of aortic stenosis, per se. Exceptions include rare instances of calcific emboli[8] and emboli arising due to associated atrial fibrillation (an infrequent arrhythmia with pure aortic stenosis but a risk factor for left atrial clots and emboli just the same). In general, embolic events are unusual, and their occurrence, therefore, should occasion a search for associated mitral valve disease, endocarditis, or a left ventricular source due to prior myocardial infarction.

Fatigue is a notoriously nonspecific symptom but may be noted in children (where the fatigue must be judged in relation to the child's peer group) or in older adults with congestive heart failure and a decreased cardiac output. It is not part of the syndrome of pure aortic stenosis with well-compensated left ventricular function.

Intestinal bleeding from a variety of vascular malformations (angiodysplasia) of the colon has been reported to be associated with valvular aortic stenosis both anecdotally and in at least one careful case-controlled study.[9] A consensus about this relationship, however, is not unanimous. Resolution of the bleeding with aortic valve replacement has also been reported,[10] but this is neither a proven cause-effect relationship nor a 100% reliable scenario. However, in patients undergoing aortic valve replacement, a history of intestinal bleeding may have important implications for the choice of prosthesis as it relates to the need for chronic postoperative anticoagulation.

PHYSICAL EXAMINATION
Venous Pulse

The mean venous pressure, venous wave form, and respiratory dynamics of the venous pulse are typically normal. On rare occasions with severe concentric left ventricular hypertrophy, the decreased compliance of the interventricular septum may contribute to a decrease in right ventricular compliance and produce an accentuated (or giant) A wave. Advanced and chronic left ventricular dysfunction and failure can cause pulmonary venous and arterial hypertension with a commensurate rise in the mean central venous pressure. Most patients, however, either die or undergo an intervention to relieve the obstruction before this occurs. In Lombard and Selzer's recent series of adults with valvular aortic stenosis, 5% and 12%, respectively, showed a mean right atrial pressure > 10 mm Hg and a mean pulmonary arterial pressure > 40 mm Hg. Both abnormalities were more frequent in those with more severe stenosis.[3]

Arterial Pulse

BLOOD PRESSURE AND PULSE VOLUME

With aortic stenosis in younger patients, the arterial pulse pressure may be narrow (e.g., < 30 mm Hg), reflecting the slowed left ventricular ejection. A reduced systolic blood pressure and arterial pulse volume (as judged by palpation of the carotid pulse) also may be present. These findings are more difficult to interpret in young patients because their blood pressures are normally low in comparison to the typical older American. In fact, however, the blood pressure and pulse pressure are frequently normal despite significant aortic stenosis, and these observations cannot be used to exclude the diagnosis. In older adults, in particular, the arterial pulse pressure and volume are typically normal or even increased, reflecting an age-related loss of arteriolar elasticity and, in some patients, superimposed atherosclerosis. Similarly, a normal, or even hypertensive, systolic blood pressure is common. As a clinical rule, though, sustained blood pressures > 175 mm Hg are unusual in patients with valvular gradients > 50 mm Hg as chronic left ventricular systolic pressures ≥ 225 mm Hg are usually not tolerated for long in the older adult. Exceptions occur, however (particularly in the elderly), and the possibility of aortic stenosis should be kept in the differential despite hypertension if other features point toward this diagnosis.

Because of the frequent association between coarctation and congenital aortic leaflet deformities, the combination of hypertension and aortic valve disease is an indication for careful simultaneous palpation of the radial and femoral pulses. A delayed femoral pulse relative to the radial pulse is almost pathognomonic of coarctation. It is also more easily obtained than trying to find an appropriate size thigh cuff to measure leg blood pressures.

ARTERIAL PULSE MORPHOLOGY (UPSTROKE AND NUMBER OF PEAKS)

The classic parvus et tardus (small and late peaking) pulse of aortic stenosis is pathognomonic of significant aortic stenosis. It is most frequent in younger patients with an elastic arterial vasculature and a well-preserved cardiac output. It is due to severe obstruction and a slowing of the left ventricular ejection rate. A fall in cardiac output as left ventricular dysfunction occurs later in the disease course can also contribute to a diminished pulse volume. In the older adult, despite significant aortic stenosis, the upstroke of the carotid pulse may appear to be well preserved to palpation.

In all age groups the arterial pulse is single unless there is associated moderate to severe aortic regurgitation. Combined aortic stenosis and regurgitation (or pure aortic regurgitation), however, may cause a bifid or bisferious arterial pulse. Occasionally with isolated aortic stenosis, the pulse may be mistakenly interpreted as bifid. This occurs when the sharp break between the arterial pulse's initial small and more normal rate of rise (the anacrotic shoulder) or the immediately following anacrotic notch are felt as an initial peak and the subsequent slow rise, as a second peak (Fig. 4.1). In fact, the older literature sometimes called this anacrotic type of pulse bisferious. As defined today, however, a bisferious arterial pulse has a brisk upstroke, wide pulse pressure, and a rapid mid-systolic collapse in marked contrast to the usual pulse of aortic stenosis.

In all age groups and independent of underlying aortic valve morphology, significant aortic stenosis frequently causes a carotid thrill or, if particularly coarse vibrations are present, a "shudder" (Fig. 4.2). These findings reflect the vibrations of the transmitted aortic valve murmur, and both are typically more prominent over the left as compared to the right carotid. This preferential transmission occurs because the left carotid, though "farther" from the murmur source, is a direct branch of the aortic arch. The right carotid, on the other hand, arises from the innominate artery and is therefore two branch points downstream. With supravalvular aortic stenosis, this pattern reverses with preferential transmission of the thrill and bruit to the right carotid. A significantly higher blood pressure in the right as compared to the left arm may also occur. When there is an irregular rhythm (e.g., premature beats or atrial fibrillation), the carotid thrill accentuates following a pause and may be palpable only at that time.

Carotid thrills are not pathognomonic of aortic stenosis as they also occur with pure aortic regurgitation and, rarely, with underlying carotid arterial stenosis. A bedside clue to the latter occurs when the bruit becomes louder as one inches the stethoscope superiorly toward the angle of the jaw. If the bruit arises from the origin of the carotid vessel, however, it may more closely mimic a transmitted aortic valvular murmur.

Precordium

The precordial findings of importance in assessing aortic stenosis include thrills and abnormalities of the apical impulse.

A systolic thrill over the upper right sternal edge

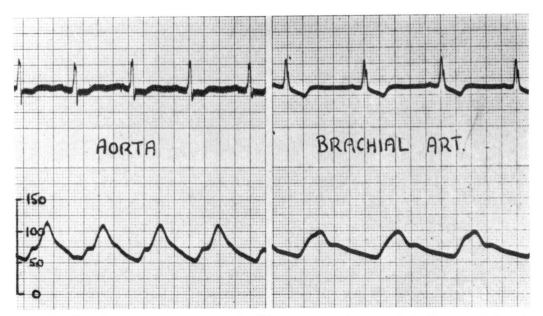

Figure 4.1. These intraarterial pressure tracings, from Wood's classic treatise, were obtained in a patient with aortic stenosis. The aortic pressure curve (AORTA) shows a low anacrotic shoulder followed by a perceptible notch and then a second slow rise to a delayed peak. In the brachial tracing (BRACHIAL ART.), the anacrotic shoulder is higher and the notch less prominent. The initial shoulder and/or the notch may be appreciated as one peak and, in concert with the second peak, lead to the mistaken impression that the pulse is bifid. (By permission from Wood P. Aortic stenosis. *Am J Cardiol Vol 1:* 553–571, 1958. Figure 10)

and in the suprasternal notch is characteristic of valvular aortic stenosis. Like the thrill over the carotid pulse, the precordial systolic thrill may be felt only after a pause in the rhythm (e.g., following a premature beat or a longer RR interval during atrial fibrillation). Palpating at the base while the patient sits up and leans forward during full expiration enhances the likelihood of appreciating the thrill.

The location and size of the apical impulse can provide valuable information about the severity of the aortic stenosis. With well-compensated aortic stenosis, the location of the apex impulse is typically normal (within 10–12 cm of the midsternal line in the fifth intercostal space). Despite a normal location, an increased size is usual, reflecting concentric ventricular hypertrophy. With decompensation (or with concomitant aortic regurgitation), the left ventricle dilates. The apex impulse, therefore, is inferolaterally displaced and further enlarged. The latter findings also may reflect concomitant processes such as ischemic or hypertensive heart disease. Obesity, lung disease, and increased muscle mass make appreciation of these changes difficult.

Whether normally located or inferolaterally displaced, the morphology of the apex impulse also changes predictably. The systolic impulse, in addition to being enlarged, becomes sustained throughout more of systole. In addition, the decreased compliance of left ventricular hypertrophy leads to more forceful atrial systole. The A wave of the apex impulse, therefore, is accentuated and becomes palpable (Fig. 4.3). An enlarged (or palpable) apical A wave, in carefully selected patients, typically correlates with a significant gradient.[11] Palpable A waves also can reflect hypertrophic or congestive cardiomyopathy, prior infarction, and preexistent/concomitant hypertension, where they are less predictive of the presence or severity of any gradient. Only rarely do patients survive long enough for their left ventricular failure to cause pulmonary venous and arterial hypertension. Precordial pulsations due to pulmonary artery dilation and right ventricular hypertrophy are uncommon.

Auscultation

FIRST AND SECOND HEART SOUNDS

The first heart sound is typically normal. Prominent splitting of the first heart sound that is well heard at the upper right sternal edge should always suggest an aortic ejection sound (see next section). With poor left ventricular function or first degree AV block, the first heart sound softens.

The behavior of the second heart sound in terms of loudness and response to respiration depends on the type and severity of the underlying aortic valve disease. In the younger age group, aortic stenosis is usually due to a congenital leaflet deformity with a mobile valve. The aortic component of the second heart sound, therefore, is well preserved or even accentuated (ejection sounds tend to be prominent as well). In the older adult whose aortic stenosis is due to progressive calcification with valve immobility, the aortic component of S_2 typically softens and is more difficult to hear (Fig. 4.2). With left ventricular decompensation and elevated pulmonary and venous arterial pres-

sures, a well-preserved or even accentuated but single S_2 not uncommonly reflects a loud pulmonary closure sound that is mistaken for a preserved aortic closure sound.

Severe aortic stenosis prolongs the left ventricular ejection time and delays A_2. If the delay is sufficient, A_2 follows P_2 and paradoxical splitting occurs. Detecting paradoxical splitting, of course, requires audible aortic and pulmonary valve closure sounds. A well-preserved aortic component is usual when the stenosis occurs with mobile leaflets (i.e., a bicuspid aortic valve with commissural fusion) or when it is subvalvular (either membranous or muscular). In older patients, unfortunately, the same factor that contributes to progressive severity (i.e., valvular calcification) also contributes to valve immobility, a decreased distal aortic pressure, and a decreased intensity of A_2.

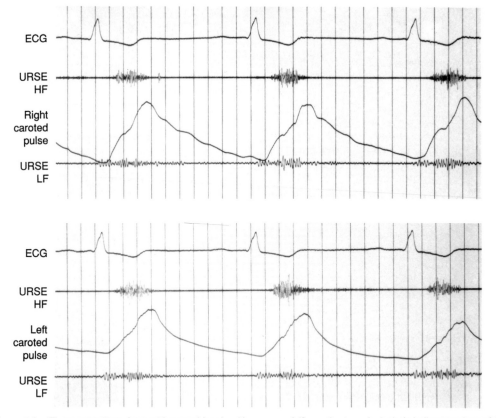

Figure 4.2. These recordings, from a 59-year-old male with severe calcific aortic stenosis, include indirect tracings of the right (panel **A**) and left (Panel **B**) carotid pulses, an ECG (lead II), and phonocardiogram from the upper right sternal edge (URSE). In comparison to the left carotid, the right carotid pulse showed a more prominent anacrotic shoulder and notch and barely detectable high frequency systolic vibrations. Clinically, a transmitted systolic murmur and faint thrill were present. The left carotid shows more obvious high frequency systolic vibrations typical of a "shudder" and clinically the transmitted aortic murmur was louder on this side. The sound recording is also typical of severe calcific aortic stenosis with no ejection sound, a long mid to late peaking murmur, and absent second heart sound. Time lines = 1.0 second; HF = high frequency; LF = low frequency

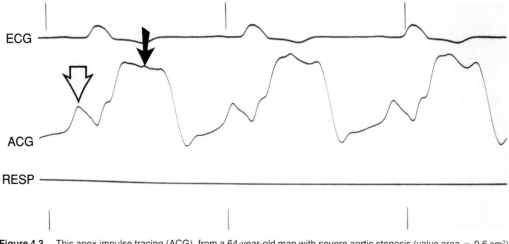

Figure 4.3.   This apex impulse tracing (ACG), from a 64-year-old man with severe aortic stenosis (valve area = 0.6 cm^2), demonstrates a prominent A wave (open arrow) followed by a sustained systolic contour (closed arrow). Clinically, the impulse also was enlarged. These findings are typical of left ventricular hypertrophy with decreased compliance. On ECG, there was left bundle branch block and a top normal PR interval. The latter separated the A wave and the following systolic component making the augmented atrial filling wave easier to feel. Time lines = 1.0 second; RESP = respirometer

Thus, paradoxical splitting is frequently more difficult (but still possible) to hear in elderly patients with severe aortic stenosis. In this age group, the combination of an aortic outflow murmur and easily detected paradoxical splitting should suggest one of two possibilities: subvalvular obstruction or less severe obstruction with concomitant left bundle branch block.

EXTRA SOUNDS/GALLOPS

With congenital aortic valvular stenosis, an ejection sound is so typical that its absence should raise the question of subvalvular or supravalvular aortic stenosis. Of course, ejection sounds can be very difficult to hear in the newborn (with their tachypnea and rapid heart rate) or in patients whose associated systolic murmur is loud. With the latter, the ejection sound occurs just at the onset of the murmur and their similar frequency content "blends" them together (Fig. 4.4). Fortunately, left-sided ejection sounds radiate well to the apex. Auscultation at the apex where the murmur may be softer, therefore, will frequently allow an aortic ejection sound to be readily appreciated (Fig. 4.4). Even loud murmurs with and without concomitant ejection sounds have a different quality and any interested observer can learn to recognize these differences through practice with appropriate feedback on accuracy. With aortic stenosis due to progressive valvular calcification and immobility,

the aortic ejection sound (as well as S_2) typically softens and is more difficult to hear.

With significant left ventricular hypertrophy, an audible fourth heart sound reflecting diminished compliance typically accompanies a palpable presystolic apical impulse. Not uncommonly, the enhanced presystolic apical impulse is easier to feel than the fourth heart sound is to hear. In patients < 40 years of age, an audible S_4 predicts a peak gradient ≥ 75 mm Hg, whereas in older patients, an audible S_4 may simply reflect concomitant disease processes.[12,13]

MURMURS

A systolic murmur is the acoustic hallmark of aortic stenosis. It is crescendo-decrescendo or diamond-shaped, mid or coarse in frequency (harsh, grating, and grunting are common descriptive terms), and typically maximal at the upper right sternal edge. With maintained left ventricular function, its length and time-to-peak are roughly proportional to severity. It is frequently grade 4 (i.e., associated with a thrill) or louder. These various features are particularly likely to be found in patients < 60 years of age (Fig. 4.5).

With increasing age, a variety of factors may combine to alter these typical findings. In patients with marked kyphosis or emphysema, the murmur may be maximal over the apex (particularly in the left lateral decubitus position) or even in the neck. The murmur also may be higher frequency at the

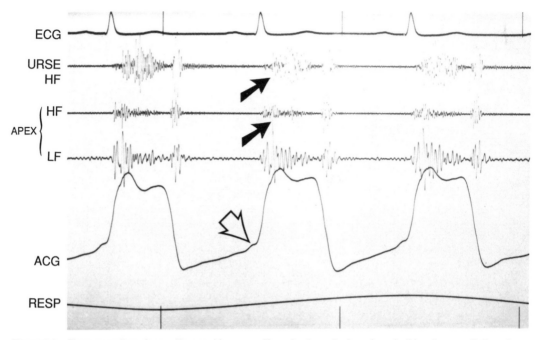

Figure 4.4. These recordings, from a 46-year-old woman with moderate aortic stenosis and mild aortic regurgitation, show a typical systolic, mid-frequency, diamond-shaped, early to mid-peaking murmur at the upper right sternal edge (URSE) and apical area (APEX). A soft diastolic blow of aortic regurgitation is present at the URSE as well (DM). An aortic ejection sound (arrows) is present in both locations, but clinically it was much easier to hear at the apex where the murmur was softer. The apex impulse (ACG) was mildly sustained, but the A wave (open arrow) was not accentuated, no fourth heart sound was present, and the aortic component (A_2) of the second heart sound was well preserved, findings also compatible with less than severe stenosis. Time lines = 1.0 second; HF = high frequency; LF = low frequency; RESP = respirometer.

apex related to the preferential radiation of these frequencies "upstream" from their site of origin, the so-called Gallavardin Phenomenon.[14] Although the contour and response of the murmur to interventions remain typical of an aortic outflow etiology, this higher frequency murmur is not infrequently mistaken for mitral regurgitation.

Left ventricular function is also an important determinant of some characteristics of the murmur. With left ventricular failure, the murmur may become unassuming with a loudness ≤ grade 2, a briefer duration, earlier peaking, and much less impressive radiation to the neck. In fact, the murmur may become inaudible, and aortic stenosis is a potential etiology in any patient with heart failure of undetermined cause with or without an aortic systolic murmur.

Although diastolic murmurs are not part of the picture of "pure" aortic stenosis, trivial aortic regurgitation accompanies aortic stenosis 30–50% of the time. In older patients with less severe stenosis, the differential between an aortic sclerosis murmur (the so-called innocent murmur of the elderly) and a murmur due to mild aortic stenosis may be difficult. An associated aortic diastolic

murmur (and/or an aortic ejection sound) is a very helpful bedside finding that identifies "true" aortic valve pathology. Steps to enhance the likelihood of hearing this murmur include pressing the diaphragm of the stethoscope firmly at the patient's lower left sternal edge. Having the patient seated, leaning forward, and the breath held during full expiration (analogous to the technique for palpating the systolic thrill) are also helpful.

Other Physical Findings

Growth and development are generally normal in both congenital and acquired aortic stenosis. Mental retardation and distinctive facies with a murmur of aortic stenosis should suggest supravalvular aortic stenosis.[15]

LABORATORY EVALUATION
Electrocardiography

LEFT VENTRICULAR HYPERTROPHY

Despite the newer, sophisticated technologies, the electrocardiogram (ECG) continues to provide valuable information in the evaluation of patients with valvular aortic stenosis. Although the ECG is insensitive to early left ventricular hypertrophy (LVH), increased QRS voltage in the left ventricular leads (R waves in leads I, II, aVL, and V_4–V_6 either alone or in combination with S waves in leads V_1–V_2) usually reliably identifies at least moderately severe LVH. Left ventricular voltage increases in combination with ST–T wave depression (without digitalis therapy) in these same leads (the so-called strain pattern) are highly predictive of even more severe left ventricular hypertrophy (Fig. 4.6).

Neither an isolated increase in left ventricular voltage (particularly in young patients) nor isolated ST–T wave changes (particularly with digoxin therapy) are sufficient for the diagnosis of LVH. Isolated voltage increases or ST–T wave changes, however, may be "summed" with a left atrial abnormality or "enlargement," abnormally prolonged intrinsicoid delay in the lateral precordial leads, and/or left axis deviation to identify hypertrophy (the Romhilt-Estes point scoring system for LVH).[16]

INTRAVENTRICULAR CONDUCTION PATTERN AND RHYTHM

Extensive aortic valvular calcification may extend into the interventricular septum; impinge on the His bundle or bundle branches; and cause PR interval prolongation, intraventricular conduction disturbances, and heart block. Left anterior hemiblock is particularly frequent, but both left and right bundle branch block may occur. Left bundle branch block also may reflect slowed left ventricular activation due to extensive left ventricular hypertrophy (i.e., a type of "peripheral" left bundle branch block). First degree AV block is more likely in the elderly patient, where it may

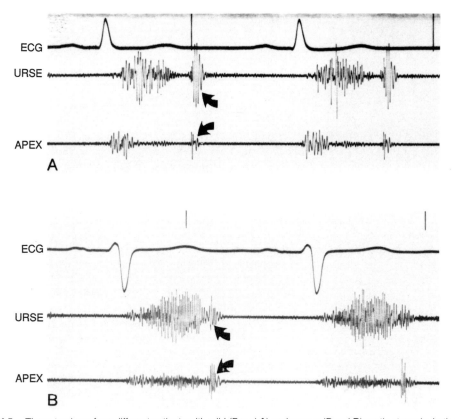

Figure 4.5.   These tracings, from different patients with mild (Panel **A**) and severe (Panel **B**) aortic stenosis, both show a systolic, mid-frequency, diamond-shaped murmur at the upper right sternal edge (URSE) and apex (APEX). In panel **A,** the mild gradient correlates with a relatively short, early peaking murmur that is very soft at the apex. The aortic component of the second heart sound (arrow) is also well preserved. In panel **B,** the severe gradient in this elderly patient correlates with a long, late peaking murmur that radiates well to the apex. What appears to be a well-preserved aortic closure sound (arrow) is actually an accentuated pulmonary closure sound that was, in turn, related to moderate pulmonary hypertension. Time lines = 1.0 second.

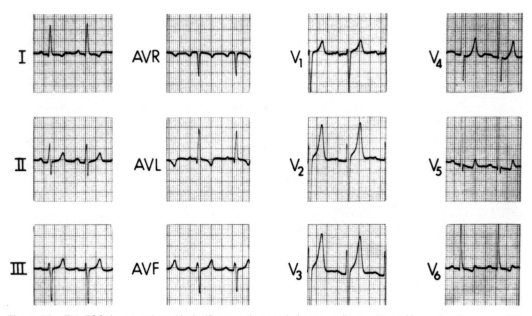

Figure 4.6.   This ECG, from a patient with significant aortic stenosis (mean gradient = 46 mm Hg, aortic valve area = 0.6 cm²), demonstrates normal sinus rhythm, a top normal PR interval, and QRS changes typical of left ventricular hypertrophy. Note the increased left ventricular voltage (the tall R waves in leads I, AVL, and V_5–V_6), the ST–T wave changes (the inverted Ts in these same leads plus ST depression in V_5 and V_6), and the borderline left axis deviation. (Standard: 1 mv = 10 mm)

reflect involvement of the His bundle or disease of the AV node due to concomitant processes. A higher degree of AV block is a rare complication.

The cardiac rhythm is usually sinus. Premature ventricular and supraventricular beats are much less frequent than in mitral valve disease. Atrial fibrillation should suggest associated mitral valve involvement. In the older age group, however, poor left ventricular function, secondary mitral regurgitation, coronary artery disease, and/or hypertension can combine to cause atrial enlargement and make atrial fibrillation more likely.

Chest Roentgenogram

Typical findings on the PA view include clear lung fields, a normal cardiothoracic ratio, and post-stenotic dilation of the proximal aortic root (Fig. 4.7A and 4.8A). On the lateral view, left ventricular enlargement displaces the left ventricular silhouette posteriorly (Fig. 4.7B). The detection of LVH may be enhanced by applying quantitative criteria such as that proposed by Hoffman and Rigler.[17] The left atrium and right-sided chambers are normal. In older patients, left ventricular enlargement is more frequent, even without heart failure.

In patients > 35 years of age with significant aortic stenosis, aortic valvular calcification may be seen on the plain film (Fig. 4.8B). Associated calcification of the mitral valve anulus is common. Calcification is noted even more frequently with fluoroscopy, a more sensitive technique. Its absence almost excludes significant aortic stenosis in this age group. Its presence, on the other hand, does not identify a significant gradient, as patients with severe aortic valve calcification may have either a mild or nonexistent gradient. In children and young adults, the gradient is not dependent on valvular calcification, and its absence does not exclude a gradient.

In all age groups, heart failure produces typical roentgenographic signs of pulmonary venous hypertension (cephalization, interstitial edema, Kerley B lines) and either the appearance of left ventricular enlargement or its progression. On the PA view, there is an increased AP diameter and inferolateral displacement of the apex. On the lateral view, more obvious posterior displacement of the left ventricle occurs. Oblique views of the heart also have characteristic changes, but more accurate techniques such as echocardiography have superseded their use.

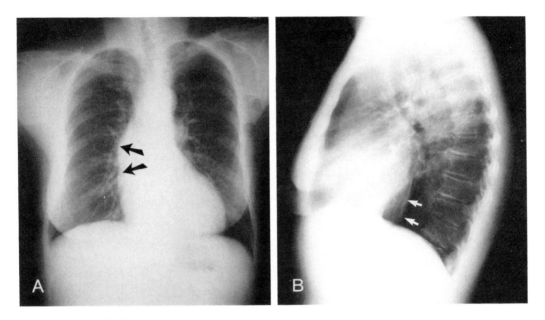

Figure 4.7. These PA (**A**) and lateral (**B**) roentgenograms are from a 58-year-old woman with a history of heart murmur since age 35 and a 6-week history of exertional presyncope and substernal tightness. The PA view shows poststenotic dilation of the ascending aorta (arrows) and a left ventricular contour with a top normal to mildly increased cardiothoracic ratio (0.52). The lateral view shows obvious ventricular enlargement (arrows) and no apparent valvular calcification (although it was present on fluoroscopy). At catheterization, the peak-to-peak valvular gradient was 102 mm Hg. (The roentgenograms used to make these illustrations were provided by James T. T. Chen, M.D., Professor of Radiology, Duke University Medical Center.)

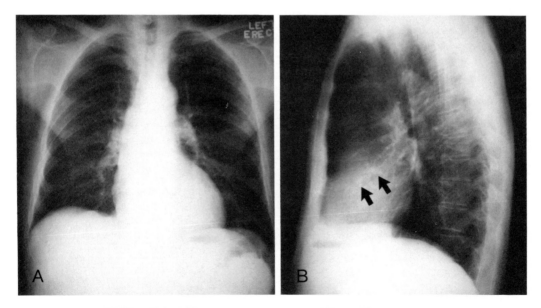

Figure 4.8. These PA (**A**) and lateral (**B**) roentgenograms are from a 72-year-old man with a 16-year history of a heart murmur and the recent onset of exertional substernal aching discomfort that radiated to the neck and left shoulder. On the PA view, the ascending aorta and cardiothoracic ratio are normal. On the lateral view, there is aortic valvular calcification (arrows) and no evidence of left ventricular hypertrophy. At catheterization, the mean gradient was 56 mm Hg. (The roentgenograms used to make these illustrations were provided by James T. T. Chen, M.D., Professor of Radiology, Duke University Medical Center.)

Other Laboratory Evaluations

In days of old, numerous additional laboratory tests were used in the evaluation of patients with known or suspected aortic stenosis. A partial list includes phonocardiography with detailed analyses of the apex contour, carotid pulse contour, heart sounds and murmurs, systolic time intervals, and comparing the patient's observed left ventricular ejection time to that predicted by left ventricular stroke volume (the difference is linearly related to aortic valve area).[18] Phonocardiography still has a valid role in teaching and in resolving confusing physical findings. As diagnostic tools, however, the precise morphological and functional data obtained by echo-Doppler cardiography and cardiac catheterization have rendered these tests obsolete in the evaluation of aortic stenosis.

Exercise stress testing has no obligatory role in the evaluation of adults with aortic stenosis regardless of the presence or absence of chest pain. It is relatively contraindicated in patients with a history of syncope and should be used with caution if at all when the stenosis is suspected to be severe. In patients whose clinical syndrome does not correlate with laboratory measurements of severity, exercise testing may be one method of inducing symptoms under controlled circumstances. The induction of ST–T wave depression/inversion during exercise stress testing has been used as an indication for intervention in asymptomatic children whose gradient is not clearly in the operative range (e.g., 40–70 mm Hg).[19]

Radionuclide imaging has no obligatory role in the evaluation of patients with aortic stenosis. It can assess ventricular function both at rest and can provide functional data during stress. Left ventricular dysfunction, however, is not a definite contraindication to surgery. Echocardiographic or angiographic measurements obtained during catheterization also provide an assessment of left ventricular systolic and diastolic function. The role of computerized tomography and magnetic resonance imaging (both static and gated) in the evaluation and management of patients with aortic stenosis remains investigational.

DIFFERENTIAL DIAGNOSIS

The differential diagnosis, particularly in the stable ambulatory patient, is essentially that of a murmur suggesting outflow track obstruction. The most frequent differential is between the murmur of aortic sclerosis (the so-called innocent murmur of the elderly) versus true aortic stenosis. This differential may be more semantic than real as the murmur of aortic sclerosis may be a harbinger of eventual aortic stenosis given a sufficient period of survival. The combination of normal carotid and apical pulses, a brief murmur, no ejection sound, no diastolic aortic murmur, and a normal ECG and chest roentgenogram, aortic sclerosis can be diagnosed with some certainty (at least at that particular point in time) even without the diagnostic coup d'état of echo-Doppler cardiography.

Not infrequently, a combination of processes confuses the picture. For example, patients with CAD and a prior apical infarction may have a prominent apical A wave and sustained contour that mimics aortic stenosis. Preexistent hypertension can do the same thing. When these findings occur with a prominent aortic sclerotic murmur, the differential becomes more difficult. Rarely, acute mitral regurgitation produces a regurgitant jet that radiates anteriorly toward the aortic root with a murmur that is prominent at the base. The murmur is typically nonholosystolic because of the rapid equilibration of left ventricular systolic pressure with that of a small, noncompliant left atrium. These findings simulate the murmur of aortic stenosis, but a host of other diagnostic clues to the real diagnosis are usually present.

The main differential is between valvular, supravalvular, and subvalvular stenosis. Table 4.1 and 4.2 list potentially important points in this differential diagnosis. In all instances, echo-Doppler cardiography can resolve the differential and pinpoint severity.

NATURAL HISTORY AND DECISIONS FOR INTERVENTION

The clinical management of adult patients with valvular aortic stenosis is straightforward. Asymptomatic patients should be followed medically until the onset of symptoms. They should be educated about good dental hygiene and, when indicated, appropriate dental referrals effected. Bacterial endocarditis prophylaxis is also indicated although the risk of endocarditis with pure aortic stenosis is small. Patients also should be advised to avoid sudden and strenuous exertion, but there is no documented contraindication to modest isotonic exercise (e.g., regular walking as part of a mild cardiovascular conditioning program) in asympto-

Table 4.1.
Differential Diagnosis of Aortic Stenosis Pulses

Conditions	Venous Pulse	Arterial Pulse	Precordial Pulse
Acute MR	Early ↑ CVP, giant A wave	Brisk upstroke, single peak	Nondisplaced, hyperdynamic, palpable S_4/S_3
Supravalvular aortic stenosis	Normal	Parvus et tardus BP R. arm > L. arm, thrill R. carotid > L. carotid	Nondisplaced, enlarged, and sustained with palpable S_4
Membranous subvalvular aortic stenosis	Normal	Parvus et tardus	Nondisplaced, enlarged, and sustained with palpable S_4
Muscular subvalvular aortic stenosis (HOCM)	Normal (occasionally giant A wave)	Brisk upstroke, spike and dome configuration	Nondisplaced,[b] enlarged, with prominent S_4 and sustained to bifid systolic (triple impulse)
Congenital and calcific aortic stenosis	Normal	Parvus et tardus,[a] thrill L. carotid > R. carotid	Nondisplaced,[b] enlarged, and sustained with palpable S_4
Aortic sclerosis	Normal	Normal	Normal

MR = mitral regurgitation; CVP = central venous pressure; HOCM = hypertrophic obstructive cardiomyopathy; L. = left; R. = right.
[a] Normal upstroke and normal to increased pulse pressure occur, particularly in the elderly.
[b] Inferolateral displacement common with chronicity/left ventricular dysfunction.

matic adults. They should be alerted to the typical symptoms of their disease and encouraged to seek early evaluation with their onset.

The view has been expressed that asymptomatic patients with severe aortic stenosis should be operated upon. This opinion stems primarily from the observation that sudden death may occur with no premonitory symptoms and that this scenario is even more likely in children. In reality, the exact risk of sudden death in truly asymptomatic patients is difficult to derive. In most series, it was a distinct rarity. Even in children, more conservative estimates have scaled down estimates of the risk of sudden death. On the other hand, in children the operation is typically a valvuloplasty of some sort including, more recently, balloon valvuloplasty. These lower risk procedures typically leave patients with their native valves intact and good initial hemodynamic results. These lower risk procedures must be balanced against the low but measurable risk of sudden death in asymptomatic patients left untreated. In the aggregate, a case can be made for an operative intervention in asymptomatic children with severe aortic stenosis (gradient > 70 mm Hg and valve area < 0.5–0.7 cm²/m²).

In asymptomatic adults, on the other hand, the risk of sudden death is even lower and the natural history is excellent. This excellent prognosis must be balanced against the higher initial operative mortality of aortic valve replacement and the subsequent morbidity and mortality of an aortic valve prosthesis. In the aggregate, reserving operation until the onset of any symptoms is a credible choice. In patients with unclear symptoms and borderline severity of the aortic stenosis, exercise studies may provide useful additional data.

The onset of any one or more of the classic three symptoms (angina, heart failure, or syncope) in the presence of a significant reduction in aortic valve area heralds a change in the prognosis for that patient and is a clear indication for intervention (Fig. 4.9).[20] There is a hierarchy of worsening prognosis, with angina having the longest mean survival (4–5 years), syncope the next longest (2–3 years), and congestive heart failure the shortest (2 years or less). This symptom-related variability in prognosis, however, should have no effect on the timing of the intervention to relieve the obstruction. Even very poor left ventricular function is not a contraindication to aortic valve surgery as the dysfuction may improve with relief of the obstruction. Once symptomatic, the risk of sudden death also increases, adding further to the urgency of proceeding to an intervention once symptoms occur. Because percutaneous aortic balloon valvuloplasty may only incompletely relieve outflow obstruction, the effectiveness of its use may be affected by underlying ventricular function.

Table 4.2.
Differential Diagnosis of Aortic Stenosis Auscultation

Condition	S_1	S_2	Ejection Sound	Gallop Sounds	Systolic Murmurs	Diastolic Murmurs
Acute MR	Preserved, (may be lost in murmur)	↑ P_2, early normal A_2, widely split S_2	None	S_3/S_4 common	Decrescendo, ± holosystolic, ↓ es with amyl nitrite	Apical mitral flow rumble
Supravalvular aortic stenosis	Normal	↑ A_2, normally split S_2	None	S_4	Mid-frequency, diamond-shaped, mid to late peaking, maximal at URSE, radiates best to R. carotid	None
Membranous subvalvular aortic stenosis	Normal	Normal A_2, normal to paradoxic splitting of S_2	None	S_4	Mid-frequency, diamond-shaped, mid to late peaking, maximal at mid to LLSE, poor radiation to carotids	Diastolic blow of AR common
Muscular subvalvular aortic stenosis (HOCM)	Normal	Normal A_2, normal to paradoxic splitting of S_2	None	S_4	Mid-frequency, diamond-shaped, mid to late peaking, maximal at mid to LLSE, ↑ es during Valsalva strain, associated MR murmur common	None
Congenital aortic stenosis (pliable leaflets)	Normal	Normal to ↑ A_2, normal to para-dox. split-ting of S_2	Loud	S_4	Mid-frequency, diamond-shaped, mid to late peak, maxi-mal at URSE radiates to L. > R. carotid	Diastolic blow of AR common
Calcific aortic stenosis	Normal	↓ A_2, single S_2 (i.e., P_2), para-dox. S_2 (if A_2 is audible)	Typically none, particu-larly if A_2 is ↓	S_4	Mid-frequency, diamond-shaped, mid to late peak, maxi-mal at URSE,[a] radiates to L. > R. carotid	Diastolic blow of AR common
Aortic sclerosis	Normal	Normal A_2, normal splitting of S_2	None	None	Mid-frequency, early to mid-peaking, maxi-mal at URSE, Gr ≤ 3, poor radiation to carotids	None

MR = mitral regurgitation; URSE = upper right sternal edge; LLSE = lower left sternal edge; HOCM = hypertrophic obstructive cardiomyopathy; L. = left; R. = right; AR = aortic regurgitation.
[a] May be maximal in neck or at apex (where it is higher frequency), particularly in older patients.

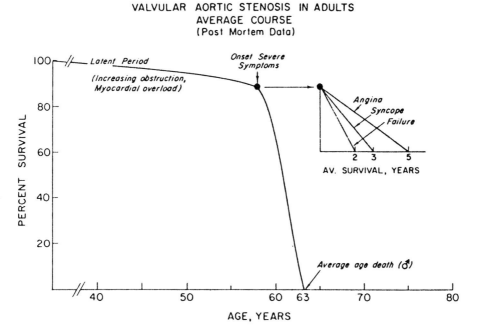

Figure 4.9. These survival data are from patients with aortic stenosis and are based on a compilation of postmortem data from the literature. Initially, the actuarial survival curve is that of the average American male. After a long latent (or asymptomatic) interval with relatively normal survival, the patient with aortic stenosis typically becomes symptomatic in his mid to late 50s. With the onset of symptoms, there is a marked acceleration in mortality with death at an average age of 63 years. The inset shows the gradation in prognosis among the three symptoms with heart failure predicting the shortest survival and angina the longest. Any of these symptoms, however, identifies a marked change in prognosis and the need for an intervention to relieve the obstruction. (By permission from Ross J and Braunwald E. Aortic stenosis. *Circulation 37–38* (Supplement 5):61–67, 1968. Figure 1).

REFERENCES

1. Selzer A. Changing aspects of the natural history of valvular aortic stenosis. *N. Engl J Med 317*:91–98, 1987.

2. Wood P. Aortic stenosis. *Am J Cardiol 1*:553–571, 1958.

3. Chizner MA, Pearle DL, deLeon AC Jr. The natural history of aortic stenosis in adults. *Am Heart J 99*:419–424, 1980.

4. Lombard JT, Selzer A. Valvular aortic stenosis: A clinical and hemodynamic profile of patients. *Ann Int Med 106*:292–298, 1987.

5. Thibault GE, DeSanctis RW, Buckley MJ. Aortic stenosis. In: *The Practice of Cardiology,* ed by RA Johnson, E Haber, and WG Austen. Boston, Little Brown, 1980.

6. Johnson AM. Aortic stenosis, sudden death, and the left ventricular baroceptors. *Br Heart J 33*:1–5, 1971.

7. Mark AL, Kioschos JM, Abboud FM, Heistad DD, Schmidt PG. Abnormal vascular responses to exercise in patients with aortic stenosis. *J Clinical Invest 52*:1138–1146, 1973.

8. Brockmeier LB, Adolph RJ, Gustin BW, Holmes JC, Sacks JG. Calcium emboli to the retinal artery in calcific aortic stenosis. *Am Heart J 101*:32–37, 1981.

9. Shoenfeld Y, Eldar M, Bedazovsky B, Levy MJ, Pinkhas J. Aortic stenosis associated with gastrointestinal bleeding. A survey of 612 patients. *Am Heart J 100*:179–182, 1980.

10. Love JW. The syndrome of calcific aortic stenosis and gastrointestinal bleeding: Resolution following aortic valve replacement. *J Thorac Cardiovasc Surg 83*: 779–783, 1982.

11. Kavalier M, Stewart J, Tavel ME. The apical a wave versus the fourth heart sound in assessing the severity of aortic stenosis. *Circulation 51*:324–327, 1968.

12. Goldblatt A, Aygen MM, Braunwald E. Hemodynamic phonocardiographic correlates of the fourth heart sound in aortic stenosis. *Circulation 26*:92–96, 1962.

13. Caulfield WH, de Leon AC Jr., Perloff JK, Steelman RB. The clinical significance of the fourth heart sound in aortic stenosis. *Am J Cardiol 28*:179–182, 1971.

14. Gallavardin L, Ravault P. Le souffle du retrecissement aortique peut changer de timbre et devenir musical dans sa propagation apexienne. *Lyon Med 35*:523–529, 1925.

15. Perloff JK. *The Clinical Recognition of Congenital Heart Disease*. 2nd ed. Philadelphia, W.B. Saunders, 1978, pp. 93–95.

16. Romhilt DW, Estes EH. Point score system for the ECG diagnosis of left ventricular hypertrophy. *Am Heart J 75*:752–758, 1968.
17. Hoffman RB, Rigler LG. Evaluation of left ventricular enlargement in the lateral projection of the chest. Radiology *85*:93–100, 1965.
18. Bache RJ, Wang Y, Greenfield JC Jr. Left ventricular ejection time in valvular aortic stenosis. *Circulation 47*:527–533, 1973.
19. Rudolph AM. *Congenital Disease of the Heart.* Chicago, Yearbook Medical Publishers, 1974, p. 327.
20. Ross J, Braunwald E. Aortic stenosis. *Circulation 37–38* (Supplement 5):61–67, 1968.

5

Echo-Doppler Evaluation of Aortic Stenosis and the Effect of Percutaneous Balloon Aortic Valvuloplasty

CATHERINE M. OTTO

Doppler and two-dimensional (2-D) echocardi-ography now is an established method for accurate noninvasive assessment of stenosis severity in patients with valvular aortic stenosis. In addition, these techniques can be utilized to evaluate left ventricular systolic function, the degree of coexist-ing aortic regurgitation, and the presence and severity of other valvular lesions. While similar information can be obtained at cardiac catheteriza-tion, most clinicians prefer to avoid the risk and cost of this invasive procedure for diagnosis alone. Thus, in elderly patients with symptoms that may be due to aortic stenosis, the noninvasive approach is of particular importance in deciding about the potential need for aortic valvuloplasty, in assessing short-term results, and in following disease severity long-term post-valvuloplasty.

ECHO-DOPPLER ASSESSMENT OF DISEASE SEVERITY IN VALVULAR AORTIC STENOSIS
Diagnosis

Since the clinical presentation of severe valvular obstruction is not always straightforward, the first step in evaluation of an adult with symptoms that may be due to aortic stenosis is establishing the correct diagnosis (Table 5.1). Symptoms of aortic stenosis—angina, syncope, heart failure—are com-mon in this elderly population and often are due to other prevalent conditions, including coronary artery disease, hypertension, conduction system abnormalities, and cardiomyopathies. A systolic murmur often is present and again may be due to a variety of causes other than valvular aortic stenosis,

including mild degenerative calcific changes of the aortic valve (without significant obstruction), hypertensive hypertrophic cardiomyopathy of the elderly, or mitral regurgitation. Other clinical findings can be misleading, since in elderly patients with severe aortic stenosis the murmur may radiate to the apex instead of the carotids. The carotid upstroke may be brisk due to increased stiffness of the vessel wall. Systolic hypertension does not exclude the diagnosis. The electrocardiogram does not always show evidence of left ventricular hypertrophy.[1]

Two-dimensional echocardiography can estab-lish the diagnosis of valvular aortic stenosis by imaging the thickened calcified leaflets with re-duced systolic mobility.[2] It may be possible to distinguish degenerative changes of a congenitally bicuspid valve from "senile" degeneration of a trileaflet valve. In addition, obstruction to left ventricular outflow at sites other than the aortic valve—supravalvular stenosis, a fixed subvalvular membranous or muscular obstruction, or dynamic subaortic obstruction due to hypertrophic cardio-myopathy—can be diagnosed reliably.

Pressure Gradient

Once the diagnosis is established, the next step is to determine the severity of outflow obstruction. While an aortic leaflet separation $\geq$ 15 mm by 2-D echocardiography indicates that severe stenosis is not present, obstruction may be mild, moderate, or severe when leaflet separation is < 15 mm[2]. Attempts to quantitate stenosis severity based on imaging of the valve itself have been of limited success given the complex three-dimensional anat-

Table 5.1.
Echo-Doppler Assessment of Aortic Stenosis

Confirm diagnosis of *valvular* AS
Determine AS severity
    Maximal velocity of aortic jet
    Mean pressure gradient
    Continuity equation for determination of the AVA
Evaluate LV systolic function
Assess severity of coexisting aortic regurgitation
Evaluate severity of other valve disease (esp. mitral
    regurgitation)

AS = aortic stenosis; LV = left ventricular; AVA = aortic valve
area.

omy of the stenotic aortic valve. Instead of
focusing on imaging, it is useful to determine the
velocity of blood flow through the narrowed
orifice since, for a constant volume flow rate,
velocity increases as the orifice narrows. The
quantitative relationship between velocity through
a stenotic valve (V_{jet} in m/sec) and the pressure
gradient across the valve (ΔP in mm Hg) is stated
in the simplified Bernoulli equation:

$$\Delta P = 4 \ (V^2_{jet} - V^2_{prox}) \qquad (1)$$

where V_{prox} = the velocity in the left ventricular
outflow tract just proximal to the valve. This
simplification of a basic principle of fluid dynamics
assumes that conversion of potential energy to
kinetic energy accounts for the major component
of the pressure drop across the valve and that
viscous losses and losses due to acceleration/
deceleration are negligible for valve areas in the
clinical range. Appropriate conversion factors for
units of measurement and the known mass density
of blood are included in the approximated constant
of 4.

Compared to jet velocity, outflow tract velocity
is relatively low (usually ≤ 1.0 m/sec) so that it
usually can be ignored in the clinical setting. Then,
the simplified Bernoulli equation becomes

$$\Delta P = 4V^2 \qquad (2)$$

In situations where the proximal velocity is elevated (such as with severe coexisting aortic insufficiency) Equation 1 should be used. Despite the
numerous assumptions of the simplified Bernoulli
equation, this relationship provides quite accurate
noninvasive pressure gradients compared to invasive data both in animal models[3,4] and in adults
with valvular aortic stenosis.[5-11]

In aortic stenosis, jet velocities are in the 3 to 6
m/sec range so that either continuous wave Dopp-

ler or high pulse repetition frequency pulsed
Doppler ultrasound must be used for accurate
velocity measurement.[12] Maximum transaortic
pressure gradient can be calculated from maximum
velocity, while mean transaortic pressure gradient
can be calculated by integrating the instantaneous
pressure gradients over the systolic ejection period
(using a microcomputer or measurement package
in the ultrasound system). It should be noted that
maximum Doppler gradients are not equivalent to
the peak-to-peak gradient measured in the
catheterization laboratory (Figure 5.1). With the
Doppler technique, the maximum velocity corresponds to the maximum instantaneous pressure

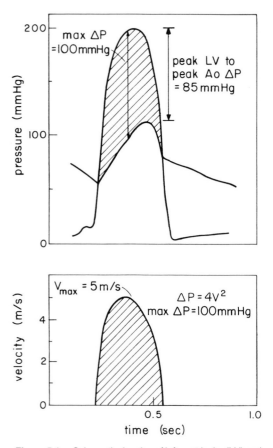

Figure 5.1. Schematic drawing of left ventricular (LV) and
aortic (Ao) pressures and corresponding continuous wave
Doppler velocity curve in valvular aortic stenosis. Note that
pressure gradient (ΔP) is related to velocity (V) as stated in
the simplified Bernoulli equation (at bottom). Also note the
relationship between the maximum instantaneous transaortic gradient and the maximum jet velocity and the lack of
correspondence with peak-to-peak gradient. Mean pressure gradient is 68 mm Hg by both techniques.

gradient across the valve. In contrast, peak left ventricular and peak aortic pressures do not occur simultaneously so that their difference does not represent the maximum instantaneous pressure gradient. It should be emphasized that mean pressure gradients by the two techniques measure the same variable and agree closely.[5-11]

There are several potential sources of error in determining Doppler pressure gradients. The Doppler technique measures a frequency shift (Δf in KHz) and velocity (V in m/sec). It is calculated using the Doppler equation:

$$V = \frac{\Delta f \times c}{2f_o \cos \theta} \qquad (3)$$

where c = the speed of sound in blood, f_o = the transducer frequency, and θ = the intercept angle between the ultrasound beam and the direction of blood flow. In cardiac Doppler applications, the sonographer attempts to align the Doppler beam parallel to blood flow so that $\cos \theta$ always is assumed to equal 1 and thus can be ignored in the calculation of velocity from frequency shift. Failure to align the beam parallel to flow results in velocity underestimation. This is an important potential problem in valvular aortic stenosis. Jet direction often is eccentric within the aortic root and cannot be predicted from 2-D imaging or determined reliably in three dimensions with color flow techniques. It is essential that the sonographer examine the patient from multiple windows (apical, suprasternal, right parasternal, and occasionally subcostal, left parasternal, supraclavicular) with optimal patient positioning and with careful angulation of the transducer from each window to obtain the "best" aortic jet signal. The highest frequency shift then obtained is assumed to represent the most parallel intercept angle with the jet and is used for subsequent velocity and pressure gradient calculations.

Because of the technical difficulty of recording optimal aortic jet signals, each sonographer and each laboratory will have a significant "learning curve" for accurate results with this technique. Each laboratory should confirm the validity of its own data before using the results to guide patient management.

However, the most important limitations of pressure gradients in evaluating stenosis severity are not technical but physiologic. In an individual patient, pressure gradients vary with transaortic volume flow rate. This accounts for many of the apparent discrepancies between noninvasive and invasive pressure gradient determinations, since heart rate and cardiac output often are different at different times.[13] Doppler and catheter gradients correspond most closely when both are recorded simultaneously.[3-5]

In comparing patients with each other, pressure gradients can vary widely for a given degree of valvular obstruction depending on the degree of coexisting aortic regurgitation (which will increase transaortic volume flow rate and pressure gradient) or the degree of left ventricular systolic dysfunction (which will lower volume flow rate and pressure gradient). Both of these conditions are common in adults with valvular aortic stenosis.[14] Severe stenosis with low transaortic volume flow is of particular concern since, based on pressure gradient or velocity data alone, it may not be recognized that severe stenosis is present in these patients. Since ventricular function may improve after relief of aortic stenosis, surgical intervention may be considered in this patient group. For these reasons, it is important to determine aortic valve areas in addition to transaortic pressure gradients, regardless of whether the data are obtained noninvasively with echo-Doppler techniques or invasively in the catheterization laboratory.

Aortic Valve Area

Aortic valve area can be determined noninvasively based on the continuity of flow in the left ventricular ouflow tract (LVOT) just proximal to the valve and in the narrowed aortic orifice (Ao) itself. When flow is laminar, stroke volume (SV in cm³) can be calculated from the cross-sectional area of flow (CSA in cm²) times the spatial-temporal mean flow velocity over the period of flow (VTI = the velocity time integral in cm):

$$SV = CSA \times VTI \qquad (4)$$

Transaortic stroke volume can be determined in the left ventricular outflow tract just proximal to the valve.[15] Given that:

$$SV_{Ao} = SV_{LVOT} \qquad (5)$$

assuming the flow in the aortic jet itself is laminar and the cross-sectional area of the narrowed orifice is aortic valve area (AVA), then:

$$AVA \times VTI_{Ao} = CSA_{LVOT} \times VTI_{LVOT} \qquad (6)$$

or: $$AVA = \frac{CSA_{LVOT} \times VTI_{LVOT}}{VTI_{Ao}} \qquad (7)$$

Outflow tract cross-sectional area (CSA_{LVOT}) is determined from the 2-D echo measurement of LVOT diameter as $\pi(D/2)^2$. Aortic valve areas calculated with the continuity equation (Fig. 5.2) have been validated in comparison to Gorlin formula valve areas obtained at cardiac catheterization (Fig. 5.3) in several clinical studies.[8–11]

The continuity equation can be simplified by substituting maximum velocities for velocity time integrals[11,16]:

$$AVA = \frac{CSA_{LVOT} \times V_{LVOT}}{V_{Ao}} \qquad (8)$$

The simplified continuity equation measures the functional area of flow (as does the Gorlin formula) and has the advantages that it is noninvasive, does not require an empiric constant for coefficients of discharge and contraction, and can

be measured reproducibly and repeatedly in an individual patient over time.

Left Ventricular Function

Disease severity in valvular aortic stenosis includes more than the severity of valve narrowing itself; complete evaluation should include assessment of left ventricular systolic and diastolic function, the degree of coexisting aortic regurgitation, and the presence and severity of other valvular lesions. The response of the left ventricle to outflow obstruction can be evaluated qualitatively by measurement of wall thickness and internal dimensions, and quantitatively by calculation of left ventricular mass.[17] More importantly, left ventricular systolic function can be assessed either qualitatively (normal or mildly, moderately, or severely reduced) or

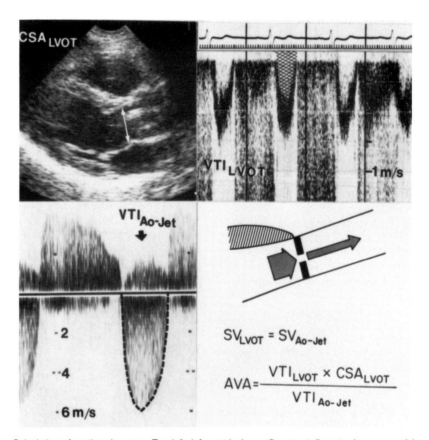

Figure 5.2. Calculation of aortic valve area. Top left, left ventricular outflow tract diameter is measured (arrows) from parasternal long-axis view and cross-sectional area (CSA_{LVOT}) calculated as π $(D/2)^2$. Top right, velocity time integral in outflow tract (VTI_{LVOT}) is recorded from apical view, shown by cross-hatching. Bottom left, velocity time integral in aortic jet ($VTI_{Ao\text{-}jet}$) is measured from approach giving highest velocity, in this case apical. Bottom right, since stroke volume (SV) in LVOT equals stroke volume in aortic jet, aortic valve area (AVA) can be determined. (From Otto et al. *Arch Intern Med* 148:2553, 1988. Copyright 1988, American Medical Association.)

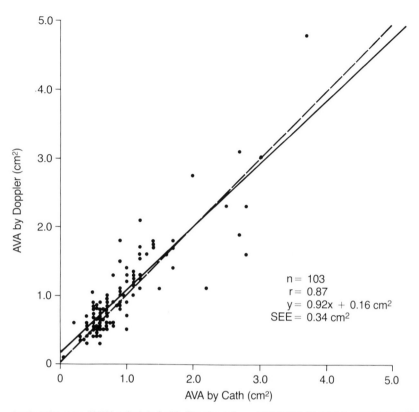

Figure 5.3. Aortic valve area (AVA) calculated with Doppler echo-cardiography (*y*-axis) is compared with aortic valve areas calculated with Gorlin and Gorlin formula at catheterization (*x*-axis). SEE indicates standard error of the estimate. (From Otto et al. *Arch Intern Med 148*:2553, 1988. Copyright 1988, American Medical Association.)

quantitatively by 2-D echocardiography.[17] As noted subsequently, the qualitative assessment of baseline left ventricular systolic function by 2-D echocardiography is an important predictor of outcome after aortic valvuloplasty. The presence and extent of segmental wall motion abnormalities due to coexisting coronary artery disease also may be helpful in patient management.

Insight into left ventricular diastolic function can also be obtained from the Doppler left ventricular inflow velocity curve[18,19] although interpretation is complicated by changes associated with aging, left ventricular systolic function, and loading conditions.[20] For example, in adults with aortic stenosis, the diastolic filling pattern is related not just to the presence of left ventricular hypertrophy, but also to left ventricular systolic function with a higher early diastolic velocity seen in patients with poor systolic function.[21] The height of the A wave is also a function of the strength of atrial contraction and this may diminish late in the disease. Mitral regurgitation also will increase early

diastolic filling velocity and alter the ratio of early to late filling velocities.

Coexisting Aortic Regurgitation

Aortic regurgitation often is present in adults with valvular aortic stenosis. Although the degree of regurgitation usually is only mild or moderate, assessment of severity is important in choosing the most appropriate therapeutic option. Several non-invasive methods are available for grading the degree of aortic regurgitation—color flow mapping in multiple tomographic planes, the diastolic slope of the continuous wave Doppler curve, evidence of diastolic flow reversal in the descending aorta, and the amount of left ventricular dilation.[22] It is useful to integrate the findings of each of these approaches in assessing regurgitant severity.

Coexisting Mitral Regurgitation

In patients with aortic stenosis due to rheumatic heart disease, mitral valve disease (either stenosis, regurgitation, or mixed) is invariably present and can be assessed using Doppler techniques. Candidates for aortic valvuloplasty more often have calcific aortic stenosis. In this population, coexisting mitral regurgitation is common due to mitral annular calcification, left ventricular systolic dysfunction, or nonspecific degenerative changes of the mitral valve leaflets. The degree of mitral regurgitation can be assessed noninvasively using either conventional pulsed Doppler or color flow imaging techniques.[22]

CLINICAL UTILITY OF ECHO-DOPPLER DATA IN AORTIC STENOSIS PATIENTS

Timing of Aortic Valve Replacement

Echo-Doppler data of the severity of valvular aortic stenosis is an accurate and cost-effective approach for determining the need for valve replacement in adults with symptomatic aortic stenosis.[9] Maximum aortic jet velocity (if recorded accurately by an experienced laboratory) is a useful screening test since valve replacement rarely is needed when jet velocity is < 3.0 m/sec, while valve replacement is usually indicated in those with a velocity > 4.0 m/sec. The utility of maximum jet velocity alone is not surprising given that maximum velocity relates to maximum pressure gradient in a predictable fashion (via the Bernoulli equation) and that maximum pressure gradients are related linearly to mean pressure gradients in aortic stenosis patients.[9]

In symptomatic patients with a maximal jet velocity between 3.0 and 4.0 m/sec, the continuity equation valve area and the assessment of the degree of coexisting aortic regurgitation can be used to guide patient management. In an occasional patient, when clinical and noninvasive data are inconsistent, it may be necessary to evaluate stenosis severity invasively. Most of these patients need coronary angiography given the high prevalence of coronary artery disease in this population.

Hemodynamic Progression of Asymptomatic Aortic Stenosis

In order to be useful for following individual patients over time, a diagnostic method must be reproducible as well as accurate. Reproducibility of Doppler measures of aortic stenosis severity includes day-to-day physiologic variability, variability in recording the data, and variability in measuring the data. Based on studies addressing the reproducibility of Doppler data,[23] a change in aortic jet velocity of 0.2 m/sec or a change in valve area greater than 0.15 cm^2 (for values in the mid-range of this patient group) is outside the limits of variability. This degree of reproducibility is comparable to other diagnostic tests, including Gorlin formula aortic valve areas.

Given that Doppler measures of aortic stenosis severity are reproducible and accurate, the hemodynamic progression of aortic stenosis severity in individual patients can be studied.[23] The rate of progression is extremely variable from patient to patient, and baseline characteristics that predict the rate of progression in an individual patient have not been identified. Thus, this technique is useful in following the asymptomatic patient or the patient with equivocal symptoms thought not due to valvular aortic stenosis.

ROLE OF ECHO-DOPPLER IN AORTIC VALVULOPLASTY PATIENTS

Evaluation of Candidates for Aortic Valvuloplasty

Echo-Doppler techniques for assessment of valvular aortic stenosis apply equally well to potential candidates for aortic valvuloplasty. This subset of patients differs from the entire group of aortic stenosis patients in that candidates for valvuloplasty are older, more often female, may have more severe symptoms (especially congestive heart failure), and often have serious comorbid diseases that preclude surgical valve replacement. In this group it is perhaps even more important than in general that evaluation of disease severity include (1) confirmation of the diagnosis of valvular aortic stenosis; (2) determination of aortic stenosis severity including maximum aortic jet velocity, mean transaortic pressure gradient, and continuity equation valve area; (3) assessment of left ventricular structure and function; and evaluation of (4) the degree of coexisting aortic regurgitation, and (5) other valvular lesions (especially mitral regurgitation).

Typically, patients undergo the initial cardiac catheterization as part of the valvuloplasty procedure itself. Doppler data are used for clinical decision making prior to catheterization in these patients. However, it must be remembered that patient selection for aortic valvuloplasty must not be based on echo-Doppler findings alone but is dependent on several other clinical parameters, including the degree of symptoms and the relative or absolute contraindications to cardiac surgery.

Echo-Doppler versus Catheterization Measures of Aortic Stenosis Severity

Concern has been raised about the variable correlation between Doppler and catheterization measures of aortic stenosis severity in valvuloplasty patients. Post-valvuloplasty it is not surprising that changes in loading conditions and possible physiologic changes (i.e., early restenosis) may result in discrepancies between the two methods. It is less clear why pre-valvuloplasty measures of stenosis severity should disagree since these patients simply represent a subset of the entire population of adults with valvular aortic stenosis.

This issue has been addressed in several studies. At first glance, the correlation coefficients for noninvasive versus invasive pressure gradients and valve areas appear to be somewhat poorer both pre- and post-valvuloplasty compared to previously published data comparing these methods in unselected series of aortic stenosis patients (Table 5.2). However, there are several reasons for these apparent discrepancies, as detailed subsequently. On more careful analysis, it is clear that the Doppler approach remains accurate in the subset of aortic stenosis patients who undergo valvuloplasty (Figs. 5.4 and 5.5).

Potential physiologic changes in loading conditions (which will affect pressure gradients more than valve areas) have been mentioned already as one reason for apparent disagreement between invasive and noninvasive data, when data are not recorded simultaneously. In addition, there may be actual changes in valve areas between the two studies due to acute stretching of the aortic anulus during valvuloplasty,[30] with early restenosis due to loss of this stretch by the time of the echo-Doppler study 24 to 72 hours after the procedure.[27, 28] In addition, both stroke volume and ejection fraction may rise in the first 3 days after the procedure.[28] Another potential source of error is the method for determining transvalvular volume flow. In the catheterization laboratory, a Fick or thermodilation cardiac output usually is substituted in the Gorlin formula. This "forward" cardiac output will underestimate transaortic volume flow if coexisting aortic regurgitation is present (as it is to some degree in 80% of adults with aortic stenosis). In contrast, stroke volume measured by echo-Doppler just proximal to the stenotic valve accurately measures transaortic volume flow[15] regardless of coexisting aortic regurgitation and thus should allow more accurate calculation of valve area.

Yet another potential source of discrepancy is the inherent inaccuracy of each of the two techniques. In valvuloplasty studies, comparison of noninvasive and invasive techniques was not the primary research goal so that less attention may have been directed toward technical details in both the echocardiography laboratory (aortic jet maximum velocity, LVOT flow, and diameter) and the catheterization laboratory (optimal pressure recordings in terms of frequency response, damping,

Table 5.2.
Correlations between Echo-Doppler and Catheterization Measures of Aortic Stenosis Severity

Study	N	Valve Area		Mean Pressure Gradient	
		r-Value	Range	r-Value	Range
Unselected Series					
Zoghbi et al.[11]	50	0.95	0.4–2.1 cm^2	0.90[a]	16–130 mm Hg[a]
Otto & Pearlman[9]	103	0.87	0.2–3.7 cm^2	0.88	2–107 mm Hg
Teirstein et al.[10]	30	0.88	0.3–1.9 cm^2	0.92	8–88 mm Hg
Oh et al.[8]	100	0.83	0.2–1.8 cm^2	0.86	8–90 mm Hg
Aortic Valvuloplasty Patients					
Come et al.[24]	40	Pre 0.71	0.2–1.1 cm^2	Pre 0.82	20–110 mm Hg
		Post 0.85	0.5–2.6 cm^2	Post 0.77	5–56 mm Hg
Nishimura et al.[25]	55	Pre 0.72	0.2–0.9 cm^2		
		Post 0.61	0.5–1.3 cm^2		
Desnoyers et al.[26]	42	0.74	0.3–1.3 cm^2	0.83	10–90 mm Hg
Kruck et al.[27]	33	—	—	0.84	—
Stoddard et al.[29]	19	Pre 0.84	0.2–0.8 cm^2	Pre 0.74	15–120 mm Hg
		Post 0.87	0.3–1.2 cm^2	Post 0.83	15–80 mm Hg

[a]Peak-to-peak gradient compared to maximum Doppler gradient

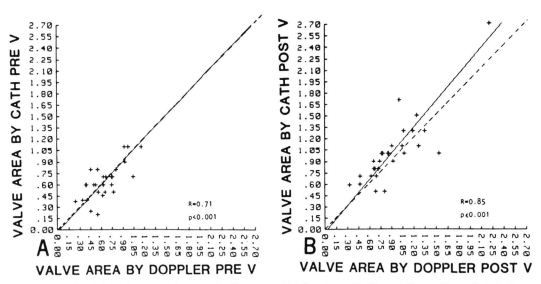

Figure 5.4. Correlations between valve area (cm²) assessed by Doppler continuity equation and by catheterization techniques before (**A**) and after (**B**) valvuloplasty (V). The solid lines represent the regression lines, and the dotted lines denote the lines of identity. (From Come et al. *Am J Cardiol 61*:1300, 1988, with permission.)

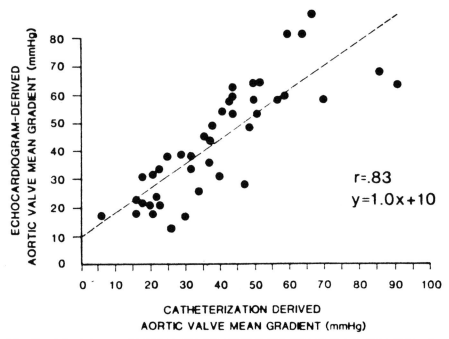

Figure 5.5. Correlation between echocardiographic and catheterization determination of mean aortic valve gradient. (From Deshoyers et al. *Am J Cardiol 62*:1078, 1988, with permission.)

transducer calibration, and accurate and simultaneous transaortic volume flow measurement). Even under conditions of optimal data recording, valve area calculations by both techniques are only accurate to approximately ± 0.2 cm².[23,31–35]

Finally, some of the apparent discrepancy is a statistical phenomenon. Calculation of a correlation coefficient assumes that the range of data sampled is representative of the entire population. In studies of unselected aortic stenosis patients, comparing invasive and noninvasive data, aortic valve areas typically ranged from 0.1 cm² to 3.0

cm². In the valvuloplasty studies the total range of valve areas typically is 0.2 to 1.3 cm². The importance of range is illustrated by one study at an experienced laboratory[24] where the correlation coefficient for Doppler versus Gorlin formula valve areas is 0.85 post-valvuloplasty (with a range of valve areas from 0.5 to 2.6 cm²), while the pre-valvuloplasty correlation coefficient in the same patients is only 0.71 (with a valve area range of only 0.2 to 1.1 cm²) (Fig. 5.4). The correlation coefficients for transaortic pressure gradients in valvuloplasty patients are similar to those in unselected series since there is a wide range of pressure gradients (Table 5.2).

Thus, echo-Doppler techniques for assessment of stenosis severity are reasonably accurate in aortic valvuloplasty patients and can be used for clinical decision making just as they are in aortic stenosis patients in general.[36]

Echo-Doppler during Aortic Valvuloplasty

Echo-Doppler recordings in the catheterization laboratory during the aortic valvuloplasty procedure have provided insight into the acute hemodynamic changes that occur during balloon inflation and the corresponding changes in Doppler velocity curves. Nishimura and his colleagues[37] noted that progressive outflow tract obstruction during balloon inflation results in an increase in peak outflow velocity, a prolongation of the ejection time, and shortening of the aortic regurgitant velocity curve deceleration time. A substantial number of patients have an increase in mitral regurgitant severity during balloon inflation, presumably due to increased afterload. These observations not only highlight the acute hemodynamic effects of balloon inflation but elegantly demonstrate the instantaneous and accurate relationship between invasive hemodynamics and Doppler velocity recordings on a beat-to-beat basis (Fig. 5.6).

Serial Changes in Aortic Stenosis Severity Post-Valvuloplasty

Echo-Doppler techniques are useful post-valvuloplasty in assessing the immediate and long-term results of the procedure. In the early post-valvuloplasty period (24–72 hours post-procedure) echo-Doppler measures of stenosis severity may be more relevant clinically than data recorded in the catheterization laboratory immediately after the procedure since (1) loading conditions are more

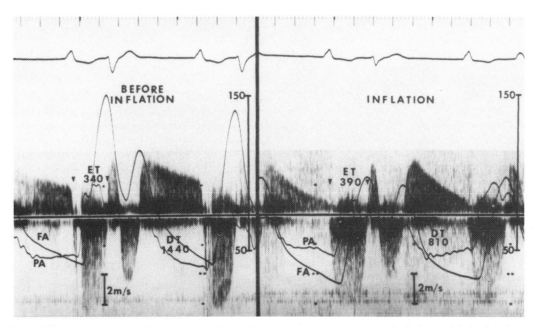

Figure 5.6. Continuous wave Doppler echocardiographic recording across the aortic valve before and during inflations, demonstrating a decrease in deceleration time (DT) of the aortic regurgitation signal during balloon inflation. There is also a prolongation of ejection time (ET). FA = femoral artery; PA = pulmonary artery. Reprinted with permission from the American College of Cardiology (*Journal of the American College of Cardiology, 11,* 1988, pp. 1219).

likely to be similar to pre-valvuloplasty, and (2) transient effects, such as stretch of the aortic anulus, will no longer be present.

Doppler valve areas typically increase from an average of 0.6 cm² pre-valvuloplasty to 0.8 cm² post-procedure. The slightly smaller average increase by noninvasive techniques versus Gorlin formula valve areas is due, at least in part, to the timing of data collection since transient increases in functional orifice area due to stretch of the aortic wall will no longer be present at the time of the echo-Doppler study.[27,30] In addition, even though the overall direction and magnitude of change as measured by the two techniques agree reasonably well, the absolute values for valve area may not correspond exactly pre- and post-procedure for the reasons discussed previously. It should be noted that the measured degree of change in valve area is nearly within the limits of measurement variability for each of these techniques. While there can be no doubt that the average valve area increases for a group of patients undergoing aortic valvuloplasty (given the statistical power of a large sample size), precise definition of the absolute change in an individual patient is more difficult.

Several studies have evaluated serial changes in aortic valve area using echo-Doppler techniques up to one year post-valvuloplasty.[25–28,38,39] Although the group mean valve area decreases only slightly, there is marked individual variability (Table 5.3) as evidenced by the increase in standard deviation for the group means. Some patients have no change in valve area over the follow-up period, while others have evidence of significant restenosis, which either can occur early or can be slowly progressive over the follow-up period. Several investigators have emphasized that restenosis occurs in one subset of patients while the remainder have a sustained improvement in aortic stenosis severity

at follow-up. While these subgroups with and without restenosis can be defined retrospectively, factors that identify these subgroups prospectively at baseline have not been defined. It should be noted that, despite the obvious selection bias in this population (i.e., patients with more severe disease may have either died or undergone valve replacement and thus are not included), a decrease in valve area at follow-up occurs even in those patients who survived and returned for a follow-up echocardiogram.

Echo-Doppler Evaluation of Coexisting Valvular Regurgitation and Left Ventricular Function Post-Valvuloplasty

Echo-Doppler evaluation has shown only a small overall increase in the severity of coexisting aortic regurgitation after aortic valvuloplasty.[40] Most often aortic regurgitation increases from trace to 1+ (mild) or, less commonly , from 1+ (mild) to 2+ (moderate) in severity. Severe aortic regurgitation has rarely been reported as a complication of valvuloplasty, and of course, patients with more severe aortic regurgitation at baseline are not candidates for the procedure.

Coexisting mitral regurgitation is common in adults undergoing aortic valvuloplasty, being present in approximately 70% and being moderate or severe in degree in about one-half of these patients. In a series of 144 valvuloplasty patients,[41] overall mean mitral regurgitation severity decreased from 1.1 ± 1.0 to 1.0 ± 1.0 ($p < 0.001$) after valvuloplasty with regurgitant severity graded on a 0 (none) to 4+ (severe) scale. While this numerical decrease is statistically significant, it is less clear whether a clinically significant decrease in mitral regurgitation occurs in most patients, although some subsets of patients do appear to benefit. For example, 20 of 25 patients (80%) with

Table 5.3.
Serial Doppler Aortic Valve Areas Post-Valvuloplasty

Study	N	Pre-	Immediate Post-	Late-Post	Mean Follow-up Duration (months)
			Aortic Valve Areas (cm²)		
Safian et al.[38]	86	0.64 ± 0.21	0.87 ± 0.30	0.86 ± 0.41	4.1
Nishimura et al.[25]	35	0.54 ± 0.15	0.85 ± 0.23	0.67 ± 0.19	6.2
Desnoyers et al.[26]	25	0.53 ± 0.03	0.76 ± 0.04	0.72 ± 0.06	8.9
Kruck et al.[27]	33	0.39 ± 0.11	0.74 ± 0.16	NA	11
Stoddard et al.[29]	19	0.52 ± 0.12	0.75 ± 0.20	0.70 ± 0.13	5.7
Balloon Valvuloplasty Registry[39]	240	0.6 ± 0.3	0.8 ± 0.3	NA	6

at least moderate mitral regurgitation and symptoms of heart failure had a decrease in mitral regurgitation severity associated with an improvement in heart failure symptoms.[41] The possible importance of decreased mitral regurgitation (due to afterload reduction after relief of aortic stenosis) as a mechanism for relief of symptoms and improved long-term clinical outcome after valvuloplasty needs further study.

Evaluation of left ventricular systolic function after aortic valvuloplasty is feasible and often utilized in the clinical setting; however, most of the published data on ventricular function after aortic valvuloplasty is based on radionuclide data. The effect of valvuloplasty on left ventricular function will be addressed in detail in a later chapter (Chapter 7), but it is clear that a carefully performed and analyzed 2-D echocardiogram can provide qualitative and quantitative information on left ventricular systolic function that is equivalent to angiographic or radionuclide data.[17] Even a qualitative evaluation of left ventricular systolic function by echocardiography provides valuable prognostic information.

Left ventricular diastolic function often is abnormal in patients with aortic stenosis and would be expected to improve after relief of outflow obstruction, especially if there is regression of left ventricular hypertrophy, and might account for clinical improvement in some patients. Stoddard et al.[29] found that in patients without mitral regurgitation, the Doppler pattern of left ventricular diastolic filling showed an increase in the early peak filling velocity (E), and in the ratio of early to late filling velocities (E:A ratio) immediately post-valvuloplasty, with a continued increase in early diastolic filling at 3–6-month follow-up, most likely reflecting more rapid and complete left ventricular relaxation (Figure 5.7). However, this improvement in diastolic filling did not correspond to the degree of clinical improvement in these patients. In patients with coexisting mitral regurgitation, there was no change in the Doppler pattern of diastolic filling immediately post-valvuloplasty, while at later follow-up there was a decrease in the early diastolic filling velocity. The role of diastolic dysfunction in the clinical manifestations of aortic stenosis patients and the possible changes after relief of outflow obstruction deserve further study.

Noninvasive Predictors of Outcome after Aortic Valvuloplasty

Perhaps the most important role of echo-Doppler evaluation in potential candidates for aortic valvu-

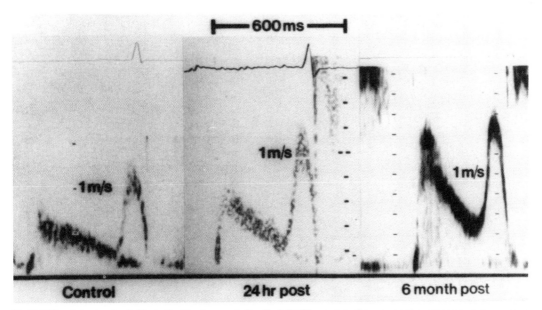

Figure 5.7. A case example illustrating the changes in the diastolic filling pattern that occurs after valvuloplasty in a patient without mitral regurgitation. Twenty-four hours after valvuloplasty (post), a small increase in peak early filling velocity occurs. Six months after valvuloplasty, the diastolic pattern appears normal. Reprinted with permission from the American College of Cardiology (*Journal of the American College of Cardiology, 14*, 1989, pp. 1218).

loplasty is in predicting the long-term results of the procedure. Initial enthusiasm for aortic valvuloplasty has been replaced by a more critical analysis of outcome in these severely ill elderly patients. While overall mortality is high, there may be specific patient subgroups that do benefit from the procedure. The challenge is to identify which patients will show sustained symptomatic improvement and improved survival based on clinical and noninvasive variables at presentation.

Preliminary univariate analysis of data from the Balloon Valvuloplasty Registry[42] identified several noninvasive factors that predicted mortality after aortic valvuloplasty. The severity of symptoms at baseline (assessed by NYHA functional class or by a functional status score) predicted a worse prognosis for a greater degree of limitation at baseline. Left ventricular systolic function at baseline—assessed qualitatively by 2-D echocardiography—was a strong predictor of outcome with a one-year survival of approximately 70% for those with normal systolic function compared to a one-year survival of approximately 30% in those with severely reduced systolic function.

Aortic stenosis jet velocity or transaortic mean pressure gradients pre-valvuloplasty also separated patients into high- and low-risk groups. Those with a high velocity (and high mean gradient) had a better survival than those with a low jet velocity. Although this finding initially appears paradoxical, it must be remembered that all these patients had severe valvular aortic stenosis. Thus, the subgroup

with a low velocity (or gradient) represents those patients with severe aortic stenosis and low transaortic volume flow—most often due to left ventricular systolic dysfunction.

Post-valvuloplasty, the degree of change in transaortic pressure gradient was related to subsequent outcome; this finding is not surprising since a better outcome would be expected in patients with a better hemodynamic result. Kruck et al.[27] also found that the post-valvuloplasty transaortic gradient was predictive of outcome and suggested that Doppler gradients recorded 24 to 72 hours later are better predictors of long-term outcome than invasive gradients recorded immediately after the procedure.

On multivariate analysis, mortality was related to poor baseline functional status, poor left ventricular systolic function, low mean transaortic pressure gradient prior to the procedure, and small valve area post-valvuloplasty. Other variables of significance were gender and the degree of coexisting mitral regurgitation.

In selection of candidates for aortic valvuloplasty, those with normal left ventricular systolic function and only mild to moderate symptoms appear to have a relatively good prognosis compared to those with abnormal ventricular function or severe symptoms. Of course, alternate therapeutic options will need careful consideration, even in patients with a relatively good prognosis after valvuloplasty, since these same patients may have an even better outcome with surgical intervention. In the patient in whom surgical intervention is contraindicated or must be deferred, baseline noninvasive criteria may be helpful in assessing the potential benefit of aortic valvuloplasty. Post-valvuloplasty echo-Doppler measures of stenosis severity may be helpful in counseling the patient and family about outcome or in deciding whether to proceed with high-risk cardiac surgery.

Table 5.4.
Role of Echo-Doppler in Aortic Valvuloplasty

Evaluation of potential candidates
    Severity of valvular AS
    LV systolic function
    Contraindications to valvuloplasty
Prediction of outcome
    Degree of symptoms
    LV systolic function
    Maximal velocity or mean pressure gradient
    Coexisting mitral regurgitation
Post-valvuloplasty follow-up
    Immediate
        Improvement in AS severity
        Baseline data for future studies
        Potential complications
    Intermediate and long-term follow-up
        Evidence of restenosis
        LV systolic and possibly diastolic function

SUMMARY

Doppler echocardiography is essential for appropriate clinical decision making in adults with symptomatic aortic stenosis. This technique has been well validated against invasive standards for determination of transaortic pressure gradients and valve areas by experienced laboratories. Given the potential technical difficulties of this method, caution should be exercised in using Doppler data from less experienced laboratories.

Echo-Doppler data is of particular importance

in potential candidates for aortic valvuloplasty (Table 5.4). Accurate diagnosis, determination of stenosis severity, assessment of coexisting valvular lesions, and evaluation of left ventricular systolic function are of particular importance for choosing appropriate therapy in this patient group. Pre-valvuloplasty echo-Doppler data provide useful prognostic information on the expected long-term outcome after the procedure. Post-valvuloplasty, long-term follow-up of stenosis severity, left ventricular systolic and diastolic function, and the severity of coexisting valvular regurgitation can be performed with echo-Doppler techniques.

Regardless of whether aortic valvuloplasty becomes standard clinical therapy, the data obtained using this noninvasive technique in aortic valvuloplasty patients have increased our understanding of the fluid dynamics of valvular aortic stenosis and have provided insight into the natural history of severe left ventricular outflow tract obstruction.

Acknowledgments

The author wishes to thank Dr. Alan S. Pearlman for critical review of the chapter, and Sharon Kemp for preparation of the manuscript.

REFERENCES

1. Rahimtoola SH, Cheitlin MD, Hutter AM Jr. Valvular and congenital heart disease. *J Am Coll Cardiol 10*:60A–62A, 1987.
2. DeMaria AN, Bommer W, Joye J, Lee G, Bouteller J, Mason DT. Value and limitations of cross-sectional echocardiography of the aortic valve in the diagnosis and quantification of valvular aortic stenosis. *Circulation 62*:304–312, 1980.
3. Callahan MJ, Tajik AJ, Su-Fan Q, Bove AA. Validation of instantaneous pressure gradients measured by continuous-wave Doppler in experimentally induced aortic stenosis. *Am J Cardiol 56*:989–993, 1985.
4. Smith MD, Dawson PL, Elion JL, Booth DC, Handshoe R, Kwan OL, Earle GF, DeMaria AN. Correlation of continuous wave Doppler velocities with cardiac catheterization gradients: An experimental model of aortic stenosis. *J Am Coll Cardiol 6*:1306–1314, 1985.
5. Currie PH, Seward JB, Reeder GS, Vlietstra RE, Bresnahan DR, Bresnahan JF, Smith HC, Hagler DJ, Tajik AJ. Continuous-wave Doppler echocardiographic assessment of severity of calcific aortic stenosis: A simultaneous Doppler-catheter correlative study in 100 adult patients. *Circulation 71*:1162–1169, 1985.
6. Hatle L: Noninvasive assessment and differentiation

7. of left ventricular outflow obstruction with Doppler ultrasound. *Circulation 64*:381–387, 1981.
8. Hatle L, Angelsen BA, Tromsdal A. Non-invasive assessment of aortic stenosis by Doppler ultrasound. *Br Heart J 43*:284–292, 1980.
9. Oh JK, Taliercio CP, Holmes DR Jr, Reeder GS, Bailey KR, Seward JB, Tajik AJ. Prediction of the severity of aortic stenosis by Doppler aortic valve area determination: Prospective Doppler-catheterization correlation in 100 patients. *J Am Coll Cardiol 11*:1227–1234, 1988.
10. Otto CM, Pearlman AS. Doppler echocardiography in adults with symptomatic aortic stenosis: Diagnostic utility and cost-effectiveness. *Arch Intern Med 148*:2553–2560, 1988.
11. Teirstein P, Yeager M, Yock PG, Popp RL. Doppler echocardiographic measurement of aortic valve area in aortic stenosis: A noninvasive application of the Gorlin formula. *J Am Coll Cardiol 8*:1059–1065, 1986.
12. Zoghbi WA, Farmer KL, Soto JG, Nelson JG, Quinones MA. Accurate noninvasive quantification of stenotic aortic valve area by Doppler echocardiography. *Circulation 73*:452–459, 1986.
13. Otto CM, Pearlman AS, Gardner CL. A comparison of high pulse repetition frequency and continuous wave Doppler echocardiography in adults with aortic stenosis or tricuspid regurgitation. *Am J Cardiac Imaging 2*:220–228, 1988.
14. Otto CM, Pearlman AS, Comess KA, Reamer RP, Janko CL, Huntsman LL. Determination of the stenotic aortic valve area in adults using Doppler echocardiography. *J Am Coll Cardiol 7*:509–517, 1986.
15. Otto CM, Pearlman AS, Comess KA, Saal AK, Janko CL, Reamer RP. Limitations of Doppler measurement of volume flow in adults with aortic stenosis. In: *Color Doppler Flow Imaging,* ed by J Roelandt, Dordrecht, Martinus Mijhoff, 1986, pp. 155–167.
16. Otto CM, Pearlman AS, Gardner CL, Enomoto DM, Togo T, Tsuboi H, Ivey TD. Experimental validation of Doppler echocardiographic measurement of volume flow through the stenotic aortic valve. *Circulation 78*:435–441, 1988.
17. Otto CM, Pearlman AS, Gardner CL, Kraft CD, Fujioka MC. Simplification of the Doppler continuity equation for calculating stenotic aortic valve area. *J Am Soc Echo 1*:155–157, 1988.
18. American Society of Echocardiography Committee on Standards, Subcommittee on Quantitation of Two-Dimensional Echocardiograms: Schiller NB, Shah PM, Crawford M, DeMaria A, Devereux R, Feigenbaum H, Gutgesell H, Reichek N, Sahn D, Schnittger I, Silverman NH, Tajik AJ. Recommendations for quantitation of the left ventricle by two-dimensional echocardiography. *J Am Soc Echo 2*:358–367, 1989.
19. Spirito P, Maron BJ. Doppler echocardiography for

assessing left ventricular diastolic function. *Ann Int Med 109*:122–126, 1988.

19. Rokey R, Kuo LC, Zoghbi WA, Limacher MC, Quinones MA. Determination of parameters of left ventricular diastolic filling with pulsed Doppler echocardiography: Comparison with cineangiography. *Circulation 71*:543–550, 1985.

20. Stoddard MF, Pearson AC, Kern MJ, Ratcliff J, Mrosek DG, Labovitz AJ. Influence of alteration in preload on the pattern of left ventricular diastolic filling as assessed by Doppler echocardiography in humans. *Circulation 79*:1226–1236, 1989.

21. Otto CM, Pearlman AS, Amsler LC. Doppler echocardiographic evaluation of left ventricular diastolic filling in isolated valvular aortic stenosis. *Am J Cardiol 63*:313–316, 1989.

22. Pearlman AS, Otto CM. Quantification of valvular regurgitation. *Echocardiography 4*:271–287, 1987.

23. Otto CM, Pearlman AS, Gardner CL. Hemodynamic progression of aortic stenosis in adults assessed by Doppler echocardiography. *J Am Coll Cardiol 13*:545–550, 1989.

24. Come PC, Riley MF, Safian RD, Ferguson JF, Diver DD, McKay RG. Usefulness of noninvasive assessment of aortic stenosis before and after percutaneous aortic valvuloplasty. *Am J Cardiol 61*:1300–1306, 1988.

25. Nishimura RA, Holmes DR Jr, Reeder RS, Orszulak TA, Bresnahan JF, Ilstrup DM, Tajik AJ. Doppler evaluation of results of percutaneous aortic balloon valvuloplasty in calcific aortic stenosis. *Circulation 78*:791–799, 1988.

26. Desnoyers MR, Isner JM, Pandian NG, Wang SS, Hougen T, Fields CD, Lucas AR, Salem DN. Clinical and noninvasive hemodynamic results after aortic balloon valvuloplasty for aortic stenosis. *Am J Cardiol 62*:1078–1084, 1988.

27. Kruck I, Spielberg C, Linderer T, Schröder R. Doppler-echocardiography can predict positive and negative medium-term results already 24–48 hours after aortic valvuloplasty. *Circulation 78* (Suppl II):II-2, 1988.

28. Davidson CJ, Skelton TN, Harpole DH, Kisslo K, Bashore TM. Analysis of the early rise in aortic transvalvular gradient following aortic valvuloplasty. *Am Heart J 117*:411–417, 1989.

29. Stoddard MF, Vandormael MG, Pearson AC, Gudipati C, Kern MJ, Deligonul U, Labovitz AJ. Immediate and short-term effects of aortic balloon valvuloplasty on left ventricualr diastolic function and filling in humans. *J Am Coll Cardiol 14*:1218–1228, 1989.

30. Waller BF, McKay CR, Erny R, Morgan R, Mohler E. Catheter balloon valvuloplasty of necropsy ste-

notic aortic valves: Etiology of aortic stenosis is a major factor in early "restenosis." *J Am Coll Cardiol 13*:16A, 1989.

31. Gorlin R, Gorlin SG. Hydraulic formula for calculation of the area of the stenotic mitral valve, other cardiac valves, and central circulatory shunts: I. *Am Heart J 41*:1–29, 1951.

32. Segal J, Lerner DJ, Miller DG, Mitchell RS, Alderman EA, Popp RL. When should Doppler-determined valve area be better than the Gorlin formula?: Variation in hydraulic constants in low flow states. *J Am Coll Cardiol 9*:1294–1305, 1987.

33. Cannon SR, Richards KL, Crawford M. Hydraulic estimation of stenotic orifice area: A correction of the Gorlin formula. *Circulation 71*:1170–1178, 1985.

34. Cannon SR, Richards KL, Crawford MH, et al. Inadequacy of the Gorlin formula for predicting prosthetic valve area. *Am J Cardiol 62*:113–116, 1988.

35. Carabello BA. Advances in the hemodynamic assessment of stenotic cardiac valves. *J Am Coll Cardiol 10*:912–919, 1987.

36. Miller FA Jr. Aortic stenosis: Most cases no longer require invasive hemodynamic study. *J Am Coll Cardiol 13*:551–553, 1989.

37. Nishimura RA, Holmes DR Jr, Reeder GS, Tajik AJ, Hatle LK. Doppler echocardiographic observations during percutaneous aortic balloon valvuloplasty. *J Am Coll Cardiol 11*:1219–1226, 1988.

38. Safian RD, Berman AD, Diver DJ, McKay LL, Come PC, Riley MF, Warren SE, Cunningham MJ, Wyman RM, Weinstein JS, Grossman W, McKay RG. Balloon aortic valvuloplasty in 170 consecutive patients. *N Engl J Med 319*:125–130, 1988.

39. Come PC (for the NHLBI Balloon Valvuloplasty Registry). Doppler-echo evaluation of aortic stenosis severity pre- and post-balloon aortic valvuloplasty. *J Am Coll Cardiol 13*:114A, 1989.

40. McKay RG, Safian RD, Lock JE, Diver DJ, Berman AD, Warren SE, Come PC, Baim DS, Mandell VE, Royal HD, Grossman W. Assessment of left ventricular and aortic valve function after aortic balloon valvuloplasty in adult patients with critical aortic stenosis. *Circulation 75*:192–203, 1987.

41. Gome PC, Riley MF, Berman AD, Safian RD, Waksmonski CA, McKay RG. Serial assessment of mitral regurgitation by pulsed Doppler echocardiography in patients undergoing balloon aortic valvuloplasty. *J Am Coll Cardiol 14*:677–682, 1989.

42. Otto CM (for the NHLBI Balloon Valvuloplasty Registry). Predictors of outcome six months after balloon aortic valvuloplasty. *Circulation 80* (Suppl II):II-74, 1989.

6

Techniques and Complications Related to Balloon Aortic Valvuloplasty

ROBERT D. SAFIAN

Since 1985, approximately 3000 balloon aortic valvuloplasty procedures have been performed worldwide in adult patients with aortic stenosis. Patients with symptomatic severe aortic stenosis who are not felt to be candidates for open heart surgery may be considered for balloon aortic valvuloplasty. Absolute contraindications to balloon aortic valvuloplasty include the presence of left ventricular thrombus and moderately severe aortic regurgitation.

There are several potential approaches to the balloon aortic valvuloplasty technique. In general, successful balloon dilation can be accomplished by the retrograde approach from either the femoral or the brachial artery, or by the antegrade approach using the transseptal technique. Aortic valves can be safely dilated with a single balloon (one balloon, one shaft), multiple balloons (two or three balloons, two or three shafts), and complex balloon configurations (two or three balloons, single shaft).

EQUIPMENT FOR BALLOON AORTIC VALVULOPLASTY

Balloon dilation catheters. In the United States, the most commonly used catheter is the single balloon configuration on a 9-French shaft (Mansfield Scientific, Inc., Watertown, MA), which was recently approved by the FDA for aortic valvuloplasty. These low profile polyethylene balloons range from 15 to 23 mm in diameter and from 3 to 5.5 cm in length (Fig. 6.1). Longer balloons are preferred because they can be seated more easily across the aortic valve and are less likely

to be ejected out of the valve orifice during inflation.

Dilating balloons measuring 23 mm in diameter can be inserted percutaneously through a 14-French sheath, and the 20-mm balloon catheter can be inserted through a 12-French sheath. Lower profile PET balloons are currently being evaluated that can be inserted through a 10-French sheath.

Since 1987, a specially designed catheter for aortic valvuloplasty has been available in Europe (Mansfield). This 9-French catheter consists of three lumens and a distal pigtail with multiple sideholes and an endhole (Fig. 6.2). The lumen proximal to the balloon can be used to monitor pressure in the central aorta, the distal lumen can be used to monitor pressure in the left ventricle and to be perform left ventriculography or supravalvular aortography, and the third lumen is for balloon inflation. The polyethylene balloon measures 5 cm in length and is available in inflated diameters of 15, 18, and 20 mm. Double-sized single balloons are also available, with a larger proximal balloon segment (20- or 23-mm diameter) tapering abruptly to a smaller distal balloon segment (15 or 18 mm diameter, respectively). The double-sized balloon measuring 23 by 18 mm must be inserted through a 14-French sheath.

Potential advantages of the pigtail design are that it may be less traumatic to the left ventricle, thus reducing the chance of perforation, and it allows for rapid pressure measurements and angiography.

Other dilating catheters with complex balloon configurations have been used in small numbers of

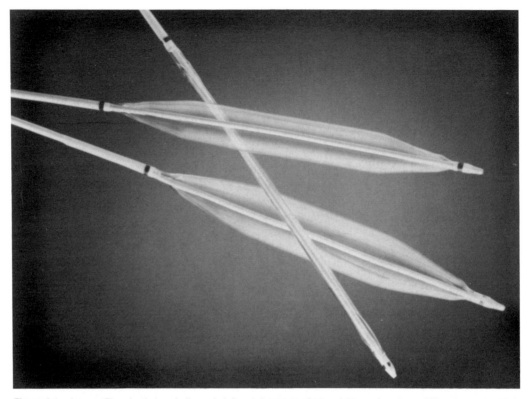

Figure 6.1. Low-profile polyethylene balloons in inflated diameters of 15 and 20 mm (courtesy of Mansfield Scientific).

patients in Europe. The bifoil and trefoil configurations (Schneider Medintag A.G., Zurich, Switzerland) consist of two (2 × 15 mm diameter) or three (3 × 10 and 3 × 12 mm diameter) modified polyvinyl chloride balloons, measuring 4 cm in length, mounted on a single 10-French shaft. The effective diameters are 23 mm for the bifoil balloon and 21 mm and 25 mm for the two trefoil balloons, respectively (Fig. 6.3).

There are several potential advantages of the bifoil and trefoil balloon configurations. Both designs may allow for continuous blood flow through the aortic valve during balloon inflations and could theoretically lead to better hemodynamic tolerance, particularly in patients with poor left ventricular function, extensive coronary artery disease, or cerebrovascular disease. Use of multiple small balloons on a single shaft may also permit use of higher inflation pressures compared to use of a single large balloon.

Despite the potential availability of pigtail balloons and of complex balloon configurations, there are no data to suggest clear superiority of any given design. Voudris and associates retrospectively evaluated acute hemodynamic results of

aortic valvuloplasty in 47 patients using monofoil balloons (19-mm diameter), bifoil balloons (2 × 15 mm, equivalent to 23-mm diameter), and trefoil balloons (3 × 10 mm, equivalent to 21-mm diameter). Although all patients had significant increases in aortic valve area following dilation, the valve area increased by 118% in the bifoil group, compared to 74% and 76% for the monofoil and trefoil balloons, respectively.[1] However, it is likely that the larger effective dilating area of the bifoil balloon, rather than the bifoil design itself, was responsible for the larger increment in aortic valve area for this group. Studies of larger numbers of patients will be needed to determine if the hemodynamic tolerance and acute complication rate are improved by use of bifoil and trefoil balloons.

Guidewires. Special guidewires for balloon aortic valvuloplasty are not required. Balloon dilation catheters are advanced over a 0.038-inch J-tip guidewire (260 cm) (Cook, Inc., Bloomington, IN) via the antegrade or retrograde approach. For transseptal left heart catheterization, a 0.032-inch or 0.035-inch (Medrad) J-tip guidewire (170 cm) is recommended for initial placement of the

Mullins sheath and dilator in the superior vena cava.

Introducer sheaths. Due to the relatively large profile of balloon dilation catheters, large bore introducing sheaths are required. In the retrograde percutaneous femoral approach, 10-, 12-, and 14-French introducing sheaths (Universal Medical Instruments Corporation, Ballston Spa, NY) may be used, depending on the preference of the operator and the size of the balloon.

The easiest method is to insert a 12-French sheath in the femoral artery after baseline hemodynamics are obtained. A low-profile 20-mm balloon catheter can readily be advanced through this sheath and can usually be withdrawn through the sheath after balloon inflation. If the balloon catheter cannot be removed through the sheath, the catheter and sheath can be removed en bloc over the guidewire, and a 12-French sheath can be reinserted in the femoral artery without significant blood loss. A 20-mm balloon can also be advanced and withdrawn through a 14-French sheath, but this may result in a higher incidence of vascular complications. Balloon catheters with diameters greater than 20 mm cannot be withdrawn through a 14-French sheath and must be inserted percutaneously without a sheath.

An alternative approach that may be useful in patients with vascular disease is to insert the 20-mm balloon dilation catheter percutaneously without a sheath. After the balloon catheter is removed, a 10-French sheath can then be inserted in the femoral artery without significant blood loss around the sheath. The disadvantage of this approach is that continuous compression of the femoral artery is required during the valvuloplasty procedure, which may result in significant patient discomfort and blood loss.

PATIENT PREPARATION

Prior to valvuloplasty and after appropriate informed consent has been obtained, patients should be premedicated in a fashion similar to that for conventional cardiac catheterization. An arterial monitor line should be inserted, and right heart catheterization should be performed with a balloon flotation catheter equipped with a bipolar

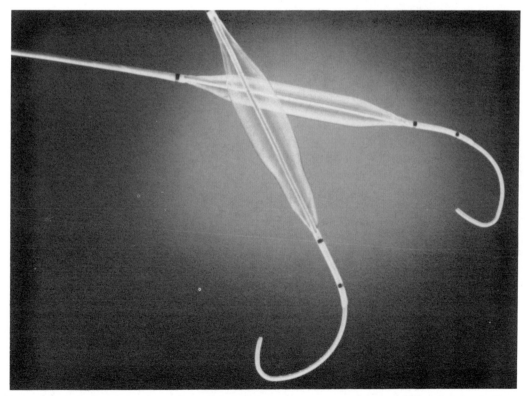

Figure 6.2. Pigtail balloon catheters for aortic valvuloplasty. The double-sized balloon (20-mm tapering to 15-mm diameter) and the single-sized balloon (15-mm diameter) are shown (courtesy of Mansfield Scientific).

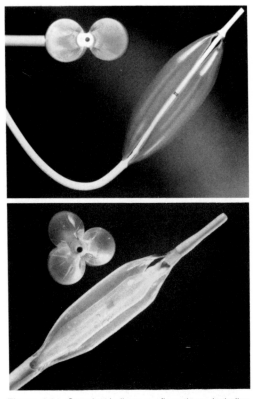

Figure 6.3. Complex balloon configurations, including the bifoil (2 × 15 mm diameter, top panel) and trefoil (3 × 10 mm diameter, bottom panel) designs (courtesy of Schneider Medintag).

pacing electrode. Initial evaluation should include direct measurement of transaortic valve gradient and estimation of aortic valve area, as well as assessment of left ventricular systolic function, aortic regurgitation, and the extent of coronary artery disease.

BALLOON CATHETER PREPARATION, INSERTION, AND INFLATION

Prior to inserting the balloon catheter in the patient, negative pressure should be applied to the balloon lumen to aspirate air, and the central guidewire lumen should be flushed. Inflation of the balloon outside the patient should be avoided in order to minimize the profile of the deflated balloon. The balloon catheter should be advanced over the guidewire under fluoroscopic guidance until the balloon is centered across the aortic valve. Once in position, the balloon should be inflated with dilute (20–30%) contrast.

During the initial balloon inflation, the balloon may become immobile when it is fully inflated and there may be a waist in the balloon, which disappears once the balloon is completely inflated. During subsequent inflations, increased mobility of the balloon across the aortic valve may indicate that satisfactory inflations have been achieved. In contrast to coronary angioplasty, special indeflators are unnecessary, and balloon inflation is readily accomplished using a hand-held syringe.

The number and duration of balloon inflations is less important than achieving full balloon inflation. Two or three 15–30-sec inflations are usually sufficient. Need for a larger balloon should be determined by the clinical response of the patient and the residual gradient and valve area. A larger balloon (or multiple balloons) may be utilized if adequate gradient reduction has not been achieved (by approximately 50%), provided the initial balloon could be maximally inflated without untoward hemodynamic consequences. Some investigators prefer to deliberately rupture the balloon during the last inflation, but this probably results in minimal incremental increase in the final aortic valve area.

RETROGRADE APPROACH TO BALLOON AORTIC VALVULOPLASTY

Percutaneous femoral approach. The retrograde femoral approach to balloon aortic valvuloplasty is the easiest and most straightforward (Fig. 6.4).[2,3] Conventional left heart catheterization is performed by percutaneous entry of the common femoral artery using the modified Seldinger technique. After intravenous administration of 5000 Units of heparin, the aortic valve is crossed by standard methods using a 0.035-inch or 0.038-inch straight-tip guidewire, and the baseline hemodynamic evaluation is obtained.

In our cardiac catheterization laboratory, left heart catheterization is usually performed with a 7-French angled pigtail catheter. Hemodynamic evaluation includes simultaneous measurement of pressures in the left ventricle, femoral artery, pulmonary artery, and pulmonary capillary wedge position. Fick cardiac output is calculated by measurement of pulmonary and systemic arterial saturations and by measurement of oxygen consumption using the Metabolic Rate Meter (Waters Instruments, Inc., Rochester, MN).

After baseline hemodynamic measurements are obtained, a 0.038-inch J-tip guidewire (260 cm)

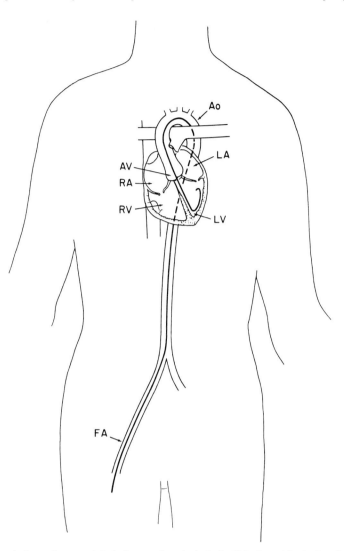

Figure 6.4. Retrograde femoral approach to balloon aortic valvuloplasty. Note the guidewire loop in the left ventricular (LV) apex. AO = aorta; AV = aortic valve; LA = left atrium; RA = right atrium; RV = right ventricle; FA = femoral artery.

should be inserted into the left ventricle. An additional curve should be placed in the guidewire so that it lies curled in the left ventricular apex (Fig. 6.5). The diagnostic left catheter should be exchanged over the guidewire, and a 12-French sheath with a sidearm adapter should be inserted in the femoral artery. The balloon catheter is advanced through the sheath over the guidewire and across the aortic valve, where one or more balloon inflations are performed.

Following valve dilation, the balloon catheter is removed over the guidewire, and the diagnostic left heart catheter is reinserted. Hemodynamic measurements are repeated, and if an adequate result has been achieved, the procedure is terminated. Although left ventricular pressure can be measured through the distal lumen of the balloon dilation catheter, the deflated balloon may partially occlude the aortic valve orifice and lead to spuriously elevated transaortic valve gradients.

The 12-French sheath may be removed 2–3 hours after the effects of heparin have worn off, or protamine may be administered and the sheath may be removed immediately. The arterial monitor line and the right heart catheter are removed the following day if the patient remains stable.

Femoral approach by cutdown. Investigators at New England Medical Center have utilized a limited cutdown over the femoral artery under local anesthesia in some patients.[4] Advantages of this approach include elimination of inadvertent placement of the 12-French arterial sheath in the superficial femoral artery, improved hemostasis, less frequent need for blood transfusion, and a lower incidence of femoral arteriovenous fistulae and pseudoaneurysms.

The major disadvantage of this approach is the requirement for a surgical procedure in all patients. Issues regarding blood loss during catheter exchanges during percutaneous procedures have been addressed by use of lower profile balloon catheters that can be passed through a 12-French sheath. However, cutdown over the femoral artery should be considered in massively obese patients in whom location of the common femoral artery may be more difficult and in whom adequate compression of the femoral artery cannot be achieved after sheath removal.

Brachial approach. Balloon aortic valvuloplasty can be performed safely via the retrograde ap-proach by cutdown entry into the brachial artery (Fig. 6.6). This approach is a reasonable alternative to the percutaneous femoral approach, particularly in patients with occlusive peripheral vascular disease, a history of prior vascular surgery, or marked vessel tortuosity. This approach has been used in 5–10% of aortic valvuloplasty patients without significant complications.[5,6]

To avoid multiple catheters in the antecubital fossa, we recommend placement of an arterial monitor line in the femoral artery or in the contralateral radial artery, and right heart catheterization via the femoral or internal jugular vein. We generally perform left heart catheterization using a 7-French Sones catheter. After baseline hemodynamic measurements are obtained, the Sones catheter is exchanged over the 0.038-inch J-tip guidewire (260 cm), with an extra curve as described previously. Standard 20-mm balloon catheters may be inserted into the brachial artery without difficulty, and with acute hemodynamic results similar to those of the retrograde femoral

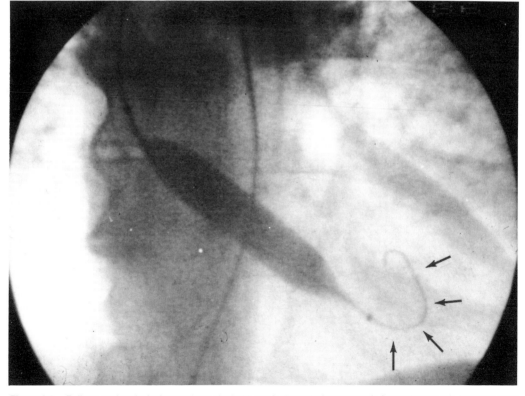

Figure 6.5. Balloon aortic valvuloplasty using a single 20-mm balloon via the retrograde femoral approach. Note the extra curve in the 0.038-inch guidewire (black arrows), which facilitates positioning the balloon catheter in a quiet position in the left ventricle.

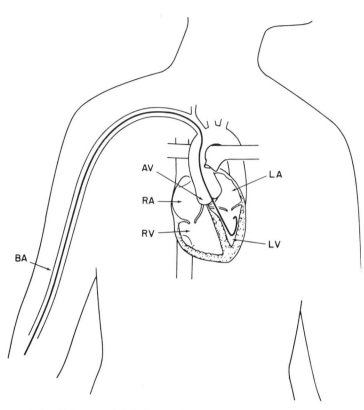

Figure 6.6. Retrograde brachial approach to balloon aortic valvuloplasty. LA = left atrium; LV = left ventricle; AV = aortic valve; BA = brachial artery; RA = right atrium; RV = right ventricle.

approach. Balloon diameters larger than 20 mm may be difficult to insert into the brachial artery because of their large deflated profile.

Once the balloon has been inflated in the aortic valve, it is imperative that negative pressure be applied to completely deflate the balloon before pulling it through the brachial artery. When the balloon is at the arteriotomy site, the balloon catheter should be removed by grasping the balloon directly and pulling it through the arteriotomy. Although the edges of the arteriotomy may be irregular, the site can be easily trimmed, and closure can be accomplished with several interrupted sutures.

ANTEGRADE APPROACH TO BALLOON AORTIC VALVULOPLASTY

General considerations. The antegrade approach to balloon aortic valvuloplasty is a reasonable alternative to the retrograde approach, particularly in patients in whom the retrograde approach

is not possible. The antegrade approach is technically more difficult since it requires skill in performing transseptal left heart catheterization (Fig. 6.7). Absolute contraindications to transseptal left heart catheterization are the presence of atrial or ventricular thrombus.

Transseptal left heart catheterization. The technique of transseptal left heart catheterization is identical to that performed for balloon mitral valvotomy.[7,8] The right common femoral vein is entered percutaneously, and an 8-French Mullins dilator and sheath with sidearm adapter (C.R. Bard, Inc., Billerica, MA) are placed in the superior vena cava over a 0.032-inch J-tip guidewire. Blood samples should be taken from the superior vena cava and from the pulmonary artery to screen for the presence of a left to right shunt.

A modified Brockenbrough needle is then inserted into the dilator approximately 1 cm from its tip, and central venous pressure is recorded. During continuous pressure monitoring, the Mullins sheath and dilator and Brockenbrough needle are pulled back into the right atrium in the AP

Figure 6.7. Antegrade transseptal approach to balloon aortic valvuloplasty. Note the guidewire loop in the left ventricular (LV) apex and the tip of the guidewire across the aortic valve (AV), in the descending aorta (AO). RFV = right femoral vein; IVC = inferior vena cava; RA = right atrium; FO = foramen ovale; LA = left atrium; MV = mitral valve.

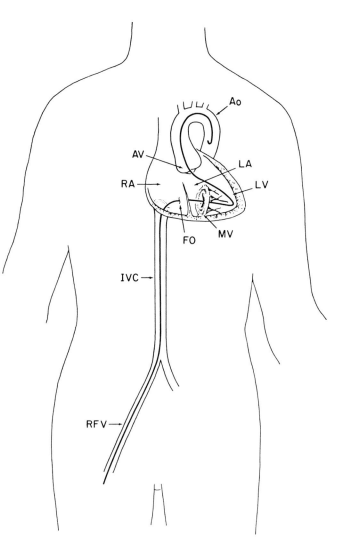

projection, with the needle directed at approximately 4 o'clock. As the assembled system is withdrawn, the tip of the dilator will ride over the lateral wall of the aorta, in close proximity to the dense calcification in the aortic valve. Further withdrawal of the assembly below the level of the aortic valve should continue along the atrial septum until the tip of the dilator "drops" into the fossa ovalis. Slight withdrawal of the system and then gentle forward pressure will confirm that the dilator is in the fossa ovalis.

Under fluoroscopic guidance and during continuous pressure monitoring, the Brockenbrough needle is advanced firmly into the atrial septum. Once the needle is fully advanced, a phasic left atrial pressure can usually be identified. However, if the pressure is damped, incomplete septal

perforation may be confirmed by gentle contrast injection through the needle, after which time the entire system may be advanced slightly (generally about 1 cm) until a phasic left atrial pressure is identified. A slight "popping" sensation may occur as the left atrial pressure appears. If there is any doubt about the position of the needle, the needle should be withdrawn, the sheath and dilator should be flushed, and the procedure repeated.

Once left atrial pressure has been confirmed, the entire assembly is advanced about 1–2 cm until the tip of the dilator traverses the atrial septum. In the LAO projection we generally inject small amounts of contrast through the needle to identify the tip of the Mullins sheath and the back wall of the left atrium. Once the Mullins sheath has been advanced into the left atrium (which may be accompanied by a second "popping" sensation), the dilator and needle are removed, left atrial pressure is recorded through the sidearm adapter, and 10,000 Units of heparin are administered.

A 7-French balloon flotation catheter that will accommodate a 0.038-inch guidewire (Arrow International, Inc., Reading, PA) is then advanced through the Mullins sheath into the left atrium. The balloon is inflated with CO_2 and floated across the mitral valve and into the left ventricle, at which time baseline hemodynamic measurements are obtained.

Frequently, the most difficult part of the antegrade procedure is negotiating the sharp turn from the left ventricular apex to the aortic valve, to gain access to the thoracic aorta. By using a 0.038-inch guidewire with a tight distal curve, the tip of the balloon-flotation catheter can be turned and directed toward the aortic valve, where it can then be passed across the aortic valve and into the ascending aorta. Another 0.038-inch J-tip guidewire (260 cm) may be advanced through the balloon-flotation catheter and placed in the de-

scending thoracic aorta. During these guidewire and catheter manipulations, it is crucial to maintain a guidewire loop in the left ventricular apex (Fig. 6.8). Without this loop, the balloon dilating catheter will be unable to make the sharp turn over the anterior leaflet of the mitral valve into the aortic valve.

Some investigators prefer use of a 400-cm guidewire, which can be snared and delivered percutaneously through a sheath in the left femoral artery.[9] However, although this technique may provide greater stability of the guidewire and balloon across the aortic valve, it requires an additional arterial puncture, increases the complexity of the procedure, and may damage the mitral apparatus by excessive traction on the guidewire.

Once the guidewire is in satisfactory position, the balloon-flotation catheter and Mullins sheath are removed. The atrial septum should be dilated with an 8-French catheter with an 8-mm balloon (Mansfield) advanced over the 0.038-inch guidewire (Fig. 6.8). The valvuloplasty balloon catheter may then be advanced over the guidewire and

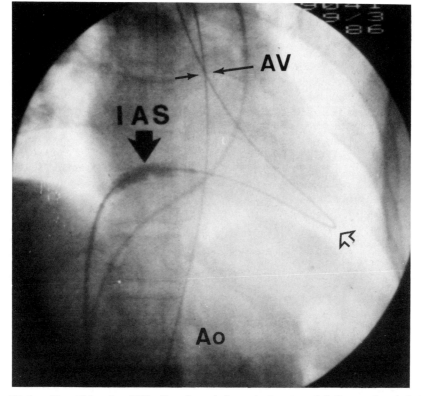

Figure 6.8.   Dilation of the atrial septum (IAS) with an 8-mm balloon prior to antegrade balloon aortic valvuloplasty. Note the position of the 0.038-inch guidewire across the aortic valve (AV) and in the descending aorta (AO), and the guidewire loop in the left ventricular apex (open arrowhead).

across the aortic valve, where one or more inflations can be performed. Balloon dilation has been accomplished with balloons measuring 20 mm in diameter, but dilation with larger balloons using the antegrade approach may be difficult.

Once the final inflation has been made, the balloon catheter should be exchanged for the balloon-flotation catheter and Mullins sheath for repeat hemodynamic measurements. A formal oximetry run should be made to assess the magnitude of the left to right shunt through the atrial septum. A 12-French sheath is placed in the right femoral vein until the effects of heparin have worn off, at which time the sheath is removed.

COMPARISON OF ANTEGRADE AND RETROGRADE BALLOON AORTIC VALVULOPLASTY

Immediate hemodynamic results. The antegrade and retrograde approaches to balloon aortic valvuloplasty should be viewed as complementary procedures. Block and Palacios compared the acute hemodynamic results of retrograde percutaneous aortic valvuloplasty to those of antegrade aortic valvuloplasty.[10] After retrograde valvuloplasty in 25 patients, the transaortic valve gradient decreased from 63 ± 4 mm Hg to 35 ± 4 mm Hg, and the aortic valve area increased from 0.4 ± 0.04 cm² to 0.7 ± 0.05 cm². Similar results were obtained in 30 patients treated with antegrade valvuloplasty in whom the transaortic valve gradient decreased from 59 ± 3 mm Hg to 29 ± 2 mm Hg, and the aortic valve area increased from 0.5 ± 0.03 cm² to 0.8 ± 0.04 cm².

Similarly, investigators at the University of Utah Medical Center found no significant differences in final aortic valve area or transaortic valve gradient among 25 patients treated with either the antegrade or retrograde techniques.[9] Therefore,

there appears to be no acute hemodynamic advantage of one approach versus the other.

Complications. The major advantage of the antegrade approach is virtual elimination of significant femoral arterial complications, as well as reduction in transfusion requirements. Block and Palacios reported significant vascular complications in 7 of 25 patients treated by the retrograde femoral approach, compared to none of the 30 patients treated by the antegrade approach. Complete heart block was more common in the antegrade group and may have been secondary to the need for more aggressive catheter manipulation to gain access to the aortic valve. The incidence of other complications, such as stroke, peripheral embolization, and aortic insufficiency is similar in both approaches.[10]

The major limitation of the antegrade technique is the risk of pericardial tamponade (which occurs in approximately 1–8% of patients undergoing transseptal left heart catheterization for balloon mitral valvuloplasty). Tamponade is usually secondary to perforation of the left atrium.[11] The incidence of pericardial tamponade during retrograde balloon aortic valvuloplasty is < 1% and is usually secondary to perforation of the left ventricle (Table 6.1). The second major limitation of the antegrade technique is difficulty crossing the aortic valve, which is usually due to technical problems maintaining a guidewire loop in the left ventricular apex to allow smooth passage of the balloon catheters. Failure to maintain an adequate loop in the left ventricular apex could potentially result in damage to the mitral valve or subvalvular apparatus.

Selection of antegrade versus retrograde technique. Most interventional cardiologists will prefer the retrograde approach because of their familiarity with the technique. Many centers have little or no experience with the transseptal tech-

Table 6.1.
Complications of Balloon Aortic Valvuloplasty (%)

Study	Number	Death	CVA	Perf	MI	AR	Vasc
Cribier[6]	334	4.5	1.4	0.6	0.3	0	13.1
Lewin[21]	125	10.4	3.2	0	1.6	1.6	9.6
Safian[5]	170	3.5	0	1.7	0.6	1.1	10
Block[27]	162	7.0	2.0	0	0	0	7.0
TOTAL	791	5.4	1.5	0.6	0.5	0.5	10.6

Abbreviations: Number = number of patients; CVA = cerebrovascular events; Perf = cardiac perforation; MI = acute myocardial infarction; AR = severe aortic regurgitation; Vasc = vascular injury.

nique. We recommend the retrograde percutaneous femoral approach for most patients. For patients with severe peripheral vascular disease, we prefer the retrograde brachial approach and reserve the antegrade approach for those patients in whom the femoral and brachial approaches are not feasible.

MULTIPLE BALLOON TECHNIQUE

In vitro studies of balloon aortic valvuloplasty have demonstrated that significant damage to the aortic valve and anulus can occur during dilation with oversized balloons.[12,13] Nevertheless, inflations of a single balloon may not result in adequate reduction of the transaortic valve gradient, necessitating use of larger balloon dilating areas, usually by multiple balloons. Yeager has reported the effective dilating diameters for a variety of double balloon combinations, as indicated in Table 6.2.[14]

Some investigators measure the dimensions of the aortic anulus in an attempt to predict the appropriate balloon size for aortic valvuloplasty. To minimize complications, Lewin and associates recommend balloon sizes to maintain the ratio of balloon area to aortic anulus area ≤ 1.2.[15] Mullins

and co-workers recommend balloon selection such that the sum of the inflated balloon diameters is equal to 1.2 to 1.3 times the diameter of the aortic anulus.[16]

Although dimensions of the aortic anulus are readily available by two-dimensional echocardiography, they may not predict the maximum safe balloon size in all patients. The baseline aortic valve area is probably more important in selecting the appropriate balloon size, since most of the reported cases of balloon-mediated disruption of the aortic valve or anulus have occurred in patients with aortic valve areas of 0.2–0.5 cm² (Table 6.3).[15,17–20] Furthermore, data in younger patients may not apply to elderly patients with calcific, degenerative aortic stenosis.[16]

The world's largest experience with multiple balloon aortic valvuloplasty was reported by Lewin and associates.[21] The multiple balloon technique was utilized in 95% of their 125 patients, including 19 patients treated with simultaneous inflation of three balloons. The double balloon technique was usually performed by retrograde catheterization of the brachial and femoral arteries, and the triple balloon technique was performed by retrograde catheterization of the brachial artery and both femoral arteries.

An alternative approach to double balloon aortic valvuloplasty is to insert both balloon catheters through the same femoral artery, using a 9-French angioplasty guiding catheter or an 8-French double lumen catheter (Mansfield), which will accommodate two 0.038-inch guidewires. This procedure has been performed successfully by percutaneous (without an introducing sheath) or cutdown entry into the femoral artery. Both balloon catheters can be advanced simultaneously or sequentially across the aortic valve, followed by

Table 6.2.
Effective Dilating Diameters (mm) for Double Balloon Combinations

		Balloon diameter (mm)			
		12	15	18	20
Balloon	12	19.6	22.1	24.8	26.5
diameter	15	22.1	24.6	27.1	28.8
(mm)	18	24.8	27.1	29.5	31.1
	20	26.5	28.8	31.1	32.7

Table 6.3.
Damage to the Aortic Valve and Anulus: Patient Characteristics and Balloon Size

Author (reference)	Complication	Age (years)	AVA (cm²)	AVG (mm Hg)	BSA (m²)	Balloon Size	Dsum (mm)	Dann (mm)	BAR	Outcome
Lewin (15)	anulus tear	70	0.48	79	NA	18,20	38	29	1.3	death
Lewin (15)	anulus tear	91	0.48	60	NA	18,18	36	26	1.4	AVR
Lembo (19)	rupture	86	0.2	120	2.08	3 × 12	36	22	1.6	death
Dean (18)	AR	88	0.3	80	NA	18	18	NA	NA	AVR
Vrolix (20)	rupture	74	0.3	80	NA	19,13	32	23	1.4	death
Safian (5)	leaflet tear	83	0.3	80	1.6	18	18	29	0.6	death

Abbreviations: AVA = aortic valve area; AVG = peak transaortic valve gradient; BSA = body surface area; Dsum = effective dilating diameter determined by the sum of the individual balloon diameters; Dann = diameter of aortic anulus; BAR = ratio of effective dilating diameter of balloons to diameter of aortic anulus; AVR = aortic valve replacement; AR = severe aortic regurgitation; NA = not available.

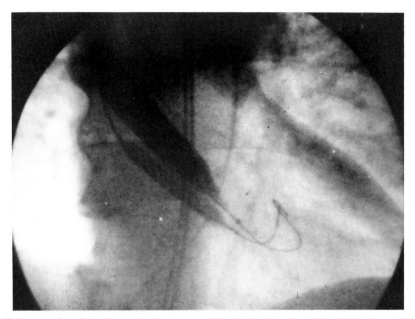

Figure 6.9. Balloon aortic valvuloplasty using the retrograde femoral approach and double balloon technique. Both balloons (20-mm + 10-mm diameter) were inserted percutaneously through the right femoral artery.

simultaneous inflation of both balloons (Fig. 6.9). After dilation, negative pressure must be applied to one balloon catheter as it is delivered through the arterial entry site.

COMPARISON OF SINGLE AND MULTIPLE BALLOON TECHNIQUES

Acute hemodynamic results and follow-up. The immediate hemodynamic results are similar for large numbers of patients with aortic stenosis treated with the single balloon or multiple balloon techniques (Table 6.4). In general, balloon aortic valvuloplasty results in a 50–70% reduction in transaortic valve gradient, a 50–70% increase in aortic valve area, and a modest increase in cardiac output.[5,6,11,21,22]

However, in those patients in whom effective gradient reduction is not achieved with single balloon techniques, better gradient reduction and larger aortic valve areas may be obtained in some patients by multiple balloon techniques. In this subgroup of patients, the final gradient and valve area achieved are similar to those obtained in patients who undergo successful valvuloplasty with a single balloon.[22,23]

Long-term follow-up studies have indicated that aortic valve restenosis is very common and occurs in at least 50% of patients at the end of one year. The incidence of late death, aortic valve replacement, and need for repeat aortic valvuloplasty is similar for patients treated by either single or multiple balloon techniques.[5,6,11,21]

Complications. The incidence of major complications appears to be similar for single and multiple balloon techniques. However, there may be slightly more morbidity associated with multiple arterial entries and repairs required for the multiple balloon technique. Use of multiple balloons has also been associated with persistent complete heart block following aortic valvuloplasty.[24]

During inflations with a 20-mm balloon, a transient fall in systolic blood pressure to 60–80 mm Hg is not unusual, but few patients become symptomatic since blood pressure increases immediately after balloon deflation. Poor hemodynamic tolerance during inflations with a single 20-mm balloon is quite unusual, except in patients with extremely narrow orifice dimensions. In these patients, the same arguments that apply to complex balloon configurations with respect to potential hemodynamic tolerance should also apply to the multiple balloon technique, provided the aortic valve is not overdilated.

Selection of single versus multiple balloon technique. In most patients, the simplest and least morbid approach is the single balloon technique, using a 20-mm balloon (Fig. 6.5). The immediate hemodynamic results of mutiple balloon procedures are not sufficiently compelling to mandate routine use of more than one balloon during the initial dilation. Morever, mild increments in aortic valve area have not been shown to be associated with a more favorable long-term outcome. However, in some cases, single balloon dilation results in inadequate gradient reduction, necessitating use of larger balloon dilating areas, usually by multiple balloons (Fig. 6.9).

For patients with extremely narrow aortic valve orifices (e.g., < 0.5 cm^2), we generally recommend initial use of relatively small effective balloon diameters (e.g., 15- or 18-mm diameter), with further increases in balloon size dictated by repeat hemodynamic assessment after each dilation. Some aortic valves cannot be effectively dilated, and deliberate oversizing of the valve may result in disruption of the aortic valve and anulus, and death of the patient.

COMBINED AORTIC AND MITRAL BALLOON VALVULOPLASTY

Select patients with severe aortic and mitral stenosis who are not felt to be candidates for cardiac surgery may be considered candidates for balloon dilation of both valves during the same procedure. The combined procedure is initiated by first performing transseptal left heart catheterization, as described earlier. Once the left atrium has been entered, heparin is administered and retrograde balloon aortic valvuloplasty is performed. Following successful dilation of the aortic valve, balloon mitral valvuloplasty may be performed, as described in Chapter 13.

Several features of this combined procedure are worth emphasis. First, transseptal catheterization is performed before aortic valvuloplasty to avoid heparinization before attempting the transseptal puncture. Second, the aortic valve is dilated first since balloon inflation across the mitral valve usually results in profound hypotension, which may be poorly tolerated if the aortic valve has not been predilated. Third, after aortic valve dilation, the balloon-flotation catheter can be placed across the mitral valve into the left ventricle. The tip of the exchange guidewire can be placed in the left ventricular apex, and the mitral valve can then be dilated. This avoids the time-consuming and technically challenging step of passing the guidewire antegrade around the apex, across the aortic valve, and into the descending aorta. Of course, if this can be accomplished easily, there is no reason why aortic and mitral valvuloplasty could not be performed using the antegrade approach alone.

Acute hemodynamic results and complications are similar to those observed during balloon valvuloplasty for isolated aortic or mitral stenosis.[25]

COMPLICATIONS OF BALLOON AORTIC VALVULOPLASTY

The early application of balloon aortic valvuloplasty to adult patients with calcific aortic stenosis was limited initially by fears of distal embolization and disruption of the valvular apparatus. Several postmortem and intraoperative studies have suggested a very low likelihood of liberating valve debris or damaging the aortic valve apparatus when appropriate size balloons are used.[12,13]

These studies have been confirmed by published reports of balloon aortic valvuloplasty in large numbers of patients.[5,6,11,21] The incidence of serious, life-threatening complications is quite low. Among four large published series with a total of nearly 800 patients, the in-hospital mortality rate

Table 6.4.
Acute Hemodynamic Results of Balloon Aortic Valvuloplasty Using Single and Multiple Balloons

Author (Reference)	Number	Method	AVA (cm^2) pre	AVA (cm^2) post	AVG (mm Hg) pre	AVG (mm Hg) post
Letac (6)	334	Single	0.54 ± 0.18	0.98 ± 0.32	72 ± 14	28 ± 12
Safian (5)	170	Single	0.6 ± 0.2	0.9 ± 0.3	71 ± 20	36 ± 14
Block (11)	162	Single	0.5 ± 0.01	0.9 ± 0.02	61 ± 2	27 ± 1
Lewin (21)	125	Multiple	0.6 ± 0.2	1.0 ± 0.3	87 ± 38	32 ± 17
Isner (22)	16	Multiple	0.45 ± 0.04	0.77 ± 0.06	79 ± 8	36 ± 4

Abbreviations: Number = number of patients; AVA = aortic valve area; AVG = peak transaortic valve gradient; pre = before balloon valvuloplasty; post = after balloon valvuloplasty.

was 5.4% (Table 6.1). In most cases, death occurred in moribund patients and was felt to be unrelated to the procedure itself. The incidence of all complications falls with increasing experience.

Cerebrovascular events, including stroke and transient ischemic episodes, are uncommon, and the incidence of clinically important cerebral events is approximately 1–2%. These events could be related to embolization of calcific debris or hypotension during balloon inflations. A prospective study using computerized tomography of the brain suggests that a bicuspid aortic valve may be a risk factor for systemic embolization during balloon valvuloplasty.[26]

Major damage to the aortic valve and anulus occurs in < 1% of patients who undergo balloon aortic valvuloplasty (Table 6.3).[5,6,21,27] The risk of these complications is certainly increased in patients in whom the ratio of the balloon dilating area to anulus area exceeds 1.2, but it may also occur in patients in whom the ratio is less than 1.1. The greatest risk is in patients of small body size

(BSA < 1.6 m²) with large gradients (peak gradients > 60 mm Hg) and small orifice dimensions (aortic valve area < 0.5 cm²).

Patients who develop severe chest pain during balloon inflation, particularly if associated with hemodynamic signs of worsening congestive heart failure, should be suspected of having an aortic annular tear or avulsion of an aortic valve leaflet, leading to sudden massive aortic regurgitation (Fig. 6.10).[5,15] Hemodynamic measurements may reveal marked elevation of left heart filling pressures and near-equalization of pressure in the left ventricle and aorta (Fig. 6.11). The presence of severe aortic regurgitation can be confirmed by supravalvular aortography or two-dimensional echocardiography. Immediate management should include the use of diuretics and vasodilators, if possible, followed by emergency surgery, if appropriate.

Transient acute severe aortic regurgitation has also been reported following balloon aortic valvuloplasty.[17] This complication may be secondary to overstretching the aortic anulus or to transient

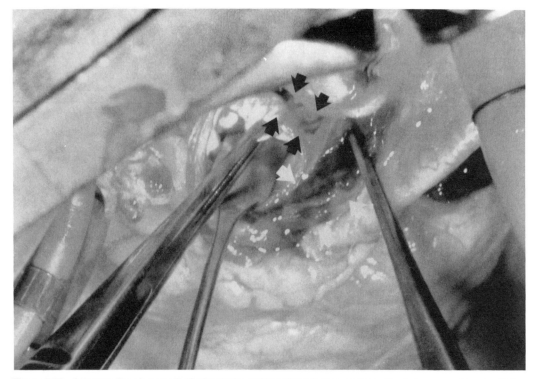

Figure 6.10.   Intraoperative photograph of a tear in the aortic anulus (black arrows) resulting in severe aortic regurgitation in a 91-year-old woman. A hematoma is evident between the aorta and the pulmonary artery (white arrow). Balloon valvuloplasty had been performed with the double balloon technique (two 18-mm balloons). (Reproduced, with permission, from Lewin RF et al. Aortic annular tear after valvuloplasty: The role of aortic annulus echocardiographic measurement. *Cathet Cardiovasc Diagn 16*:123, 1989.)

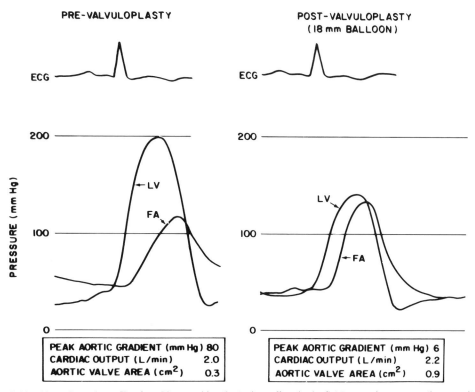

Figure 6.11.   Hemodynamic profile of an 83-year-old patient who suffered a leaflet tear and severe aortic regurgitation following aortic valvuloplasty with a single 18-mm balloon. Note the marked fall in the peak transaortic valve gradient and the rise in left ventricular diastolic pressure, leading to near-equalization of pressures in the left ventricle (LV) and femoral artery (FA). ECG = electrocardiogram.

cusp eversion, leading to incomplete leaflet closure and aortic regurgitation. Two-dimensional echocardiography is useful in evaluating patients with severe aortic regurgitation following balloon aortic valvuloplasty, but failure to identify a structural abnormality of the valve or anulus is reassuring only if the patient shows immediate improvement with diuretics and vasodilators. Patients who fail to improve immediately should be considered for surgery even if a structural abnormality cannot be identified.[18]

Sudden hemodynamic collapse immediately following balloon aortic valvuloplasty should raise suspicion for aortic rupture (Fig. 6.12)[19,20] or cardiac perforation,[5,6] each of which occurs in < 1% of patients. The finding of immobile heart borders is further presumptive evidence for pericardial tamponade, which frequently requires emergency pericardiocentesis before the diagnosis can be confirmed by two-dimensional echocardiography.

Rupture of the aorta is usually fatal. Pericardiocentesis may be difficult, and even if a pericardial drain can be placed, blood loss into the pericardium may continue.

If guidewire perforation of the left ventricle occurs, the sudden increase in left ventricular pressure during balloon inflations may result in extravasation of blood into the pericardium and tamponade. Some of these patients can be managed by immediate pericardiocentesis without surgery, particularly if the aortic valve was successfully dilated. A more serious problem is cardiac perforation due to the balloon catheter, which usually requires emergency pericardiocentesis followed by surgery.

Acute myocardial infarction occurs in < 1% of patients treated by balloon aortic valvuloplasty. Non-Q-wave myocardial infarction may occur in the presence of severe coronary artery disease and may be secondary to a combination of diminished coronary blood flow and increased myocardial oxygen demands during periods of elevated left ventricular wall stress. Embolization of calcific debris could potentially lead to Q-wave myocardial infarction, but this appears to be a very rare event.

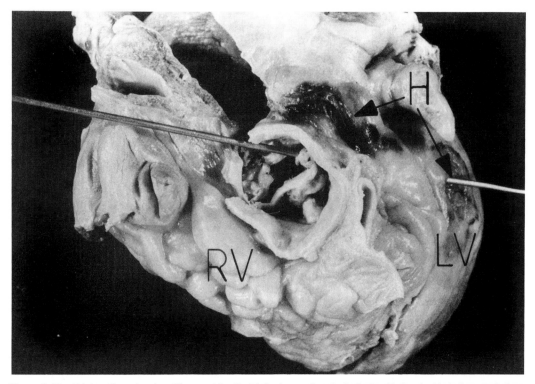

Figure 6.12. Fatal aortic rupture in a 74-year-old patient following aortic valvuloplasty with the double balloon technique (19-mm + 13-mm balloons). A probe identifies the site of rupture just above the left sinus of Valsalva, with an associated hematoma (H) overlying the left main coronary artery. LV = left ventricle; RV = right ventricle. (Reproduced, with permission, from Vrolix M et al. Fatal aortic rupture: An unusual complication of percutaneous balloon valvuloplasty for acquired valvular aortic stenosis. *Cathet Cardiovasc Diagn 16*:119, 1989.)

The presence of angina and severe coronary artery disease is not a contraindication to balloon aortic valvuloplasty. The majority of patients have significant coronary disease, and tolerance of the procedure is usually excellent. However, balloon aortic valvuloplasty should be performed cautiously in patients with ostial stenoses of the left or right coronary arteries. During balloon inflations, large calcified nodules on the valve leaflets may occlude the coronary ostia and may lead to ischemia or significant left ventricular dysfunction. In selected individuals, coronary angioplasty and balloon valvuloplasty may be performed concurrently, if clinically indicated.[28]

The most common complication of balloon aortic valvuloplasty is injury to the femoral artery, which occurs in 10–15% of patients. These arterial complications may be due to hemorrhage, thrombosis, perforation, pseudoaneurysm formation, or the development of arteriovenous fistulae and may require blood transfusion or surgical repair of the vessel (Fig. 6.13). The incidence of vascular complications seems to be falling with increasing operator experience and with use of lower profile balloon catheters and smaller diameter introducing sheaths. As mentioned, a potential advantage of the transseptal approach to aortic valvuloplasty is the virtual elimination of arterial complications.

Transient dysrhythmias are common during balloon aortic valvuloplasty.[29] Nonsustained ventricular tachycardia frequently occurs during manipulation of the guidewire and balloon catheter and is not clinically important. Transient intraventricular conduction delay occurs in 18% of patients and is probably secondary to direct mechanical effects of the guidewire and balloon. Transient complete heart block, lasting minutes to several hours, occurs in approximately 1% of patients and generally requires a temporary pacemaker.

Isolated case reports of other complications include mitral valve rupture (during retrograde valvuloplasty),[30] bacterial endocarditis,[31] and atrial septal defect (after antegrade valvuloplasty) requiring surgical repair.[32]

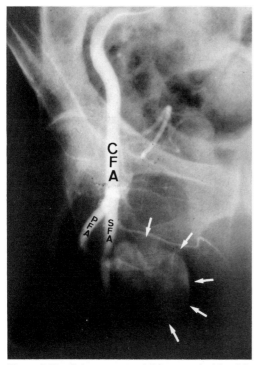

Figure 6.13. False aneurysm (white arrows) of the right superficial femoral artery (SFA) after removal of the 12-French arterial sheath, requiring surgical repair under local anesthesia. The arterial puncture was too low, as shown by the position of the common femoral artery (CFA) and the profunda femoral artery (PFA).

SUMMARY

Balloon aortic valvuloplasty is a reasonable palliative procedure for elderly patients with symptomatic aortic stenosis who are not candidates for aortic valve replacement. The procedure may be performed via the retrograde femoral or brachial approach, or via the antegrade transseptal approach.

The retrograde femoral approach is the easiest procedure and the retrograde brachial approach may be used in the presence of severe peripheral vascular disease. The antegrade approach is technically the most difficult approach and should probably be reserved for patients who cannot be approached by the retrograde technique and should be performed at centers with extensive experience with transseptal left heart catheterization.

Retrograde balloon aortic valvuloplasty can be performed with a variety of different balloons, including single balloons (one balloon, one shaft),

mutiple balloons (two or three balloons on two or three shafts), and complex balloon configurations (bifoil or trefoil balloons). The immediate hemodynamic results and long-term outcome are similar for large numbers of patients treated with single balloons, multiple balloons, and complex balloon configurations. Some patients who have insufficient gradient reduction with the single balloon technique may benefit from dilation with catheters with larger effective dilating areas (mutiple balloons or complex balloons).

Life-threatening complications are uncommon during balloon aortic valvuloplasty. In-hospital mortality is approximately 5%, and death usually occurs in moribund patients. Damage to the aortic valve and anulus occurs in < 1% of patients and is more common in patients with extremely narrow orifice dimensions (valve area < 0.5 cm^2). Cerebrovascular events are also uncommon and occur in 1–2% of patients. The most common complication is vascular injury, which occurs in 10–15% of patients, but may become less common with improvements in equipment and enhanced operator experience.

REFERENCES

1. Voudris V, Drobinski G, L'Epine Y, Sotirov I, Moussallem N, Canny M. Results of percutaneous valvuloplasty for calcific aortic stenosis with different balloon catheters. *Cath Cardiovasc Diag 17*: 80–83, 1989.
2. Cribier A, Savin T, Berland J, et al. Percutaneous transluminal balloon valvuloplasty of adult aortic stenosis: Report of 92 cases. *J Am Coll Cardiol 9*: 381–386, 1987.
3. McKay RG, Safian RD, Lock JE, et al. Balloon dilatation of calcific aortic stenosis in elderly patients: Postmortem, intraoperative, and percutaneous valvuloplasty studies. *Circulation 74*:119–125, 1986.
4. Isner JM, Salem DN, Desnoyers MR, et al. Treatment of calcific aortic stenosis by balloon valvuloplasty. *Am J Cardiol 59*:313–317, 1987.
5. Safian RD, Berman AD, Diver DJ, et al. Balloon aortic valvuloplasty in 170 consecutive patients. *N Engl J Med 319*:125–130, 1988.
6. Cribier A, Gerber LI, Letac B. Percutaneous balloon aortic valvuloplasty: The French experience. In: *Textbook of Interventional Cardiology*, ed by EJ Topol, Philadelphia, WB Saunders, 1990, pp. 849–867.
7. McKay RG, Lock JE, Keane JF, Safian RD, Aroesty JM, Grossman W. Percutaneous mitral valvuloplasty in an adult patient with calcific rheumatic mitral stenosis. *J Am Coll Cardiol 7*:1410–1415, 1986.
8. Palacios IF, Lock JE, Keane JF, Block PC. Percuta-

neous transvenous balloon valvotomy in a patient with severe calcific mitral stenosis. *J Am Coll Cardiol* 7:1416–1419, 1986.

9. Orme EC, Wray RB, Barry WH, Krueger SK, Mason JW. Comparison of three techniques for percutaneous balloon aortic valvuloplasty of aortic stenosis in adults. *Am Heart J* 117:11–17, 1989.

10. Block PC, Palacios IF. Comparison of hemodynamic results of anterograde versus retrograde percutaneous balloon aortic valvuloplasty. *Am J Cardiol* 60: 659–662, 1987.

11. Block PC, Palacios IF. Aortic and mitral balloon valvuloplasty: The United States experience. In: *Textbook of Interventional Cardiology*. ed by EJ Topol, Philadelphia, WB Saunders, 1990, pp. 831–848.

12. Safian RD, Mandell VS, Thurer RE, et al. Postmortem and intraoperative balloon valvuloplasty of calcific aortic stenosis in elderly patients: Mechanisms of successful dilation. *J Am Coll Cardiol* 9: 655–660, 1987.

13. Letac B, Gerber LI, Koning R. Insights on the mechanism of balloon valvuloplasty in aortic stenosis. *Am J Cardiol* 62:1241–1247, 1986.

14. Yeager SB. Balloon selection for double balloon valvotomy. *J Am Coll Cardiol* 9: 467–468, 1987.

15. Lewin RF, Dorros G, King JF, Seifert PE, Schmahl TM, Auer JE. Aortic annular tear after valvuloplasty: The role of aortic annulus echocardiographic measurement. *Cathet Cardiovasc Diagn* 16:123–129, 1989.

16. Mullins CE, Nihill MR, Vick GW, III, et al. Double balloon technique for dilation of valvular or vessel stenosis in congenital and acquired heart disease. *J Am Coll Cardiol* 10:107–114, 1987.

17. Sadaniantz A, Malhotra R, Korr KS. Transient acute severe aortic regurgitation complicating balloon aortic valvuloplasty. *Cathet Cardiovasc Diagn* 17: 186–189, 1989.

18. Dean LS, Chandler JW, Saenz CB, Baxley WA, Bulle TM. Severe aortic regurgitation complicating percutaneous aortic valve valvuloplasty. *Cathet Cardiovasc Diagn* 16:130–132, 1989.

19. Lembo NJ, King SB, III, Roubin GS, Hammami A, Niederman AL. Fatal aortic rupture during percutaneous balloon valvuloplasty for valvular aortic stenosis. *Am J Cardiol* 60:733–735, 1987.

20. Vrolix M, Piessens J, Moerman P, Vanhaecke J, DeGeest H. Fatal aortic rupture: An unusual complication of percutaneous balloon valvuloplasty for acquired valvular aortic stenosis. *Cathet Cardiovasc Diagn* 16:119–122, 1989.

21. Lewin RF, Dorros G, King JF, Mathiak L. Percutaneous transluminal aortic valvuloplasty: Acute outcome and follow-up of 125 patients. *J Am Coll Cardiol* 14:1210–1217, 1989.

22. Isner JM, Salem DN, Desnoyers MR, et al. Dual balloon technique for valvuloplasty of aortic stenosis in adults. *Am J Cardiol* 61:583–589, 1988.

23. Midei MG, Brennan M, Walford GD, et al. Double vs. single balloon technique for aortic balloon valvuloplasty. *Chest* 94:245–250, 1988.

24. Plack RH, Porterfield JK, Brinker JA. Complete heart block developing during aortic valvuloplasty. *Chest* 96:1201–1203, 1989.

25. Berman AD, Weinstein JS, Safian RD, Diver DJ, Grossman W, McKay R. Combined aortic and mitral balloon valvuloplasty in patients with critical aortic and mitral valve stenosis: Results in six cases. *J Am Coll Cardiol* 11:1213–1218, 1988.

26. Davidson CJ, Skelton TN, Kisslo KB, et al. The risk for systemic embolization associated with percutaneous balloon valvuloplasty in adults. *Ann Intern Med* 108:557–560, 1988.

27. Block PC, Palacios IF. Percutaneous aortic balloon valvuloplasty (PAV) in the elderly: Update of immediate results in follow-up. *Circulation* (abstract) 78 (Suppl II): II-593, 1988.

28. McKay RG, Safian RD, Berman AD, et al. Combined percutaneous aortic valvuloplasty and transluminal coronary angioplasty in adult patients with calcific aortic stenosis and coronary artery disease. *Circulation* 76:1298–1306, 1987.

29. Carlson MD, Palacios I, Thomas JD, et al. Cardiac conduction abnormalities during percutaneous balloon mitral or aortic valvotomy. *Circulation* 79: 1197–1203, 1979.

30. de Ubago JLM, Vazquez JA, Moujir F, Olalla JJ, Figuerao A, Colman T. Mitral valve rupture during percutaneous dilation of aortic valve stenosis. *Cathet Cardiovasc Diagn* 16:115–118, 1989.

31. Cujec B, McMeekin J, Lopez J. Bacterial endocarditis after percutaneous aortic valvuloplasty. *Am Heart J* 115:178–179, 1988.

32. Lemmer JH Jr, Winniford MD, Ferguson DW. Surgical implications of atrial septal defect complicating aortic balloon valvuloplasty. *Ann Thorac Surg* 48:295–297, 1989.

7

Acute Hemodynamic Effects of Percutaneous Balloon Aortic Valvuloplasty

THOMAS M. BASHORE and CHARLES J. DAVIDSON

The acute hemodynamic effects observed after balloon aortic valvuloplasty are complex and further complicated by the difficulty in measuring systolic and diastolic properties in the face of the abnormal loading conditions posed by outflow obstruction. A brief review of the pathophysiology of aortic stenosis (AS) and the effect of AS on measures of left ventricular performance is important to better understand the manner in which aortic valvuloplasty alters these properties. This chapter will review this basic physiology and attempt to put the acute and early hemodynamic changes reported from the balloon aortic valvuloplasty (BAV) procedure in perspective.

The development of AS results in resistance to left ventricular (LV) outflow and the appearance of a gradient across the diseased aortic valve. The magnitude of this gradient is dependent on both the amount of flow through the valvular orifice (i.e., the cardiac output) and the size of the valvular orifice (i.e., the aortic valve area). The relationship between flow, valve area, and gradient is nonlinear and can best be represented by a family of curves (Fig. 7.1).

This basic relationship becomes quite relevant for interpretation of the effect of interventions such as aortic valve replacement or BAV. For instance, if a heart rate of 75 bpm and a cardiac output of 4.5 liters / min are assumed present, the mean aortic valve gradient with an aortic valve area (AVA) of 0.5 cm² would be 77 mm Hg. If, after BAV, the AVA improves by an increment of 0.3 cm² to 0.8 cm², the gradient will fall to 30 mm Hg—a 47 mm Hg change. But if the AVA at baseline is 0.8 cm² and BAV increases the AVA by 0.3 cm²

to 1.1 cm², the gradient will fall only 14 mm Hg to a mean of 16 mm Hg. Thus, the same incremental change in AVA is associated with a strikingly different final aortic valve gradient depending on the baseline and the subsequent orifice size and cardiac output. Figure 7.1 emphasizes these observations. In patients with severe AS, a small change in either the AVA or the cardiac output is translated into a much greater change in the gradient than is seen in patients with milder AS. To interpret the effects of aortic valvuloplasty or aortic valve replacement using the AVA only or the gradient only obviously does not relay the whole story.

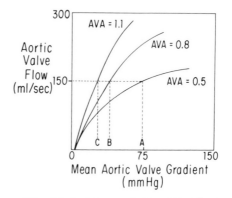

Figure 7.1. Effect of changes in the aortic valve area (AVA) on the transvalvular aortic valve gradient. The relationship between cardiac output (flow), the aortic valve gradient, and the aortic valve area (AVA) is represented by a family of curves. A 0.3 cm² AVA change from 0.5 cm² to 0.8 cm² (**A** to **B**) results in a much greater change in gradient than a similar change from 0.8 cm² to 1.1 cm² (**B** to **C**).

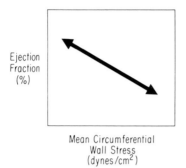

Ejection
Fraction
(%)

Mean Circumferential
Wall Stress
(dynes/cm^2)

Figure 7.2.   Effect of increasing wall stress on ejection fraction. This inverse relationship occurs in patients with preserved contractile performance and emphasizes the afterload dependence of measures of ejection such as the ejection fraction, (Modified from Carabello et al. *Circulation* 59:679, 1979, with permission.)

In addition, the ability to accurately measure the aortic valve area using the Gorlin formula or similar methods has recently been strongly challenged.[1-3] The measurement of the aortic valve area is particularly a problem in low output states where even a small gradient may be translated into "clinically significant" stenotic AVA.[3] This has raised the question as to which approach best clinically describes aortic valve stenosis severity. A review of this entire topic is provided in Chapter 3 by Dr. Kass and will not be discussed further here.

IMPACT OF AORTIC VALVE STENOSIS ON VENTRICULAR FUNCTION

The pressure overload that results from LV outflow obstruction increases systolic wall stress. This increased stress, or afterload, opposes cardiac muscle shortening and can profoundly affect measures of ejection, such as the ejection fraction (Fig. 7.2). Ejection fraction is inversely related to mean circumferential wall stress[4] and directly related to inherent contractility. It is less influenced by preload changes.

The response of the LV to the increased afterload is to develop concentric hypertrophy and to increase wall thickness. While the mechanisms responsible for this response are not well understood, the effect is a reduction in wall stress through the Laplace relationship:

$$\text{Wall stress} = \frac{\text{Pressure} \times \text{Radius}}{\text{Wall Thickness}}$$

The hypertrophic response is not uniform either throughout the ventricle or among patients,

however. A wide variability in afterload is observed in patients with AS. In each patient, for instance, the myocardial wall at the LV apex lacks the concentric muscle bundles seen throughout the remainder of the LV, and the apex is thus inherently much thinner than the remainder of the heart. This results in less long axis shortening relative to short axis shortening during systole. The variability in the degree of hypertrophy present among patients is perhaps best exemplified by the "excessive" hypertrophy that often occurs in children with AS in whom the ejection fraction is often greater than normal.[5] This is in contrast to adults in whom the ejection fraction may be depressed solely due to the effects of the increased afterload.[4]

Interpretation of the ejection fraction in AS is therefore difficult due to the counterbalancing effects of afterload and hypertrophy. While it is known that the ejection fraction may rise in many patients after aortic valve replacement,[6] others with the same baseline ejection fraction may not improve following relief of the outflow obstruction because myocardial muscle dysfunction has now ensued. Thus, at some point, hypertrophy appears to become pathologic. In fact, recent evidence suggests that the hypertrophied myocardial cell exhibits both systolic and diastolic dysfunction.[7] Hypertrophy of the nonmyocyte supporting cells in the heart may also contribute to the reduction in LV function observed.[8]

Given the uncertainty of ejection fraction measurements in AS, a variety of other means have been sought to decipher whether contractile function is impaired in these patients. Measures of isovolumic indices,[9] of the mean circumferential fiber shortening rate,[10] of the stress-ejection fraction relationship,[11] and of the end-systolic stress-volume relationship[12] have all been used with some limited success. As most of these measures are fraught with difficulties either in acquiring the necessary data or in interpreting the results, they have yet to be widely adopted in most invasive catheterization laboratories.

In AS it can be argued that diastolic function should be of equal or greater importance than systolic function since symptoms of congestion and possibly angina due to reduced coronary reserve[13] are primarily a result of abnormalities in diastolic properties. Pressure overload of the LV due to AS is associated with a reduction in both early relaxation and LV chamber compliance that is translated as a higher diastolic pressure at any particular volume.[14] Early relaxation can be grossly quantitated using the time constant (tau) of isovolumic relaxation, while chamber compliance can be similarly estimated using a constant derived from the slope of the late diastolic pressure-volume curve (Kp—the modulus of chamber stiffness). The effects of aortic valvuloplasty on these measures will be discussed later. Figure 7.3 outlines the diastolic variables that have been measured in clinical studies following aortic valvuloplasty.

While it is still controversial whether increased stiffness of the LV chamber is due to actual myocardial stiffness or simply to the effects of hypertrophy on the chamber dynamics,[14] the result is an increase in filling pressures and the production of pulmonary congestion—especially when preload increases, such as during exercise. A reduction in LV hypertrophy following relief of outflow obstruction might be expected to have a favorable effect on diastolic function.

HEMODYNAMIC OBSERVATIONS DURING BALLOON AORTIC VALVULOPLASTY

Inflation of a balloon or balloons in the stenotic aortic valve results in an acute decline in systemic pressure and a rise in the LV systolic and diastolic pressure. Using transseptal catheter pressure

measurements, Bittl et al.[15] found that the LV systolic pressure may rise as high as 386 mm Hg during the procedure. A significant range in the generated LV peak pressure was noted, however (Fig. 7.4). The magnitude of the LV pressure rise during valvuloplasty was shown to inversely correlate with the status of LV systolic and diastolic performance measures and with a measure of LV geometry (mass:volume ratio). Data from this study also suggested that a clinical correlation existed between symptoms related to congestive heart failure and the ability of the LV to generate a high systolic pressure during the valvuloplasty procedure.

Using simultaneous Doppler measurements, Nishimura et al.[16] found that the ejection time increased by 30% and peak velocity increased 26% during balloon occlusion of the LV outflow tract. Aortic regurgitation deceleration time actually decreased, though, as the LV diastolic pressure rose to even greater levels than aortic diastolic pressure in some instances. In fact, the authors noted forward end-diastolic flow in a few patients. Using contrast angiography, Cribier et al.[17] reported in 10 patients that aortic regurgitation actually worsens during the procedure, though. Thus, the reduction in the Doppler aortic regurgi-

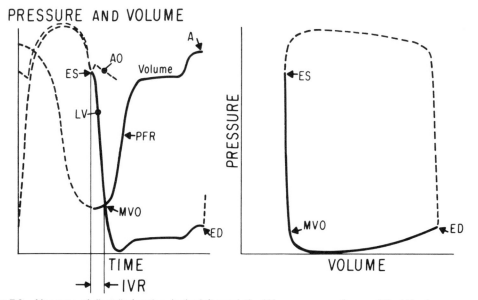

Figure 7.3. Measures of diastolic function. In the left panel, the LV pressure waveform and the LV volume curve are superimposed. The time from aortic valve closure (ES = end systole) to mitral valve opening (MVO) defines an isovolumic relaxation period (IVR). Pressure fall during this period is exponential, and the time for the pressure to fall 1/e is referred to as tau or the time-course of LV relaxation. Once the mitral valve opens (MVO), LV filling begins, and the peak filling rate (PFR) can be measured from angiography. In the right panel, the pressure-volume relationship is shown with similar points of interest labeled as in the left panel. The shape of the late diastolic portion of the P-V curve can be modeled and a constant Kp derived that provides some quantitative data regarding chamber stiffness. ED = end-diastole.

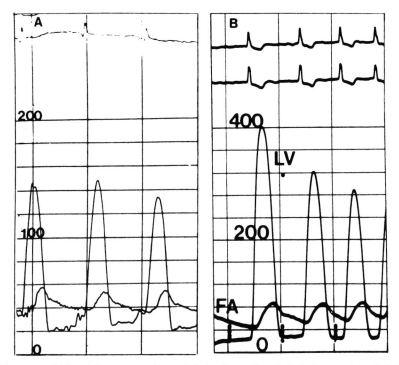

Figure 7.4. The range of LV systolic pressure observed during the aortic valvuloplasty procedure. Data from panel **A** reveals a representative patient in whom a peak systolic pressure of 154 ± 7 mm Hg was observed, while the patient in panel **B** developed a peak pressure of 386 ± 22 mm Hg during the aortic valvuloplasty procedure. (From Bittl et al. *J Am Coll Cardiol 14*:135–142, 1989, with permission.)

tation velocity during the valvuloplasty procedure appears to be a reflection of a reduction in the aortic to LV diastolic gradient.

Using the mitral inflow pattern from Doppler, Nishimura et al.[16] also reported that a significant reduction in the deceleration time occurred in association with the elevation in LV diastolic pressure during valvuloplasty. This suggested that an acute increase in LV chamber stiffness becomes manifest during the procedure. In 10 of 16 patients with mitral regurgitation, the authors also noted increased mitral insufficiency during the aortic balloon inflation.

Rousseau and colleagues[18] measured coronary flow, myocardial O_2 uptake, and lactate handling in 17 patients undergoing balloon aortic valvuloplasty. During inflation, coronary blood flow decreased from 272 ± 111 to 166 ± 92 milliliters/min, myocardial oxygen uptake fell, and lactate extraction shifted to lactate production—all consistent with low flow myocardial ischemia. These changes were not affected by the presence of associated coronary artery disease. This acute reduction in coronary flow may result in "stun-

ning" of the myocardium. Fortunately, recovery of oxidative metabolism and coronary flow appeared to occur quickly after the procedure. Smucker et al.,[19] in fact, using isoproterenol as a "stress test" before and after aortic valvuloplasty, noted an improvement in coronary sinus blood flow and an apparent beneficial effect of aortic valvuloplasty on the myocardial oxygen supply:demand ratio immediately following valvuloplasty.

The acute rise in ventricular and atrial pressures and the acute decrease in systemic arterial pressures have also been shown to stimulate the release of a variety of humoral factors. A rise in atrial natriuretic factor and vasopressin but no rise in renin have been reported in two separate studies.[20,21] It is likely that LV baroreceptor stimulation and subsequent reflex vasodilation[22] also occur. In addition, reflex catecholamine release and blood loss during the catheterization procedure may also contribute to the immediate hemodynamic response.

In an effort to reduce the hemodynamic severity resulting from often total occlusion of LV outflow by single balloons during valvuloplasty, dual or trefoil balloons have been evaluated. These arrangements allow for flow around the balloons themselves[23–26] and may allow for a larger final AVA to be achieved. When balloon sizes greater than the aortic anulus are used, however, severe aortic regurgitation has been reported.[27,28] While echocardiographic measurements may help prevent this serious complication by allowing sizing of balloons to the anulus,[29] the beneficial role of multiple balloons remains unclear. Since adverse hemodynamic consequences are rarely attributable to the use of single balloons, and since the single balloon technique is technically easier, most active laboratories are now primarily using a single balloon approach.

ACUTE HEMODYNAMIC RESPONSE TO BALLOON AORTIC VALVULOPLASTY

Despite reports of little, if any, change in the appearance of the diseased aortic valve either at surgery[30] or in vitro[31] following balloon inflation, an acute improvement in outflow hemodynamics is certainly observed in most patients. Table 7.1 provides an overview of recent series from a variety of institutions.[17,32–47] From these data it is clear that one can expect to see an acute reduction in the aortic valve gradient of about 50% and an acute rise in the AVA of about 50% as well. The "typical" aortic peak-to-peak gradient falls from 70 to 35 mm Hg and the "typical" aortic valve area increases from 0.6 to 0.9 cm^2. Little change or only a small increase is usually observed in the ejection fraction (when measured) or in the cardiac output.

The manner in which the outflow obstruction is reduced appears dependent on the substrate of the diseased valve itself. While relief of commissural fusion may occur in some patients, perhaps most often in those with a rheumatic etiology,[48] this is not true for the majority of patients. Patients with bicuspid aortic valves may have a more intense distribution of calcific deposits throughout the valve than those with senile calcific AS,[49] and less improvement in the gradient has been reported in bicuspid valve stenosis. In most elderly patients, the aortic valve has three cusps, the calcific deposits virtually "weigh down" the leaflets, and there is a variable amount of commissure fusion.[50] Pathologic studies of these trileaflet calcific valves after valvuloplasty suggest that fracture of these

Table 7.1.
Acute Hemodynamic Results in Adults

Author	Year	Ref	# Pts	Mean Age (Yrs)	Aortic Gradient Before (mm Hg)	Aortic Gradient After (mm Hg)	AO Valve Area Before (cm^2)	AO Valve Area After (cm^2)	Ejection Fraction Before (%)	Ejection Fraction After (%)	Cardiac Output Before (liters/min)	Cardiac Output After (liters/min)
Cribier	1987	17	92	75	75	30	0.49	0.93	48	51	NA	NA
McKay	1987	32	32	79	77	39	0.60	0.90	NA	NA	NA	NA
Safian	1988	33	170	77	71	36	0.60	0.90	NA	NA	4.6	4.8
Litvak	1988	34	24	80	70	36	0.50	0.70	NA	NA	4.0	3.9
Grollier	1988	35	30	75	82	45	0.37	0.60	NA	NA	3.6	3.3
Block	1988	36	81	79	(61)	(30)	0.4	0.8	NA	NA	3.6	3.9
Desnoyers	1988	37	47	79	70	32	0.5	0.9	NA	NA	3.5	3.9
Letac	1988	38	218	74	72	29	0.52	0.93	49	52	NA	NA
Serruys	1988	39	25	75	84	41	0.47	0.72	42	NA	176*	208*
Berland	1989	40	55	77	66	28	0.47	0.83	29	34	[2.3]	[2.4]
Sherman	1989	41	36	86	(46)	(23)	0.5	0.9	NA	NA	3.9	3.9
Leonard	1989	42	193	77	71	36	0.6	1.0	NA	NA	4.4	4.8
Lewin	1989	43	125	76	87	32	0.6	1.0	57	NA	4.3	4.6
Letac	1989	44	92	84	71	27	0.48	0.91	47	51	2.5	2.6
Erdmann	1989	45	67	78	88	37	0.39	0.73	NA	NA	4.2	4.1
Davidson	1990	46	81	76	70	34	0.57	0.83	46	49	4.2	4.2
Bashore	1990	47	671	79	(55)	(29)	0.5	0.8	47	NA	4.0	4.1

The aortic gradient reported is the peak-to-peak gradient unless otherwise bracketed. AO = aortic; * = milliliters/sec rather than liters/min; ( ) = mean valvular gradient; [ ] = cardiac index rather than cardiac output.

calcific deposits substantially improves leaflet mobility and allows a hinge-like effect to occur.[51–55]

To better define the hemodynamics after valvuloplasty, we have used a dual sensor, high-fidelity micromanometer catheter system to simultaneously track the LV and aortic pressures before and after the valvuloplasty procedure. By coupling these pressure data with computerized, digital-subtraction angiographic information, a variety of systolic and diastolic variables can be derived

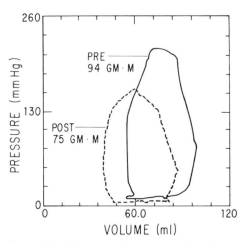

LV STROKE WORK
PRE AND POST AORTIC VALVULOPLASTY

Figure 7.5. Representative pressure-volume loops before and after the valvuloplasty procedure. A fall in the height of the loop and a shift toward the left is evident. The area of the loop is reduced and is consistent with a reduction in stroke work.

immediately before and after the procedure. Simultaneous pressure and volume data permit construction of pressure-volume loops. The effect of aortic valvuloplasty on the pressure-volume loop of a representative patient is shown in Figure 7.5. The addition of echo-Doppler information at the time of catheterization also permits an evaluation of Doppler flow patterns and of wall thickness—the latter incorporated with the pressure-volume data to derive wall stress measurements.

Using this systematic approach, Table 7.2 outlines representative changes we have observed on a variety of systolic variables.[56,57] In general, the LV systolic pressure acutely falls in association with a reduction in the aortic valve gradient (Fig. 7.6A). The aortic pressure usually does not change, though wide patient-to-patient variability has been noted. In fact, at times the LV systolic pressure has been observed to remain elevated with the aortic valve gradient reduction resulting solely from a rise in aortic pressure (Fig. 7.6B). Analysis of aortic ejection dynamics in this setting reveals that a substantial increase in aortic impedance occurs when this phenomenon is present.[58]

The ejection fraction after valvuloplasty is only rarely measured in most studies due to concern regarding serial ventriculography in these generally frail patients (Table 7.1). In our own series, the ejection fraction appears to increase slightly due almost entirely to a fall in end-systolic rather than end-diastolic volume. This increase in the ejection fraction occurs primarily due to a reduction in afterload. Measures of both peak and end-systolic stress are consistent with that concept (Table 7.2).

Table 7.2.
Effect of Percutaneous Aortic Valvuloplasty on Acute Measures of LV Systolic Function

	Pre-BAV	Post-BAV	p
Heart rate (bpm)	74 ± 16	77 ± 16	NS
LV peak systolic pressure (mm Hg)	215 ± 36	182 ± 31	< 0.05
Aortic peak systolic pressure (mm Hg)	146 ± 33	145 ± 33	NS
Cardiac output (liters/min)	4.3 ± 1.2	4.4 ± 1.3	NS
LV ejection fraction (%)	52 ± 18	55 ± 17	< 0.05
LV end-systolic volume (milliliters)	66 ± 50	63 ± 46	<0.05
Peak positive dP/dt (mm Hg/sec)	1650 ± 460	1500 ± 490	< 0.05
Peak systolic wall stress ($\times 10^3$ dynes/cm^2)	171 ± 71	142 ± 58	< 0.05
End-systolic wall stress ($\times 10^3$ dynes/cm^2)	98 ± 52	84 ± 46	< 0.05

Modified from Harrison et al.[56]
BAV = balloon aortic valvuloplasty.

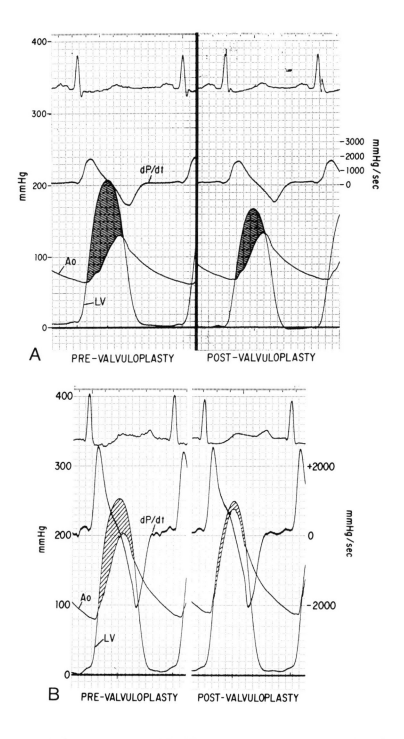

Figure 7.6. Variability in the acute response of the LV pressure to balloon aortic valvuloplasty. In panel **A**, aortic valvuloplasty has resulted in a reduction in the aortic valve gradient, a rise in the aortic systolic pressure, and a fall in the LV systolic pressure. In panel **B**, the aortic valve gradient has fallen and the aortic systolic pressure has risen, but the LV systolic pressure has not declined. *dP/dt* = first derivative of LV pressure.

Associated with a reduction in afterload, the pressure-volume loop shifts to the left and modestly downward (Fig. 7.5). The area of this loop (stroke work) decreases accordingly. Peak positive dP/dt also falls, likely due to a combination of transient myocardial "stunning" with reduced contractility and to changes in loading conditions.[59]

Table 7.3 outlines the effects of aortic valvuloplasty on a variety of diastolic variables.[57] After valvuloplasty there is clear evidence for acute diastolic dysfunction. While the LV end-diastolic pressure changes little, there is a consistent and significant prolongation of the time-course of LV pressure fall (tau), implying an acute reduction in active LV relaxation.[60] The most likely explanation for this change is that myocardial ischemia has occurred.[61] The studies cited regarding the reduction in coronary blood flow and the effect of balloon occlusion on metabolism during valvuloplasty are consistent with that notion.[18,19] If such "stunning" occurs, it might be expected to persist for minutes to days.[62] Stoddard et al.[63] also noted a prolongation of tau immediately after valvuloplasty, but Paulus et al.[64] reported no change following aortic valvuloplasty alone. This latter group noted a prolongation in isovolumic relaxation only when nitroprusside was added post-valvuloplasty. The reason for this discrepancy is unclear, but sample size, only nine patients were studied with combined pressure and angiography in the latter study, may have contributed. Diver et al.[65] have shown that nitroprusside infusion in AS changes neither tau nor the peak filling rate despite lowering both the end-diastolic pressure and volume.

Reductions in peak negative dP/dt, in peak filling rate, and in the previously discussed measure of LV chamber compliance (Kp) are also seen after the valvuloplasty procedure. Using Doppler diastolic mitral flow patterns, Nishimura et al.[66] have observed a restriction of flow consistent with an acute worsening of LV diastolic compliance. The observation that the LV end-diastolic pressure is unchanged despite a fall in the LV end-diastolic volume also suggests that a change in the LV diastolic pressure-volume relationship takes place. After the procedure, a change in the severity of aortic insufficiency only rarely occurs,[67] and aortic regurgitation is not implicated in the overall results. Variable degrees of aortic regurgitation or of mitral regurgitation[68] could impact on the hemodynamics observed in individual patients, however.

In summary, the acute effects of aortic valvuloplasty are complex and include afterload reduction, preload reduction, acute "stunning" of the LV with both a negative inotropic and lusitropic effect, and a worsening of LV chamber compliance. With all these disparate effects interacting on LV function, it is little wonder that a rather wide variability in hemodynamics has been reported after the procedure.

EARLY POST-VALVULOPLASTY HEMODYNAMICS

Given the rather sudden shock of the valvuloplasty procedure on LV function and the shifts in fluid and reflexes that occur immediately after aortic

Table 7.3.
Effect of Percutaneous Aortic Valvuloplasty on Acute Measures of LV Diastolic Function

	Pre-BAV	Post-BAV	p
LV end-diastolic pressure (mm Hg)	22 ± 9	20 ± 9	NS
Mean pulmonary pressure (mm Hg)	26 ± 10	24 ± 10	NS
LV end-diastolic volume (milliliters)	130 ± 42	123 ±	< 0.05
Peak negative dP/dt (mm Hg)	− 1602 ± 420	− 1473 ± 421	< 0.05
Tau (msec)	78 ± 29	96 ± 40	< 0.05
Kp (modulus of chamber stiffness)	0.107 ± 0.071	0.141 ± 0.083	< 0.05
End-diastolic wall stress ($\times 10^3$ dynes/cm^2)	22 ± 16	19 ± 14	NS
Peak filling rate (milliliters/sec)	247 ± 80	226 ± 78	< 0.05

Modified from Sheikh et al.[57]
BAV = balloon aortic valvuloplasty

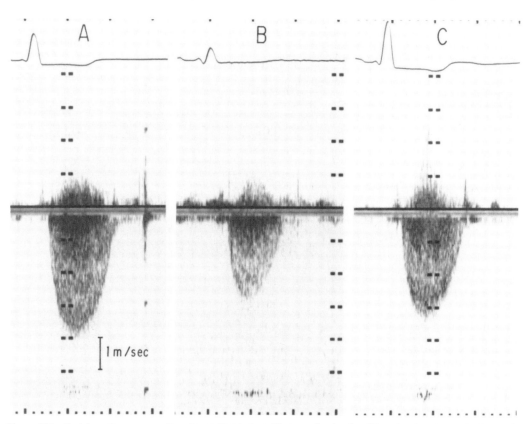

Figure 7.7. Serial continuous wave Doppler profiles before (**A**), immediately after (**B**) and at two days following aortic valvuloplasty (**C**). A return in the gradient is routinely seen. (From Davidson et al. *Am Heart 117*:411, 1989, with permission.)

valvuloplasty, a serial change in many of these variables would be expected to occur over the following several hours to days afterward. These dynamic changes probably contribute to the weaker correlation between catheterization and Doppler gradients post-valvuloplasty ($r = 0.77$) versus pre-valvuloplasty ($r = 0.82$).[69] We have observed, for instance, that the Doppler aortic velocity profile almost invariably increases progressively during the 2–4-day period following the procedure (Fig. 7.7). First-pass radionuclide angiography done at the same time as the echo-Doppler studies has revealed that this increase in the transvalvular gradient can be explained almost entirely by an increase in stroke volume[70] and does not necessarily represent early restenosis.

To further define the apparent early improvement in LV hemodynamics that occurs after aortic valvuloplasty, serial measurements of radionuclide angiography were obtained immediately before and after the procedure[71] and then serially at 2 hours, 4 hours, 6 hours, and 3 days.[72] As shown in Figure 7.8, the decline in LV end-diastolic volume observed acutely continues over the next 3 days. The LV ejection fraction, however, continues to rise during this interval with the LV end-systolic volume falling accordingly.

Given all the vagaries in the measurement of many of these variables, care must be taken in over-interpreting these results. Taken as a whole, however, these data do suggest that the afterload reduction provided by aortic valvuloplasty results in a gradual improvement in LV hemodynamics during the initial 72 hours after the procedure. It is likely that the inotropic and lusitropic impact from balloon occlusion of LV outflow wears off during this period, and the effect of the reduction in LV afterload gradually becomes apparent. Since the majority of patients experience early symptomatic improvement after the procedure, there does appear to be a clinical correlate to these hemodynamic findings.

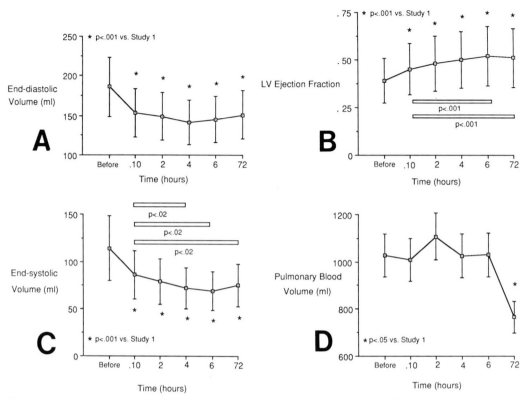

Figure 7.8. Serial data following aortic valvuloplasty obtained using first-pass radionuclide angiography immediately before, acutely following (0.10) and at 2, 4, 6, and 72 hours after the procedure. Associated with a progressive decline in the LV end-diastolic and end-systolic volume, the LV ejection fraction continually improves. Measurement of stroke volume reveals a progressive improvement as well and helps explain the early increase in gradient observed in Figure 7.7. (From Harpole et al. *Am Heart 119*:130–135 1990, with permission.)

REFERENCES

1. Carabello BA. Advances in the hemodynamic assessment of stenotic cardiac valves. *J Am Coll Cardiol 10*:912–919, 1987.

2. Flachskampf FA, Weyman AE, Guerrero JL, Thomas JD. Influence of orifice geometry and flow rate on effective valve area: An *in-vitro* study. *J Am Coll Cardiol 15*:1173–1180, 1990.

3. Segal J, Lerner DJ, Miller DC, Mitchell S, Alderman EA, Popp RL. When should Doppler determined valve area be better than the Gorlin formula? Variation in hydraulic constants in low flow states. *J Am Coll Cardiol 9*:1294–1305, 1987.

4. Gunther S, Grossman W. Determinants of ventricular function in pressure-overload hypertrophy in man. *Circulation 59*:679–688, 1979.

5. Donner R, Carabello A, Black I, Spann JF. Left ventricular wall stress in compensated aortic stenosis in children. *Am J Cardiol 51*:946–951, 1983.

6. Smith N, McNuly JH, Rahimtoola SH. Severe aortic stenosis with impaired left ventricular function and clinical heart failure: Results of valve replacement. *Circulation 58*:255–262, 1978.

7. Grossman W. Diastolic dysfunction and congestive heart failure. *Circulation 81* (Suppl III):III-1–III-17, 1990.

8. Covell JW. Factors influencing diastolic function. Possible role of the extracellular matrix. *Circulation 81* (Suppl III):III-155–III-158, 1990.

9. Fifer MA, Gunther S, Grossman W, Mirsky I, Carabello B, Barry WH. Myocardial contractile function in aortic stenosis as determined from the rate of stress development during isovolume systole. *Am J Cardiol 44*:1318–1325, 1979.

10. Liedtke AJ, Gentzler RD, Babb JK, Hunter AS, Gault JH. Determinants of cardiac performance in severe aortic stenosis. *Chest 69*:192–197, 1976.

11. Carabello BA, Green LH, Grossman W, Cohn LH, Koster JK, Collins J Jr. Hemodynamic determinants of prognosis of aortic valve replacement in clinical aortic stenosis and advanced congestive heart failure. *Circulation 62*:42–48, 1980.

12. Spann JF, Bove AA, Natarasan G, Kreulen T. Ventricular performance, pump function and compensatory mechanisms in patients with aortic stenosis. *Circulation 62*:576–583, 1980.

13. Marcus ML, Doty DB, Hiratzka LF, Wright CB, Eastham CL. Decreased coronary reserve. A mecha-

nism for angina pectoris in patients with aortic stenosis and normal coronary arteries. *N Engl J Med* 307:1362–1367, 1982.

14. Carabello BA, Grossman W. Pressure overload: Human studies. In: *The Ventricle: Basic and Clinical Aspects*. ed by HJ Levine and WH Gaasch. Martinus Nijhoff Publishing, 1985, pp. 225–236, Chap. 11.

15. Bittl JA, Bhatia SJ, Plappert T, Ganz P, St. John Sutton MG, Selwyn AP. Peak left ventricular pressure during percutaneous aortic balloon valvuloplasty: Clinical and echocardiographic correlations. *J Am Coll Cardiol* 14:135–142, 1989.

16. Nishimura RA, Holmeds DR, Reeder GS, Tajik AJ, Hatle LK. Doppler echocardiographic observations during percutaneous aortic balloon valvuloplasty. *J Am Coll Cardiol* 11:1219–1226, 1988.

17. Cribier A, Savin T, Berland J, Rocha P, Mechmeche R, Saoudi N, Behar P, Letac B. Percutaneous transluminal balloon valvuloplasty of adult aortic stenosis: Report of 92 cases. *J Am Coll Cardiol* 9: 381–386, 1987.

18. Rousseau MF, Wyns W, Hammer F, Caucheteux D, Hue L, Pouleur H. Changes in coronary blood flow and myocardial metabolism during aortic balloon valvuloplasty. *Am J Cardiol* 61:1080–1084, 1988.

19. Smucker ML, Tedesco CL, Manning SB, Owen RM, Feldman MD. Demonstration of an imbalance between coronary perfusion and excessive load as a mechanism of ischemia during stress in patients with aortic stenosis. *Circulation* 78:573–582, 1988.

20. Suarez-de-Lezo-J, Montilla P, Pan M, Romero M, Sancho M, Ruiz-de Castroviejo J, Tejero I, Arizon J, Carrasco JL. Abrupt homeostatic responses to transient intracardiac occlusion during balloon valvuloplasty. *Am J Cardiol* 64:491–497. 1989.

21. Lewin RF, Raff H, Findling JW, Skelton MM, Cowley AW Jr, King JF, Dorros G. Stimulation of atrial natriuretic peptide and vasopressin during percutaneous transluminal valvuloplasty. *Am Heart J* 118(2): 292–298, 1989.

22. Mark AL, Kioschos JM, Abboud FM, Heistad DD, Schmid PG. Abnormal vascular responses to exercise in patients with aortic stenosis. *J Clin Invest* 52: 1138–1146, 1973.

23. Midei MG, Brennan M, Walford GD, Aversano T, Gottlieb SO, Brinker JA. Double vs single balloon technique for aortic balloon valvuloplasty. *Chest* 94: 245–250, 1988.

24. Orme EC, Wray RB, Barry WH, Krueger SK, Mason JW. Comparison of three techniques for percutaneous balloon aotic valvuloplasty of aortic stenosis in adults. *Am Heart J* 117:11–17, 1989.

25. Voudris V, Drobinski G, Lepine Y, Sotirov I, Moussallem N, Canny M. Results of percutaneous valvuloplasty for calcific aortic stenosis with different balloon catheters. *Cathet Cardiovasc Diagn* 17:80–83, 1989.

26. Meier B, Friedli B, Oberhansli I. Trefoil balloon for aortic valvuloplasty. *Br Heart J* 56:292–293, 1986.

27. Sadaniantz A, Malhotra R, Korr KS. Transient acute severe aortic regurgitation complicating balloon aortic valvuloplasty. *Cathet Cardiovasc Diagn* 17:186–189, 1989.

28. Vrolix M, Piessens J, Moerman P, Vanhaecke J, De-Geest H. Fatal aortic rupture: An unusual complication of percutaneous balloon valvuloplasty for acquired valvular aortic stenosis. *Cathet Cardiovasc Diagn* 16:119–122, 1989.

29. Lewin RF, Dorros G, King JF, Seifert PE, Schmahl TM, Auer JE. Aortic annular tear after valvuloplasty: The role of aortic annulus echocardiographic measurement. *Cathet Cardiovasc Diagn* 16:123–129, 1989.

30. Robicsek F, Harbold NJ Jr. Limited value of balloon dilatation in calcified aortic stenosis in adults: Direct observations during open heart surgery. *Am J Cardiol* 60:857–864, 1989.

31. Robicsek F, Harbold NB, Slotten LN, Walker DK. Balloon dilatation of the stenosed aortic valve: How does it work? Why does it fail? *Am J Cardiol* 65: 761–766, 1990.

32. McKay RG, Safian RD, Lock JE, Diver DJ, Berman AD, Warren SE, Come PC, Baim DS, Mandell VE, Royal HD, et al. Assessment of left ventricular and aortic function after aortic balloon valvuloplasty in adult patients with critical aortic stenosis. *Circulation* 75:192–203, 1987.

33. Safian RD, Berman AD, Diver DJ, McKay LL, Come PC, Riley MF, Warren SE, Cunningham MJ, Wyman RM, Weinstein JS, et al. Balloon aortic valvuloplasty in 170 consecutive patients. *N Engl J Med* 319:125–130, 1988.

34. Litvak F, Jakubowski AT, Buchbinder NA, Eigler N. Lack of sustained clinical improvement in an elderly population after percutaneous aortic valvuloplasty. *Am J Cardiol* 62:270–275, 1988.

35. Grollier G, Commeau P, Sesboue B, Huret B, Potier JC, Foucault JP. Short-term clinical and haemodynamic assessment of balloon aortic valvuloplasty in 30 elderly patients. Discrepancy between immediate and eighth-day haemodynamic values. *Eur Heart J* 9: 155–162, 1988.

36. Block PC, Palacios IF. Clinical and hemodynamic follow-up after percutaneous aortic valvuloplasty in the elderly. *Am J Cardiol* 62:760–763, 1988.

37. Desnoyers MR, Isner JM, Pandian NG, Wang SS, Hougen T, Fields CD, Lucus AR, Salem DN. Clinical and noninvasive hemodynamic results after aortic balloon valvuloplasty for aortic stenosis. *Am J Cardiol* 62:1078–1084, 1988.

38. Letac B, Cribier A, Koning R, Bellefleur JP. Results of percutaneous transluminal valvuloplasty in 218 adults with valvular aortic stenosis. *Am J Cardiol* 62: 598–605, 1988.

39. Serruys PW, Luijten HE, Beatt KJ, DiMario C, de-Feyter PJ, Essed CE, Roelandt JR, van-den-Brand M. Percutaneous balloon valvuloplasty for

calcific aortic stenosis. A treatment 'sine cure'? *Eur Heart J 9*:782–794, 1988.

40. Berland J, Cribier A, Savin T, Lefebvre E, Koning R, Letac B. Pecutaneous balloon valvuloplasty in patients with severe aortic stenosis and low ejection fraction. Immediate results and 1-year follow-up. *Circulation 79*:1189–1196, 1989.

41. Sherman W, Hershman R, Lazzam C, Cohen M, Ambrose J, Gorlin R. Balloon valvuloplasty in adult aortic stenosis: determinants of clinical outcome. *Ann Int Med 110*:421–425, 1989.

42. Leonard BM, Grossman W. Aortic valvuloplasty— How beneficial is it? *Choices in Cardiology 3*:82–84, 1989.

43. Lewin RF, Dorros G, King JF, Mathiak L. Percutaneous transluminal aortic valvuloplasty: Acute outcome and follow-up of 125 patients. *J Am Coll Cardiol 14*:1210–1217, 1989.

44. Letac B, Cribier A, Koning R, Lefebvre E. Aortic stenosis in elderly patients aged 80 or older. *Circulation 80*:1514–1520, 1989.

45. Erdmann E, Von Scheidt W, Werdan K, Hormann M. Percutaneous balloon valvuloplasty or aortic stenosis in 67 patients over 70 years of age. *Geriatric Cardiovasc Med 1*:259–262, 1988.

46. Davidson CJ, Harrison JK, Leithe ME, Kisslo KB, Bashore TM. Failure of balloon aortic valvuloplasty to result in sustained clinical improvement in patients with depressed left ventricular function. *Am J Cardiol 65*:72–77, 1990.

47. Bashore TM, Davidson CJ, Berman AD, Kennedy JW, Davis KB, for the NHLBI Balloon valvuloplasty Registry Participants. Percutaneous balloon aortic valvuloplasty: The acute and 30 day follow-up results in 671 patients. *Circulation 82*:(Suppl III)-III 79, 1990.

48. Ribeiro PA, Al-Zaibag M, Rajendran V. Double balloon aortic valvotomy for rheumatic aortic stenosis; *in-vivo* studies. *Eur Heart J 10*:417–422, 1989.

49. Isner JM, Chokshi SK, DeFranco A, Braimen J, Slovenkai GA. Contrasting hitoarchitecture of calcified leaflets from stenotic bicuspid versus stenotic tricuspid aortic valves. *J Am Coll Cardiol 15*:1104–1108, 1990.

50. Normand J, Loire R, Zambartas C. The anatomical aspects of adult aortic stenosis. *Eur Heart J 9*:31–36, 1988.

51. McKay RG, Safian RD, Lock JR, Mandell VS, Thurer RL, Schnitt SJ, Grossman W. Balloon dilatation of calcific aortic stenosis in elderly patients: Postmortem, intraoperative, and percutaneous valvuloplasty studies. *Circulation 74*:119–125, 1986.

52. Berdoff RL, Strain J, Crandall C, Ghali V, Goldman B. Pathology of aortic valvuloplasty: Findings after postmortem successful and failed dilatations. *Am Heart J 117*:688–690, 1989.

53. Kalan JM, Mann JM, Leon MB, Pichard A, Kent KM, Roberts WC. Morphologic finding in stenotic aortic valves that have had "successful" percutaneous balloon valvuloplasty. *Am J Cardiol 62*:152–154, 1988.

54. Kennedy KD, Hauck AJ, Edwards WD, Holmes DR Jr, Reeder GS, Nishimura RA. Mechanism of reduction or aortic valvular stenosis by percutaneous transluminal balloon valvuloplasty: Report of five cases and review of the literature. *Mayo Clin Proc 63*:769–776, 1988.

55. Isner JM, Samuels DA, Slovenkai GA, Halaburka KR, Hougen TJ, Desnoyers MR, Fields CD, Salem DN. Mechanism of aortic balloon valvuloplasty: Fracture of valvular calcific deposits. *Ann Intern Med 108*:377–380, 1988.

56. Harrison JK, Davidson CJ, Leithe ME, Kisslo KB, Skelton TN, Bashore TM. Serial left ventricular performance evaluated by cardiac catheterization before, immediately after and at 6 months after balloon aortic valvuloplasty. *J Am Coll Cardiol 16*:1351–1354, 1990.

57. Sheikh KH, Davidson CJ, Honan MB, Skelton TN, Kisslo KB, Bashore TM. Changes in left ventricular diastolic performance after aortic balloon valvuloplasty: Acute and late results. *J Am Coll Cardiol 16*:795–803, 1990.

58. Pasipoularides A, Thomas DC, Dandrea CL, Harrison JK, Spero LA, Harding MB, Bashore TM. Ventricular ejection load changes after balloon aortic valvuloplasty (abstract). *Circulation* (Suppl III)-III-724, 1990.

59. Quinones MA, Gaasch WH, Alexander JK. Influence of acute changes in preload, afterload, contractile state and heart rate on ejection and isovolumic indices of myocardial contractility in man. *Circulation 53*:293–299, 1976.

60. Weiss JL, Frederiksen JW, Weisfeldt ML. Hemodynamic determinants of the time-course of fall in canine left ventricular pressure. *J Clin Invest 58*:751–763, 1976.

61. Hess OM, Osakaoa G, Lavelle JF, Gallagher KP, Kemper WS, Ross J Jr. Diastolic myocardial wall stiffness and ventricular relaxation during partial and complete coronary occlusions in the conscious dog. *Circ Res 52*:387–393, 1983.

62. Braunwald E, Kloner RA. The stunned myocardium: prolonged, postischemic ventricular dysfunction. *Circulation 61*:436–440, 1982.

63. Stoddard M, Vandormael M, Pearson A, et al. Immediate and short-term effects of aortic valvuloplasty in left ventricular systolic and diastolic function and filling in humans. *J Am Coll Cardiol 4*:1218–1228, 1989.

64. Paulus WJ, Heyndrickx GR, Buyl P, Goethals MA, Andries E. Wide-range load shift of combined aortic valvuloplasty—arterial vasodilation slows isovolumic relaxation of the hypertrophied left ventricle. *Circulation 81*:886–898, 1990.

65. Diver DJ, Royal HD, Aroesty JM, et al. Diastolic function in patients with aortic stenosis: Influence of

ventricular load reduction. *J Am Coll Cardiol 12*: 642–648, 1988.

66. Nishimura RA, Holmes DR Jr., Reeder GS, Tajik AJ, Hatle LK. Doppler ecocardiographic observations during percutaneous aortic balloon valvuloplasty. *J Am Coll Cardiol 11*:1219–1226, 1988.

67. Davidson CJ, Kisslo K, Burgess R, Bashore TM. Quantification of aortic regurgitation after balloon aortic valvuloplasty using videodensitometric analysis of digital subtraction angiography. *Am J Cardiol 63*:585–588, 1989.

68. Come PC, Riley MF, Berman AD, Safian RD, Wakmonski CA, McKay RG. Serial assessment of mitral regurgitation by pulsed Doppler echocardiography in patients undergoing aortic valvuloplasty. *J Am Coll Cardiol 14*:677–682, 1989.

69. Come PC, Riley MF, Safian RD, Ferguson JF, Diver DD, McKay RG. Usefulness of noninvasive assessment of aortic stenosis before and after percutaneous aortic valvuloplasty. *Am J Cardiol 61*:1300–1306, 1988.

70. Davidson CJ, Harpole DA, Kisslo KB, Skelton TN, Kisslo J, Jones RH, Bashore TM. Analysis of the early rise in aortic transvalvular gradient after aortic valvuloplasty. *Am Heart J 117*:411–417, 1983.

71. Harpole DH, Davidson CJ, Skelton TN, Kisslo KB, Jones RH, Bashore TM. Changes in left ventricular systolic performance immediately after percutaneous aortic balloon valvuloplasty. *Am J Cardiol 65*: 1213–1218, 1990.

72. Harpole DH, Davidson CJ, Skelton TN, Jones RH, Bashore TM. Serial evaluation of ventricular function after percutaneous aortic balloon valvuloplasty. *Am Heart J 119*:130–135, 1990.

8

Late Clinical and Hemodynamic Follow-up after Balloon Aortic Valvuloplasty

CHARLES J. DAVIDSON and THOMAS M. BASHORE

Data describing long-term (i.e., 5 to 10 years) outcome after balloon aortic valvuloplasty are not yet available. However, intermediate-term results have been detailed in numerous publications.[1–10] This chapter will review these data describing the clinical and hemodynamic outcome following percutaneous balloon aortic valvuloplasty (BAV). Specific attention will be focused on the intermediate-term effects of balloon valvuloplasty on the transvalvular gradient and aortic valve area, including a discussion of the impact of the procedure on systolic and diastolic left ventricular function. Restenosis evaluated clinically and hemodynamically will be described, as well as the results of repeat balloon aortic valvuloplasty for the treatment of restenosis. Finally, the predictors of patient outcome following BAV will be reviewed.

CLINICAL OUTCOME AFTER INITIAL AORTIC VALVULOPLASTY PROCEDURES

Although acute improvement in symptoms of congestive heart failure and angina generally occurs following BAV, recurrent symptoms commonly develop within months following the procedure.[1–10] Table 8.1 summarizes representative studies describing the overall intermediate-term clinical outcome of patients undergoing BAV.

Although all series must be interpreted in light of the patient population undergoing this procedure, it is clear that restenosis is common and improvement in valvular hemodynamics is often only moderate. Since the final aortic valve area achieved with BAV is often unrelated to procedural factors including balloon diameter,[5,8] it

would appear that the mechanism of valvuloplasty and the pathology of valvular stenosis itself best describe successful BAV. In the most optimistic study to date, Letac and co-workers have reported follow-up at a mean of 8 months in 144 patients, in whom there was symptomatic improvement in 84% of patients with death in 27 (11%).[3] Conversely, others have reported an incidence from 38 to 64% of recurrent symptoms or death within 5 to 9 months following initial balloon dilation.[1,2,4,5,7,8] Thus, while there are little data to suggest that prolongation of survival occurs following successful BAV, improvement in overall functional status generally does occur for a variable period. Due to the overall disability and comorbid disease of the patient population undergoing BAV, noncardiac deaths account for approximately 5 to 15% of all late deaths.[1,5] However, as might be expected, cardiovascular death due to progressive congestive heart failure is the predominant cause of death. Other common cardiovascular causes include sudden death and stroke.

INVASIVE HEMODYNAMIC FOLLOW-UP

Systematic recatheterization has not generally been performed following BAV. However, several groups have been able to obtain repeat catheterization in selected subsets of patients.[2,3,12–14] Evaluation of invasive hemodynamics at follow-up incorporates data regarding both valvular function and left ventricular performance. The available data suggest that restenosis at 6 months is a frequent occurrence.

Letac and co-workers studied 37 of 218

Table 8.1.
Summary of studies describing patient outcome following BAV

	Reference	Number of Patients	Follow-up Interval (Mos) (mean)	Improved N (%)	Death N (%)	AVR N (%)	Re-BAV N (%)
Safian et al.	1	157	9.1	103 (66)	25 (16)	17 (11)	15 (10)
Block & Palacios	2	81	5.5	36 (44)	23 (28)	NA	15 (18)
Desnoyers et al.	6	44	10.2	38 (86)	2 (5)	3 (7)	NA
Letac et al.	3	144	8	101 (84)	24 (17)	NA	NA
Davidson et al.	4	81	6	35 (43)	13 (16)	4 (5)	14 (17)
Holmes et al.	7	79	7.8	39 (49)	19 (24)	16 (20)	7 (9)
Sherman et al.	8	33	7	14 (43)	10 (30)	4 (12)	1 (3)
Lewin et al.	5	112	12	57 (51)	40 (36)	7 (6)	10 (9)
TOTAL		731	8.4	423 (58)	156 (21)	51 (10)	62 (11)

AVR = aortic valve replacement; Re-BAV = repeat balloon aortic valvuloplasty.

patients at a mean of 5 months post-valvuloplasty.[3] Although all 37 patients were clinically improved, restenosis, defined as a loss of 50% of more of the benefit in valve area obtained by dilation, was noted in 9 (24%). In the 28 patients without restenosis, the mean aortic valve area at follow-up was 0.85 cm². This was similar to the immediately post-valvuloplasty valve area of 0.88 cm² in these patients. In the 9 patients with restenosis, the mean aortic valve area at follow-up was 0.69 cm², compared with 0.90 cm² immediately after dilation. Factors that related to this difference between the groups were unclear.

Other investigators have found a higher incidence of valvular restenosis at recatheterization. Block and Palacios restudied 15 patients from a group of 84 patients at 5.6 months after initial BAV.[2] All 15 demonstrated complete return of the transvalvular gradient and an aortic valve area similar to the baseline values prior to valvuloplasty. These investigators stated that if one combines all patients with class IV congestive heart failure, those incurring cardiac death and those who have documented restenosis by catheterization, the overall restenosis rate would be 45 of 81 (56%) at 5.6 months. Safian et al. also reported restenosis in 29 of 35 patients (83%) evaluated by recatheterization at 6.4 months.[1] All 21 of the patients in this series who returned due to recurrent symptoms had restenosis, whereas only 8 of the 17 patients without symptoms demonstrated restenosis. These data suggested a 44% "clinical" rate of restenosis based on recurrent symptoms and death.

In the Mansfield Valvuloplasty Registry, 95 patients (18%) returned for follow-up catheterization.[13] Thirty-nine (41%) of these patients were

improved and 56 (59%) had recurrent symptoms at time of recatheterization. At follow-up, the improved group had a greater aortic valve area (0.70 ± 0.32 cm² vs. 0.58 ± 18 cm², $p = 0.02$) and higher ejection fraction (59 ± 19% vs. 48 ± 20%, $p = 0.07$) than the symptomatic group. No baseline or post-procedural hemodynamic parameter predicted restenosis at recatheterization, although the less symptomatic group at 6 months had a larger valve area achieved immediately after valvuloplasty (0.70 ± 0.32 cm² vs. 0.58 ± 18 cm², $p < 0.02$). Restenosis occurred in many patients prior to recurrent symptoms, and symptoms recurred in some patients without evidence of restenosis. This study is limited, however, by its observational nature and by the fact that only 18% of all eligible patients underwent recatheterization. Thus, generalization of these results to the overall population undergoing aortic valvuloplasty is difficult.

In the largest group of patients who were systematically recatheterized, 41 of 71 patients at Duke Medical Center underwent invasive evaluation immediately pre, post, and at 6 months after BAV.[12] High-fidelity aortic and left ventricular micromanometer pressure and digital subtraction angiography were obtained in all. Stroke work was derived from calculation of the area within the pressure-volume loop. Demographics and baseline valvular and left ventricular parameters were similar between the recatheterization cohort and the total group of patients undergoing aortic valvuloplasty at this institution. At the time of recatheterization, the mean transvalvular gradient had returned near baseline in most, although it was slightly less than before the valvuloplasty (53 ± 17 mm Hg at late recath vs. 60 ± 18 mm Hg before valvuloplasty, $p < 0.002$). Similarly, the valve area remained minimally increased in comparison to the pre-valvuloplasty value (0.58 ± 16 cm² vs. 0.51 ± 0.14 cm², $p < 0.0001$). Fick cardiac output was unchanged (Table 8.2).

Table 8.3 describes the parameters of left ventricular performance before, immediately after, and at 6-month recatheterization in these patients. The left ventricular and aortic peak systolic pressure and aortic diastolic pressure as well as left ventricular end-systolic volume at late recatheterization were similar to baseline values. Despite the fact that the left ventricular end-diastolic pressure was unchanged

at 6 months compared to pre-BAV, left ventricular end-diastolic volume was significantly reduced (136 ± 52 vs. 111 ± 40, $p = 0.003$). Peak positive and peak negative dP/dt were similar to the pre-valvuloplasty values. There was also a statistically insignificant trend toward a decrease in stroke work at 6-month recatheterization (14 ± 6 erg × 10^3 vs. 16 ± 7 erg × 10^3, $p = 0.095$).

When paired ventriculograms are obtained at the time of BAV, a clinically small, yet statistically significant, increase in left ventricular ejection fraction was noted.[3,4] However, at late recatheterization, the ejection fraction generally returned to pre-valvuloplasty levels. Rarely, some patients

Table 8.2.
Hemodynamic variables observed before, immediately after, and at 6-month recatheterization following balloon aortic valvuloplasty (BAV) ($N = 41$)

	Pre-BAV	Post-BAV	6-month recath
Mean aortic gradient (mm Hg)	59.7 ± 18.4	35.6 ± 12.7[a]	53.1 ± 16.5
Cardiac output (liters/min)	4.3 ± 1.1	4.5 ± 1.2	4.4 ± 1.2
Aortic valve area (cm²)	0.51 ± 0.14	0.81 ± 0.19[a]	0.58 ± 0.16[a]
LV systolic pressure (mm Hg)	215 ± 36	182 ± 31	211 ± 40
Aortic systolic pressure (mm Hg)	146 ± 33	145 ± 33	156 ± 31
Aortic diastolic pressure (mm Hg)	64 ± 13	63 ± 16	64 ± 13

[a]$p < 0.05$ compared with pre-BAV

Table 8.3.
Further indices of left ventricular performance before, immediately after, and 6 months after balloon aortic valvuloplasty (BAV) ($N = 41$)

	Pre-BAV	Post-BAV	6-month recath
LV ejection fraction (%)	51.9 ± 18.0	55.0 ± 17.3[a]	54.4 ± 15.6
LV end-diastolic volume (milliliters)	136 ± 52	134 ± 51	111 ± 40[a]
LV end-systolic volume (milliliters)	66 ± 50	63 ± 46[a]	54 ± 36
LV end-diastolic pressure (milliliters)	19 ± 9	15 ± 8[a]	20 ± 9
Stroke work (ergs × 10^3)	16.3 ± 6.9	14.0 ± 5.1[a]	13.8 ± 5.9
Peak positive dP/dt (mm Hg/sec)	1650 ± 460	1500 ± 490[a]	1750 ± 670
Peak negative dP/dt (mm Hg/sec)	−1440 ± 270	−1290 ± 410[a]	−1450 ± 670
Heart rate (bpm)	74 ± 16	77 ± 16	77 ± 17

[a]$p < 0.05$ compared with pre-BAV

demonstrated a sustained and dramatic improvement in ejection fraction at late recatheterization. Nine of 15 patients in this latter series with a baseline ejection fraction < 50% had an increase in ejection fraction at the 6-month study.[12] Thus, at 6 months, some remodeling of the left ventricle appears to have occurred. Despite valvular restenosis, the left ventricle is less dilated and is able to maintain cardiac output at a reduced preload. Wall stress is reduced, potentially diminishing myocardial oxygen demand as well.

The issue as to which patients demonstrate improvement in left ventricular ejection fraction after valvuloplasty has been addressed by Safian and co-workers.[9] The authors examined 28 patients with a radionuclide angiographically defined ejection fraction of less than 55%. As an entire group, the mean ejection fraction increased from $37 \pm 11\%$ to $44 \pm 14\%$ immediately after the valvuloplasty, then to $49 \pm 13\%$ at 3 months ($p < 0.001$ vs. baseline). These investigators noted a heterogeneity of response. Thirteen patients displayed greater than a 10 ejection fraction unit increase at the 3-month study, while 15 patients had no change observed. The two groups of patients did not appear to differ with respect to any demographic variable or baseline ejection fraction measurement. Likewise, baseline and immediate post-procedural valvular hemodynamics were similar (i.e., aortic valve area, transvalvular gradient, cardiac output, and left ventricular peak systolic pressure were all similar). Left ventricular end-diastolic volume was higher at all three study intervals for the group of patients who did not increase their ejection fraction compared to those who did. Conversely, prior to valvuloplasty, left ventricular peak systolic wall stress was higher in those whose ejection fraction did not improve. They speculated that the late sustained improvement in left ventricular ejection fraction may be due to improvement in contractile function as a result of hypertrophy regression or relief of subendocardial ischemia, although there are no definite data to support these assumptions at this time.

Studies from our institution have examined the relationship between afterload and LV systolic ejection phase indices after BAV in 16 patients who underwent 6-month recatheterization.[14] Immediately after BAV, ejection fraction and velocity of circumferential fiber shortening (Vcf) are increased, and the LV mean systolic stress is decreased proportionally. At 6 months, mean systolic stress has returned to baseline along with the ejection fraction and Vcf. Based on these data, there is little evidence to support a change in myocardial contractility at 6 months. In fact, it appears that the ejection fraction changes seen reflect altered loading conditions as defined by the mean systolic stress.

Unfortunately, prospective determination of patients likely to demonstrate improved left ventricular performance has not been possible with the data that are currently available. Valvuloplasty itself can be used as a "diagnostic intervention" to predict potential changes in ventricular function as measured by these systolic ejection phase indices. In the end, this may be the only way to learn which patients benefit from the procedure.

Diastolic left ventricular performance has also been reported at 6-month follow-up in a study of 26 patients who underwent initial balloon aortic valvuloplasty.[15] Baseline and follow-up catheterization data were obtained with simultaneous digital ventriculography and high-fidelity micromanometer catheters. Two-dimensional and Doppler echocardiography were also obtained at baseline, immediately after BAV, and at the repeat catheterization. At follow-up, 16 of the patients were symptomatically improved (Group 1), and 10 had developed recurrent symptoms (Group 2). Aortic valve area, cardiac output, and left ventricular ejection fraction had returned to baseline for both groups. However, left ventricular diastolic indices and mass were both improved in the symptomatically improved group, while these variables were worse in patients with recurrent symptoms. Parameters evaluated included peak filling rate (Group 1: +8% vs. Group 2: −20%, $p = 0.001$); Tau, the time course of LV relaxation (used as a measure of active relaxation), (Group 1: −11% vs. Group 2: +35%, $p = 0.008$); Kp, the modulus of chamber stiffness (used as a measure of LV compliance), (Group 1: −27% vs. Group 2: +26%, $p = 0.001$); and LV mass (Group 1: −9% vs. Group 2: +6%, $p = 0.004$). Figure 8.1 summarizes these results. Based on these data, it appears that symptomatic status at 6 months is more closely tied to improved diastolic performance than to either the calculated valve area or the gradient at recatheterization. The decrease in LV wall stress with its potential effect on subendocardial blood flow[16] and the improvement observed in LV compliance may contribute to this observed symptomatic improvement. These observations may help explain why symptoms do not seem to correlate with either valve area or gradient at follow-up.

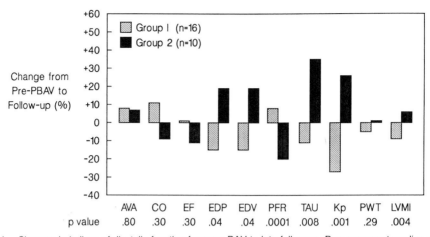

Figure 8.1. Changes in indices of diastolic function from pre-BAV to late follow-up. Bars represent median percentage changes from pre-BAV to late follow-up for Group 1 (Improved) versus Group 2 (Recurrent Symptoms). Figures below the variable represent p values which compare the significance of changes in Group 1 versus Group 2.
     AVA = aortic valve area; CO = cardiac output; EF = LV ejection fraction; EDP = LV end-diastolic pressure; EDV = LV end-diastolic volume; PFR = peak filling rate; Tau = time constant of isovolumic relaxation; Kp = modulus of chamber stiffness; PWT = LV posterior wall thickness; LWMI = LV mass index. (Reprinted with permission from author and *J Am Coll Cardiol* 16:795–803, 1990.)

ECHOCARDIOGRAPHIC FOLLOW-UP

Left ventricular diastolic functional measurements have also been reported in a group of 19 patients evaluated by serial echocardiography obtained at 3 ($N = 2$) and 6 ($N = 17$) months after balloon aortic valvuloplasty.[17] At the 3- to 6-month follow-up, patients without mitral regurgitation ($N = 12$) had an increase in peak early filling velocity versus baseline, (66 ± 21 baseline to 93 ± 31 cm/sec at follow-up, $p < 0.02$), an improved peak early to late atrial filling velocity ratio (0.6 ± 0.2 to 0.9 ± 0.4, $p < 0.02$), and the early time-velocity integral (9 ± 4 vs. 16 ± 6 cm, $p < 0.002$). In patients with mitral regurgitation ($N = 7$), significant decreases occurred in the peak early filling velocity and peak early to late atrial filling velocity ratio at follow-up.

Thus, the diastolic filling pattern in patients without mitral regurgitation is often normalized within 3 to 6 months after the valvuloplasty procedure. In this study, functional class at follow-up did not correlate with changes in aortic valve area, transvalvular gradient, ejection fraction, or diastolic filling. In contrast to the invasive study by Sheikh and co-workers,[15] improved functional class at follow-up was not related to improved echo-Doppler diastolic function or filling measurements. Differences between the conclusions of these two studies are likely related to the methods used to define diastolic functional status and to noncomparable patient populations.

Noninvasive evaluation of valvular function by Doppler echocardiography has been the preferred method of follow-up in this often elderly population who are reluctant to undergo invasive evaluation. The transvalvular gradient is obviously a function of both left ventricular stroke volume and the aortic valve area. Thus, changes in peak or mean aortic valve gradients at late follow-up may be attributed to either restenosis or to altered LV contractility and stroke volume. Since aortic valve area, as determined by the continuity equation, may be less dependent on LV function,[18] it provides a useful noninvasive parameter with which to evaluate BAV. The Doppler-derived continuity equation has been shown to correlate with catheterization measurements of aortic valve area before and after BAV,[19] while Doppler estimates of the aortic valvular gradient at 2–4 days after aortic valvuloplasty are greater than catheterization-derived valvular gradients.

One explanation for this discrepancy was described in the study of Davidson and co-workers.[20] Using Doppler ultrasound combined with radionuclide angiographic determined stroke volumes performed before, immediately after, and at 2–4 days after BAV, the authors noted that both valvular remodeling and an increase in left ventricular stroke volume contributed to a rise in aortic transvalvular gradient observed within this early post-BAV period. Thus, the echocardiographic increase in transvalvular gradient observed early after valvuloplasty likely is due to both restenoses and improved flow. It is speculative, but aortic recoil may partially contribute. The improved stroke volume is not related to increasing aortic regurgitation.

In another report, Doppler echocardiography was obtained on 35 of 42 patients surviving to a mean of 6.2 months following BAV.[21] Thirty patients had data collected before, after, and at late follow-up. As a group, aortic valve mean gradient pre-procedure was 48 ± 18 mm Hg, decreasing to 33 ± 12 mm Hg immediately after, and rising to 46 ± 16 mm Hg at late follow-up. Aortic valve area at baseline was 0.57 ± 0.15 cm², increasing to 0.85 ± 0.23 cm² immediately after, and falling back to 0.67 ± 0.19 cm² at follow-up. When compared to pre-BAV, there was a significant decrease in aortic valve gradient 2–4 days after the procedure. At late follow-up, the mean gradient was higher than after the procedure, but lower than pre-BAV. Similarly, aortic valve area rose immediately after and decreased toward baseline at follow-up. Restenosis (loss of > 50% of improvement in AVA) was noted in 63% of patients. Since patients dying prior to follow-up are not included within this analysis, these data, and the invasive follow-up data are inherently highly selected. Thus, the true incidence of restenosis for the entire group is likely higher than reported.

In another report, 25 of 42 patients followed for a mean of 8.9 months underwent serial Doppler echocardiography. Mean aortic valve gradient decreased from 64 ± 4 mm Hg to 40 ± 3 mm Hg after BAV and increased to 46 ± 5 mm Hg at 3 months, which then remained stable for 9 months and trended upward following this. Aortic valve area initially was 0.53 ± 0.03 cm², increasing to 0.76 ± 0.04 cm² after dilation, and declining to 0.68 ± 0.06 cm² at 3 months and 0.72 cm² at 9 months. Thirteen of 25 patients demonstrated restenosis, 5 of whom were symptomatic. No variable, including patient characteristics, valvular descriptions, or technical factors, distinguished patients with restenosis from those without restenosis.[6]

At Duke Medical Center, 3-month follow-up echocardiograms were obtained in 56 patients and 6-month follow-up data were available in 53 of these 56. The valvular hemodynamics from Doppler are listed in Table 8.4. Within 3 months, partial restenosis had occurred as evidenced by partial return of both the transvalvular gradient and the aortic valve area toward baseline. By the 6-month follow-up, the aortic valve area and the transvalvular gradient returned to baseline in the majority of patients. Restenosis, defined as return of aortic valve area within 0.1 cm² of baseline, occurred in 44 of 53 (83%) patients, although many of these patients remained symptomatically improved at the follow-up evaluation.

RADIONUCLIDE ANGIOGRAPHIC FOLLOW-UP

Serial radionuclide angiography has also been performed with simultaneous high-fidelity micromanometer pressure immediately before and after and at 6 months following BAV and reported in a group of 17 patients.[22] Pressure-volume loop and systolic wall stress data were assessed. At the 6-month study, restenosis occurred in most patients despite evidence for sustained clinical improvement. The hemodynamics determined at each interval are shown in Table 8.5. Left ventricular meridional end-systolic wall stress initially

Table 8.4.
Echocardiographic-determined variables of transvalvular stenosis at baseline and at various follow-up intervals

	Baseline (N = 106)	Immediate Post-BAV (N = 100)	3-month Post-BAV (N = 56)	6-month Post-BAV (N = 53)
Mean gradient (mm Hg)	48 ± 16	39 ± 14[a]	42 ± 14	48 ± 15
Peak instantaneous gradient (mm Hg)	79 ± 25	64 ± 22[a]	68 ± 21	78 ± 22
AVA (cm²)	0.48 ± 0.21	0.63 ± 0.28[a]	0.55 ± 0.18	0.50 ± 0.19

[a] $p < 0.05$ vs. Baseline
AVA = aortic valve area; BAV = balloon aortic valvuloplasty.

Table 8.5.
LV function determined by radionuclide angiography performed at baseline, immediately after, and 6 months following BAV ($N = 17$)

	Pre-BAV	Immediate Post-BAV	6-month Post-BAV
LVEF (%)	0.48 ± 0.16	0.54 ± 0.18	0.49 ± 0.16^a
Wall stress (dynes $\times$ 10^3/cm^2)	81 ± 45	62 ± 34	84 ± 44^a
LVEDV (milliliters)	161 ± 29	143 ± 27	159 ± 41^b
LVESV (milliliters)	87 ± 39	68 ± 36	85 ± 47^a
LVEDP (mm Hg)	17 ± 8	13 ± 6	21 ± 10^a
LV stroke work (erg $\times$ 10^6)	17.5 ± 7.3	14.7 ± 7.1	16.3 ± 7.1^a
dP/dt (mm Hg/sec)	1616 ± 420	1465 ± 220	1737 ± 457
ESPVR (mm Hg/milliliter)	2.9 ± 1.3	3.2 ± 1.6	3.1 ± 1.7

$^a p < 0.05$ vs. Post-BAV
$^b p < 0.07$ vs. Post-BAV
LVEF = left ventricular ejection fraction; LVEDV = left ventricular end-diastolic volume; LVESV = left ventricular end-systolic volume; LVEDP = left ventricular end-diastolic pressure; ESPVR = end-systolic pressure:volume ratio.

lar meridional end-systolic wall stress initially declined then returned to baseline. Conversely, left ventricular ejection fraction rose immediately after BAV then fell at late follow-up. Ejection fraction appeared to be inversely related to wall stress. Interestingly, end-diastolic volume progressively decreased at each time interval. Left ventricular stroke work (the area of the pressure-volume loop) decreased immediately post-BAV then also returned to baseline at 6 months. The pressure-volume loop, which had initially shifted to the left and downward immediately after BAV, returned toward baseline by the 6-month evaluation (Fig. 8.2). These data resemble those observed with contrast angiography under similar conditions.[14]

REPEAT BALLOON AORTIC VALVULOPLASTY

Repeat BAV has been utilized in an attempt to treat recurrent symptoms and aortic valve restenosis after initial BAV.[1,2,11] Candidates for repeat dilation often represent patients in whom all medical therapy and even a prior BAV have failed to improve symptoms and aortic valve replacement is not considered a reasonable option. Thus, as anticipated, clinical outcome in this exceptionally high risk group may be poor. In a study of 17 patients undergoing repeat dilation, there were 10 (59%) cardiac events within 2 months of the second procedure, including 8 (47%) cardiac deaths.[11]

Thus, the value of repeat BAV as a method to improve long-term survival is unclear. Short-term symptomatic and functional status may improve in

certain patients similar to that observed after the initial procedure. However, symptoms appear to occur within an even shorter time interval than following the first procedure. Cardiac mortality after repeat procedures appears to be primarily associated with poor left ventricular pump function.[11] Repeat BAV is, therefore, limited in its application in these latter patients and probably represents little more than a treatment of last resort.

To assess the acute hemodynamic events and clinical outcome of patients undergoing repeat balloon aortic valvuloplasty, 17 of the first 138 patients at our institution returned for repeat dilation.[11] Prior to initial and repeat BAV, there was no significant difference in any hemodynamic parameter, including aortic valve area, mean transvalvular gradient, ejection fraction, stroke work, cardiac output, or peak ($+$) or peak ($-$) dP/dt. During both interventions, the acute change in hemodynamics created by the valvuloplasty procedure was similar for all variables measured (Fig. 8.3).

In 10 of the 17 patients, the use of a larger balloon at repeat BAV provided no additional improvement in LV and aortic valve hemodynamics. Most disturbingly, cardiac events occurred within a mean of 2 months of the second BAV in 10 of 17 patients, including 8 cardiac deaths. Thus, repeat BAV resulted in similar hemodynamic changes as the initial procedure, even when larger balloon diameters were used. Mortality in patients undergoing repeat BAV was approximately 50% within 2 months in this small series.

Block and Palacios have also reported on 15 patients undergoing repeat balloon valvuloplasty for symptomatic restenosis.[2] Similar to our own series, despite larger balloons and double balloons the final aortic valve area at the repeat procedure was similar to the initial procedure. No clinical follow-up data were reported.

PREDICTORS OF PATIENT OUTCOME AFTER BALLOON AORTIC VALVULOPLASTY

Although long-term follow-up studies are not yet available, certain clinical and hemodynamic factors have been identified that help predict clinical outcome following BAV.

Clinical factors that predict mortality within 6 months have been identified from preliminary data from the National Heart, Lung, and Blood Institute (NHLBI) Balloon Valvuloplasty Registry.[23] In 331 patients eligible for 6-month follow-up, overall mortality was 30%. Univariate analysis revealed that poor survival was predicted by poor clinical functional status, low transvalvular gradi-

ent, moderate to severe mitral regurgitation, or poor left ventricular function assessed qualitatively. Multivariate analysis indicated that poor clinical functional status, low transvalvular gradient at baseline, severity of mitral regurgitation, and a smaller aortic valve area after BAV were predictive of survival.

Symptomatic status at 6-month follow-up was multivariately predicted by clinical functional status, qualitative LV function before BAV, and the aortic valve area obtained by echocardiography at 24–72 hours after BAV, with the poorest outcome in patients with New York Heart Association functional class IV symptoms, a poor EF, and severely stenotic aortic valve.

The data from the NHLBI Balloon Valvuloplasty Registry, however, were limited in their ability to quantitatively assess LV function since post-procedural ejection fraction data were not generally available.

Numerous other studies, describing smaller populations of patients, have also concluded that baseline left ventricular function is a strong predictor of 3- and 6-month clinical outcome, including

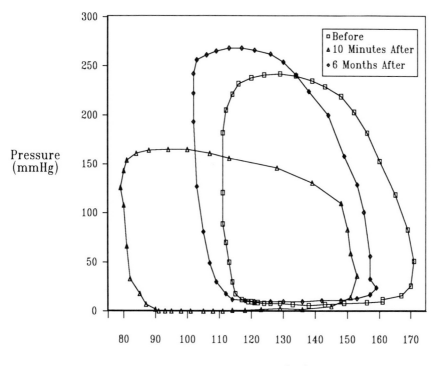

Figure 8.2.   Pressure-volume data are demonstrated from a representative patient before, 10 min, and 6 months after BAV. (Reprinted with permission from author and *Am J Cardiol 66*:327–332, 1990.)

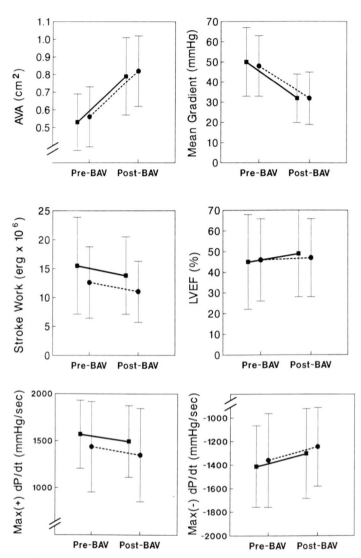

Figure 8.3. The acute LV hemodynamics in patients undergoing repeat BAV compared to the initial procedure. ($N = 17$) Solid Line = Initial BAV; Dashed Line = Repeat BAV.

death and symptomatic status.[4,5,7] Utilizing a Cox proportional hazards model, Holmes and co-workers evaluated the association of various clinical and hemodynamic variables with mortality.[7] Factors associated with subsequent cardiac death were more severe impairment of New York Heart Association functional class for heart failure at baseline ($p < 0.004$), smaller initial aortic valve area ($p < 0.003$), and lower baseline cardiac output ($p = 0.005$).

Similarly, hemodynamic data from our laboratory have indicated that despite its afterload dependence, the left ventricular ejection fraction is the only independent predictor of overall status at 3 months ($p = 0.002$).[4] Eighty-four percent of patients with a baseline ejection fraction $> 45\%$ were improved at 3 months. In the group with an ejection fraction $\leq 45\%$, less that half of the patients demonstrated improved symptoms at short-term follow-up (Fig. 8.4). Univariate analysis revealed that patients with recurrent symptoms had a lower cardiac output (3.8 ± 1.2 vs. 4.5 ± 1.3 liters/min, $p = 0.007$), a higher LV end-systolic volume both at baseline (98 ± 55 vs. 68 ± 51 milliliters, $p = 0.004$) and after valvuloplasty (93 ± 49 vs. 63 ± 47 milliliters, $p = 0.001$), a decreased baseline LV ejection fraction (35 ± 17 vs. $52 \pm 17\%$, $p = 0.0002$), a low LV stroke work (11 ± 8 vs. $14 \pm$

6 erg × 10^6, p = 0.007), and a decreased peak positive dP/dt (1397 ± 481 vs. 1765 ± 499 mm Hg/sec, p = 0.003).

Various measures of LV performance were used to assess systolic performance in this latter study. Despite the known effect of afterload on ejection phase indices, the LV ejection fraction was still the best independent predictor of patient outcome. While more sophisticated measures of LV function including stroke work and peak positive dP/dt were univariably associated with short-term patient outcome, no other baseline hemodynamic parameter added to the predictive value of ejection fraction. Thus, it appears that short-term clinical outcome after BAV is primarily related to underlying LV function rather than any measurable variable derived following the procedure.

Lewin reported that univariate predictors of mortality after BAV included Functional Class IV congestive heart failure (relative risk = 5.1), male sex (relative risk = 3.5), low cardiac output (relative risk = 2.0 per 1-liter decrease in cardiac output), age (relative risk = 1.8 per increase in 10 years), and the ejection fraction (relative risk = 1.5 per 10-point decrease).[5] Multivariate analysis demonstrated that only baseline ejection fraction and baseline cardiac output were predictors of mortality. Similar to the previous study, aortic valve area determined immediately post-procedure measured by the Gorlin formula was not associated with eventual survival.

Sherman identified predictors of adverse events at 2 months in 33 patients.[8] Ejection fraction, pulmonary artery systolic pressure, pulmonary vascular resistance, and right ventricular end-diastolic pressure were determinants of adverse events. At 6 months, all factors remained predictive except ejection fraction. The association of ejection fraction with 2-month and not 6-month outcome is unclear. However, given the small patient population reported, a Type II error is likely. Once again, aortic valve area post-BAV was not a determinant of clinical outcome. Although other preliminary studies have suggested that a final aortic valve area >1.0 cm^2 portends a good outcome from BAV, this finding has not been consistently demonstrated.[24] Long-term follow-up with a sufficient number of patients who achieve a final aortic valve area greater than 1.0 cm^2 will be necessary to settle this issue.

Berland and co-workers compared clinical initial hemodynamic and valvuloplasty results between patients who died (N = 25) and survivors (N = 30).[10] Univariate analysis showed that valve area and ejection fraction before and after the procedure were not different for the two groups and that cardiac index was the only variable significantly different. No multivariate analysis was reported in this study.

Predictors of one-year outcome have recently been analyzed in 108 consecutive patients who underwent BAV at our institution.[25] Using Cox multivariate analysis, major events, defined as cardiac death (N = 30), aortic valve replacement (N = 21), or repeat BAV (N = 13) were predicted by advanced age, baseline CHF class, and echocardiographically determined LV diameter. The only multivariate predictor of cardiac death was the baseline ejection fraction (p = 0.002). Absolute post-BAV values including stroke work, dP/dt, aortic valve area, end-systolic volume, Fick cardiac

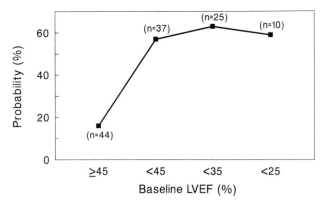

Figure 8.4. Probability of recurrent symptoms based on baseline LV ejection fraction (LVEF). (Reprinted from *Am J Cardiol* 65:72–77, 1990, with permission.)

output, transvalvular gradient, and the acute changes measured by catheterization or echocardiography were not predictive of one-year outcome. Similarly, valve area by echocardiography at 3 or 6 months added no further prognostic information. With an ejection fraction $\geq 45\%$ ($N = 63$), cardiac survival at one year was 80%, irrespective of age, sex, severity of coronary disease, or CHF class.

From these data, it was concluded that prognosis can be determined by noninvasive clinical and echocardiographic data obtained prior to cardiac catheterization. Despite advanced age and co-morbid disease, BAV patients with an ejection fraction $\geq 45\%$ have an excellent one-year cardiac survival.

Waller and co-workers have suggested that the etiology of aortic stenosis is a potential predictor of successful balloon dilation.[26] In a study of 30 stenotic necropsy aortic valves, they noted that in all 16 nonrheumatic valves, superficial and minor cuspal cracks did little to improve cuspal mobility. Aortic wall stretching was noted at the nonfused cusp sites during balloon inflation. In contrast, the 4 rheumatic aortic valves had commissural splitting with and without cuspal cracks, which markedly improved aortic valve mobility. It was concluded that overstretched walls of nonrheumatic aortic stenosis likely have recoil and are thus prone to early restenosis. Whereas, dilation of rheumatic aortic stenosis results in maximal cuspal injury, minimal aortic wall stretching, and could result in a lower incidence of early restenosis. Based on these data, the clinical recognition of aortic stenosis etiology may help predict long-term therapeutic success.

REFERENCES

1. Safian RD, Berman AD, Diver DJ, et al. Balloon aortic valvuloplasty in 170 consecutive patients. *N Eng J Med 319*:125–130, 1988.
2. Block PC, Palacios IF. Clinical and hemodynamic follow-up after percutaneous aortic valvuloplasty in the elderly. *Am J. Cardiol 62*:760–763, 1988.
3. Letac B, Cribier A, Koning R. Bellefleur JP. Results of percutaneous transluminal valvuloplasty in 218 adults with valvular aortic stenosis. *Am J Cardiol 62*: 598–605, 1988.
4. Davidson CJ, Harrison JK, Leithe ME, Kisslo KB, Bashore TM. Failure of balloon aortic valvuloplasty to result in sustained clinical improvement in patients with depressed left ventricular function. *Am J Cardiol 65*:72–77, 1990.
5. Lewin RF, Dorros G, King JF, Mathiak L. Percutaneous transluminal aortic valvuloplasty: Acute outcome and follow-up of 125 patients. *J Am Coll Cardiol 14*:1210–1217, 1989.
6. Desnoyers MR, Isner JM, Pandian NG, et al. Clinical and noninvasive hemodynamic results after aortic balloon valvuloplasty for aortic stenosis. *Am J Cardiol 62*:1078–1084, 1988.
7. Holmes DR, Nishimura RA, Wagner PJ, Illstrup DM. Clinical follow-up after percutaneous aortic balloon valvuloplasty. *Arch Intern Med 149*:1405–1409, 1989.
8. Sherman W, Hershman R, Lazzam C, Cohen M, Ambrose J, Gorlin R. Balloon valvuloplasty in adult aortic stenosis determinants of clinical outcome. *Annals Int Med 110*:421–425, 1989.
9. Safian RD, Warren SE, Berman AD, et al. Improvement in symptoms and left ventricular performance after balloon aortic valvuloplasty in patients with aortic stenosis and depressed left ventricular ejection fraction. *Circulation 78*:1181–1191, 1988.
10. Berland J, Cribier A, Savin T, LeFebvre E, Koning B, Letac B. Percuaneous balloon valvuloplasty in patients with severe aortic stenosis and low ejection fraction. Immediate results and 1-year follow-up. *Circulation 79*:1189–1196, 1989.
11. Davidson CJ, Harrison JK, Leithe ME, Kisslo K, Bashore TM. Left ventricular performance and clinical outcome after repeat balloon aortic valvuloplasty. *Annals Int Med 113*:250–252, 1990.
12. Harrison JK, Davidson CJ, Leithe ME, Kisslo KB, Skelton TN, Bashore TM. Serial left ventricular performance evaluated by cardiac catheterization before, immediately after, and at 6 months after balloon aortic valvuloplasty. *J Am Coll Cardiol 16*:1351–1358, 1990.
13. Bashore TM, Davidson CJ, and the Mansfield Scientific Aortic Valvuloplasty Registry Investigators. Follow-up recatheterization after percutaneous aortic valvuloplasty. *J Am Coll Cardiol* 1991 (In press).
14. Harrison JK, Hanemann D, Leithe ME, Davidson CJ, Kisslo K, Bashore TM. Acute and chronic measures of left ventricular contractile performance, corrected for afterload, are unchanged following balloon aortic valvuloplasty. *J Am Coll Cardiol 15* (Suppl 2):42A, 1990.
15. Sheikh KH, Davidson CJ, Honan MB, Skelton TN, Kisslo KB, Bashore TM. Changes in left ventricular diastolic performance following aortic balloon valvuloplasty: Acute and late effects. *J Am Coll Cardiol 16*:795–803, 1990.
16. Smucker MC, Tedesco CL, Manning SB, Owen RM, Feldman MD. Demonstration of an imbalance between coronary perfusion and excessive load as a mechanism of ischemia during stress in patients with aortic stenosis. *Circulation 78*:573–582, 1988.
17. Stoddard MF, Van dormael MG, Pearson AC, et al. Immediate and short-term effects of aortic balloon valvuloplasty on left ventricular diastolic function and filling in humans. *J Am Coll Cardiol 14*: 1218–1228, 1989.
18. Skjaerpe T, Hegrenaes L, Hatle L. Noninvasive estimation of valve area in patients with aor-

tic stenosis by Doppler ultrasound and two-dimensional echocardiography. *Circulation 72*:810, 1985.

19. Come PC, Riley MF, Safian RD, Ferguson JF, Diver DD, McKay RG. Usefulness of noninvasive assessment of aortic stenosis before and after percutaneous aortic valvuloplasty. *Am J Cardiol 61*:1300–1306, 1988.

20. Davidson CJ, Harpole DA, Kisslo K, et al. Analysis of the early rise in aortic transvalvular gradient after aortic valvuloplasty. *Am Heart J 117*:411–417, 1989.

21. Nishimura RA, Holmes DR, Reeder GS, et al. Doppler evaluation of results of percutaneous aortic balloon valvuloplasty in calcific aortic stenosis. *Circulation 78*:791–799, 1988.

22. Harpole DH, Davidson CJ, Skelton TN, Kisslo KB, Jones RH, Bashore TM. Early and late changes in left ventricular systolic performance after percutane-ous aortic balloon valvuloplasty. *Am J Cardiol 66*: 327–332, 1990.

23. Otto CM for the NHLBI Balloon Valvuloplasty Registry. Predictors of outcome six months after balloon aortic valvuloplasty. *Circulation 80* (Suppl II):II-73, 1989.

24. Berland J, Cribier A, Savin T, et al. Postvalvuloplasty follow-up of elderly patients with severe aortic stenosis and low ejection fraction. *J Am Coll Cardiol 11*:15A, 1988.

25. Davidson CJ, Harrison JK, Pieper KS, Kisslo K, Harding MJ, Bashore TM. Balloon aortic valvuloplasty: What constitutes a successful one year outcome? *Circulation 82*:III-80, 1990.

26. Waller BF, McKay CR, Erny R, Morgan R, Mohler E. Catheter balloon valvuloplasty of necropsy stenotic aortic valves; etiology of aortic stenosis is a major factor in early restenosis. *J Am Coll Cardiol 13*:17A, 1989.

9

Aortic Valvuloplasty: A Surgical Perspective

PAUL J. HENDRY and JAMES E. LOWE

The invasive management of aortic valvular stenosis has been evolving since the first surgical procedure was performed in 1914. At that time, Tuffier used finger dilation via an aortotomy to open a stenotic aortic valve.[1] This technique was refined by others in the 1950s when aortic valvotomy was performed through an aortotomy or left ventriculotomy.[2,3] With the advent of cardiopulmonary bypass, more effective procedures have been made possible including valvuloplasty and valvular replacement (AVR) with either mechanical or bioprosthetic valves. The most recent technique under clinical investigation is percutaneous balloon aortic valvuloplasty (BAV). With these various interventions available, cardiologists and surgeons treating patients with aortic stenosis (AS) must be made aware of the advantages and disadvantages of each. In general, none of these procedures has proved to be the ideal cure for AS, as one set of risks is replaced by another. This chapter discusses the current state of surgical treatment of AS and attempts to put into perspective the role of BAV.

The etiology of AS may be congenital, rheumatic, degenerative, or calcific. With a decrease in rheumatic valvular disease and the longer survival of the population in general, calcific AS has become the most common pathologic finding in patients requiring intervention.[4] Once AS has been recognized, the rate of progression of the disease is not predictable.[4–6] Thus, the ideal timing for intervention is not easily discerned for all patients. Natural history studies have indicated that survival is limited to 5 years once symptoms begin.[7] Mortality in the first year after onset of symptoms is 22–43%, 75% at 3 years, and 91% at 10 years.[5,8] More specifically by symptom, 5-year survival with angina is 37%, with syncope 30%, and with

congestive heart failure 0%.[5] Thus, symptomatology is the major determinant for timing of surgical intervention.

SURGICAL PROCEDURES

Indications and risk factors. Surgery is generally considered to be the only effective treatment for both congenital and acquired AS,[4] and it serves as the standard against which any new technique must be compared. Since patients with AS can remain asymptomatic for some time, surgical intervention is usually considered only after symptoms of angina, syncope, or congestive heart failure occur. In addition, left ventricular hypertrophy, an ejection fraction less than 50%, an aortic valve area less than 0.8 cm^2, and a ventricular/aortic gradient greater than 50 mm Hg identified at cardiac catheterization should prompt intervention. Once these criteria are met, surgical intervention is indicated for most patients. Numerous studies have identified risk factors for increased mortality following aortic valve procedures, and these form the objective basis for rejecting a minority of patients for surgery.

Increasing age has been identified as a predictor of operative mortality in many studies assessing results of AVR in the general population.[9–16] However, in recent studies assessing risk factors within the elderly subset, increasing age was not a significant determinant of mortality or morbidity.[17,18] In other words, an 80-year-old was at no greater risk than a 70-year-old undergoing AVR. However, most would agree that mortality following AVR increases in the elderly compared to younger patients.[19–21] This is thought to be due to a greater fragility of the elderly vascular bed,[22] a more rapid development of ventilator dependence,[23] and a higher incidence of subsequent pneumonia and respiratory failure.[24] Increasing age also leads to a general decline in the overall reserve of multiple organ systems.[13,25] Elderly patients are less likely to recover from perioperative complications,[26] which implies a decreased resiliency after surgery compared to younger patients. In addition, they are more likely to have coronary artery disease complicating their valvular heart disease.[14] The older patient is therefore more likely to develop complications due to deterioration of other organ systems, and this in turn increases the risk of death following surgery. This is likely to hold true for any intervention that may affect hemodynamics. In the elderly population, a low level of activity may delay the manifestation of symptoms. Physicians who are wary of aggressive treatment in the elderly may postpone referral for surgery until there has been significant clinical deterioration.[26] The latter two factors may lead to an increased risk for surgery since left ventricular function will have deteriorated.

In contrast to the increased risks of surgery in the elderly, there are benefits to be gained. Aortic valve replacement has been shown to improve survival in elderly patients with AS, with the actuarial survival curve after AVR approaching that of the normal age-matched population.[17,19,27] Many of the late deaths seen in the elderly are noncardiac in origin[12,22] and reflect the higher mortality in this population due to malignancy and other illnesses.

Assuming that all patients in published series fulfilled indications for AVR, other details of their clinical status are not particularly clear. It is therefore difficult to deduce the clinical condition of the patients presented. Were they so-called "good" 80-year-olds or were they moribund? There is likely a selection bias in the surgical results[24] that favors the healthier elderly patient and may be a limiting factor when trying to compare results with BAV. Since BAV has been recommended for moribund individuals or those at high risk for surgery, a more detailed profile of patients undergoing AVR would be beneficial if a valid comparison with BAV is to be made. The benefits of AVR outweigh the risks in most elderly patients, and the data to be presented generally support the conclusion that AVR may be offered to elderly patients, resulting in a reasonable long-term survival. Age alone should not be used as a contraindication for AVR.[24,28,29]

Other risk factors for AVR relate directly to the status of the heart at the time of surgery. Patients with severe congestive heart failure (NYHA III–IV) are at greater risk for operative mortality[6,10,11,13,26,30] presumably because of inherent poor ventricular function. Removal of the stenosis leads to an overall improvement of cardiac function,[4] and those patients with poor left ventricular function may do very well with AVR.[4,21,31] In patients with ventricular dysfunction after surgery, other causes for myocardial dysfunction not directly related to AS or the AVR procedure may be the cause.[22] While not attributable to AVR, technical problems leading to stunned or infarcted myocardium can be addressed by changes in cardioplegic techniques or greater attention to revascularization procedures. The presence of coronary artery disease increases the risk of AVR.[10,11,26] In addition, patients requiring emergency AVR have a higher mortality.[13,26] Acute decompensation implies the presence of advanced ventricular dysfunction and underscores the importance of appropriate early intervention in these patients.

These risk factors are not contraindications to surgery. In determining operability, the surgeon must make a subjective and objective assessment as to whether or not the patient is a reasonable risk. With today's surgical and anesthetic techniques, there are fewer patients in whom surgery would be denied based on status of ventricular function or age. The presence of additional medical problems must be taken into consideration when evaluating a patient for surgery. In terminally ill patients, predicted longevity is a major factor in determining the advisability of AVR. The ethical question concerning the appropriateness of a given procedure deserves discussion between cardiologist, surgeon, patient, and family.

There are two surgical options to improve valvular function. The *first* is to repair the native valve using an open or closed valvotomy or valvuloplasty[32–42] or to debride the valve of calcium either manually, using ultrasound or laser technology.[43–45] The *second* and most common technique is to resect the dysfunctional valve and replace it with either a homograft,[46,47] a mechanical,[12,22,48,49] or a bioprosthetic[20,50–55] valve. A comparison of valve gradients and area among mechanical and bioprosthetic valves is presented in Table 9.1. These data are approximate values taken from in vivo measurements of valve gradients and areas, which may be used for comparison with post-BAV values (Table 9.4). Aortic valve replacement can offer substantial improvement in valve characteristics. Large series that review experience

Table 9.1.
Approximate in vivo valve gradients and valve areas for commonly used mechanical and bioprosthetic valves for comparison with results from BAV[114–116]

Valve Type	Valve Gradient (mm Hg)				
Mechanical	19m	21m	23m	25m	27m
Starr-Edwards		29	18	13	13
Bjork-Shiley (Std)	16	22	13.8	9.3	10.7
St. Jude	11	5	2.6	2.5	0.8
Medtronic-Hall		11.0	6.2	2.3	5.3
Biological					
Hancock		15	16	14	10
Carpentier-Edwards		13	16	13	10

	Valve Area (cm²)				
Mechanical	19m	21m	23m	25m	27m
Starr-Edwards		1.0	1.1	1.3	1.8
Bjork-Shiley (Std)	1.1	1.3	1.7	2.2	2.4
St. Jude	1.5	2.2	2.9	2.9	3.6
Medtronic-Hall		1.7	2.2	2.3	2.4
Biological					
Hancock		1.2	1.4	1.6	1.8
Carpentier-Edwards		1.3	1.5	1.6	2.1

with over 1000 patients followed over 10 years have proven the safety and efficacy of AVR.[10,13,53,54]

The elderly patient and AVR. Balloon aortic valvuloplasty has been used most extensively in two patient groups: the elderly with calcified AS and in neonates with congenital AS. Results of AVR will be presented so that they may be contrasted with those of BAV. Table 9.2 summarizes contemporary studies that assessed the results of AVR in the elderly. All the series presented have been published since 1980 and reflect the surgical and anesthetic techniques from 1970 to 1988. It is not uncommon for BAV series to quote older AVR studies for comparison. This may not be valid since operative conditions have changed significantly in recent years, which has led to decreased operative mortality and morbidity. In a study comparing early surgical experience in the 1970s to more recent procedures performed later than 1980 at the same institution, there was an increasing number of elderly patients undergoing AVR, while there was a decreasing number of patients with moderate to severe impairment of left ventricular function.[10] Overall hospital mortality appears to be decreasing in recent years (e.g., 10.67% from 1970 to 1976 and 2% from 1980 to 1985).[11]

The series outlined in Table 9.2 represents the cumulative experience of 11 centers performing AVR on 1831 elderly patients ranging in age from 61 to 97 years. Major complications included thromboembolic events, anticoagulant-related hemorrhage, infections of the prostheses, and valve failure. Comparison of series using either mechani-

Table 9.2.
Results of series for aortic valve replacement in elderly patients

Ref	#Pts	Study Year	Mean Age (y)	Age Range (y)	% pure AS	CHF FC III-IV (%)	A (%)	S (%)	Grad (mm Hg)	BIO (%)	Mech (%)
19	98	74–82	73	70–83	37	40	27			93	7
20	635	75–87		>65						100	
22	131	80–85	71	65–84	79						100
23	33	76–87	83	80–97	86					73	27
24	64	74–87	82	80–89	48	53	53	31	61		
25	55	78–81	68								
26	315	82–86	74		57	89				87	13
27	68	70–85	74	70–91	79	71	62				100
	73		75		67	48	60			100	
29	61	83–88	67	61–78		92					100
117	219	72–86	75	70–88	48.9	99			88	92	8
118	62	70–82	73	70–79	65	100	55	31	96		100

A = angina; S = syncope; CHF = congestive heart failure; y = years; m = months; py = patient years; Grad = preoperative valve gradient; BIO = bioprosthetic valve; Mech = mechanical valve; Thrombo = thromboembolic phenomenon; Anticoag = anticoagulant-related morbidity; INF = valve prosthesis infection; Mort = mortality; Comp = complications; FU = duration of follow-up; Morbid. = morbidity.

cal or bioprosthetic valves cannot identify a clear superiority of one valve type over the other in terms of survival.[56] Morbidity may be less when using bioprosthetic valves (10.7%) compared to mechanical valves (17.6%).[27] The major complication rates are not different from those seen in younger patients; however, the elderly have a higher incidence of postoperative psychosis and tend to have longer hospital stays.[19] Early mortality ranges from 5 to 30% with a mean of 10%. Five-year survival rates vary from 61 to 93% (mean of 72%). Late mortality rates are either expressed as percentages or in percent patient years with length of follow-up varying between studies, making comparison difficult. Most of the mortality rates presented are acceptable, and the differences may be partly explained by patient selection.[21,24] It must be assumed that various centers have somewhat different thresholds for accepting elderly patients for surgery, criteria which are not identified in published series.

Congenital aortic stenosis and surgery. Neonates and children with congenital AS have also been treated surgically. This condition is less common than acquired AS, resulting in fewer patients for analysis (Table 9.3). At the present time, open valvotomy is the most commonly performed procedure for congenital AS,[32,33,37–42,57] while aortic homografts are being used more frequently when valve replacement becomes necessary in the very young.[46,47] The closed approach for valvotomy is less invasive but also is less effective.[33] When the general pediatric population is considered, early mortality rates vary between 2 and 12.4%. Late mortality varies between 0 and 26% with a 25-year survival approaching 84%. Approximately 10 to 50% of patients require further surgery (either repeat valvotomy or valve replacement), with an overall freedom from re-operation of 94% and 65% at 10 and 25 years, respectively.[32]

Unfortunately, results are less favorable for neonates requiring surgery for AS. One group reports an excellent early mortality of 9% in a small series of 10 patients.[41] The latter results stand out from the majority of series where the 30-day mortality rates vary between 25% and 58%.[33,42] Many of these neonates have other cardiac anomalies, including hypoplastic left ventricles and endocardial fibroelastosis, that increase their risk for surgery.[32,37,40,41,57] In addition, neonates frequently require surgical intervention urgently, which increases the likelihood for early death.

Left ventricular function improves following surgery[58] with left ventricular wall stress and ejection fraction returning to normal levels after valvotomy. With the exception of neonates, in whom mortality remains exceedingly high, surgical treatment of AS is effective in the management of children with congenital AS.

Table 9.2.
Results of series for aortic valve replacement in elderly patients *(Continued)*

Thromb. Morbidity	Anti-Coag Morbid.	INF	Valve Failure	Mort. (%)	FU	Late Mort.	Other Comp.	% Survival (estimated)
—	—	1%	—	5	24 m	22%	14%	
2.3%py	0.3%py	0.2%py	0.44%py	6	3.5 y	5.2%py		(5 y 74)
1.8%py	0.2%py	0.2%py	0.1%py	6	4.3 y	6.9%py		(5 y 66)
				30	40.9 m	18%		
				9.4	28 m	18.9%		5 y 67
				5.5	—	—		
				7.6				
4.8%py	9.2%py	0.7%py	0	17.6	4.3 y	41		5 y 61
5.3%py	2.3%py	1.0%py	0	19.1		25		67
0	2.0%py	2%py	0	13.1	1.6 y	1.3%py	2.6%py	5 y 93
1.4%	4.2%	0	0	12.1	58.2 m	4.82%py	35%	7 y 77.2 (5 y 76)
1.6%	1.6%			8	26 m	22.6%		7 y 69.4 10 y 49

Table 9.3.
Results from series evaluating surgical results for congenital aortic stenosis

Ref	#Pts	Yr	Age (mean)	Age (Range)	Grad (mm Hg) Pre	Post	EF (%) Pre	Post	% AVR	Procedure % Open Valve	% Closed Valve	% Early Mort	FU	% Late Mort.	% Reop
32	177	55–86		1 d–25 y	53 -103	13 -19				100		12.4	12.1 y	11	21
33	40	65–85		< 28 d	55 -68		34 57		0	55	45	58	9.4 y	19	33
37	120	62–84		2 d–19 y					2	98		5	8.7 y	3.5	23
38	104	57–86	10.1 y	1 d–19 y	85	35				100		2	5.2 y	0	13
	30		20 d	0–56 d						50	50	60	—	3	—
39	33	72–86		< 6 m	75 -79		43 -51			100		42	4.1 y	5	26
40	10	83–84	21.2 d	1–38 d	42	18					100 (TV)	30	8.7 m	14	14
41	11	76–81	9.9 d	1–24 y	77					100		9	2.2 y	0	10
42	8			2 d–7 m						100		25	6–28 m	0	50
57	36	65–85	14.7 y	3 m–19 y					100			8	45 m	26	—
119	41	58–74	11.4 y	2–17 y	93					100		0	15.1 y	19.5	17
120	162	56–75	1–20 y							100		1.9	7.1 y	19	12.7
	25		< 1 y							100		52	4.1 y	17	8

Yr = year; Grad = gradient; EF = ejection fraction; Mort = mortality; Rcop = reoperation; FU = duration of follow-up; TV = transventricular; d = day; m = month; y = years.

RESULTS OF PERCUTANEOUS BALLOON AORTIC VALVULOPLASTY

Indications and mechanisms. In addition to the symptomatic and hemodynamic criteria for intervention in AS outlined previously, BAV is recommended for patients who are elderly, those at increased risk for surgery including patients with other medical or terminal illnesses, those who have congenital AS, when AS becomes symptomatic during pregnancy, for those who refuse AVR, or as a bridge for urgent cardiac and noncardiac surgery.[59–72] Most centers now performing BAV do so on patients who are not surgical candidates due to advanced age or medical illness (68–96% of BAV patients) or who refuse surgery (4–32%).[60,73] The latter group raises several questions concerning reasons for refusal since these patients may be otherwise good surgical candidates. Was a surgeon involved in discussing the options with the patient? How were risks and results of both procedures presented? While the reasons for denying surgery may be varied, information and advice provided by the cardiologist or surgeon may be presented in a biased fashion that favors one approach over the other.

While pathology and intervention can both be assessed directly during surgery, the cardiologist performing BAV has less control over the procedure during valve dilation. Autopsy studies and assessment of valves at AVR have shown that BAV results in fracture of calcium deposits within the valve, separation of fused commissures, and/or stretching of the valve orifice and anulus, which results in an increase in cusp mobility.[74–81] Valves can undergo healing with thrombus formation at the fracture sites, or they may reapproximate soon after the procedure[77,82] leading to restenosis. In BAV patients who later developed restenosis and require AVR, the valve is frequently found to be intact without any lesion attributable to BAV.[6,82] There may be some differences in the underlying pathological basis of stenosis that make some lesions less amenable to BAV, but this is not discernable at the time of the procedure.[83]

If success of the procedure is defined by a 50% increase in valve area, the method by which this is calculated must be examined. Aortic valve areas (AVA) are determined using the Gorlin formula from data collected at cardiac catheterization. Echocardiography can also be used to calculate AVA using the continuity equation. Correlation between the two has been variable with regression coefficients (r values) ranging between 0.56 and 0.86.[84,85] The preoperative AVA calculated using the Gorlin formula has been shown frequently to be smaller than the actual valve area measured at surgery.[6,82,86,87] The AVA may be smaller than calculated post-BAV due to elasticity of the aortic valve.[88] The acute changes in hemodynamics following BAV may lead to inaccurate measurements of AVA especially at low flow states.[84,87,89] Despite finding decreased gradients and increased AVA, hemodynamics seen several days after BAV are similar to those seen with severe AS.[6] The individual responses to BAV are quite variable,[90,91] which may be related to unpredictable changes in AVA with BAV.[80]

Despite the less invasive nature of BAV, the procedure is not without complications. The most common are arterial complications arising from the trauma caused by insertion of the large sheath through which the BAV catheter is advanced.[92–95] Hematomas and transfusions are common, and operative repair of femoral arterial trauma is required in 4 to 25% of patients.[96–99] Emergency cardiac surgery has been required less frequently for perforation of the left ventricle,[60,90,100,101] anular disruption,[102,103] aortic rupture,[86,104] and creation of a large ASD.[105] Embolic phenomena, myocardial infarction, and endocarditis have been reported.[94–96,106–108] Although AVR is associated with significant complications, BAV cannot be presented as an innocuous alternative.

Results in the elderly. The results of 18 recent studies consisting of 20 or more patients are presented in Table 9.4. There were 1207 patients reported who underwent BAV between 1985 and 1988. The mean ages indicate that the majority of patients were in the elderly age group, with most having symptoms of severe congestive heart failure. Major complications included new or worsened aortic regurgitation; embolic events; and arterial (transfusions were not considered major complications for the purposes of this review), ventricular, or aortic trauma that required operative intervention. Complication rates ranged from 8 to 32% and the early mortality (less than 30 days) varied from 0 to 14% (mean of 6.3%). Follow-up has been brief for most studies, ranging from 4 to 14 months. Late mortality for these short periods may not adequately reflect the long-term success of this procedure. Most groups have encountered a high restenosis rate ranging from 37 to 100%. The variable rates may reflect differing follow-up protocols. Some centers perform echocardiography or catheterization on

Table 9.4.
Results from series assessing the results of percutaneous balloon aortic valvuloplasty for acquired aortic stenosis

Ref#	#Pts	Study Years	Mean Age (y)	Age Range (y)	CHF FC III-IV (%)	A (%)	S (%)	Mean Gradient (mmHg) Pre	Post	Peak Gradient (mmHg) Pre	Post
28	33	—	74	60–84						84	40
59	125	86–88	76	37–94	70	4	14	70	30	87	32
60	170	85–88	77	35–94	78	42	36	56	31	71	36
61	90	86–87	79	52–95	98		2	61	30		
73	47		79	65–97	80	39	28	49	24	70	32
88	56	86–87	79		93			59	40		
95	37	85–86	75	60–88	65	11	19	64	32	80	37
96	245	85–88	74	30–98	71	23	38			72	29
97	88		80	60–103	75	49	40	58	32	65	30
98	24	86–87	80	51–91	92			66	40	70	36
99	36	86–88	77		94	5		48	23		
121	81	86–89	76	53–89	91	63		57	18	70	34
122	22		78	68–93				57	32		
123	26	87–88	86	80–94	77	35	35	59	31		
124	20	86–87	74	54–90	90	10				70	35
125*	24	—	77	59–85	100	33	33			76	30
			80	75–89	100	42	33			73	23
126	58	86–87	66	40–89						93	51
127	25	86–87	75	60–88	88	52	28	73	43	84	41

*Upper row = results with 19-mm balloon; lower row = results with 25-mm balloon

y = years; CHF = congestive heart failure; A = percentage of patients with angina; S = syncope; CO = cardiac output (L/min); CI = cardiac index (L/min/m²); EF = ejection fraction; Compl = complications; FU = length of follow-up; AVR = percentage of patients requiring aortic valve surgery.

all patients, whereas others investigate only those who become symptomatic. Asymptomatic patients have been shown to have restenosis rates as high as 50 to 75%, which emphasizes the need for complete hemodynamic follow-up.[59,60]

BAV for congenital aortic stenosis. Balloon aortic valvuloplasty in the pediatric population seems to have greater promise. Reports from 12 recent articles describing BAV in 212 patients with ages between 1 day and 39 years are summarized in Table 9.5. While complication rates are high (mostly new or worsened aortic regurgitation), the early mortality is generally low. The BAV experience with neonates parallels that of surgery, which both lead to high mortality rates. One report that described BAV in neonates (ages 2 to 34 days) had an early mortality of 30%.[109] Patients with cardiac anomalies such as hypoplastic left ventricles and fibroelastosis are at particularly high risk.[109,110] Follow-up of these patients has been insufficient to comment on the late mortality or long-term hemodynamic and functional results. However, in this brief period, the restenosis rate has been 0% in most series, which is in striking contrast to the adult BAV results. The mechanism of BAV in congenital AS appears to be the separation of fused commissures. The valve pathology may lend itself better to this technique than the adult form of acquired AS.

Other indications. There have been limited reports detailing experiences with BAV for patients in whom AS complicates other conditions. Pregnancy may precipitate decompensation in patients with AS. In two reports, six patients underwent BAV with good initial results leading to the delivery of healthy infants.[66,67] Unfortunately, during two years of follow-up, three of four patients had fatal or near-fatal events. Surgery had been postponed by the mother due to a decrease in symptomatology and a desire to spend time with the newborn.

Balloon aortic valvuloplasty has been used as a bridge to AVR or preoperatively prior to noncardiac surgery. Patients presenting in cardiogenic shock due to severe AS have been palliated with BAV followed by uncomplicated AVR.[68,69] Balloon aortic valvuloplasty allowed the discontinuance of

Table 9.4.
Results from series assessing the results of percutaneous balloon aortic valvuloplasty for acquired aortic stenosis *(Continued)*

AVA (cm²)		CO or (CI)		EF (%)		Major Compl. %	Early Mort. %	FU	Late Mort. %	AVR %	Restenosis (estimated) %
Pre	Post	Pre	Post	Pre	Post						
0.39	0.74							17m	30	36	(79)
0.6	1.0	4.3	4.6			18	9	12m	36	6	46
0.6	0.9	4.6	4.8			14	4	9m	15	10	(83)
0.4	0.8	3.6	3.9				9	6m	28	—	56
0.5	0.9	3.5	3.9				6	10m	10	4	52
0.49	0.75					21	7	4m	28	9	(53)
0.39	0.78	3.5	3.7			11	5	6m	10	14	—
0.53	0.95	(2.79)	(2.86)	48	51	6	4.9	18m	33	11	37
0.48	0.74					8	10	8m	24	18	(53)
0.5	0.7	(2.5)	(2.4)			29	4	10m	21	29	—
0.5	0.9	3.9	3.9			14	9	7m	55	11	(44)
0.57	0.83			46	49		0	6m	16	5	(57)
0.51	0.85					14	14	—	—	—	—
0.45	0.67	3.6	3.6			15	8	6m	21	4	—
0.51	0.73	4.0	3	52	55	10	0	—	—	—	—
0.4	0.57	(2.4)	(2.3)	44	46	13	13	5m	19	—	—
0.47	0.88	(2.2)	(2.3)	43	47						
								8m	—	—	(100)
0.47	0.72					32	8	13m	0	20	—

inotropic support and improvement in overall end-organ function. Subsequent surgery was performed on an elective basis. In patients who refuse AVR surgery or who are not surgical candidates initially, BAV can be used to improve hemodynamics for a brief period to allow noncardiac procedures.[70,71,111,112] Primary surgical procedures such as hip replacement, gastrectomy, colectomy, and so forth or diagnostic procedures may be performed with greater safety for the patient. The decision to perform AVR may be made once the outcome from the other procedure is determined.

Stenosis of bioprosthetic valves has been treated by BAV with unpredictable results.[113] Two patients had unsuccessful attempts at BAV. One underwent AVR for continued symptoms, but another patient died with severe BAV-induced aortic regurgitation before AVR could be performed. The technique is contraindicated in patients with vegetations, thrombus, or degenerative prosthetic valve regurgitation.

Results of AVR following BAV. At Duke University, 137 patients underwent 158 BAV procedures from January 1987 to February 1990. Of this group, 33 patients (24%) with a mean age of 71.7 ± 1.5 years required subsequent AVR during a 7.5 ± 1.3 month follow-up period. The hemodynamic results post-BAV were similar to those presented in other series. The initial indications for BAV included 11 patients for age alone, 8 refused surgery, 11 were high risk or had other medical contraindications for surgery, and 2 BAVs were performed as bridges to AVR. The operative mortality for this selected group was 3% with a 1-year survival of 90.6% during a mean 7.1-month follow-up period. The overall mortality for the BAV group was 39.4% during a mean of 5.6 months of follow-up. Eight surgical patients (24%) had complications including coagulopathies, arrhythmias, pneumothorax, perivalvular leak, and ileus. The patients with coagulopathy and aortic regurgitation both died prior to discharge from the hospital. These results indicate that AVR may be performed with a low morbidity and mortality rate in selected patients who have undergone BAV.

DISCUSSION

There is no ideal intervention that may be performed for AS that results in a risk-free cure. Surgical valvuloplasty and valve replacement re-

Table 9.5.
Results from series evaluating results of percutaneous balloon aortic valvuloplasty for the treatment of congenital aortic stenosis

Ref	#Pts	Study Year	Mean Age (y)	Age Range	Mean Grad (mmHg) Pre	Post	Peak Grad (mmHg) Pre	Post
64	8	85–86		3m–14y			74	38
65	23	82–83	9y	2–17y			113	32
81	34	86–88		16m–17y			71	28
109	10	85–87		2–34d	61	20		
128	26	85–87		3m–21y			80	38
129	27	82–84	9y	20m–17y			108	32
130	9	85–87		4m–16y			88	41
131	75	84–87	9y	1d–39y	76	34		

Grad = gradient; AVA = aortic valve area; Comp = complication; Mort = mortality; Surg = percentage of patients requiring aortic valve surgery (valvotomy/replacement); y = years; m = months; d = days.

quire continued surveillance for native or prosthetic valve failure and infection, anticoagulant-related problems, and thromboembolic phenomena. Percutaneous balloon aortic valvuloplasty has been developed recently, but the results have not been impressive in the adult. Therefore for AS, BAV has been restricted to those cases in which surgery is not advisable or possible, but when some intervention is desirable.

Of the indications listed previously, most patients undergoing BAV are either elderly or refuse surgery. Since restenosis rates are high and limited short-term follow-up indicates that late mortality is high, should surgery not be strongly recommended to these patients? If BAV is presented as a viable alternative, then patients who might benefit greatly from surgery may be less well treated by proceeding with valvuloplasty. Since long-term follow-up is scant, the effect of persisting or recurrent stenosis on left ventricular function and mortality is not known. Predictably however, if the stenosis is not adequately relieved, then cardiac function will deteriorate with or without symptomatology to warn of impending decompensation. It is clear that restenosis may occur without the development of symptoms.[60]

Conversely, it may be argued that BAV should be attempted prior to AVR since it is less invasive and seems to result in symptomatic relief in many patients. Provided that adequate follow-up is pursued using serial echocardiograms or catheterizations to evaluate restenosis and cardiac function, then AVR may be offered to these patients at a later date with good results. It is difficult to quantify the net gain or loss in long-term survival that this approach might create.

Patients who are extreme surgical risks because of concomitant medical illnesses or who are terminally ill may be palliated by BAV. When a major surgical intervention such as valve replacement may not be advisable, BAV may be a good alternative due to its less invasive nature. Selection of patients fulfilling these criteria is important. Different centers are willing to undertake surgery on patients in varying medical conditions. Whether or not a patient is accepted for surgery will depend on the aggressiveness of the cardiac surgeon. Intuitively, multi-system failure would likely result in high mortality after AVR. Due to the many combinations of system dysfunction that may be possible, no series evaluating AVR results is large enough to predict outcome for any given combination. Therefore, decisions concerning high-risk patients must be made on an individual basis without the benefit of statistical data. Ethical questions must be raised in many of these high-risk cases or in patients with terminal illnesses.

Balloon aortic valvuloplasty as a primary intervention appears to have a role in the treatment of congenital AS and as a bridge to AVR. The initial results of BAV in children have paralleled operative valvotomy. The advantages are that gradients are reduced resulting in normalization of left ventricular function, which can either eliminate or postpone surgery until growth allows for valve replacement using an appropriate size of prosthesis.

Bridging to AVR is an attractive use for BAV since there are patients who are pregnant or suffering from various medical conditions that warrant other forms of management prior to a major operation. It must be stressed that the relief of symptoms after BAV may give the patient a false

Table 9.5.
Results from series evaluating results of percutaneous balloon aortic valvuloplasty for the treatment of congenital aortic stenosis *(Continued)*

AVA (cm²)		Compl Rate	Early Mort %	FU	Late Mort %	Surg %	Restenosis %
Pre	Post						
0.48	0.65	40	0	2–8m	0	—	0
		43	0	1–9m	0	9	0
		41	0	13m	0	3	0
		40	30	16m	0	40	0
		31	0	—	—	—	—
		37	0	7m	0	7	0
		30	0	1.5y	0	11	0
		50	4	7–8m	0	3	0

sense of security and result in a reluctance to undergo valve surgery. This will likely lead to an increased mortality in this group.

SUMMARY

Due to the variability in patient selection, acceptable outcome criteria, and follow-up, comparisons between AVR and BAV are difficult. Allowing for this, the following conclusions can be drawn:

1. BAV has a limited role in treating select elderly patients with AS in whom AVR has been shown to be an effective therapeutic modality.
2. BAV may be the primary intervention for symptomatic patients with congenital AS or as a temporary bridge to AVR in adults.
3. BAV in the adult patient offers short-term palliation only. The patient must be aware that close follow-up is required, and future intervention is necessary in most cases.
4. BAV has a high restenosis rate and resultant high late mortality due to incomplete relief of valve stenosis.
5. BAV should only be undertaken following consultation with both cardiologist and cardiac surgeon. Risks and benefits of both procedures must be fairly presented to the patient.
6. Concomitant severe medical or terminal illnesses warrant careful deliberation with patient and family prior to any intervention for AS.
7. AVR following BAV appears to be safe with low morbidity and mortality.
8. Long-term results of BAV are pending and will be essential to further delineate the role of BAV.

REFERENCES

1. Tuffier T. Etude experimentale sur la chirurgie des valves de coeur. *Bull Acad Med Paris 71*:293–295, 1914.

2. Ellis FH Jr, Kirklin JW. Aortic stenosis. *Surg Clin North Am 35*:1029–1034, 1955.
3. Bailey CP, Ramirez HP, Larselere HB. Surgical treatment of aortic stenosis. *JAMA 150*:1647–1652, 1952.
4. Selzer A. Changing aspects of the natural history of valvular aortic stenosis. *N Engl J Med 317*:91–98, 1987.
5. Turina J, Hess O, Sepulcri F, Krayenbuehl HP. Spontaneous course of aortic valve disease. *Eur Heart J 8*:471–483, 1987.
6. Grollier G, Commeau P, Sesboue B, Huret B, Potier JC, Foucault JP. Short-term clinical and haemodynamic assessment of ballon aortic valvuloplasty in 30 elderly patients. Discrepancy between immediate and eighth-day haemodynamic values. *Eur Heart J 9 (Suppl E)*:155–162, 1988.
7. Rappaport B. Natural history of aortic and mitral valve disease. *Am J Cardiol 35*:221–227, 1975.
8. O'Keefe JH Jr, Vlietstra RE, Bailey KR, Holmes DR Jr. Natural history of candidates for balloon aortic valvuloplasty. *Mayo Clin Proc 62*:986–991, 1987.
9. Teoh KH, Ivanov J, Weisel RD, Darcel IC, Rakowski H. Survival and bioprosthetic valve failure. Ten-year follow-up. *Circulation 80* (Suppl I):I-8–I-15, 1989.
10. Lytle BW, Cosgrove DM, Taylor PC, Goormastic M, Stewart RW, Golding LAR, Gill CC, Loop FD. Primary isolated aortic valve replacement. Early and late results. *J Thorac Cardiovasc Surg 97*:675–694, 1989.
11. Di Lello F, Flemma RJ, Anderson AJ, Mullen DC, Kleinman LH, Werner PH. Improved early results after aortic valve replacement: Analysis by surgical time frame. *Ann Thorac Surg 47*:51–56, 1989.
12. Flemma RJ, Mullen DC, Kleinman LH, Werner PH, Anderson AJ, Weirauch E. Survival and "event-free" analysis of 785 patients with Bjork-

Shiley spherical-disc valves at 10 to 16 years. *Ann Thorac Surg 45*:258–272, 1988.

13. Scott WC, Miller DC, Haverich A, Dawkins K, Mitchell RS, Jamieson SW, Oyer PE, Stinson EB, Baldwin JC, Shumway NE. Determinants of operative mortality for patients undergoing aortic valve replacement. Discriminant analysis of 1,479 operations. *J Thorac Cardiovasc Surg 89*:400–413, 1985.

14. Christakis GT, Weisel RD, Fremes SE, Teoh KH, Skalenda JP, Tong CP, Azuma JY, Schwartz L, Mickleborough LL, Scully HE, Goldman BS, Baird RJ. Can the results of contemporary aortic valve replacement be improved? *J Thorac Cardiovasc Surg 92*:37–46, 1986.

15. Acar J, Luxereau Ph, Ducimetiere P, Cadilhac M, Jallut H, Vahanian A. Prognosis of surgically treated chronic aortic valve disease. Predictive indicators of early postoperative risk and long-term survival, based on 439 cases. *J Thorac Cardiovasc Surg 82*:114–126, 1981.

16. MaGovern JA, Pennock JL, Campbell DB, Pae WE, Bartholomew M, Pierce WS, Waldhausen JA. Aortic valve replacement and combined aortic valve replacement and coronary artery bypass grafting: Predicting high risk groups. *J Am Coll Cardiol 9*: 38–43, 1987.

17. Fishman NH, Roe BB. Cardiac valve replacement in patients over 65 during a 10-year period. *J Gerontol 33*:676–680, 1978.

18. Bessone L, Pupello DF, Blank RH, Lopez-Cuenca E, Hiro SP, Ebra G. Valve replacement in the elderly: A long-term appraisal. *J Cardiovasc Surg* (Torino) *26*:417–425, 1985.

19. Craver JM, Goldstein J, Jones EL, Knapp WA, Hatcher CR Jr. Clinical, hemodynamic, and operative descriptors affecting outcome of aortic valve replacement in elderly versus young patients. *Ann Surg 199*:733–741, 1984.

20. Jamieson WRE, Burr LH, Munro AI, Miyagishima RT, Gerein AN. Cardiac valve replacement in the elderly: Clinical performance of biological prostheses. *Ann Thorac Surg 48*:173–185, 1989.

21. Smucker ML, Manning SB, Stuckey TD, Tyson DL, Nygaard TW, Kron IL. Preoperative left ventricular wall stress, ejection fraction, and aortic valve gradient as prognostic indicators in aortic valve stenosis. *Cathet Cardiovasc Diagn 17*:133–143, 1989.

22. Antunes MJ. Valve replacement in the elderly. Is the mechanical valve a good alternative? *J Thorac Cardiovasc Surg 98*:485–491, 1989.

23. Edmunds LH Jr, Stephenson LW, Edie RN, Ratcliffe MB. Open-heart surgery in octogenarians. *N Engl J Med 319*:131–136, 1988.

24. Levinson JR, Akins CW, Buckley MJ, Newell JB, Palacios IF, Block PC, Fifer MA. Octogenarians with aortic stenosis. Outcome after aortic valve replacement. *Circulation 80* (Suppl I):I-49–I-56, 1989.

25. Santinga JT, Flora J, Kirsh M, Baublis J. Aortic valve replacement in the elderly. *J Am Geriatric Soc 31*:211–212, 1983.

26. Fremes SE, Goldman BS, Ivanov J, Weisel RD, David TE, Salerno T. Valvular surgery in the elderly. *Circulation 80* (Suppl I):I-77–I-90, 1989.

27. Borkon AM, Soule LM, Baughman KL, Baumgartner WA, Gardner TJ, Watkins L, Gott VL, Hall KA, Reitz BA. Aortic valve selection in the elderly patient. *Ann Thorac Surg 46*:270–277, 1988.

28. Spielberg Ch, Kruck I, Schroder R. Die balloon-valvuloplastie der kalzifizierten aortenstenose ist keine realistische alternative zur operation: Klinische und invasive ergebnisse 17 monate nach 1. oder evtl. 2. dilatation. *Z Kardiol 78*:86–94, 1989.

29. Dietrich MS, Nashef SAM, Bain WH. Heart valve replacement with the Bjork-Shiley monostrut valve in patients over 60 years of age. *Thorac Cardiovasc Surgeon 37*:131–134, 1989.

30. Meurs AAH, Grundemann AM, Bezemer PD, Geldof ChP, Zienkowicz BS, Ong ST, de Jong IH. Early and 8 year results of aortic valve replacement: A clinical study of 232 patients. *Eur Heart J 6*: 870–881, 1985.

31. Carabello BA, Green LH, Grossman W, Cohn LH, Koster JK, Collins JJ Jr. Hemodynamic determinants of prognosis of aortic valve replacement in critical aortic stenosis and advanced congestive heart failure. *Circulation 62*:42–48, 1980.

32. Tveter KJ, Foker JE, Moller JH, Ring WS, Lillehei CW, Varco RL. Long-term evaluation of aortic valvotomy for congenital aortic stenosis. *Ann Surg 206*:496–503, 1987.

33. Pelech AN, Dyck JD, Trusler GA, Williams WG, Olley PM, Rowe RD, Freedom RM. Critical aortic stenosis. Survival and management. *J Thorac Cardiovasc Surg 94*:510–517, 1987.

34. Rees JR, Holswade GR, Lillehei CW, Glenn F. Aortic valvuloplasty for stenosis in adults. *J Thorac Cardiovasc Surg 67*:390–394, 1974.

35. Lewis FJ, Shumway NE, Niazi SA, Benjamin RB. Aortic valvulotomy under direct vision during hypothermia. *J Thorac Surg 32*:481–492, 1956.

36. Weinstein GS, Reed WA, Killen DA. Aortic valvuloplasty for calcific aortic stenosis in the adult. *J Cardiovasc Surg* (Torino) *21*:675–680, 1980.

37. Wheller JJ, Hosier DM, Teske DW, Craenen JM, Kilman JW. Results of operation for aortic valve stenosis in infants, children, and adolescents. *J Thorac Cardiovasc Surg 96*:474–477, 1988.

38. Brown JW, Stevens LS, Holly S, Robison R, Rodefeld M, Grayson T, Marts B, Caldwell RA, Hurwitz RA, Girod DA, King H. Surgical spectrum of aortic stenosis in children: A thirty-year experience with 257 children. *Ann Thorac Surg 45*: 393–403, 1988.

39. Hammon JW, Lupinetti FM, Maples MD, Merrill WH, Frist WH, Graham TP Jr, Bender HW Jr.

Predictors of operative mortality in critical valvular aortic stenosis presenting in infancy. *Ann Thorac Surg 45*:537–540, 1988.

40. Duncan K, Sullivan I, Robinson P, Horvath P, de Leval M, Stark J. Transventricular aortic valvotomy for critical aortic stenosis in infants. *J Thorac Cardiovasc Surg 93*:546–550, 1987.

41. Messina LM, Turley K, Stanger P, Hoffman JIE, Ebert PA. Successful aortic valvotomy for severe congenital valvular aortic stenosis in the newborn infant. *J Thorac Cardiovasc Surg 88*:92–96, 1984.

42. Sink JD, Smallhorn JF, Macartney FJ, Taylor JFN, Stark J, de Leval MR. Management of critical aortic stenosis in infancy. *J Thorac Cardiovasc Surg 87*:82–86, 1984.

43. Hill DG. Long-term results of debridement valvotomy for calcific aortic stenosis. *J Thorac Cardiovasc Surg 65*:708–711, 1973.

44. Enright LP, Hancock EW, Shumway NE. Aortic debridement—Long-term follow-up. *Circulation 53*:I-68–I-72, 1971.

45. Isner JM, Michlewitz H, Clarke RH, Donaldson RF, Konstam MA, Salem DN. Laser-assisted debridement of aortic valve calcium. *Am Heart J 109*:448–452, 1985.

46. Matsuki O, Robles A, Gibbs S, Bodnar E, Ross DN. Long-term performance of 555 aortic homografts in the aortic position. *Ann Thorac Surg 46*:187–191, 1988.

47. Angell WW, Oury JH, Lamberti JJ, Koziol J. Durability of the viable aortic allograft. *J Thorac Cardiovasc Surg 98*:48–56, 1989.

48. Thulin LI, Bain WH, Huysmans HH, van Ingen G, Prieto I, Basile F, Lindblom DA, Olin CL. Heart valve replacement with the Bjork-Shiley monostrut valve: Early results of a multicenter clinical investigation. *Ann Thorac Surg 45*:164–170, 1988.

49. Arom KV, Nicoloff DM, Kersten TE, Northrup WF III, Lindsay WG, Emery RW. Ten years' experience with the St. Jude medical valve prosthesis. *Ann Thorac Surg 47*:831–837, 1989.

50. Spencer FC, Grossi EA, Culliford AT, Baumann FG, Galloway AC. Experiences with 1643 porcine prosthetic valves in 1492 patients. *Ann Surg 203*:691–700, 1986.

51. Jamieson WRE, Rosado LJ, Munro AI, Gerein AN, Burr LH, Miyagishima RT, Janusz MT, Tyers GFO. Carpentier-Edwards standard porcine bioprosthesis: Primary tissue failure (structural valve deterioration) by age groups. *Ann Thorac Surg 46*:155–162, 1988.

52. Milano AD, Bortolotti U, Mazzucco A, Guerra F, Stellin G, Talenti E, Thiene G, Gallucci V. Performance of the Hancock porcine bioprosthesis following aortic valve replacement: Considerations based on a 15-year experience. *Ann Thorac Surg 46*:216–222, 1988.

53. Pelletier LC, Carrier M, Leclerc Y, Lepage G,

deGuise P, Dyrda I. Porcine versus pericardial bioprostheses: A comparison of late results in 1,593 patients. *Ann Thorac Surg 47*:352–361, 1989.

54. Cohn LH, Collins JJ, DiSesa VJ, Couper GS, Peigh PS, Kowalker W, Allred E. Fifteen-year experience with 1678 Hancock porcine bioprosthetic heart valve replacements. *Ann Surg 210*:435–443, 1989.

55. Lindbolm D. Long-term clinical results after aortic valve replacement with the Bjork-Shiley prosthesis. *J Thorac Cardiovasc Surg 95*:658–667, 1988.

56. Hammond GL, Geha AS, Kopf GS, Hashim SW. Biological versus mechanical valves. *J Thorac Cardiovasc Surg 93*:182–198, 1987.

57. Robbins RC, Bowman FO, Malm JR. Cardiac valve replacement in children: A twenty-year series. *Ann Thorac Surg 45*:56–61, 1988.

58. Dorn GW II, Donner R, Assey ME, Spann JF Jr, Wiles HB, Carabello BA. Alterations in left ventricular geometry, wall stress, and ejection performance after correction of congenital aortic stenosis. *Circulation 78*:1358–1364, 1988.

59. Lewin RF, Dorros G, King JF, Mathiak L. Percutaneous transluminal aortic valvuloplasty: Acute outcome and follow-up of 125 patients. *J Am Coll Cardiol 14*:1210–1217, 1989.

60. Safian RD, Berman AD, Diver DJ, McKay LL, Come PC, Riley MF, Warren SE, Cunningham MJ, Wyman RM, Weinstein JS, Grossman W, McKay RG. Balloon aortic valvuloplasty in 170 consecutive patients. *N Engl J Med 319*:125–130, 1988.

61. Block PC, Palacios IF. Clinical and hemodynamic follow-up after percutaneous aortic valvuloplasty in the elderly. *Am J Cardiol 62*:760–763, 1988.

62. Lababidi Z. Aortic balloon valvuloplasty. *Am Heart J 106*:751–752, 1983.

63. Lababidi Z, Weinhaus L. Successful balloon valvuloplasty for neonatal critical aortic stenosis. *Am Heart J 112*:913–916, 1986.

64. Choy M, Beekman RH, Rocchini AP, Crowley DC, Snider AR, Dick M II, Rosenthal A. Percutaneous balloon valvuloplasty for valvar aortic stenosis in infants and children. *Am J Cardiol 59*:1010–1013, 1987.

65. Lababidi Z, Wu J, Walls JT. Percutaneous balloon aortic valvuloplasty: Results in 23 patients. *Am J Cardiol 53*:194–197, 1984.

66. Easterling TR, Chadwick HS, Otto CM, Benedetti TJ. Aortic stenosis in pregnancy. *Obstet Gynecol 72*:113–117, 1988.

67. Angel JL, Chapman C, Knuppel RA, Morales WJ, Sims CJ. Percutaneous balloon aortic valvuloplasty in pregnancy. *Obstet Gynecol 72*:438–440, 1988.

68. Friedman HZ, Cragg DR, O'Neill WW. Cardiac resuscitation using emergency aortic balloon valvuloplasty. *Am J Cardiol 63*:387–388, 1989.

69. Desnoyers MR, Salem DN, Rosenfield K, Mackey

W, O'Donnell T, Isner JM. Treatment of cardiogenic shock by emergency aortic balloon valvuloplasty. *Ann Int Med 108*:833–835, 1988.

70. Levine MJ, Berman AD, Safian RD, Diver CJ, McKay RG. Palliation of valvular aortic stenosis by balloon valvuloplasty as preoperative preparation for noncardiac surgery. *Am J Cardiol 62*:1309–1310, 1988.

71. Hayes SN, Holmes DR Jr, Nishimura RA, Reeder GS. Palliative percutaneous aortic balloon valvuloplasty before noncardiac operations and invasive diagnostic procedures. *Mayo Clin Proc 64*: 753–757, 1989.

72. Nishimura RA, Holmes DR Jr, Reeder GS, Orszulak TA, Bresnahan JF, Ilstrup DM, Tajik AJ. Doppler evaluation of results of percutaneous aortic balloon valvuloplasty in calcific aortic stenosis. *Circulation 78*:791–799, 1988.

73. Desnoyers MR, Isner JM, Pandian NG, Wang SS, Hougen T, Fields CD, Lucas AR, Salem DN. Clinical and noninvasive hemodynamic results after aortic balloon valvuloplasty for aortic stenosis. *Am J Cardiol 62*:1078–1084, 1988.

74. Ferguson JJ III, Bush HS, Riuli EP. Doppler echocardiographic assessment of the effect of balloon aortic valvuloplasty on left ventricular systolic function. *Am Heart J 117*:18–24, 1989.

75. Kennedy KD, Hauck AJ, Edwards WD, Holmes DR Jr, Reeder GS, Nishimura RA. Mechanism of reduction of aortic valvular stenosis by percutaneous transluminal balloon valvuloplasty: Report of five cases and review of literature. *Mayo Clin Proc 63*:769–776, 1988.

76. Safian RD, Mandell VS, Thurer RE, Hutchins GM, Schnitt SJ, Grossman W, McKay RG. Postmortem and intraoperative balloon valvuloplasty of calcific aortic stenosis in elderly patients: Mechanisms of successful dilation. *J Am Coll Cardiol 9*: 655–660, 1987.

77. Berdoff RL, Strain J, Crandall C, Ghali V, Goldman B. Pathology of aortic valvuloplasty: Findings after postmortem successful and failed dilatations. *Am Heart J 117*:688–690, 1989.

78. Kalan JM, Mann JM, Leon MB, Pichard A, Kent KM, Roberts WC. Morphologic findings in stenotic aortic valves that have had "successful" percutaneous balloon valvuloplasty. *Am J Cardiol 62*: 152–154, 1988.

79. Isner JM, Samuels DA, Slovenkai GA, Halaburka KR, Hougen TJ, Desnoyers MR, Fields CD, Salem DN. Mechanism of aortic balloon valvuloplasty: Fracture of valvular calcific deposits. *Ann Int Med 108*:377–380, 1988.

80. Letac B, Gerver LI, Koning R. Insights on the mechanism of balloon valvuloplasty in aortic stenosis. *Am J Cardiol 62*:1241–1247, 1988.

81. Sullivan ID, Wren C, Bain H, Hunter S, Rees PG, Taylor JFN, Bull C, Deanfield JE. Balloon dilatation of the aortic valve for congenital aortic stenosis in childhood. *Br Heart J 61*:186–191, 1989.

82. Robicsek F, Harbold NB Jr, Daugherty HK, Cook JW, Selle JG, Hess PJ, Gallagher JJ. Balloon valvuloplasty in calcified aortic stenosis: A cause for caution and alarm. *Ann Thorac Surg 45*:515–525, 1988.

83. Di Mario C, Serruys PW, Luijten HE, de Feyter PJ, van den Brand M, Essed CE, Beatt KJ, Hugenholtz PG. Percutaneous balloon valvuloplasty in adult aortic stenosis: A palliative treatment but not without risk. *Cardiologia 32*:535–543, 1987.

84. Nishimura RA, Holmes DR Jr, Reeder GS, Ilstrup DM, Small RS, Tajik AJ. Hemodynamic results of percutaneous aortic balloon valvuloplasty as assessed by sequential Doppler echocardiographic studies. *Int J Cardiol 20*:317–326, 1988.

85. Come PC, Riley MF, McKay RG, Safian R. Echocardiographic assessment of aortic valve area in elderly patients with aortic stenosis and of changes in valve area after percutaneous balloon valvuloplasty. *J Am Coll Cardiol 10*:115–124, 1987.

86. Lembo NJ, King SB III, Roubin GS, Hammami A, Niederman AL. Fatal aortic rupture during percutaneous balloon valvuloplasty for valvular aortic stenosis. *Am J Cardiol 60*:733–736, 1987.

87. Segal J, Lerner DJ, Miller DC, Mitchell RS, Alderman EA, Popp RL. When should Doppler-determined valve area be better than the Gorlin formula?: Variation in hydraulic constants in low flow states. *J Am Coll Cardiol 9*:1295–1305, 1987.

88. Acar J, Vahanian A, Slama M, Cormier B, Michel PL, Luxereau P, Farah E, Leborgne O, Dermine P. Treatment of calcified aortic stenosis: Surgery or percutaneous transluminal aortic valvuloplasty? *Eur Heart J 9* (Suppl E):163–168, 1988.

89. Gaspar J, Cohn LH, Collins JJ Jr, Barry WH, Kern M, Mudge GH Jr. Overestimation of aortic stenosis with the Gorlin equation in low flow states. (abstract) *J Am Coll Cardiol 1*:639, 1983.

90. McKay RG, Safian EG, Lock JE, Diver DJ, Berman AD, Warren SE, Come PC, Baim DS, Mandall VE, Royal HD, Grossman W. Assessment of left ventricular and aortic valve function after aortic balloon valvuloplasty in adult patients with critical aortic stenosis. *Circulation 75*:192–203, 1987.

91. McKay RG, Safian RD, Berman AD, Diver DJ, Weinstein JS, Wyman RM, Cunningham MJ, McKay LL, Bain DS, Grossman W. Combined percutaneous aortic valvuloplasty and transluminal coronary angioplasty in adult patients with calcific aortic stenosis and coronary artery disease. *Circulation 76*:1298–1306, 1987.

92. Alexopoulos D, Sherman W. Unusual hemodynamic presentation of acute aortic regurgitation following percutaneous balloon valvuloplasty. *Am Heart J 116*:1622–1623, 1988.

93. Davidson CJ, Kisslo K, Burgess R, Bashore TM. Quantification of aortic regurgitation after balloon aortic valvuloplasty using videodensitometric analysis of digital subtraction aortography. *Am J Cardiol 63*:585–588, 1989.

94. Dean LS, Chandler JW, Saenz CB, Baxley WA, Bulle TM. Severe aortic regurgitation complicating percutaneous aortic valve valvuloplasty. *Cathet Cardiovasc Diagn 16*:130–132, 1989.

95. Drobinski G, Lechat Ph, Metzger J Ph, Lepailleur Cl, Vacheron A, Grosgogeat Y. Results of percutaneous catheter valvuloplasty for calcified aortic stenosis in the elderly. *Eur Heart J 8*:322–328, 1987.

96. Letac B, Cribier A, Koning R. Le traitement du retrecissement aortique acquis de l'adulte par valvuloplastie percutanee par catheter a ballonnet. *Arch Mal Coeur 82*:17–25, 1989.

97. Holmes DR Jr, Nishimura RA, Reeder GS, Wagner PJ, Ilstrup DM. Clinical follow-up after percutaneous aortic balloon valvuloplasty. *Arch Intern Med 149*:1405–1409, 1989.

98. Litvack F, Jakubowski AT, Buchbinder NA, Eigler N. Lack of sustained clinical improvement in an elderly population after percutaneous aortic valvuloplasty. *Am J Cardiol 62*:270–275, 1988.

99. Sherman W, Hershman R, Lazzam C, Cohen M, Ambrose J, Gorlin R. Balloon valvuloplasty in adult aortic stenosis: Determinants of clinical outcome. *Ann Int Med 110*:421–425, 1989.

100. Jackson G, Thomas S, Monaghan M, Forsyth A, Jewitt D. Inoperable aortic stenosis in the elderly: Benefit from percutaneous transluminal valvuloplasty. *Br Med J 294*:83–86, 1987.

101. Sievert H, Kramer P, Kober G, Bussmann WD, Kaltenbach M. Restenosis is a common feature of the angiographic follow-up after balloon valvuloplasty of calcified aortic stenoses. *Int J Cardiol 23*:179–183, 1989.

102. Seifert PE, Auer JE. Surgical repair of annular disruption following percutaneous balloon aortic valvuloplasty. *Ann Thorac Surg 46*:242–243, 1988.

103. Lewin RF, Dorros G, King JF, Seifert PE, Schmahl TM, Auer JE. Aortic annular tear after valvuloplasty: The role of aortic annulus echocardiographic measurement. *Cathet Cardiovasc Diagn 16*:123–129, 1989.

104. Vrolix M, Piessens J, Moerman P, Vanhaecke J, De Geest H. Fatal aortic rupture: An unusual complication of percutaneous balloon valvuloplasty for acquired valvular aortic stenosis. *Cathet Cardiovasc Diagn 16*:119–122, 1989.

105. Lemmer JH Jr, Winniford MD, Ferguson DW. Surgical implications of atrial septal defect complicating aortic balloon valvuloplasty. *Ann Thorac Surg 48*:295–297, 1989.

106. Davidson CJ, Skelton TN, Kisslo KB, Kong Y, Peter RH, Simonton CA, Phillips HR, Behar VS, Bashore TM. The risk for systemic embolization

associated with percutaneous balloon valvuloplasty in adults. *Ann Int Med 108*:557–560, 1988.

107. Deligonul U, Kern MJ, Bell SR, Gabliani G, Labovitz A, Vandormael M. Acute myocardial infarction during percutaneous aortic balloon valvuloplasty. *Cathet Cardiovasc Diagn 15*:164–168, 1988.

108. Cujec B, McMeekin J, Lopez J. Bacterial endocarditis after percutaneous aortic valvuloplasty. *Am Heart J 115*:178–179, 1988.

109. Kasten-Sportes CH, Piechaud JF, Sidi D, Kachaner J. Percutaneous balloon valvuloplasty in neonates with critical aortic stenosis. *J Am Coll Cardiol 13*:1101–1105, 1989.

110. Rupprath G, Neuhaus KL. Percutaneous balloon valvuloplasty for aortic valve stenosis in infancy. *Am J Cardiol 55*:1655–1656, 1985.

111. Roth RB, Palacios IF, Block PC. Percutaneous aortic balloon valvuloplasty: Its role in the management of patients with aortic stenosis requiring major noncardiac surgery. *J Am Coll Cardiol 13*: 1039–1041, 1989.

112. Levine MJ, Berman AD, Safian RD, Diver DJ, McKay RG. Palliation of valvular aortic stenosis by balloon valvuloplasty as preoperative preparation for noncardiac surgery. *Am J Cardiol 62*:1309–1310, 1988.

113. McKay CR, Waller BF, Hong R, Rubin N, Reid CL, Rahimtoola SH. Problems encountered with catheter balloon valvuloplasty of bioprosthetic aortic valves. *Am Heart J 115*:463–465, 1988.

114. Rashtian MY, Stevenson DM, Allen DT, Yoganathan AP, Harrison EC, Edmiston A, Faughan P, Rahimtoola SH. Flow characteristics of four commonly used mechanical heart valves. *Am J Cardiol 58*:743–752, 1986.

115. Morgan RJ, Davis JT, Fraker TD. Current status of valve prostheses. *Surg Clin North America 65*: 699–720, 1985.

116. Fernandez J. Surgical aspects of valve implantation. In: *Guide to Prosthetic Cardiac Valves.* ed by D Morse, R Steiner, and J Fernandez, New York, Springer-Verlag, 1985.

117. Bessone LN, Pupello DF, Hiro SP, Lopez-Cuenca E, Glatterer MS Jr, Ebra G. Surgical management of aortic valve disease in the elderly: A longitudinal analysis. *Ann Thorac Surg 46*:264–269, 1988.

118. Glock Y, Pecoul R, Cerene A, Laguerre J, Puel P. Aortic valve replacement in elderly patients. *J Cardiovasc Surg* (Torino) *25*:205–210, 1984.

119. Jones M, Barnhart GR, Morrow AG. Late results after operations for left ventricular outflow tract obstruction. *Am J Cardiol 50*:569–579, 1982.

120. Sandor GGS, Olley PM, Trusler GA, Williams WG, Rowe RD, Morch JE. Long-term follow-up of patients after valvotomy for congenital valvular aortic stenosis in children. *J Thorac Cardiovasc Surg 80*:171–176, 1980.

121. Davidson CJ, Harrison JK, Leithe ME, Kisslo KB,

Bashore TM. Failure of balloon aortic valvuloplasty to result in sustained clinical improvement in patients with depressed left ventricular function. *Am J Cardiol 65*:72–77, 1990.

122. Orme EC, Wray RB, Barry WH, Krueger SK, Mason JW. Comparison of three techniques for percutaneous balloon aortic valvuloplasty of aortic stenosis in adults. *Am Heart J 117*:11–17, 1989.

123. Brady ST, Davis CA, Kussmaul WG, Laskey WK, Hirshfeld JW, Herrmann HC. Percutaneous aortic balloon valvuloplasty in octogenarians: Morbidity and mortality. *Ann Int Med 110*:761–766, 1989.

124. Dodek A, Hooper RO, Kiess M. Percutaneous balloon valvuloplasty for aortic stenosis: Improved quality of life for elderly patients. *Can J Cardiol 4*: 223–227, 1988.

125. Rocha P, Baron B, Lacombe P, Bernier A, Kahn JC, Liot F, Bourdarias JP. Aortic percutaneous transluminal valvuloplasty in elderly patients by balloon larger than aortic anulus. *Cathet Cardiovasc Diagn 15*:81–88, 1988.

126. Vogt A, Rupprath G, Tebbe U, Neuhaus KL. Verlaufsbeobachtung nach dilatation angeborener und erworbener aortenstenosen. *Dtsch Med Wschr 113*:1956–1959, 1988.

127. Serruys PW, Luijten HE, Beatt KJ, Di Mario C, De Feyter PJ, Essed CE, Roelandt JRTC, Van Den Brand M. Percutaneous balloon valvuloplasty for calcific aortic stenosis. A treatment "sine cure"? *Eur Heart J 9*:782–794, 1988.

128. Beekman RH, Rocchini AP, Crowley DC, Snider AR, Serwer GA, Dick M II, Rosenthal A. Comparison of single and double balloon valvuloplasty in children with aortic stenosis. *J Am Coll Cardiol 12*: 480–485, 1988.

129. Walls JT, Lababidi Z, Curtis JJ, Silver D. Assessment of percutaneous balloon pulmonary and aortic valvuloplasty. *J Thorac Cardiovasc Surg 88*: 352–356, 1984.

130. Meliones JN, Beekman RH, Rocchini AP, Lacina SJ. Balloon valvuloplasty for recurrent aortic stenosis after surgical valvotomy in childhood: Immediate and follow-up studies. *J Am Coll Cardiol 13*: 1106–1110, 1989.

131. Sholler GF, Keane JF, Perry SB, Sanders SP, Lock JE. Balloon dilation of congenital aortic valve stenosis. Results and influence of technical and morphological features on outcome. *Circulation 78*:351–360, 1988.

PERCUTANEOUS MITRAL VALVOTOMY

10

Mitral Stenosis: The Anatomic Lesion and the Physiologic State

CHARLES F. WOOLEY, ELIZABETH A. SPARKS, and HARISIOS BOUDOULAS

Knowledge of mitral stenosis parallels the history of modern medicine and the development of cardiology as a discipline. From the earliest days of cardiac physical diagnosis (with inspection, palpation, percussion, and auscultation) to the most recent imaging technology, mitral stenosis might be called the cardiologist's touchstone.

Medical trainees have been indoctrinated with the clinical hallmarks of mitral stenosis for two centuries. Diagnostic methods have changed during this time, but the clinical consequences of the lesion are still devastating on a worldwide basis. The need for diagnostic precision is greater than ever as medical care comes to populations that have never received any care, the rheumatic fever scourge continues unabated in most of the world, and the therapeutic options for patients with mitral stenosis have increased.

From the pathophysiologic viewpoint, mitral stenosis makes sense. To be sure, there are gaps in precise understanding of the pathogenesis of the valve lesion involving the period from the initiating episode of rheumatic fever to the development of the stenotic lesion. Once the obstructive lesion has developed, however, there is a logic that forms an intellectual framework for modern understanding of almost all of the clinical consequences of mitral stenosis.

BACKGROUND

Richard C. Cabot wrote *Facts on the Heart* in 1926.[1] The book was based on 1906 necropsy records of patients with cardiac disease from the Massachusetts General Hospital between 1896 and 1919. Cabot then "worked back" into the corresponding clinical records. The result was the format that became internationally famous as the Case Records of the Massachusetts General Hospital published in *The New England Journal of Medicine*.

Cabot noted that the mitral valve was involved in 85% of patients with rheumatic heart disease and in over one-half of the cases mitral involvement occurred without any other valve lesion. The association of mitral stenosis with atrial fibrillation was clearly documented, and the fact that over half the cases were not recognized in life was a matter of great concern. Cabot was puzzled by the following: "The fact that only 55 out of 107 'pure-mitral' patients are known to have had any dyspnea at all before entering the hospital is surprising, indeed almost incredible." Another three decades would pass before the clear-cut definition of the role of pulmonary vascular resistance would become an integral part of the clinical understanding of symptoms in mitral stenosis.

Each diagnostic era produced original contributions and furthered our understanding. Documentation that acute rheumatic fever preceded the development of carditis, streptococcal pharyngitis was an etiologic link between the throat and the heart, and mitral stenosis was a late sequela of these events took the better part of three centuries.

The auscultatory era began in the early 19th century and proceeded at its own pace. The basic auscultatory tenets were developed long before the rheumatic carditis-mitral stenosis pathogenesis was clearly defined. Twentieth century cardiovascular technology in the form of the electrocardiogram showed abnormal P waves and clarified the state of the cardiac rhythm with the definition of sinus rhythm and atrial fibrillation. The chest x-ray and cardiac fluoroscopy provided objective evidence of significant disease with criteria for left atrial enlargement, pulmonary venous congestion, pulmonary artery hypertension, and right ventricular enlargement.

Phonocardiography provided an objective basis for the auscultatory phenomena that previously had been a purely descriptive art, transmitted from teacher to apprentice in the clinical setting. Accentuation and delay of the mitral component of the first heart sound (M_1), splitting of the second heart sound (S_2), the mitral opening snap (MOS), the interval between the aortic closure sound (A_2), and the mitral opening snap (A_2-MOS interval), the diastolic rumble, and the presystolic murmur all became part of the clinical diagnostic repertoire as a result of the auscultatory-phonocardiographic interface.

Pathogenesis

The chain that links the throat and the heart took centuries to identify. Streptococcal pharyngitis, acute rheumatic fever, rheumatic carditis, criteria for these diagnoses, and awareness of the valvular sequelae from these events in certain individuals were major steps in our understanding of the pathogenesis of rheumatic mitral stenosis.

Increased severity of the initial carditis has been associated with a poorer prognosis. Prospective cooperative studies showed that the frequency of mitral stenosis at 5 years after the initial carditis was related to the severity of the initial attack. The analysis at 10 years showed the emergence of another group of patients, predominantly female, whose initial mitral lesion was considered to be relatively mild but showed slow and progressive mitral stenosis without evidence of acute rheumatic fever or streptococcal disease. Stollerman[2] interpreted these observations to indicate undefined host factors that influence the course of valvular sclerosis once the mitral deformity has occurred, and that progression of rheumatic heart disease may be related to factors other than the rheumatic inflammation.

Clinical Pathologic Correlates

Just as the early surgical mitral commissurotomy experience stimulated a more critical assessment of basic mitral stenosis pathology, so too the valvulo-plasty and valvular repair era requires reconciliation of current clinical, physical diagnostic, graphic, imaging, hemodynamic, and pathologic thought.

Wallach, Borgatta, and Angrist presented an extensive pathology experience in 1962 from 509 autopsy identified patients with rheumatic heart disease.[3] The study originated in New York City, extended from 1936 to 1950, and the data were analyzed for their clinical implications in terms of morbidity and mortality. This pathologic study considered mitral valve disease during three individual time periods: prior to any medical therapy for rheumatic fever, during the time sulfa drugs were available, and during the time that penicillin was introduced. Clinically significant morbidity and mortality in the entire group came from heart failure, infectious endocarditis, atrial thrombi, and valvular and atrial sources of emboli.

Emphasis was placed on the large number of older patients, which is quite pertinent to current clinical experiences. While most clinical studies showed a preponderance of younger patients, studies based on autopsies indicated a higher incidence of older patients.

Severe mitral involvement increased with age and was present without calcification in 260 patients, 51% of the group, and with calcification in 36 patients, 7% of the group. Infectious endocarditis occurred in individuals with mild rheumatic mitral involvement. Nonbacterial thrombotic endocardial lesions (NBTE) occurred in 251 patients with severe mitral involvement without calcification and in 33 with calcification. Thrombi and infarcts in the kidney, brain, and spleen were more likely with severe mitral valvular involvement and occurred in 260 patients without calcification and in 36 with calcification.

The overall experience provides a window through which the transition from the nontherapeutic era of the rheumatic heart disease may be analyzed. The large number of elderly patients in this study has clinical relevance since the clinical presentation may be atypical and the diagnosis may not be considered in the older patient.

Latent Period

Davis[4] commented on the two major postulates about the latent period (Fig. 10.1) between the acute carditis and symptomatic chronic valve lesions—either a long period of "persistent grumbling valvulitis," or disease progression as a "purely hemodynamic effect . . . on a damaged and

LIFE HISTORY - MITRAL STENOSIS

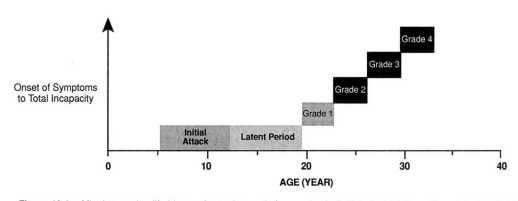

Figure 10.1. Mitral stenosis—life history. Acute rheumatic fever episode (initial attack) followed by a latent period. The onset, duration, and progression of symptoms from grade 1 to grade 4 clinical status are illustrated. Figure constructed from data of Wood.[6]

morphologically abnormal valve." He concluded that both views may be true in part, the former in young people developing symptoms within 10 years of the acute episode, the latter in patients with a prolonged latent period up to 40 years.

Clinical Awareness of Stages of Valvular Pathology

The stages of valvular pathology have assumed even greater significance in recent times. Pure commissural fusion, commoner in younger patients, results in a mobile diaphragm with minimal cusp thickening without calcification. Clinical correlates include classical auscultatory findings with an accentuated first heart sound and a prominent opening snap from a valve that is amenable to valvotomy.

Conversely, dense cusp fibrosis results in a thickened stenotic valve with reduced cusp mobility and a propensity for calcification. Auscultatory phenomena that depend on valve mobility—the accentuated M_1 and the MOS—are diminished or, with severe involvement, may be absent.

Calcification occurs at the commissures as dense, solid masses and along the closure lines as bands or linear patterns.[5] Eruption of calcium through the endothelial surface produces ulcerated areas, which can be sites of thrombus formation. The thrombi may be a source for emboli and may also provide a mechanism for supplying additional

calcium to the dynamic calcification process within the stenotic valve. Chordal fibrosis and fusion may also result in subvalvular obstruction as a result of a fixed fibrous tunnel below the fused mitral cusps.

The overall clinical assessment of the patient with mitral stenosis requires awareness of the multiple aspects and stages of valve involvement—mitral cusp thickening, commissural fusion, commissural or leaflet calcification, endothelial and valve surface phenomena, chordal fusion with subvalvular obstruction, and the resultant degrees of mobility or rigidity of the stenotic valve unit.

MEDICAL HISTORY AND CLINICAL SYMPTOMS—AN APPRECIATION OF PAUL WOOD

It is a bit humbling to read Paul Wood's 1954 classic "An Appreciation of Mitral Stenosis,"[6] which probably should be required reading for anyone interested in the diagnosis and management of patients with mitral stenosis. This was written at the beginning of the modern era in cardiovascular medicine and surgery, a time of great ferment in cardiovascular disease. Wood studied 300 patients with mitral disease "intensively" with emphasis on clinical features, and hemodynamic and surgical correlates and left a powerful legacy for clinicians. The 150 patients who had mitral valvotomy constituted the surgical group and provided Wood with an independent analysis of diagnostic data, one of the first such experiences in modern cardiology.

Wood classified patients into groups based on the anatomic lesion and the physiologic state, stressing that the combined approach was best. The spectrum of anatomic mitral stenosis lesions and certain of the clinical correlates were considered earlier. Physiologically, Wood found the most important factor was the pulmonary vascular resistance which to a large extent determined the course and pattern of the disease.

Effort intolerance due to dyspnea was an important symptom that Wood used for grading patients and relating the symptom progression to the severity of disease. Introduction of a functional classification with hemodynamic and surgical correlates provided a partial answer to Cabot's 1926 query and a rational basis for natural history studies and assessment of therapy (Fig. 10.1). Breathlessness was closely associated with pulmonary venous congestion. Orthopnea and paroxysmal cardiac dyspnea were frequent with significant disease; however, 78% of patients with high pulmonary vascular resistance had neither orthopnea nor paroxysmal cardiac dyspnea. This led Wood to the conclusion that if extreme pulmonary vascular resistance developed in mitral stenosis, it did so at a relatively early stage.

Pulmonary edema tended to occur in relatively young women with tight stenosis when the pulmonary vascular resistance was usually low and the potential for developing extremely high pressures in the pulmonary venous system existed. In this situation, hemoptysis was a relatively early symptom while it was rare when the pulmonary arterial resistance was high. Blood-streaked sputum associated with attacks of severe dyspnea was common in patients coming to valvular surgery. Dyspnea and pulmonary venous congestion were closely related, and the degree of radiographic pulmonary venous congestion was proportional to left atrial pressure.

Wood was aware of Gorlin's work published in 1951,[7] which changed the way cardiologists thought about mitral stenosis and valvular disease in general. Gorlin's approach to the calculation of a stenotic valve orifice area from hemodynamic data using hydraulic principles brought cardiac valve dynamics to clinical consciousness. Measurement of transvalvular pressure gradients, cardiac output, and transvalvular flow became part of the hemodynamic revolution in valvular heart disease and was of particular import to the study of mitral stenosis. As a result of the introduction of cardiac catheterization techniques and the use of careful measurements of cardiovascular variables, mitral stenosis was described in universally accepted hemodynamic terms and moved from a pathologic entity with auscultatory, radiographic, and electrocardiographic expressions to a dynamic entity described in terms of left atrial hypertension, a pressure gradient across the mitral valve, reduced cardiac output at rest or with effort, a calculated mitral valve area, and altered pulmonary vascular resistance.

Angina pectoris was present in 12% of Wood's patients, mostly young women in the surgery group; the symptom was associated with extreme valvular stenosis or high pulmonary vascular resistance. Wood believed that the pain was due to functional insufficiency of coronary blood flow from limitation of cardiac output. The coexistence of coronary artery disease and mitral stenosis should be considered in other patient populations who experience angina pectoris as part of their symptom complex, particularly those with high-risk coronary disease profiles and the older patient group.

Systemic embolization occurred in 14% of the surgical group. Emboli were classified as cerebral, peripheral, visceral, or both cerebral and peripheral. The cardiac rhythm was atrial fibrillation in two-thirds of the patients with embolic phenomena. No correlation was found between the incidence of embolism and the pulmonary vascular resistance, cardiac output, or the mitral valve area. Embolism was the first symptom in 13% of the patients with emboli. At surgery, clots were found in the left atrium in 21% of those with a history of emboli and 22% with no history of emboli. Embolism was an immediate complication of mitral valvotomy in 10% of the surgical patients. The tragic consequences of cerebral emboli in a group composed predominantly of young women have long been a devastating part of the mitral stenosis legacy.

Winter bronchitis was a common phenomenon in Wood's British series, was usually not a feature of mild cases, and was probably related to a state of chronic pulmonary venous congestion. Respiratory illnesses continue to produce onset or aggravation of symptoms in patients with mitral stenosis, and recovery time may be prolonged.

Chronic atrial fibrillation occurred in 41% of the surgical patients in Wood's series. These patients were older than those in sinus rhythm, 41 years versus 33 years of age, with larger left atrial size, lower cardiac output, and higher pulmonary vascular resistance. The mitral orifice size did not correlate with the presence of atrial fibrillation. Atrial fibrillation with rapid ventricular response may cause the onset of severe symptoms in previously mildly symptomatic patients, with development of intense dyspnea or congestive heart failure, as well as contributing to morbidity and mortality from embolic phenomena.

The symptom pattern that results from the onset of atrial fibrillation depends on a variety of factors and not merely on the degree of stenosis. With normal pulmonary vascular resistance, the onset of rapid ventricular response interfering with left ventricular diastolic filling will increase pulmonary venous congestion. Conversely, with high pulmonary vascular resistance, the onset of atrial fibrillation may contribute to right ventricular failure, which then dominates the clinical picture. Recent studies of the role of atrial natriuretic factor (ANF) in mitral stenosis have shown that ANF secretion is different in patients with atrial fibrillation when compared with patients in sinus rhythm, so that neurohumoral factors may also be operative.

Mitral stenosis is a heterogeneous disorder with multiple anatomic and physiologic features. The informed clinical history from the patient with mitral stenosis is the source of a great deal of information about the patient's pathophysiologic state, which in turn forms the basis for a rational classification. Careful analysis of the clinical history should provide answers to the eternal questions—Why is this patient here? And, why now?

MITRAL STENOSIS—SOME PHYSICAL DIAGNOSTIC PEARLS

The mitral facies described by Wood[6] referred to the presence of peripheral cyanosis in the face (and hands) and occurred in patients with high pulmonary vascular resistance, low and fixed cardiac output, and peripheral vasoconstriction. It is probably related to the consequences of marked pulmonary hypertension and may be seen with other causes of these physiologic responses.

The arterial pulse may be regular and normal, or it may be irregular and reveal the presence of atrial fibrillation. The differential diagnosis of atrial fibrillation should bring mitral stenosis to the mind of the examiner at this stage of the examination.

Jugular venous pulse dynamics are normal when right heart dynamics are normal, or altered with pulmonary arterial hypertension with a prominent A wave (reflecting elevated right ventricular end diastolic pressure), or with a prominent V wave when tricuspid regurgitation occurs. As with the examination of the arterial pulse, an irregular jugular pulse with absence of A waves should trigger thoughts of atrial fibrillation and, by association, of mitral stenosis.

The apex impulse may be striking, with a palpable loud first heart sound preceded by a diastolic thrill. These findings may be best appreciated with the patient in the left lateral recumbent position.

Bimanual precordial palpation, an extremely valuable diagnostic technique in all circumstances, is particularly so in combined left heart—right heart disorders such as mitral stenosis. With the examiner's right hand at the left ventricular apex impulse, slip the examining left hand along the lower left sternal border—the abnormal and forceful right ventricular impulse will be felt with the fingertips.

Now slide the left hand over the pulmonary artery impulse, feel for the pulmonic closure sound, then move the right hand from the apical impulse over the right ventricular impulse, watching the jugular venous pulse all the while. Simultaneous palpation of the sustained right ventricular impulse and a palpable pulmonary valve closure sound are consistent with right ventricular and pulmonary artery hypertension. Conversely, absence of these phenomena suggests normal right heart pressures.

This complete right heart survey requires the examiner to consider the presence or absence of pulmonary artery hypertension and elevates the physical examination to the physiologic level. It is quite possible to make the clinical diagnosis of mitral stenosis by palpation combined with thoughtful inspection and to arrive at an estimate of pulmonary vascular resistance in most patients with hemodynamically significant mitral stenosis and a mobile valve unit.

STETHOSCOPE: THE INSTRUMENT OF FIRST RESORT

Barlow, Lakier, and Pocock[8] described auscultation as "an accurate, convenient, practicable, and inexpensive method of diagnosing mitral stenosis." The auscultator's intent should include the evaluation of the degree of mitral stenosis, the mobility of the mitral complex, and the presence of mitral regurgitation or pulmonary hypertension. The use of postural maneuvers, particularly the left lateral recumbent position, with auscultation at the apex impulse and gentle application of the bell of the stethoscope, remains an important part of the auscultatory approach to the diastolic murmurs of mitral stenosis.

Wood[6] found the first heart sound to be loud in 90% of patients with pure mitral stenosis in sinus rhythm and considered the finding excellent evidence of mitral stenosis but of limited indication as to degree. The presystolic murmur was also a valuable sign of mitral stenosis but not its degree. Both auscultatory findings were evidence against significant mitral regurgitation. When the pulmonic component of the second sound was normal, pulmonary vascular resistance was normal in 80% of the patients, while two-thirds of patients with accentuated pulmonic closure sound had high pulmonary vascular resistance. The mitral opening snap signified stenosis, was one of the most important signs of dominant stenosis, and, like the loud first heart sound, was considered an excellent talisman against serious mitral regurgitation.

Generally speaking, auscultation as part of a careful, thoughtful cardiovascular examination is highly accurate in the identification of those mitral stenosis patients with preservation of the mitral valve unit mobility, a reasonably normal cardiac output, and sinus rhythm. Auscultatory precision is diminished in patients with valvular calcification, rigid and immobile valve cusps, atrial fibrillation, high pulmonary vascular resistance, and low cardiac output. Auscultatory precision is further enhanced when graphic methods such as phonocardiography (Fig. 10.2) or echophonocardi-

ography methods are used to provide an objective benchmark for a descriptive clinical skill.

M_1 and the Mitral Opening Snap

The auscultatory phenomena associated with mitral stenosis had been defined for the most part by the 19th-century clinicians who used pathologic correlations as the benchmark. Auscultation was a descriptive clinical skill until the advent of phonocardiography in the early 20th century.

Thomas Lewis[9] recorded heart sounds and murmurs in patients with mitral stenosis using the method of Einthoven, which added a second string galvanometer to the one used for the ECG, and the images of the two strings that recorded the ECG and the heart sounds were projected, side by side, upon the same camera. Lewis's paper contained records (Fig. 10.3) of remarkable clarity and dealt primarily with murmur timing and dynamics.

The recording and timing of these physiologic events with graphic methods marked a transition period in cardiology. Auscultation was linked to phonocardiography, and the technology that was used to determine the time relations for heart sounds and murmurs brought physiology from the laboratory to the bedside.

In 1922, Yandell Henderson[10] examined a postmortem excised stenotic mitral valve preparation with intact chordae, performed mechanical studies, and observed that the stenosed valve formed a funnel "which after being pushed down toward the ventricle during auricular systole, must

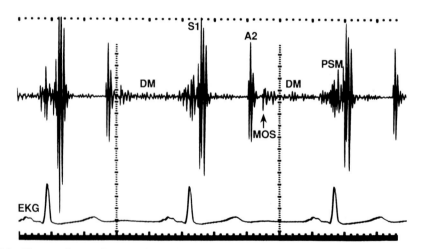

Figure 10.2. Phonocardiogram from a patient with mitral stenosis. S1 = accentuated mitral component of first heart sound; A2 = aortic component, second heart sound; MOS = mitral opening snap; DM = diastolic murmur; PSM = presystolic murmur.

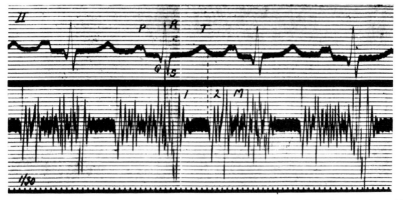

Figure 10.3. Early phonocardiogram from the work of Thomas Lewis, published in 1913.[9] Top panel: Lead II of the ECG with P, Q, R, S, and T waves. Lower panel: Phonocardiogram with S_1 (1), S_2 (2), and diastolic murmur (m). See text for details.

inevitably be subject to a considerable backlash or upthrow toward the auricle, at the onset of ventricular contraction." Henderson contrasted these motions with the dynamics of normal valves, which he and Johnson had been studying. He referred to the "terminal jerk of the . . . funnel as it comes taut," described and illustrated the systolic and diastolic positions of the mitral funnel in a fluid system (Fig. 10.4), and speculated on the association of the funnel dynamics and the auscultatory events. We will return to this observation shortly.

Margolies and Wolferth[11] published a fundamental article in 1932 that incorporated a historical review of the mitral opening snap that began with the original descriptions by the 19th-century French auscultators through the ECG-phonocardiographic studies of the first three decades of the 20th century. They traced the origins of the hypothesis that the opening snap was a sound of valvular origin due to limitation of the opening movement of the stenosed mitral valve and not part of the reduplicated second heart sound. Their own meticulous recordings led to graphic and temporal definition of the A_2-MOS interval; variations in this interval during atrial fibrillation; and a clear differentiation of the MOS from reduplication of S_2, gallop sounds, and systolic clicks. They concluded that all available evidence confirmed Rouches' 1988 hypothesis that the MOS was identified in time with sudden curtailment of the opening movement of the stenotic mitral valve.

The matter rested there for the most part until the mid-20th century when cardiac catheterization, angiography, and surgery transformed cardiology in ways that have yet to be completely analyzed. Correlative cineangiographic heart sound studies,[12] intracardiac manometer sound and pressure studies at surgery[13] and in the cardiac catheterization laboratory,[14] and echophonocardiographic studies,[15] which related cineangiographic and echophonocardiographic data, provided the basis for much of our current understanding. Advances in echo-Doppler techniques[16–20] extended, amplified, and, in certain instances, clarified these observations.

M_1, the MOS, the diastolic murmur, and the presystolic murmur were related to left atrial pressure pulse morphology, the timing of left atrial-left ventricular pressure pulse crossover, motion of the stenosed mitral valve unit, and the mitral valve diastolic pressure gradient.

Mitral Dome Excursion at M_1 and the MOS—The Concept of Reciprocal Heart Sounds

As Henderson[10] noted, the fused, stenotic yet mobile mitral complex frequently assumes a characteristic domed shape during diastole (Fig. 10.4). The MOS occurs in early ventricular diastole when movement of the mitral dome into the left ventricle terminates abruptly at the limit of the valve complex excursion. Conversely, the delayed and accentuated M_1 occurs in early ventricular systole when the excursion of the fused mitral complex toward the left atrium terminates abruptly. These observations led to the concept that the delayed and accentuated M_1 and the MOS of mitral stenosis were paired or reciprocal heart sounds,[13] which were explainable in terms of abrupt termination of the fused mitral complex.

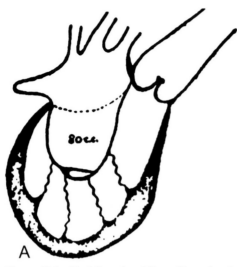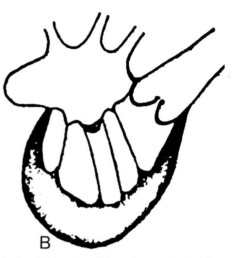

Figure 10.4. Diastolic and systolic positions of a stenotic mitral valve in a fluid system. Schematic reconstructed from mechanical studies by Henderson[10] of an excised stenotic mitral valve. Left; **A,** the stenosed mitral valve formed a "funnel," which was pushed down toward the ventricle during auricular systole; 80 cc: estimated volume in funnel. Right; **B,** movement of the stenosed mitral valve toward the auricle at the onset of ventricular contraction.

Figure 10.5. Echophonocardiograms recorded in the parasternal long-axis view. Top: labeled PLA - S_1. At the time of M_1, the mitral component of the first heart sound, S_1; LV = left ventricle; MV = mitral valve; LA = left atrium; Ao = aorta. Arrow indicates phonocardiogram at M_1. Bottom: At the time of the mitral opening snap labeled PLA - OS. Arrow indicates phonocardiogram at OS, the mitral opening snap.

The stenotic mitral valve (MV) motion toward the left atrium terminated at M_1 (top). The mitral valve dome shape may be appreciated (bottom); the MOS was recorded at termination of mitral dome motion into the left ventricle.

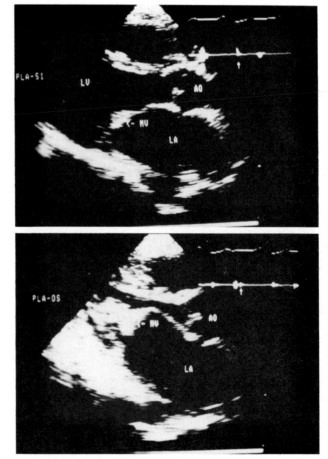

Henderson's mechanical studies and insights, together with the studies referenced previously, provided Barrington[21] with an approach to the mechanisms of the accentuated, delayed M_1, and the MOS, using echophonocardiographic methods. These studies confirmed the simultaneity of MOS with termination of mitral dome movement into the left ventricle and of M_1 with termination of mitral complex excursion toward the left atrium (Fig. 10.5).

When the distinctive left atrial and mitral dome conformational and dimensional changes at M_1 and MOS were quantitated, significant, dynamic changes in mitral dome area and length occurred from M_1 to MOS. The converse, a decrease in mitral dome area and length, occurred from MOS to M_1 (Fig. 10.6). The conformational and dimensional changes that terminated abruptly at the MOS

reversed and terminated abruptly at the time of the delayed and accentuated M_1. These findings strengthen the hypothesis that the hemodynamic and dome motion mechanisms are paired or reciprocal in nature, and that the delayed, accentuated M_1 and MOS are reciprocal cardiovascular sounds.

Dynamic Pressure and Sound Correlates in Mitral Stenosis

LEFT ATRIUM

The left atrial response to mitral stenosis includes left atrial hypertension, left atrial enlargement, increased left atrial volume, alterations in the left atrial contraction-relaxation pattern, and abnormalities in the left atrial pressure pulse.

Analysis of the left atrial pressure pulse in patients with mitral stenosis in sinus rhythm

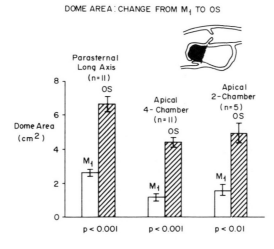

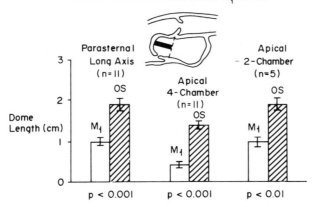

Figure 10.6. Change in dome area (cm²) from the mitral component (M_1) of the first heart sound to the mitral opening snap (OS) is shown on the left. Change in dome length (cm) from M_1 to OS is shown on the right. See text for further details.

recorded with manometer catheters (Fig. 10.7) showed that the height of the A wave was greater than normal, the peak A wave pressure was reached later, and the atrial relaxation phase was interrupted by the initial left ventricular pressure rise.[22] This prolongation of the mechanographic left atrial contraction time is consistent with prolongation of atrial systole in mitral stenosis. This observation in patients is also consistent with experimental models of mitral stenosis in dogs[23] where augmented atrial activity was manifested by elevated left atrial pressure and increased magnitude of left atrial contraction, "indicating the increased vigor and duration of atrial contraction secondary to augmented outflow resistance."[24]

In addition to the prominent A wave, there was fusion of the "A" wave and the "C" wave, with a brisk descent following C peak, and a broader,

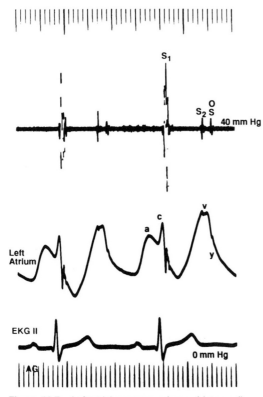

Figure 10.7. Left atrial pressure pulse and intracardiac phonocardiogram from a patient with severe mitral stenosis. Intracardiac manometer recording of: phonocardiogram, (top) S_1 = mitral component of first heart sound; S_2 = aortic component, second heart sound; OS = mitral opening snap; left atrial pressure pulse (left atrium) with A, C, V waves, y descent; bottom: electrocardiogram, lead II. Scale 0–40 mm Hg at right. Time lines = 40 msec. Note fusion of A–C waves, interruption of A wave descent by C wave. See text.

occasionally taller V wave (Fig. 10.7). M_1 began with the C peak and accompanied the rapid fall in atrial pressure following C peak. Normally the left ventricle does not contract until left atrial systole is completed, and the left atrial A and C waves are separate events. Fusion of the atrial A-C waves in mitral stenosis reflects the overlap of the prolonged atrial contraction-relaxation process with initial ventricular contraction.[22] As will be seen, these temporal relationships have a significant effect on clinical phenomena that are related to atrial performance, the presystolic murmur, the initial left ventricular contraction pattern, and late ventricular diastolic filling, which paradoxically extends into the early ventricular systole.

The aortic component of the second heart sound, A_2, occurred with a notch at the V wave peak of the left atrial pressure pulse. After ventricular systole, the left atrial pressure fell from the peak of the V wave in a relatively rapid fashion and terminated abruptly at the opening snap notch, which coincided with the MOS. These temporal relationships are an integral part of the left heart dynamics in mitral stenosis and reflect the mitral dome dynamics during the A_2-MOS interval.

Left atrial dynamics are an integral part of the hemodynamic background for understanding the left atrial, mitral valve, and left ventricular interrelationships that underlie the clinical phenomena of mitral stenosis and form a basis for studying left atrial dysfunction in chronic mitral stenosis.

LEFT VENTRICLE

The time interval from the Q wave of the ECG to the onset of left ventricular pressure pulse rise was normal (avg = 33 msec) in patients with mitral stenosis (Fig. 10.8). However, from this time on the left ventricular pressure pulse rise was abnormal. The left ventricular pressure pulse consisted of a two-phase pressure rise—an initial slow phase from initial pressure rise to the time of the M_1 (avg = 70 msec) followed by a brief interval of rapid pressure rise prior to ventricular ejection[13] (Fig. 10.8).

The delayed, accentuated M_1 was recorded with the break in the ventricular pressure pulse rise. The diastolic portion of the ventricular pressure pulse was characterized by absence of the atrial A wave, that is, absence of the atrial kick. The diastolic murmur was localized to discrete areas within the left ventricle. When the presystolic murmur was recorded, this portion of the murmur occurred during the initial left ventricular pressure pulse rise and extended into the M_1.

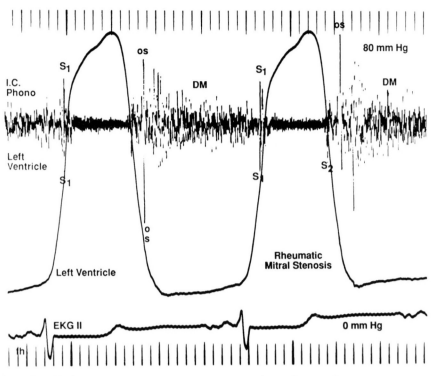

Figure 10.8.   Left ventricular pressure pulse and intracardiac phonocardiogram from a patient with severe mitral stenosis. Intracardiac manometer recording of: Top: Intracardiac phonocardiogram - IC phono from the left ventricle, with S_1 = mitral component of first heart sound, OS = mitral opening snap; DM = diastolic murmur. Middle: Left ventricular pressure pulse. Bottom: Electrocardiogram, lead II. Scale: 0–80 mm Hg at right. Time lines = 40 msec. Note change in left ventricular pressure pulse at S_1, also, timing of S_1 and OS. Diastolic murmur was recorded in the left ventricle. See text; also Figures 10.9 and 10.11.

The simultaneity of the break in the rise of the ventricular pressure pulse and the recording of the accentuated M_1 can be demonstrated as part of the clinical evaluation with simple graphic recordings of the apex impulse and the simultaneous phonocardiogram (Fig. 10.9).

MITRAL VALVE—PHYSICAL PROPERTIES

Certain fundamental differences in physical properties exist between the normal mitral valve and the stenotic mitral valve, and between the noncalcific stenotic valve and the calcific stenotic mitral valve.[5] These are illustrated in graphic form in Figure 10.10. There was a significant and progressive increase in weight from normal mitral valves to stenotic, noncalcific valves, and from stenotic, noncalcific valves to stenotic valves with advanced calcification. Similarly, there were progressive increases in volume, specific gravity, and weight per area, with corresponding decreases in fixed orifice size with each comparison. Fixed orifice size was inversely related to the extent of calcification, and measured orifice areas in advanced calcific

stenotic valves were quite small with an average of 0.5 cm².

The altered physical properties of the stenotic mitral valves influence clinical expression in a variety of ways. The obvious clinical implications include alterations in valve mobility and mobility-related phenomena such as intensity and presence of the M_1 and MOS at auscultation, more severe obstruction with very small fixed orifice size in the heavily calcified valves, and regional changes in mitral dome dynamics with progressive calcification that may be appreicated with imaging techniques.

LEFT ATRIAL, LEFT VENTRICULAR, AND MITRAL VALVE INTERACTIONS

Certain of the temporal and hemodynamic changes that occur during the cardiac cycle between the left atrium and the left ventricle with the stenotic mitral valve at the interface are shown in a schematic form in Figure 10.11. The left atrial (LA) pressure pulse tracing is shown, and the A, C,

Mitral Stenosis

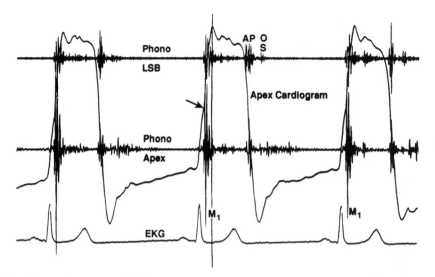

Figure 10.9. Apex cardiogram recorded from a patient with moderately severe mitral stenosis. Top to bottom: External phonocardiogram (phono) at left sternal border (LSB); external phonocardiogram (phono) at cardiac apex; apex cardiogram, an external pulse tracing of left ventricular dynamics; and bottom—electrocardiogram. M_1 = mitral component of the first heart sound; A-P = aortic and pulmonic components of second heart sound; OS = mitral opening snap. Arrow indicates the change in left ventricular pressure rise at the time of M_1.

Figure 10.10. Mitral stenosis—physical characteristics of mitral valves. Control = normal mitral valve; no calcification = stenotic mitral valve, noncalcific; calcification = stenotic mitral valve, calcific. Comparison of weight in grams top left; mitral valve volume (cm^3) top right; specific gravity (g cm^{-3}) bottom left; mitral valve area (orifice) (cm^2) bottom right.

Note significant, progressive increase in weight, volume, and specific gravity from control to mitral stenosis (no calcification) to mitral stenosis (calcification). Mitral valve area was significantly decreased in stenotic, calcified valves.

Mitral Stenosis
Physical Characteristics

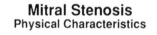

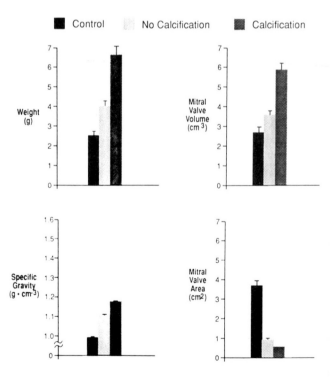

and V waves and x and y descents are labeled. The left ventricular (LV) pressure pulse is indicated. Below the pressure pulses is a representation of the heart sounds with M_1, A_2, and the MOS.

The cardiac pressure and sound relations are based on intracardiac double manometer tracings and may be thought of as a simple superimposition of the atrial and ventricular pressure pulses analyzed previously.

Left ventricular pressure crossed left atrial pressure on the upstroke of the left atrial C wave. M_1 occurred after the pressure crossover when left ventricular pressure was appreciably higher than left atrial pressure. The change in the rise of the left ventricular pressure pulse, the maximal vibrations of M_1, and the rapid pressure fall in the atrial pressure after C peak were practically simultaneous.

A_2 occurred at the appropriate time during left ventricular pressure fall and was simultaneous with the V wave peak of the atrial pressure pulse. Ventricular pressure fell below atrial pressure between the V peak and the opening snap notch of the left atrial pressure pulse. Following pressure crossover, left ventricular and left atrial pressure fell together until the left atrial pressure fall was

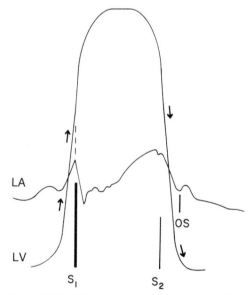

Figure 10.11. Mitral stenosis—pressure pulse and sound correlates. Schematic illustration that incorporates elements of Figures 10.7, 10.8, and 10.9. Top to bottom: LA = left atrial pressure pulse; LV = left ventricular pressure pulse; phonocardiogram; S_1 = mitral component of first heart sound; S_2 = aortic component of second heart sound; OS = mitral opening snap.

Arrow indicates break in left ventricular pressure pulse rise; dotted lines indicate near-simultaneity of this change in left ventricular pressure pulse, rapid deflections in left atrial pressure pulse, and S_1, mitral component of the first heart sound.

checked at the opening snap notch. Left atrial pressure was appreciably higher than left ventricular pressure at the time of the opening snap notch and the MOS.

Left Ventricular-Left Atrial Crossover Dynamics

Left ventricular-left atrial crossover dynamics (Figs. 10.11 and 10.12) involve the time domain, an area that has been neglected in the contemporary imaging era.[13] The time interval from the Q wave of the ECG to the onset of left ventricular pressure rise is normal; however, from that point on left ventricular pressure pulse dynamics are altered in mitral stenosis. The left ventricle spends an inordinate amount of time during its initial phases of contraction driving the mitral dome or fused membrane from the left ventricle toward the left atrium, and it does so against the resistance from the mitral dome and the elevated left atrial pressure.[13–21] It takes approximately 70 msec for the left ventricle to exceed left atrial pressure, complete the movement of the fused, stenotic mitral unit, and generate the accentuated M_1. The pressure differential at this time is approximately 14 mm Hg, ventricle exceeding atrium.[13]

Conversely, following the aortic valve closure, indicated by A_2, the mitral dome or fused unit moves toward the ventricle as left ventricular pressure falls, crosses left atrial pressure at a point between left atrial V wave peak, continues to fall below atrial pressure, and is approximately 14 mm Hg below atrial pressure at the time of the MOS.[13]

The left ventricular and left atrial pressure, time relationships, and crossover dynamics are of clinical interest since they provide the basis for understanding the genesis and timing of the abnormal heart sounds and murmurs of mitral stenosis, and an explanation for certain aspects of left atrial and left ventricular dysfunction that occur in patients with mitral stenosis.

SOUNDS OF MITRAL STENOSIS

Correlation of Barrington's echophonocardiographic mitral dome excursion studies[21] with pressure pulse-crossover studies[13,22] and the accumulated wisdom from the investigators mentioned previously permits improved understanding of the heart sounds of mitral stenosis (Fig. 10.13).

M_1 DELAY

Prolongation of the Q-M_1 interval, the time from the Q wave of the ECG to the mitral component of the first heart sound, is related primarily to the delay in the left ventricular pressure rise associated with movement of the mitral dome or fused membrane toward the left atrium in the presence of left atrial hypertension, influenced by the inertia of the mitral dome or fused membrane.

M_1 ACCENTUATION

In the presence of a left ventricular-left atrial pressure gradient, M_1 accentuation is associated with termination of stenotic valve excursion with rapid deflections in left atrial and ventricular pressure pulses at a time when left atrial and ventricular pressures are much higher than normal. The physical characteristics of the stenosed mitral valve are also important contributing factors since the stenotic valve is heavier, with increased volume and specific gravity. These characteristics doubtless contribute initially to dome inertia and later to valve tension changes at the end of the valve excursion toward the left atrium.

MITRAL OPENING SNAP

The circumstances that occur with the MOS are similar yet opposite to those at M_1. The MOS occurs at a discrete time interval after left ventricular-left atrial pressure crossover with a pressure gradient approximately equal in magnitude and opposite in direction to that occurring at M_1. MOS occurs at a time of abrupt changes in left atrial and left ventricular pressure pulse dynamics with rapid fluctuations in mitral dome tension that occur when the stenotic mitral valve reaches the limit of excursion toward the left ventricle.

Thus clinical auscultation of the sounds of mitral stenosis provides the examiner with a series of insights into the mitral valve physical characteristics, as well as left atrial and left ventricular dynamic performance in patients with mitral stenosis. When these auscultatory phenomena are recorded with graphic methods such as echo- or Doppler phonocardiography, the auscultator's diagnostic precision improves significantly.

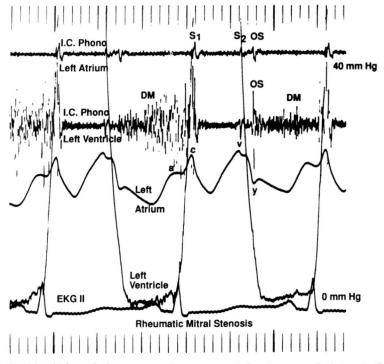

Figure 10.12.   Left atrial and left ventricular pressure pulse crossover relations in severe mitral stenosis. Two-manometer study, first manometer recording sound and pressure in left atrium, second manometer recording sound and pressure in the left ventricle. Top to bottom: Intracardiac sound (IC phono) in left atrium—S_1 = mitral component first heart sound; S_2 = aortic component of S_2; OS = mitral opening snap. Intracardiac sound (IC phono) left ventricle—DM = diastolic murmur; OS = mitral opening snap. Left atrial pressure pulse (left atrium)—A, C, V waves and y descent. Left ventricular pressure pulse. Bottom: Electrocardiogram lead II. Scale 0–40 mm Hg, right border. Time lines 40 msec.

Note the diastolic murmur was recorded in the left ventricle; in the first two complexes the diastolic murmur continued into a "presystolic" murmur.

See text under left ventricular-left atrial crossover dynamics.

Mitral Stenosis
Pressure Pulse, Sound, Echo Correlates

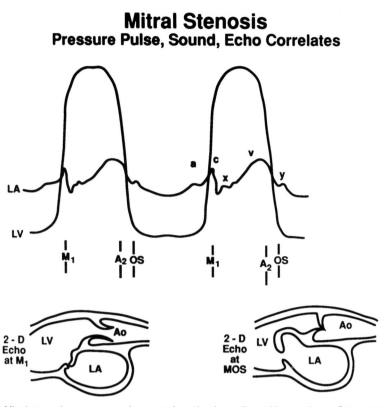

Figure 10.13. Mitral stenosis—pressure pulse, sound, and echocardiographic correlates. Schematic incorporating elements of Figures 10.5, 10.7, 10.8, 10.11, and 10.12. LA = left atrial pressure pulse with A, C, V waves, x and y descents; LV = left ventricular pressure pulse.
    Heart sounds: M_1 = mitral component of first heart sound; S_2 = aortic component of second heart sound; OS = mitral opening snap.
    Bottom left: Two-dimensional echo at M_1. Bottom right: Two-dimensional echo at OS. LA = left atrium; LV = left ventricle; Ao = aorta. See text under the sounds of mitral stenosis.

Murmurs of Mitral Stenosis

The loud first heart sound, M_1, the intensity of the pulmonary valve closure sound, P_2, and the MOS provide the auscultatory framework for the timing and recording of the mitral diastolic murmur and the mitral presystolic murmur (Figs. 10.2, 10.8, and 10.12).

Wood[6] placed emphasis on the length as well as the intensity of the mitral diastolic murmur. A prolonged mitral diastolic murmur reflects persistence of the pressure gradient across the mitral valve throughout a longer portion of diastole (Fig. 10.12). The diastolic murmur is related to turbulent blood flow across the stenotic mitral orifice, and the duration and intensity are affected by the severity of the obstruction and the volume of flow across the valve, factors that are also the basis for hemodynamic calculations of the mitral valve area. The externally recorded diastolic murmur follows the mitral opening snap and occurs during maxi-

mal ventricular filling. Craige[25] used echophonocardiography with other noninvasive pulse recordings such as the carotid pulse and apexcardiogram to mesh electrical, mechanical, acoustic, and imaging techniques to demonstrate the "characteristic galaxy of physical signs in mitral stenosis," and these approaches are adaptable to echo-Doppler studies as well.

The mitral presystolic murmur (Figs. 10.2, 10.8 and 10.12) occurs in a complex setting as can be appreciated from the atrial, valvular, and ventricular dynamics described previously. Criley[26,27] analyzed ventricular filling in mitral stenosis, which continues during the initial ventricular pressure rise until ventricular pressure exceeds atrial pressure and the fused mitral unit or dome has reached the termination of excursion toward the left atrium and M_1 has occurred. High velocity flow through a narrow orifice valve that is moving toward a "closed" position provides the setting for the "presystolic" murmur,[28] which is dependent on atrial and ventricular dynamics for its genesis and also may be present in patients in atrial fibrillation.[26]

CLINICAL DETERMINANTS IN MITRAL STENOSIS (Fig. 10.14)
Impact on the Clinical Evaluation

LEFT ATRIAL FUNCTION

Davies[4] noted that the left atrial size in mitral stenosis was variable in pathologic studies, with a complete spectrum from normal size to massive left atrial enlargement. Radiographic (chest x-ray) criteria for left atrial enlargement are dependent on displacement of adjacent tissue and are being replaced with criteria from other imaging techniques such as echocardiography with quantitative and dimensional capabilities. Echo-Doppler analysis of atrial size and function have also furthered our understanding of atrial dysfunction in mitral stenosis.

Atrial dysfunction in mitral stenosis is related to the effects of progressive and chronic left atrial hypertension, with increased left atrial volume, prolonged left atrial systole, interruption of the left atrial contraction-relaxation phase by ventricular systole, increased left atrial work, the gradual development of an atrial myopathic state, and the eventual onset of atrial fibrillation.

Analysis of left atrial volume dynamics and distribution of atrial emptying fractions provide additional insights into left atrial dysfunction. Blood flow from the left atrium to the left ventricle is normally biphasic. The first phase is passive, begins with mitral valve opening, and ends with the beginning of left atrial systole. The second phase, which begins with left atrial systole and ends with mitral valve closure, is active.

All left atrial volumes—maximal, minimal, and at the beginning of atrial systole—are increased in patients with mitral stenosis (Fig. 10.15). When compared to normal subjects, left atrial passive emptying volume is not different in patients with mitral stenosis, while the left atrial active emptying volume is larger. The net result is a normal left atrial total emptying volume (maximal minus minimal volume). In contrast, the left atrial emptying fractions (passive, active, and total) are significantly decreased in mitral stenosis. The increased left atrial volumes in patients with mitral stenosis in sinus rhythm compensate for the decreased left atrial emptying fractions and maintain left atrial total emptying volume.[29]

Friedberg[30] spoke of the stage of left atrial failure when the dilated left atrial chamber fails to eject or accommodate the excess blood behind the mitral obstruction and pulmonary congestion

Figure 10.14. Mitral stenosis: clinical determinants. Left atrium—grey area and arrows indicate hemodynamic changes related to increased left atrial pressure and volume transmitted to pulmonary circulation and right ventricle. Orifice area = black arrow. Stenotic mitral valve labeled and indicated in black. See text for details.

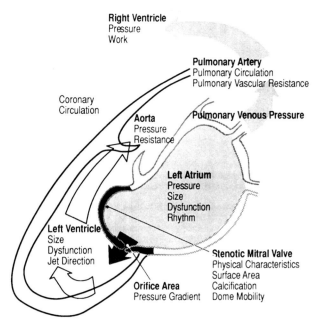

MITRAL STENOSIS: CLINICAL DETERMINANTS

Right Ventricle
Pressure
Work

Pulmonary Artery
Pulmonary Circulation
Pulmonary Vascular Resistance

Coronary
Circulation

Aorta
Pressure
Resistance

Pulmonary Venous Pressure

Left Atrium
Pressure
Size
Dysfunction
Rhythm

Left Ventricle
Size
Dysfunction
Jet Direction

Stenotic Mitral Valve
Physical Characteristics
Surface Area
Calcification
Dome Mobility

Orifice Area
Pressure Gradient

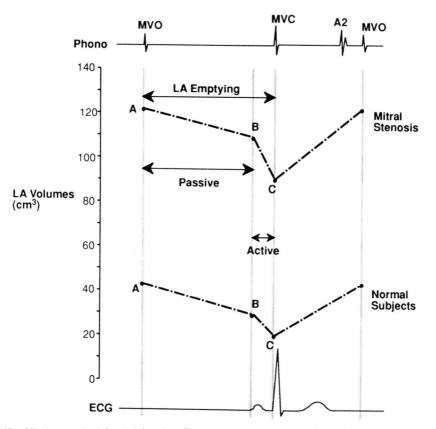

Figure 10.15. Mitral stenosis: left atrial function. Phonocardiogram (phono), left atrial (LA) volumes, and electrocardiogram (ECG), schematic presentation. **A,** LA maximal volume (mitral valve opening). **B,** LA volume at onset of atrial systole, at ECG P wave. **C,** LA minimal volume (mitral valve closure). Changes of LA volume from **A** to **B** represent the LA passive emptying volume, changes of LA volume from **B** to **C** represent the LA active emptying volume, and changes of LA volume from **A** to **C** represent the LA total emptying volume. A_2 = aortic component of the second heart sound; MVC = mitral valve closure; MVO = mitral valve opening. See text under left atrial function.

further aggravates the already altered mechanics of respiration, increasing the force and work of breathing. Traditionally, attention has been directed toward left ventricular function in mitral valve disease; however, left atrial myopathy and left atrial failure are concepts that are vital to understanding the natural history of mitral valve disease.

Atrial natriuretic factor (ANF) secretion is regulated by atrial stretch; ANF is increased in patients with mitral stenosis in sinus rhythm without congestive heart failure, depending on left atrial pressure.[31] Atrial natriuretic factor secretion is also high in patients with mitral stenosis and atrial fibrillation but does not respond appropriately to changes in left atrial pressure. The pathophysiologic role of ANF in mitral stenosis is gradually being defined and may involve regulation of the pulmonary circulatory response to elevated left atrial pressure through increased plasma cyclic GMP in the pulmonary circulation.

Longitudinal clinical evaluation of the patient with mitral stenosis will include correlation of anatomic, physiologic, and functional states with neurohumoral factors as a routine matter in the near future.

LEFT VENTRICULAR FUNCTION

The existence of a significant myocardial factor in mitral stenosis, as contrasted to the mechanical factors associated with the stenotic valve, has been a source of controversy for almost a century. The myocardial factor was "conspicuous by its absence" in Wood's classic study.[6] Since that time, left ventricular function in mitral stenosis has been evaluated by a variety of techniques, and subtle evidence of left ventricular dysfunction has accumulated gradually.

The mitral stenosis left ventricle is small, with greater systolic emptying and inferoposterior systolic wall motion abnormalities. Evidence of systolic dysfunction includes the abnormally prolonged left ventricular pressure rise time described previously, the loss of ventricular efficiency related to movement of the mitral dome toward the left atrium in the presence of left atrial hypertension, and alterations in left ventricular function related to disturbances of ventricular filling. Left ventricular isovolumetric contraction time is markedly decreased since ventricular filling continues during early ventricular systole as a result of prolonged atrial systole extending well into early ventricular systole.

Evidence of left ventricular diastolic dysfunction in mitral stenosis is more apparent. The diastolic pressure gradient at the stenotic valve, abnormal patterns of left ventricular dimensional change, absence of the atrial kick in the ventricular pressure pulse, altered diastolic inflow patterns, and the configurations of color flow jets through the mitral orifice from the mitral dome either as central-apical or eccentric jets are significant factors affecting or reflecting left ventricular diastolic dysfunction.

Diastolic regional left ventricular wall motion abnormalities associated with a significantly reduced peak filling rate have been analyzed by Gibson and associates.[32] Striking nonuniformity and asynchrony of wall motion are present; regional asynchrony includes abnormal outward wall movement during isovolumic relaxation. The dissociation of regional wall motion from left ventricular filling and the constant finding that left ventricular anterior free wall motion preceded that elsewhere raises the possibility that both phenomena may represent disorganization of the "highly specialized restoring forces whose action is the basis of coordinate filling in the normal heart."[32]

PULMONARY CIRCULATION: THE SECOND STENOSIS

Grossman[33] discussed the "second stenosis" in mitral stenosis—the first stenosis occurs at the mitral valve, the second at the level of the precapillary pulmonary arterioles of the lung. This concept dates back to the early work by Dexter and Gorlin. Left atrial pressure reaches approximately 25 mm Hg (mean) when the mitral orifice is reduced to about 1.0 cm^2, and it is after this point that pulmonary arteriolar reactive changes develop. With progressive pulmonary vascular obstruction, pulmonary arterial hypertension develops with eventual right ventricular hypertension, hypertrophy, and dysfunction.

The classification of patients with mitral stenosis on a hemodynamic basis with determination

of the mitral valve area and the pulmonary vascular resistance provides a rational basis for clinical staging and for clinical decision making. As outlined by Grossman[33] patients may present with symptoms, tight mitral stenosis and normal vascular resistance; or relatively asymptomatic with more severe stenosis, a marked increase in pulmonary vascular resistance, and cardiomegaly with left atrial enlargement and right ventricular hypertrophy. Eventually, terminal mitral stenosis with extreme pulmonary hypertension, right ventricular failure, tricuspid regurgitation, and cachexia occurs. Obviously, clinical staging based on precise anatomic and pathophysiologic data must precede rational therapy.

Cheitlin and Byrd[34] reviewed the pathogenesis of the pulmonary responses to left atrial hypertension. Movement of fluid from the capillary bed as a result of left atrial-pulmonary venous hypertension leads to increased lung water and stiffening from interstitial fluid, reduced dynamic lung compliance, increased respiratory muscle work, the sensation of dyspnea, and with the gradual increased resistance to the right ventricle, pulmonary and right ventricular systolic pressures increase. Passive or active increases in pulmonary artery pressure modulated by the changes in pulmonary vascular resistance then become major determinants in symptom production, clinical course, complications, and the potential for reversibility. Right ventricular hypertrophy, dilation, and dysfunction with pulmonary regurgitation, tricuspid regurgitation, and the syndrome of right heart failure represent the end stages of this process.

From the clinical viewpoint, this sequence means that the differential diagnosis of patients who present with dyspnea, evidence to suggest pulmonary artery hypertension, right ventricular hypertension, and tricuspid regurgitation must include mitral stenosis.

THROMBOTIC CALCIFIC MITRAL STENOSIS—CLINICAL IMPLICATIONS

Fundamental differences exist between the physical properties of the noncalcific stenotic mitral valve and the calcific stenotic mitral valve[5] (Fig. 10.10). Moderate to heavily calcified stenotic mitral valves have greater weight, volume, specific gravity, weight per area, with smaller orifice size compared to noncalcific stenotic mitral valves. Leaflet mobility is obliterated in the heavily calcified valves.

The most striking difference in calcific stenotic

mitral valves involves surface morphology (Fig. 10.16). Surface ulceration is due to eruption of the underlying calcific focus through the valvular endothelium (Fig. 10.17). Thrombus formation in the areas of ulceration is associated with symptomatic arterial embolization. Whisker formation, filamentous stalks along the line of valve closure, is also present. The moderately to heavily calcified stenotic mitral valve also has a small fixed mitral valve orifice.

From the clinical viewpoint, distinctions between noncalcific stenotic valves and calcific stenotic valves include the altered auscultatory phenomena noted earlier, the restrictive effects on dome or valve mobility with resultant imaging correlates, and the altered valve surface characteristics with thrombus formation and subsequent arterial embolization from the valve surface thrombi.

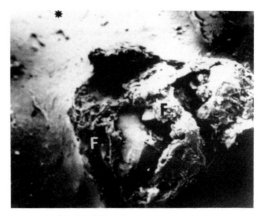

Figure 10.17. Calcific mitral stenosis, surface morphology. Scanning electron micrograph of an ulcer. Intact nonulcerated endothelial surface appears smooth as marked by asterisk (*). The jagged border of an irregularly shaped surface ulcer is shown. The ulcer base is covered with fibrin (F). ($\times$ 30)

CLINICAL ASSESSMENT OF THE STENOTIC MITRAL VALVE

Thus far, emphasis has been placed on the nuances of patient symptoms, physical diagnosis, valvular anatomic substrate, and pathophysiology. The fundamentals and complexities of calculating the area of a stenotic valve has been reviewed by Carabello,[35] who has emphasized that the Gorlin formula for calculating a stenotic valve area requires that the pressure gradient across the valve be examined in light of the cardiac output passing through the orifice. Thus an accurately obtained pressure gradient, an accurate cardiac output, and an accurate formula are requisites for diagnostic precision. The techniques reviewed by Carabello are fundamental to contemporary understanding of valvular heart disease, and the article is recommended reading for those concerned with diagnostic precision in mitral stenosis.

Gorlin's editorial comment[36] on Carabello's paper places appropriate emphasis on the issue of the quality of hemodynamic data, particularly when a decision concerning surgery or valvuloplasty is in the offing.

MITRAL STENOSIS—MIMICS

"Rheumatic-type" valve pathology without a history of acute rheumatic fever has been a long-term concern as regards etiology. The pathologic changes in chronic rheumatic valvular disease have no absolute specificity to link them to acute rheumatic fever. This has led to the supposition that there may be other causes, e.g, viruses, of chronic rheumatic-type valve disease. We concur with Davies[4] that it may be more accurate to describe rheumatic-type valves without a history of acute rheumatic fever as postinflammatory or, simply, rheumatic-type.

Congenital mitral stenosis is rare. The majority of patients are young and have associated cardiac anomalies. Juvenile mitral stenosis is a term that has been used to describe a severe form of rheumatic mitral stenosis in adolescents. We are not aware of clear-cut clinical imaging criteria that separate these two entities.

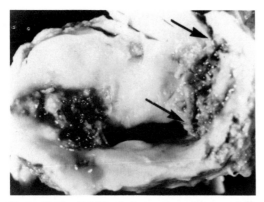

Figure 10.16. Calcific mitral stenosis, surface morphology. Gross appearance of a calcified and ulcerated mitral valve that has been surgically resected. The anterolateral commissure (on the left) shows a gross thrombus over an ulcer. The posteromedial commissure (on the right) shows an ulcer formed by eruption of a calcific mass through the surface endothelium. This ulcer is free of gross thrombus. Arrows show the extent of calcification and ulceration. ($\times$ 2.5)

Cor triatriatrum, essentially a third left atrial chamber, usually produces symptoms in early life and is rare in adult life. Membranous supravalvular mitral stenosis and other left atrial membranous lesions may mimic certain aspects of mitral stenosis. These lesions have distinctive clinical, hemodynamic, and imaging characteristics that permit discrimination from rheumatic mitral stenosis.[34,37]

Left atrial myxomas are pedunculated lesions that arise within the left atrium. The clinical profile may include constitutional symptoms, dyspnea, syncope, congestive failure, and embolic phenomena. Auscultatory findings may mimic mitral stenosis or regurgitation. Atrial fibrillation and significant left atrial enlargement are uncommon. Imaging techniques permit differentiation from rheumatic mitral stenosis.[34,37]

MITRAL STENOSIS—
ASSOCIATION WITH ANOMALOUS
PULMONARY VEINS

Partial anomalous pulmonary venous drainage occurred in approximately 1% of patients with mitral stenosis when sensitive shunt detection techniques were used at cardiac catheterization. Although uncommon, the combination may produce a clinically confounding picture, since part of the pulmonary venous return may be to the high pressure left atrium, part to the low pressure right heart, with corresponding differences in regional pulmonary vascular resistance.[38]

MITRAL STENOSIS—CLINICAL
RECOGNITION

Patients with mitral stenosis may present with a progressive symptom complex, with evidence of pulmonary hypertension, or with a complication of mitral stenosis, the evaluation of which leads the clinician back to the underlying diagnosis. The diagnosis may be quite straightforward in a young woman with appropriate symptoms, a history of rheumatic fever, clear-cut physical findings, and confirmatory laboratory studies.

The real life questions for the clinician are more complicated. When do you suspect mitral stenosis? When should you think of mitral stenosis? Some representative scenarios include

Patients who are short of breath with effort. Young women who are pregnant and short of breath. All breathless patients.

Elderly patients with atrial fibrillation. All patients with atrial fibrillation. Patients with strokes or arterial emboli, particularly those with atrial fibrillation.

Patients with hemoptysis. All patients with pulmonary congestion.

What next? Examine the patient carefully. Perform a proper physical examination, or send them to someone who will—a highly cost-effective approach.

Now, based on the physical examination, which patients should trigger thoughts about mitral stenosis?

Patients with a loud first heart sound. Patients with peculiarities of second heart sound "splitting." Is that really a widely split second heart sound, or could it be an opening snap?

Patients with an apical systolic murmur—be sure to auscult with the patient on their left side. The apical systolic murmur may be all you hear in the recumbent position in the patient with a heavily calcified stenotic valve and a fixed orifice that permits mitral regurgitation. Be sure to roll all patients on their left side as part of a thinking clinician's physical examination.

Patients with a palpable right ventricular impulse, with a loud P_2, and with a prominent A wave in the jugular venous pulse. Anyone with evidence of pulmonary hypertension.

And so on down the line. With the ECG, the chest x-ray, the echocardiogram.

The diagnosis of mitral stenosis is a ride on the carrousel—if you miss the diagnosis, i.e., the brass ring, on the first trip around, i.e., the history, you should make it on the next trip, the physical examination, from laboratory data, etc.

INDICATIONS FOR DIAGNOSTIC
PROCEDURES AND
INTERVENTIONS

Somewhere in the land of cardiology make-believe, in never-never land, there is a repository for all the slides, articles, and chapters produced during the past 50 years labeled "Indications for . . . (procedures, therapy)." Concepts, instrumentation, and technology changed so rapidly that the slides, articles, and chapters were outmoded and irrelevant at production. We will attempt to spare the reader this type of obsolescence.

Most of the natural history studies about mitral stenosis were written in the 1950s and 1960s and reflected the European and North American experiences from another time in medicine. Are these studies still valid as a benchmark? A more recent natural history study from Greece extended into the diuretic-antibiotic era. There were significant parallels with Wood's earlier study[6]; no striking differences were detected between patients with and without a history of rheumatic fever.

One hundred and seventy-six patients with mitral stenosis hospitalized in the University Hospital Medical Clinic, Aristotelian University of Thessaloniki, Greece, from 1963 to 1972 were analyzed.[39] Patients with a history of rheumatic fever (93 patients) were compared to those without a history of rheumatic fever (83 patients). The average age at symptom onset was similar in the two groups (history of rheumatic fever 36.5 ± 14 years, no history of rheumatic fever 36.7 ± 13 years). However, there was a wide distribution in the age of the beginning of symptoms in both groups as the large standard deviation indicates. The frequency of major symptoms was also similar in both groups (Fig. 10.18). The time interval from the beginning of symptoms (functional class II) to total incapacitation (functional class IV) was approximately 10 years in both groups (Fig. 10.19). This time interval varied significantly from patient to patient as the large standard deviation indicates.

Acute rheumatic fever incidence and severity changes of the favorable type have occurred in parts of the world, while other regions have experienced variations in rheumatic malignancy and severity with recognition of early, fulminant forms of rheumatic fever and valvulitis. Medical and interventional therapy have remained rudimentary in many parts of the world.

The effects on natural history of the introduction of several classes of diuretics and antibiotics; multiple cardiovascular drugs including antiarrhythmics, vasodilators, adrenergic blockers, and anticoagulants; and techniques of cardioversion have not been critically analyzed. Surgical modalities have progressed from closed to open commissurotomy, valve replacement, and repair into the era of cardiac transplantation. A variety of techniques for valvuloplasty, including percutaneous balloon valvotomy, have been, or are being, introduced.

Given this incredible diversity, how should we proceed? What is the clinician to do?

There are several basic concepts that should be stated:

Rheumatic mitral stenosis is a lifelong disease process. All diagnostic and therapeutic decisions should be made with this inexorable fact in mind. The potential for incorrect decisions rises exponentially with lifelong diseases.

MITRAL STENOSIS: Frequency of Symptoms

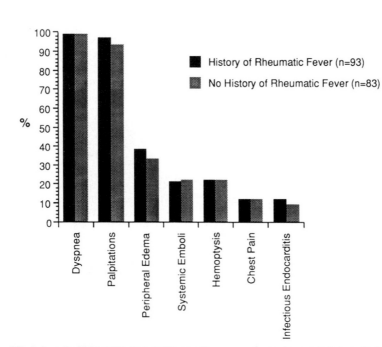

Figure 10.18. Mitral stenosis: 1963–1972 study in Greece. Frequency of symptoms-events in patients with and without history of rheumatic fever. Note the similarity between the two groups.[39]

MITRAL STENOSIS: Time Course From Beginning of Symptoms (FC II) To FC IV

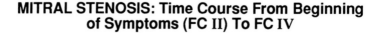

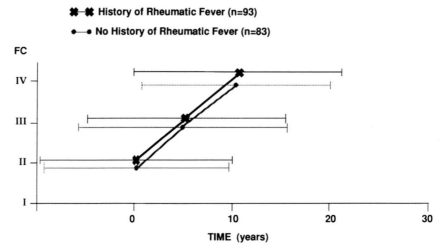

Figure 10.19. Mitral stenosis: 1963–1972 study in Greece. Time intervals from the beginning of symptoms (functional class, FC II) to total incapacitation (FC IV) in patients with mitral stenosis with and without history of rheumatic fever (mean values ± 1 standard deviation). Note the large standard deviation and the similarities between the two groups.[39]

Secondly, medical nosology and medical literature require that patients with disease be classified and considered as groups of patients. Given the individuality of humans and the way individuals experience disease, this type of classification has significant limitations. Individuals experience disease within their own unique genetic makeup, within their unique environmental setting.

Thirdly, the disease designated as rheumatic mitral stenosis is a spectrum—anatomic, physiologic, pathophysiologic, neurohumoral, and clinical. Clinical expressions vary.

Lastly, decision making should be based on the most precise data available.

Individual Patient Profiles

Clinicians are concerned with individual patients. Each patient with mitral stenosis should be analyzed individually, and a graphic presentation (Figs. 10.20 and 10.21) of the patient symptoms or events should be plotted against time, patient age, and functional classification.

Individual Patient Analysis

The Individual Patient Profile illustrates (Fig. 10.22) the unique nature of each patient's response

to rheumatic mitral stenosis. The Individual Patient Analysis presents a logical approach to the analysis of the diagnostic process. Emphasis is placed on the diagnostic process and the Individual Patient Profile.

Diagnostic methods vary. Much depends on the clinician's experience, physical facilities, and available technology. Although the methods or test availability may vary in your institution or area, precise definition of the anatomic lesion and the physiologic state should remain as the ultimate standards.

As Gorlin stated it:

"In truth, it is the integration of cardiac laboratory data of high quality with information from the physical examination and modern ultrasound imaging that permits the most accurate diagnosis possible."[36]

Acknowledgment

The authors are pleased to acknowledge the contributions of Dennis Mathias (graphics preparation) and Dawn Serafini (manuscript preparation).

Financial support was received from the Overstreet Cardiovascular Teaching and Research Lab-

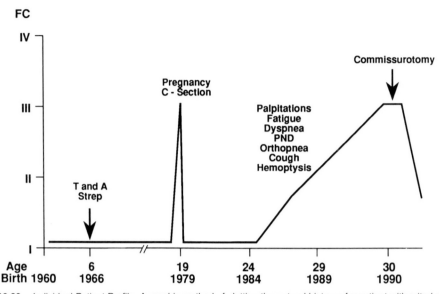

Figure 10.20. Individual Patient Profile. A graphic method of plotting the natural history of a patient with mitral stenosis. Symptoms or events, patient age and calendar year, and functional classification are shown.

Progressive symptoms began at age 24. Young woman with severe mitral stenosis, normal pulmonary vascular resistance.

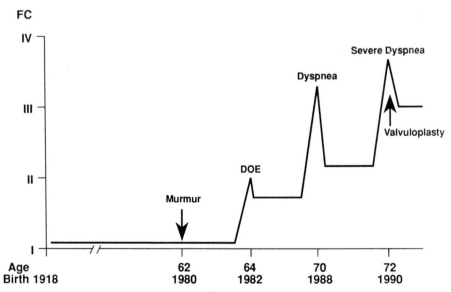

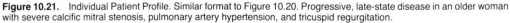

Figure 10.21. Individual Patient Profile. Similar format to Figure 10.20. Progressive, late-state disease in an older woman with severe calcific mitral stenosis, pulmonary artery hypertension, and tricuspid regurgitation.

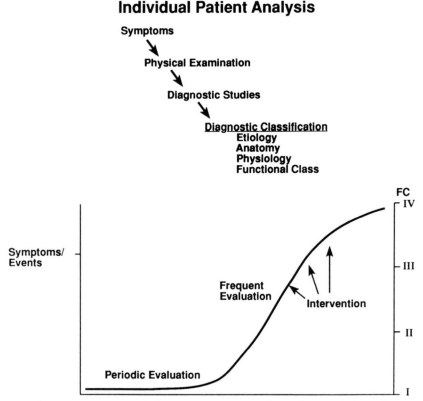

Figure 10.22. Individual Patient Analysis. Schematic incorporates the diagnostic steps—history, physical examination, diagnostic studies—necessary to develop a diagnostic classification.
    An Individual Patient Profile plots symptoms, events, time, patient age, and functional classification (FC), as in Figures 10.20, and 10.21.
    Periodic evaluation is replaced by more frequent evaluation with the development of symptoms or events.
    Intervention indicated by multiple arrows, may involve medical therapy, or valvuloplasty by surgical procedure or with angioplasty at varying times during the course of the disease.

oratory, Division of Cardiology, The Ohio State University College of Medicine, and The Columbus Foundation Columbus, Ohio.

REFERENCES

1. Cabot RC. *Facts on the Heart.* Philadelphia, W. B. Saunders Company, 1926, pp. 30–44.
2. Stollerman EH. Rheumatic and heritable connective tissue disorders of the cardiovascular system. In: *Heart Disease.* ed by E. Braunwald, Philadelphia, W. B. Saunders Company, 1984, pp. 1653–1654.
3. Wallach JB, Borgatta EF, Angrist AA. *Rheumatic Heart Disease.* Springfield, Charles C Thomas, 1962, pp. 3–92.
4. Davies MJ. *Pathology on Cardiac Valves.* London, Butterworths, 1980, pp. 110–114.
5. Wooley CF, Baba N, Kilman JW, Ryan JM. Thrombotic calcific mitral stenosis: Morphology of the calcific mitral valve. *Circulation 49*:1167–1174, 1974.

6. Wood P. An appreciation of mitral stenosis. *Br Med J 1*:1051–1063; 1113–1124, 1954.
7. Gorlin R, Gorlin SG. Hydraulic formula for calculation of the area of the stenotic mitral valve, other cardiac valves, and central circulatory shunts. *Am Heart J 41*:1–29, 1951.
8. Barlow JB, Lakier JB, Pocock JA. Mitral stenosis. In: *Perspectives on the Mitral Valve.* ed by JB Barlow, Philadelphia, FA Davis Company, 1987, pp. 151–180.
9. Lewis T. The time relations of heart sounds and murmurs with special reference to the acoustic signs in mitral stenosis. *Heart 4*:241–258, 1913.
10. Henderson Y. A neglected feature of the mechanics of mitral stenosis. *JAMA 78*:1046–1049, 1922.
11. Margolies A, Wolferth C. The opening snap (Claquement D'ouverture de la mitrale) in mitral stenosis, its characteristics, mechanism of production and diagnostic importance. *Am Heart J 7*: 443–470, 1932.

12. Ross RS, Criley JM. Cineangiocardiographic studies of the origin of cardiovascular physical signs. *Circulation 30*:255–261, 1964.

13. Wooley CF, Klassen KP, Leighton RF, Goodwin MS, Ryan JM. Left atrial and left ventricular sound and pressure in mitral stenosis. *Circulation 38*: 295–307, 1968.

14. Thompson ME, Shaver JA, Heidenreich FP, Leon DF, Leonard JJ. Sound, pressure and motion correlates in mitral stenosis. *Am J Med 49*:436–450, 1970.

15. Salerni R, Reedy PS, Sherman ME, O'Toole JD, Leon DF, Shaver JA. Pressure and sound correlates of the mitral valve echocardiogram in mitral stenosis. *Circulation 58*:119–125, 1978.

16. Craige E. On the genesis of heart sounds (Editorial). *Circulation 53*:31–33, 1976.

17. Naito M, Morganroth J, Mardelli TJ, Chen CC, Dreifus LS. Rheumatic mitral stenosis: Cross-sectional echocardiographic analysis. *Am Heart J 100*:34–40, 1980.

18. Tani M, Murayama A, Ohnishi S, et al. Evaluation of mitral valve, subvalvular structures and valvular flexibility in mitral stenosis by two-dimensional echocardiography. *J Cardiography 12*:11–12, 1982.

19. Yamamoto T. Two-dimensional echocardiographic assessment of mitral stenosis: Preoperative detection of organic change in the mitral valve apparatus. *J Cardiovasc Ultrasonography 2*:273–283, 1983.

20. Kalmanson D, Veyrat C, Bernier A, Witchitz S, Chiche P. Opening snap and isovolumic relaxation period in relation to mitral valve flow in patients with mitral stenosis: Significance of A2-OS interval. *Br Heart J 38*:135–146, 1976.

21. Barrington WW, Boudoulas H, Bashore T, Olson S, Wooley CF. Mitral stenosis: Mitral dome excursion at M_1 and the mitral opening snap. The concept of reciprocal heart sounds. *Am Heart J 115*:1280–1290, 1988.

22. Wooley CF, Klassen KP, Leighton RF, et al. The left atrial pressure pulse of mitral stenosis in sinus rhythm. *Am J Cardiol 25*:395–400, 1970.

23. Katz LN, Sigel ML. The cardiodynamic effects of acute experimental mitral stenosis. *Am Heart J 6*: 672–682, 1931.

24. Moscovitz HL, Donoso E, Gelb IJ. *An Atlas of Hemodynamics of the Cardiovascular System*. New York, Grune and Stratton, 1963, pp. 60–70.

25. Craige E. Echophonocardiography and other non-invasive techniques to elucidate heart murmurs. In: *Heart Disease*. ed by E Braunwald, Philadelphia, WB Saunders Company, 1988, pp. 65–82.

26. Criley JM, Herner AJ. Crescendo presystolic murmur of mitral stenosis with atrial fibrillation. *N Engl J Med 285*:1284, 1971.

27. Criley JM, Feldman JM, Meredith T. Mitral valve closure and the crescendo presystolic murmur. *Am J Med 51*:456, 1971.

28. Fortuin NJ, Craige E. Echocardiographic studies of genesis of mitral diastolic murmurs. *Br Heart J 35*: 75, 1973.

29. Triposkiadis F, Wooley CF, Boudoulas H. Mitral stenosis: Left atrial dynamics reflect altered passive and active emptying. *Am Heart J 120*:124, 1990.

30. Freidberg CK. Clinical features in mitral stenosis. In: *Diseases of the Heart*. ed by CK Friedberg, Philadelphia, WB Saunders Company, 1956, pp. 652–682.

31. Dussaule JC, Vahanian A, Michel PL, et al. Plasma atrial natriuretic factor and cyclic GMP in mitral stenosis treated by balloon valvulotomy. *Circulation 78*:276–285, 1988.

32. Hui WKK, Lee PK, Chow JSF, Gibson DG. Analysis of regional left ventricular wall motion during diastole in mitral stenosis. *Br Heart J 50*: 231–239, 1983.

33. Grossman W. *Cardiac Catheterization and Angiography*. Philadelphia, Lea & Febiger, 1986, pp. 360–364.

34. Cheitlin MD, Byrd RC. Mitral valve disease. In: *Valvular Heart Disease*. ed by BH Greenberg, and E Murphy, Littleton, PSB Publishing Company, Inc., 1987, pp. 92–120.

35. Carabello BA. Advances in the hemodynamic assessment of stenotic cardiac valves. *JACC 10*:912–919, 1987.

36. Gorlin R. Calculations of cardiac valve stenosis: Restoring an old concept for advanced applications. *JACC 10*:920–922, 1987.

37. Dalen JE, Alpert JS. Mitral stenosis. In: *Valvular Heart Disease*. ed by JE Dalen, and JS Alpert, Boston, Little, Brown and Company, 1981, pp. 69–70.

38. Wilson MR, Fontana ME, Wooley CF. Routine use of the hydrogen platinum electrode system in shunt detection. *Cathet Cardiovasc Diagn 1*:207–221, 1975.

39. Boudoulas H. Kontopoulos A, Parcharidis G, Metaxas P, Valtis DJ. The natural history of rheumatic valvular heart disease. Comparison of patients with a history of rheumatic fever to those without history of rheumatic fever. *Helliniki Latriki (Greek Medicine) 43*:107–115, 1974.

11

Echo-Doppler Evaluation of Mitral Stenosis and the Effect of Mitral Valvotomy

KHALID H. SHEIKH

One of the first clinical applications of echocardiography was in the evaluation of mitral valve structure and movement, and the changes in structure and movement that occurred in mitral stenosis.[1,2] As echo-Doppler technology has evolved to its current level in providing high-quality imaging of cardiac structures and blood flow, it is not surprising that echo-Doppler now plays an integral part in nearly all phases of percutaneous balloon mitral valvotomy (PMV). Echo-Doppler assessment is a reliable, noninvasive means for the diagnosis of mitral stenosis. In most cases, an echo-Doppler evaluation will eliminate the need for a separate pre-PMV diagnostic catheterization. Thus, patients suitable for PMV can be identified and admitted to the hospital specifically for PMV, without having to undergo an additional catheterization, with its associated cost and morbidity. Additionally, patients who are not candidates for PMV because of either contraindications or anatomic features that would predict a low likelihood of procedural success may be identified from the echo-Doppler examination. During PMV, echocardiography may also be useful, for instance, in guiding the selection of the appropriate balloon size for dilation. Finally, echo-Doppler provides a convenient and reliable means to assess and follow the serial changes in mitral valve area, mitral regurgitation, and hemodynamic variables that occur both immediately after, as well as in late follow-up after, PMV.

As PMV continues to evolve and its long-term results are evaluated, echo-Doppler will likely play an increasingly important role. For these reasons, clinical involvement in PMV requires a thorough understanding of the principles and limitations of the echo-Doppler evaluation of mitral stenosis and the effects of PMV.

ECHO-DOPPLER EVALUATION OF MITRAL STENOSIS
Anatomic Findings

M-MODE ECHOCARDIOGRAPHY

The pathologic changes of the mitral valve occurring in mitral stenosis are easily identified by echocardiography. The initial echocardiographic findings of mitral stenosis were reported using M-mode echocardiograms.[2] This technique pro-

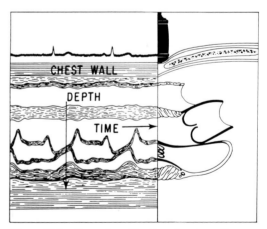

Figure 11.1. Generation of the M-mode echocardiogram. M-Mode recording from the parasternal transducer position at the level of the mitral valve leaflets. The strip chart displays depth and time. The cardiac structures are displayed by recording ultrasound reflections. Movement of cardiac structures can be visualized and timed to the cardiac cycle with the ECG.

vides a dynamic, one-dimensional ultrasonic image of cardiac structures obtained from the transmission and reflection of a single line of ultrasound (Fig. 11.1). Echo reflections of cardiac structures are displayed so that their movements in time can be recorded on a moving strip chart. Solid structures reflect ultrasound and thus generate echo signals. Blood transmits ultrasound, and thus the cardiac chambers containing blood are echolucent.

The M-mode examination is usually performed from the parasternal transducer position. An M-mode image of a normal mitral valve and its surrounding structures obtained from this location is shown in Figure 11.2A. The echocardiogram displays the structures encountered by the ultrasound beam along its path into the heart from the chest. The chest wall (CW) is nearest the transducer, shown at the top of the image. At this level, encountered in sequence from anterior to posterior, are the right ventricular cavity (RV), interventricular septum (IVS), the left ventricular cavity containing the mitral valve leaflets (MVL), and the posterior left ventricular wall. The anterior (a) and posterior (p) mitral valve leaflets can be identified. During diastole, the open mitral valve leaflets display an M shape, indicating early diastolic opening, followed by partial mid-diastolic closure and then reopening due to atrial systole. The anterior and posterior leaflets move in opposite directions during diastole, with the anterior leaflet displaying a greater excursion than the posterior leaflet. During systole, both leaflets are apposed.

An M-mode echocardiogram of mitral stenosis is shown in Figure 11.2B. The increased echogenicity of these leaflets compared to normal is due to leaflet thickening and/or calcification. Reduced leaflet mobility can be appreciated as a decrease in diastolic leaflet separation compared to normal. Commissural fusion alters the motion of the posterior leaflet. Rather than moving in the opposite direction to the anterior leaflet, the posterior leaflet is pulled forward when the mitral valve opens at the beginning of diastole, causing it to move in parallel with the anterior leaflet. Impaired early diastolic filling of the left ventricle causes the initial downslope of the M shape of the anterior mitral leaflet (designated as the "E-F slope") to be reduced in mitral stenosis. With loss of atrial systole in atrial fibrillation, the mitral leaflet reopening, indicated by the second upstroke of the M, is lost.

TWO-DIMENSIONAL ECHOCARDIOGRAPHY

The geometric configuration and spatial movements of the diseased valve leaflets are not accurately determined using M-mode echocardiography because the single echo beam intercepts moving leaflet structures at different portions of the leaflet surface as the apparatus moves in synchrony with the cardiac cycle. Furthermore, because two-dimensional echocardiography is bet-

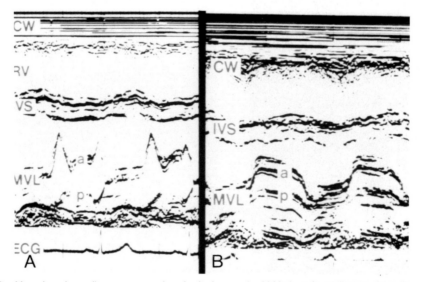

Figure 11.2. M-mode echocardiograms: normal and mitral stenosis. M-Mode echocardiogram from the parasternal position at the level of the mitral valve leaflets. **A,** Normal. **B,** Mitral stenosis. Abbreviations: CW = chest wall; ECG = electrocardiogram; IVS = interventricular septum; MVL = mitral valve leaflets (a = anterior leaflet, p = posterior leaflet); RV = right ventricle.

ter able to define spatial anatomic relationships and movement of structures relative to one another, it is superior to M-mode techniques for assessment of mitral leaflet pathology.[3] Features of mitral stenosis on the two-dimensional echocardiogram are shown in Figure 11.3. There is an increase in the echogenicity of the valve leaflets due to leaflet thickening and/or calcification. Commissural fusion is indicated by the assumption of a dome shape in diastole, with the anterior leaflet forming a characteristic "elbow" due to its tethering to the posterior leaflet. Abrupt halting of the early diastolic opening motion coincides with the opening snap evident on auscultation.

ECHOCARDIOGRAPHIC PARAMETERS OF STENOSIS SEVERITY

Not only may echocardiography be used to diagnose mitral stenosis, but an estimation of its severity may also be obtained. While the Doppler examination is now the mainstay in the evaluation of stenosis severity, structural abnormalities detected by both M-mode and two-dimensional imaging may still be useful in an overall assessment of stenosis severity.

M-Mode echocardiography. The primary M-mode parameter of stenosis severity has been the "E-F slope." A reduction in the E-F slope signifies an increased severity of stenosis (Fig. 11.4). Early work with this measurement indicated good correlations with invasively obtained mitral valve areas.[4,5] However, further experience indicated that this method was largely unsatisfactory because the E-F slope is influenced by factors other than the severity of the stenosis, such as cardiac output and left ventricular compliance.[6,7]

Two-dimensional echocardiography. As was the case for evaluation of mitral valve morphology, two-dimensional echocardiography is also superior to M-mode for assessment of stenosis severity. The mitral valve orifice may be directly visualized in diastole. From the parasternal short-axis view, it is possible to differentiate between various orifice shapes that are indistinguishable by M-mode

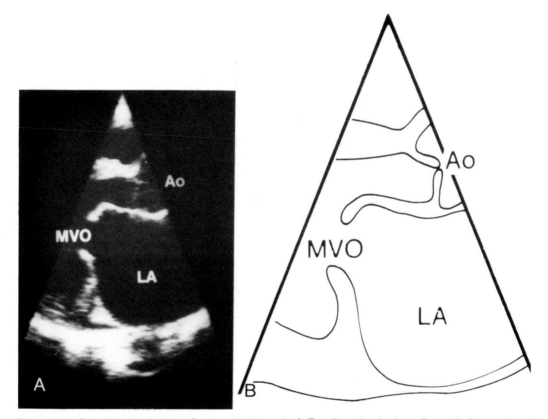

Figure 11.3.   Two-dimensional echocardiogram: mitral stenosis. **A,** Two-dimensional echocardiogram in the parasternal long-axis view, visualizing the mitral valve. **B,** Schematic of **A.** Abbreviations: Ao = aorta; LA = left atrium; MVO = mitral valve orifice.

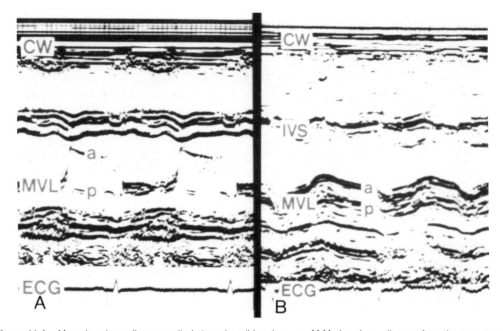

Figure 11.4. M-mode echocardiogram: mitral stenosis: mild and severe. M-Mode echocardiogram from the parasternal position at the level of the mitral valve leaflets. **A,** Mild mitral stenosis. **B,** Severe mitral stenosis. Abbreviations: As in Figure 11.2.

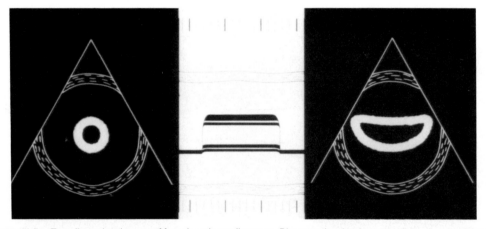

Figure 11.5. Two-dimensional versus M-mode echocardiograms. Diagram showing how two-dimensional echocardiograms (left and right panels) can differentiate between mitral valve orifices of various shapes that would appear identical on an M-mode recording (center).

echocardiography (Fig. 11.5). From a still frame parasternal short-axis image of the mitral valve leaflets, the mitral valve area may be directly measured by planimetry of the mitral orifice (Fig. 11.6). To do this properly, great care must be exercised to ensure the image selected is adequate. If the scan plane transects the valve obliquely, if the

wrong part of the cardiac cycle is used, or if there is either echo-dropout in the mitral valve or excessive image gain, measurements obtained with this method will be erroneous. Other technical difficulties arise from limitations in lateral resolution and from reverberations produced by valve calcification. In spite of these problems, in the hands of

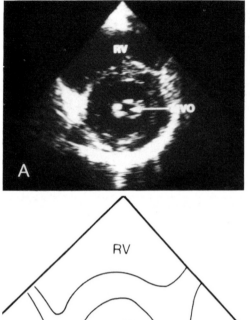

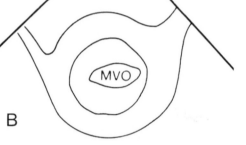

Figure 11.6. Two-dimensional echocardiogram to measure mitral valve area. **A,** Two-dimensional echocardiogram from the parasternal short-axis position, at the level of the mitral valve. The mitral valve orifice (MVO) can be visualized and planimetered to measure mitral valve area. **B,** Schematic of **A**. Abbreviations: MVO = mitral valve area; RV = right ventricle.

experienced operators, two-dimensional echocardiography is a valuable and accurate method for estimation of mitral valve area.[2,8,9]

Doppler Findings

BASIC DOPPLER PRINCIPLES

Doppler echocardiography can provide information regarding the direction, speed, and character of blood flow. It is a reliable, noninvasive means to determine mitral valve gradient as well as to estimate valve orifice area. The Doppler signal is generated by computerized analysis of the change in frequency of ultrasound that is reflected from moving red blood cells (Fig. 11.7). The Doppler principle states that the change in frequency of incident ultrasound that results when the ultrasound encounters moving red blood cells (frequency shift) is related to the direction of red

blood cell movement and is directly proportional to the velocity with which the red blood cells are moving.

Measurement of Doppler velocity requires generation of a spectral display of the Doppler signal, as is shown in Figure 11.7. This means that the measured Doppler frequency shift is converted to velocity data through the Doppler equation (Fig. 11.8) and displayed so that the flow-velocity profile of the column of blood interrogated can be examined. When obstructions to flow are present, velocity of flow increases. The increase in velocity requires a pressure drop across the obstruction. The approximate pressure drop can be calculated using the modified Bernoulli equation, which states that:

$$p_1 - p_2 = 4 \, V^2$$

where, p_1 = pressure distal to the obstruction, p_2 = pressure proximal to the obstruction, and V = the velocity of blood flow across the obstruction.

Since Doppler velocities across a stenosis are generally elevated, they are usually best measured using continuous-wave Doppler techniques, which can reliably measure higher velocities than pulsed-wave Doppler. This, however, often requires use of a special nonimaging continuous-wave transducer so that the Doppler signal of flow across the mitral valve is obtained without direct visualization of the orifice. As indicated in the Doppler equation, optimal measurement of the peak Doppler velocity requires minimizing the angle of interception of the Doppler beam with blood flow. This is usually best obtained using a transducer position at the apex of the left ventricle and positioning the Doppler beam to record diastolic flow through the mitral valve (Fig. 11.9). This flow is recognized on the spectral display as diastolic flow toward the transducer, displayed by convention as a Doppler signal above the baseline, with a measurable velocity. Accurately obtaining a peak Doppler velocity without the aid of an anatomic image requires considerable skill and experience.

DOPPLER PARAMETERS OF STENOSIS SEVERITY

The Doppler examination has largely supplanted both M-mode and two-dimensional echocardiography as the primary method for the estimation of mitral stenosis severity. Doppler techniques can provide information about transvalvular gradients as well as estimates of mitral valve area. However, each technique has limitations in certain clinical settings. Therefore, an echocardiographic estima-

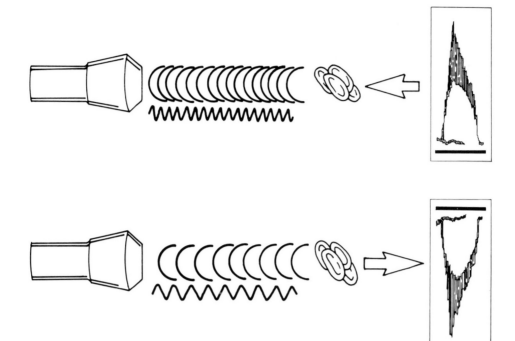

Figure 11.7. Doppler shift. The Doppler shift is measured by a change in the frequency of ultrasound returning to the transducer following reflection from red blood cells. It is based on the direction and speed of red blood cell movement. This Doppler shift can be displayed in spectral format.

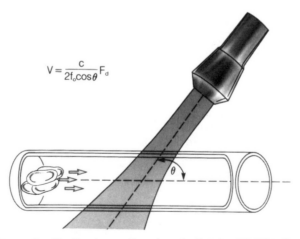

$$V = \frac{c}{2f_o \cos\theta} F_d$$

Figure 11.8. The Doppler equation. The Doppler equation relates the Doppler shift (F_d) to the velocity of red blood cell movement (V). By minimizing the incident angle of ultrasound to blood flow (θ), V may be calculated directly from F_d if transducer frequency (f_o) is known. Abbreviations: c = speed of ultrasound in tissue; F_d = Doppler shift; f_o = transducer frequency; V = velocity of flow; θ = angle of intercept of incident ultrasound to blood flow.

tion of mitral stenosis severity should not be performed purely on the basis of one single parameter, but rather from critically reviewing information derived from several Doppler techniques, as well as anatomic imaging.

Transmitral gradients. Using the modified Bernoulli equation, an estimate of the pressure gradient that exists between the left atrium and the left ventricle causing diastolic flow across the mitral valve may be obtained from Doppler echocardi-

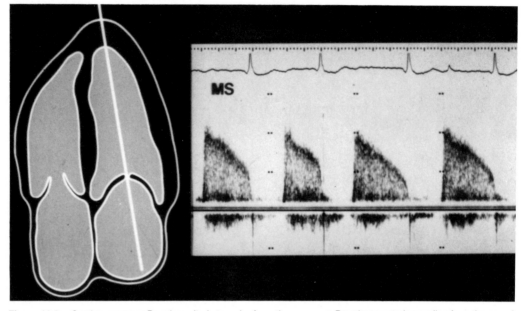

Figure 11.9. Continuous-wave Doppler: mitral stenosis. A continuous-wave Doppler spectral recording from the apex in a patient with mitral stenosis (MS). The velocity scale is on the vertical axis, with each hash mark representing 1 m/sec.

ography. By measuring either the peak velocity of flow or the mean velocity of flow (through planimetry of the flow-velocity integral), it is possible to calculate the respective peak and mean transmitral pressure gradients. Normally peak velocity is less than 1.7 m/sec and decreases rapidly as diastole proceeds, with a second peak at the time of atrial systole (Fig. 11.10). As indicated in Fig. 11.9, the spectral Doppler waveform of mitral stenosis shows elevated velocities and a progressive but slowed diastolic descent. The secondary increase in diastolic velocity may be absent either because of atrial fibrillation or, even if sinus rhythm is maintained, because the contribution to early diastolic filling may be much more prominent than the atrial contribution to left ventricular filling. In Figure. 11.9, the peak velocity is 2 m/sec and decreases more slowly than normal. Planimetry of the flow-velocity integral facilitates automated measurement of multiple instantaneous peak diastolic velocities during diastole, usually at 40–100 msec intervals. Such a computerized analysis is possible in all commercially available ultrasound systems and, for the waveform in Figure 11.9, yields a mean velocity of 1.5 m/sec. Based on the modified Bernoulli equation, these values would predict peak and mean transmitral gradients of 16 mm Hg and 9 mm Hg, respectively.

Published data indicate good correlations between Doppler-derived gradients and those measured at cardiac catheterization when the studies are performed simultaneously.[10] However, when performed at remote times, the correlations are not as good.[11] This may have to do with changes in heart rate altering the diastolic filling period, particularly in the presence of atrial fibrillation, as well as changes in flow across the valve due to changes in cardiac output and mitral regurgitation. Accurate Doppler determinations also require averaging multiple (at least 10) Doppler profiles and minimizing the Doppler angle relative to flow, both of which may be a source of variability and error, particularly when examinations are performed at different times or by examiners of different experience levels.

Mitral valve area by pressure half-time method. A low or high pressure drop across the valve may be found whether the severity of obstruction is mild or severe, depending on the flow across the valve (Fig. 11.11). Thus, use of the mitral valve area is preferable over transmitral pressure gradients as a flow-independent parameter of stenosis severity. The mitral pressure half-time method was originally described in the catheterization laboratory as an alternative to the Gorlin formula for the estimation of mitral valve area.[12] It is defined as the time interval in milliseconds (msec) required for the transmitral diastolic pressure gradient to fall to one-half of its initial value. Initial studies indicated that mitral

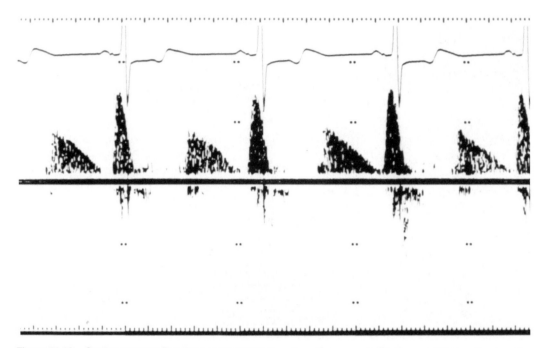

Figure 11.10. Continuous-wave Doppler: normal mitral inflow. A continuous-wave Doppler spectral recording from the apex of normal mitral inflow. The velocity scale is on the vertical axis, with each hash mark representing 1 m/sec.

valve area derived by this method correlated well with the Gorlin formula and that the method was relatively insensitive to changes in heart rate and cardiac output.[12] Subsequently, Hatle et al. applied the relationship between Doppler velocity and pressure gradients described by the modified Bernoulli equation to a Doppler method to measure mitral valve pressure half-time[13] and demonstrated good correlations with invasively obtained measures of mitral valve area. They also demonstrated the Doppler method to provide results that were independent of heart rate, cardiac output, and mitral regurgitation.[13]

The transmitral pressure gradient and the outline of the corresponding Doppler spectral envelope in a patient with mitral stenosis are indicated in Figure 11.12. The initial peak pressure gradient is 25 mm Hg, which, according to the modified Bernoulli equation, corresponds to a peak initial Doppler velocity of 2.5 m/sec ($25 = 4x(2.5)^2$). Time is indicated on the horizontal axis. The time it takes for the initial pressure gradient to drop by one-half (12.5 mm Hg) is 125 msec. The same value would be obtained using the Doppler spectral outline. However, because velocity relates to the square root of the pressure gradient, to obtain one-half of the initial velocity, 2.5 m/sec

Relationship of Gradient to Flow

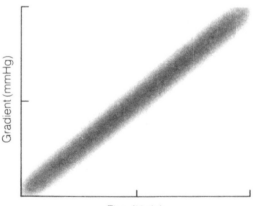

Figure 11.11. Relationship of gradient to flow. Representation of the relationship of transvalvular pressure gradient to transvalvular flow.

should be divided by the square root of two (1.4), which yields 1.79 m/sec as the half-time velocity. The time interval from the initial velocity to this half-time velocity is the pressure half-time, which is once again measured as 125 msec.

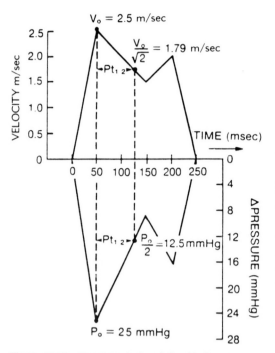

Figure 11.12. Doppler velocity relationship to pressure gradient. Simultaneous recording of Doppler velocity and invasively measured transvalvular pressure gradient in a patient with mitral stenosis. The relationship of velocity and pressure gradient is predicted by the modified Bernoulli equation. The pressure half-time ($Pt_{1/2}$) can be calculated from either method as an index of the severity of mitral stenosis.

The empirically derived relationship between mitral valve area and the pressure half-time is described by the equation:

$$\text{Mitral Valve Area (cm}^2) = \frac{220}{\text{Pressure half-time (msec)}}$$

In normal subjects, pressure half-time ranges between 20 and 60 msec.[13] In mitral stenosis, there is a marked delay and a strong correlation between pressure half-time estimated from Doppler and hemodynamic data, as well as between mitral valve area calculated from Doppler pressure half-time and the Gorlin formula using invasively obtained parameters. A pressure half-time value of 220 msec would be equivalent to a mitral valve area of 1.0 cm^2, with longer pressure half-times in patients with more severe mitral stenosis.

As an index of the severity of mitral stenosis, the pressure half-time offers a number of advantages over other echocardiographic and invasive methods. As previously discussed, the accuracy of both M-mode parameters such as the E-F slope as well as planimetry of the mitral valve orifice from

two-dimensional echocardiography for estimation of mitral valve area is highly dependent on scan plane, image quality, and resolution. In general, it is easier to obtain a good quality transmitral Doppler signal than it is to consistently obtain images of the mitral valve suitable for M-mode measurements or for planimetry.

As noted in Figure 11.11, pressure gradient, whether obtained invasively or by Doppler techniques, and flow are directly related. Figure 11.13 shows a low transmitral pressure gradient in a patient at rest, which becomes markedly elevated with exercise. Thus, despite an unchanged mitral valve area, the transmitral pressure gradient increased during exercise. However, mitral valve pressure half-time remains constant with exercise,[13] so providing a flow-independent parameter of mitral stenosis severity. Yet another advantage of pressure half-time over Doppler-derived pressure gradients is the dependence of an accurate pressure gradient determination on the Doppler angle of intercept with flow. Because pressure half-time measures the time between two velocity points, it is less sensitive to changes in the Doppler angle of intercept.[13,14]

The Gorlin formula for the determination of mitral valve area is also subject to error in the presence of a small mitral valve orifice area,[12,15] a very low cardiac output, [13–16] or when significant mitral regurgitation exists.[17] In these circumstances mitral valve area derived from the Gorlin formula usually underestimates true orifice size, whether or not mitral regurgitant flow is taken into account.[17] The mitral pressure half-time is not notably altered in mitral regurgitation,[13,14] thus under these circumstances it may be a more accurate descriptor of the mitral valve area than that obtained using the Gorlin formula.

Despite its many advantages over other methods, the pressure half-time has a number of limitations. By its nature, it is time consuming and requires experience and expertise. Improper angling may result in the detection of flow from aortic regurgitation, which has many Doppler spectral characteristics in common with mitral stenosis. Thus an erroneous diagnosis or estimation of severity may be rendered. Furthermore, in the presence of significant aortic regurgitation, because left ventricular diastolic pressure is elevated, there may be a lowering of the transmitral pressure gradient, which is unrelated to the severity of mitral stenosis. It has recently been demonstrated that significant aortic regurgitation causes the pressure half-time to overestimate mitral valve area (and thus underestimate the severity of stenosis).[18]

Central to the issue of validation and use of the pressure half-time has been the belief that it varies inversely with mitral valve area and is relatively unaffected by hemodynamic variables such as heart rate, cardiac output, left atrial pressure, and mitral regurgitation. Recent observations, particularly among patients having PMV, in whom a poor correlation between immediately post-PMV mitral valve areas derived by Doppler pressure half-time and invasive methods has been noted, have challenged this notion.[19-22] Certainly some of the discrepancy between the various methods to derive mitral valve area may be accounted for by the fact that regardless of which method is used, no "gold standard" for measurement of mitral valve area currently exists. Nevertheless, the observations of Thomas et al., using mathematical and in vitro modeling, are important in demonstrating that while the pressure half-time varies inversely with mitral valve area, it also varies directly with left atrial compliance and the initial transmitral pressure gradient.[23] The implications for these observations are that while the pressure half-time method is still valid for most clinical settings, in certain settings, such as immediately post-PMV, in aortic regurgitation, or when there is decreased left ventricular compliance due to left ventricular hypertrophy or ischemia, the pressure half-time may be less accurate.

Mitral valve area determination by continuity equation. An alternative to measurement of mitral valve area by the pressure half-time method is mitral

Gradient Variability in Mitral Stenosis

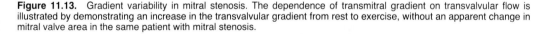

Figure 11.13. Gradient variability in mitral stenosis. The dependence of transmitral gradient on transvalvular flow is illustrated by demonstrating an increase in the transvalvular gradient from rest to exercise, without an apparent change in mitral valve area in the same patient with mitral stenosis.

Continuity Equation

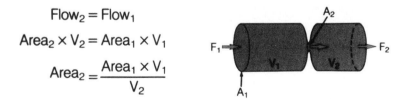

$$\text{Flow}_2 = \text{Flow}_1$$

$$\text{Area}_2 \times V_2 = \text{Area}_1 \times V_1$$

$$\text{Area}_2 = \frac{\text{Area}_1 \times V_1}{V_2}$$

Figure 11.14. Continuity equation. The continuity equation states that flow (F) at any two points in a conduit must be equal. Flow may be represented as a product of cross-sectional area (Area) of the conduit and the velocity of flow (V). Abbreviations: Area_1 = area at nonobstructed site; Area_2 = area at obstruction; Flow_1 = flow at nonobstructed site; Flow_2 = flow at obstruction; V_1 = velocity of flow at nonobstructed site; V_2 = velocity of flow at obstruction.

valve area determination using the "continuity equation." The principle of continuity of flow states that the volume flow at any point in a closed conduit will be equivalent, irrespective of a change in area of the conduit (Fig. 11.14). If flow passes from an area with a large orifice to an area with a smaller orifice, the velocity of flow in the region with the smaller orifice will increase to maintain continuity of flow. Since the Doppler examination measures flow velocity, it is well suited for mitral valve area determination using this method.

In mitral stenosis, without mitral regurgitation, a flow volume through the mitral anulus during one cardiac cycle should be equal to stroke volume. The stroke volume can be expressed as the product of the cross-sectional area of the aortic anulus and the time-velocity integral of aortic flow. Thus, in the equation in Figure 11.14, mitral valve area ($Area_2$) can be calculated as the product of aortic anular cross-sectional area ($Area_1$), obtained from the two-dimensional echocardiogram, and the aortic Doppler time-velocity integral (V_1), divided by the mitral Doppler time-velocity integral (V_2).

The continuity method has previously been validated for determination of aortic valve areas,[24,25] and recent reports indicate that it yields accurate results for mitral valve area determinations as well.[18] The continuity method may be most valuable in situations in which the pressure half-time method is subject to error, such as aortic regurgitation or after PMV. However, there are limitations to the continuity method, particularly when adequate two-dimensional images or Doppler signals cannot be obtained or if significant mitral regurgitation exists.

SELECTION OF VALVULOPLASTY CANDIDATES GUIDED BY ECHO-DOPPLER EXAMINATION

Identification of Coexistent Pathology

While echo-Doppler examination is useful in evaluating the presence and severity of mitral stenosis, it is also valuable for the evaluation of coexisting pathology. Depending on the specific finding, the results may influence the decision to perform PMV or direct a specific approach.

MITRAL REGURGITATION

The presence of severe mitral regurgitation is generally considered a contraindication to PMV. Thus, its pre-PMV echo-Doppler identification and accurate estimation are critical in the proper selection of patients for PMV.

Identification and characterization. On the spectral Doppler tracing, mitral regurgitation will be recognized as systolic flow away from an apical transducer position (Fig. 11.15). Although mitral regurgitation may be detected by continuous-wave Doppler, its severity is best estimated using either pulsed-wave sampling or Doppler color flow mapping. The severity of mitral regurgitation is based on the size of the mitral regurgitant jet detected by these techniques. Using pulsed-wave sampling, mitral regurgitation is assessed by methodically placing the Doppler cursor at various sites in the left atrium (Fig. 11.16) and examining the region for the characteristic spectral Doppler signal. The severity of regurgitation is based on the size of the regurgitant jet, as mapped by the sampling of multiple sites within the left atrium. If a signal of regurgitation is confined only to the immediate vicinity of the atrial side of the mitral valve, the regurgitation is mild. However, if the signal can be detected throughout the atrium, the regurgitation is severe. Using color flow examination, this same principle is used to provide an instantaneous color representation of the regurgitant jet in the left atrium, permitting an immediate assessment of its direction and size (Fig. 11.17). In most cases, the severity of regurgitation assessed by Doppler methods correlates closely with that detected by cardiac catheterization.[26–28] Therefore, patients with significant mitral regurgitation may be identified prior to a catheterization and so excluded from consideration for PMV.

Transesophageal echocardiography. When mitral anular or valve calcification exists, an accurate anatomic and Doppler examination from the chest wall is often not possible. In the same manner that a mitral valve prosthesis would "mask" the ultrasound signal in the left atrium,[29] the presence of calcification in the mitral valve prevents adequate ultrasound examination of the left atrium. In these circumstances, the assessment of mitral regurgitation is rendered either impossible or inaccurate using standard echo-Doppler techniques, and transesophageal echocardiography may be useful. By performing both anatomic and Doppler imaging from the esophagus, using a specially designed probe with ultrasound imaging and Doppler capabilities, the left atrium, which rests immediately anterior to the esophagus, can be specifically examined, without interference from the echogenic material within the mitral valve apparatus (Fig. 11.18).

Doppler assessment of mitral regurgitation from the transesophageal approach is performed in the same manner as from the standard chest approach. The size of the Doppler jet relates to the

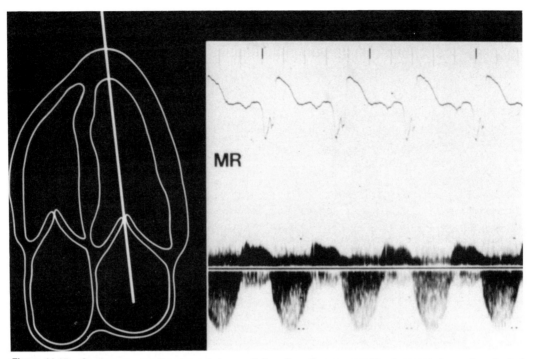

Figure 11.15. Continuous-wave Doppler: mitral regurgitation. A continuous-wave Doppler spectral recording of mitral regurgitation from the apex. The velocity scale is on the vertical axis, with each hash mark representing 1 m/sec.

severity of mitral regurgitation. Using a grading scheme such as the one indicated in Figure 11.19, experience in our laboratory[30] and others[31] indicates an excellent correlation between transesophageal Doppler and catheterization estimates of mitral regurgitation.

LEFT ATRIAL THROMBI

Left atrial thrombi are found in 10–25% of patients undergoing surgical mitral commissurotomy.[32–34] Given the frequency with which they occur and the danger of systemic embolization during transseptal puncture and manipulation of catheters within the left atrium, it becomes mandatory that all patients be assessed for left atrial thrombi before undergoing PMV. The presence of left atrial thrombi are an absolute contraindication to standard PMV.

Characterization. Echocardiography is the most sensitive and specific technique available for the identification of left atrial thrombi.[32–34] In one study, left atrial thrombi were detected in 8% of patients referred for PMV by chest echocardiography, thus excluding them from PMV.[35] As shown in Figure 11.20, left atrial thrombi are characterized as echogenic masses of variable morphology. While

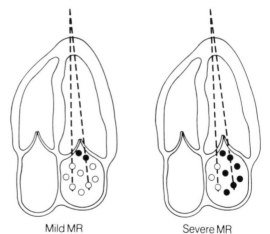

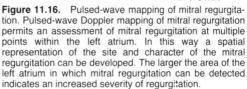

Figure 11.16. Pulsed-wave mapping of mitral regurgitation. Pulsed-wave Doppler mapping of mitral regurgitation permits an assessment of mitral regurgitation at multiple points within the left atrium. In this way a spatial representation of the site and character of the mitral regurgitation can be developed. The larger the area of the left atrium in which mitral regurgitation can be detected indicates an increased severity of regurgitation.

most are commonly found on the posterior left atrial wall or within the atrial appendage, they may occur at any site in the left atrium.

Transesophageal echocardiography. After chest echocardiography, a recent large series of

Direction and Size of Regurgitant Jets

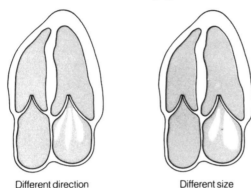

Different direction   Different size

Figure 11.17. Detection and size of regurgitant jets. By performing either tedious pulsed-wave sampling or color flow mapping, the direction and size of mitral regurgitant jets can be assessed.

patients undergoing PMV reported a 2% incidence of thromboembolic symptoms during or after PMV.[36] Recent reports indicate that both the sensitivity and specificity for detection of left atrial thrombi can be improved by transesophageal echocardiography.[37,38] Not only are ultrasound "masking" problems circumvented by transesophageal imaging, but also the left atrial appendage (Fig. 11.21) is better visualized from the transesophageal approach.[32,37,38]

ATRIAL SEPTAL ABNORMALITIES

As PMV involves transseptal puncture of the atrial septum, a pre-PMV examination of atrial septal structure and morphology may be valuable. This is best accomplished from either a subcostal or apical transducer position. In patients in whom chest wall imaging is unsatisfactory, again the transesophageal echocardiogram may be a valuable way to interrogate the atrial septum.

Atrial septal defects. Echo-Doppler examination can be used to identify atrial septal defects using either Doppler color flow imaging or a microcavitation examination using agitated saline to create microbubbles as a right-sided contrast agent. If present, the Doppler examination may be used to accurately characterize the direction and magnitude of the shunt.[39] Although the combination of mitral stenosis and atrial septal defect (Lutembacher's syndrome) is relatively uncommon, if a large left-to-right shunt is present, not only may the hemodynamics of mitral stenosis be

altered, but complete hemodynamic improvement may not be achieved unless the atrial septal defect is surgically repaired.[40] Furthermore, because atrial septal shunts may occur post-PMV, it is important to be aware of the presence and magnitude of a pre-PMV atrial septal shunt. Creation of a large left-to-right shunt in a patient who already has elevated right-sided pressures may cause serious hemodynamic consequences.[41]

Atrial septal thickness. Pathologic studies of the left atrium in mitral stenosis indicate that gross as well as cellular hypertrophy and fibrosis of the atrial walls and septum occur commonly.[42,43] Atrial septal thickening can be diagnosed echocardiographically, thus identifying patients in whom PMV may be technically difficult (Fig. 11.22).[44] Furthermore, resistance to passage of balloon dilation catheters for PMV can occur either at the atrial septum or the mitral valve orifice. By fluoroscopy it may be difficult to determine the site of resistance due to the relatively short distance and sharp bend from the fossa ovalis to the mitral valve orifice. In these situations, an echocardiogram performed during the procedure may help to identify the source of resistance.[45]

OTHER ABNORMALITIES

Other abnormalities such as rheumatic aortic or tricuspid involvement, pulmonary hypertension, and left ventricular dysfunction may all influence the decision to perform PMV. All are easily and reliably diagnosed by standard echo-Doppler techniques.

Coexistent rheumatic valve disease. Combined rheumatic mitral plus aortic or mitral plus tricuspid disease may also occur in patients referred for PMV. Failure to diagnose these before PMV may not only result in inadequate relief of symptoms but may also increase the risk of procedural complications. Occurrence of these may also influence technical aspects of the performance of PMV. With both coexistent aortic or tricuspid stenosis, combined valvuloplasty of both mitral and aortic[46,47] or tricuspid valves is an option.[48]

Echo-Doppler examination is an accurate means to identify and characterize the severity of both aortic and tricuspid stenoses. Echocardiographically, both aortic and tricuspid stenoses are characterized by abnormal valve leaflet morphology, diminished leaflet mobility, and elevated transvalvular Doppler flow velocities, indicative of elevated transvalvular gradients. The gradients, and thus severity of stenosis, may be estimated

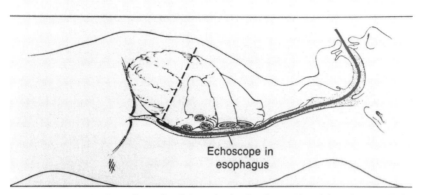

Figure 11.18. Transesophageal echocardiography. Schematic showing the position of the echoscope in the esophagus. From a position posterior to the heart, posterior cardiac structures can be easily imaged. Courtesy of De Bruijn NP, Clements FM. *Transesophageal Echocardiography.* Boston, Martinus Nijhoff, 1987, p. 6.

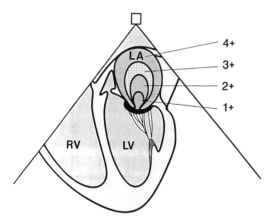

Figure 11.19. Mitral regurgitation: transesophageal approach. Long axis imaging of the left atrium from the transesophageal approach permits Doppler assessment of the severity of mitral regurgitation. In the same way that regurgitant jet direction and size can be mapped from the chest wall, it is also possible to do this from the transesophageal approach.

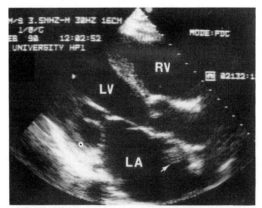

Figure 11.20. Left atrial thrombus. Left atrial thrombus (arrow) visualized on the two-dimensional echocardiogram from the parasternal long axis view. Abbreviations: LA = left atrium; LV = left ventricle; RV = right ventricle.

using the modified Bernoulli equation, as previously described for estimation of transmitral gradients.

The clinical signs of combined mitral and aortic or mitral and tricuspid disease may be quite different than mitral stenosis alone. When both severe mitral and aortic stenoses coexist, the mitral stenosis masks the clinical manifestations and electrocardiographic and radiographic signs of aortic stenosis.[49] Likewise, clinical signs of tricuspid stenosis may also be masked by coexisting mitral stenosis. Furthermore, tricuspid stenosis may be difficult to detect by cardiac catheterization because it is usually associated with low gradients and requires placement of a catheter across the

tricuspid valve, which may alter the measured gradient. Thus, it is mandatory that all candidates for PMV have a thorough echo-Doppler evaluation of both aortic and tricuspid valves.

Left ventricular dysfunction. Left ventricular dysfunction usually occurs due to coexistent coronary artery disease. Its presence and severity may be estimated echocardiographically. When severe, this may be a relative contraindication to PMV. If significant coronary artery disease is present, the patient may be better served by a combined coronary artery bypass and mitral valve operation rather than PMV.

Pulmonary hypertension. Elevation of pulmonary artery pressures is relatively common in mitral stenosis. While not a contraindication to PMV per se, its presence does identify patients at higher risk

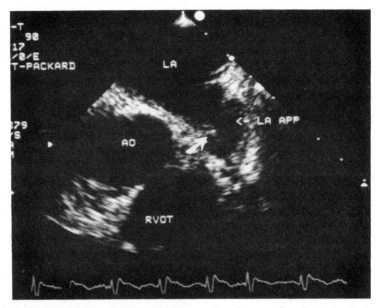

Figure 11.21.   Transesophageal echocardiogram: left atrial appendage thrombus. Two-dimensional echocardiogram from the transesophageal approach permits visualization of the left atrial appendage. The arrow identifies an echogenic target within the appendage, which at surgery was confirmed to be an atrial thrombus. Abbreviations: AO = aorta; LA = left atrium; LA APP = left atrial appendage; RVOT = right ventricular outflow tract.

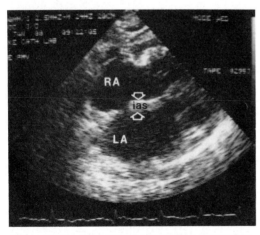

Figure 11.22.   Mitral stenosis: interatrial septal thickening. Subcostal four-chamber view shows a thickened atrial septum (arrows) in a patient with mitral stenosis. LA = left atrium; RA = right atrium; ias = interatrial septum. Courtesy of Sheikh KH et al. *Am Heart J 117*:206–210, 1989.

for complications of PMV. In particular, the combination of elevated pulmonary artery pressures and creation of a significant left-to-right shunt through an atrial septal defect during PMV may cause serious hemodynamic deterioration.[48]

The magnitude of pulmonary artery pressures may be estimated using a variety of echo-Doppler methods. This is most easily and commonly done if tricuspid regurgitation can be identified by continuous-wave Doppler examination. According to the modified Bernoulli equation, the peak Doppler velocity of the tricuspid regurgitant jet relates to the pressure difference between the right ventricle and the right atrium. The right atrial pressure can be estimated from the jugular venous pressure (JVP) by adding 5 cm to the estimated JVP to account for the distance from the clavicle to the right atrium and then converting to mm Hg by dividing by 1.3. Thus, right ventricular systolic pressure equals the transtricuspid systolic gradient plus the right atrial pressure. In Figure 11.23, a continuous-wave Doppler tracing of tricuspid regurgitation is shown, with a peak velocity of 2.4 m/sec. If the estimated JVP is 10 cm, the predicted right ventricular systolic pressure would be: $(JVP + 5)/1.3 + 4 (V)^2$ or $((10 + 5)/1.3) + 4(2.4)^2$, or 34 mm Hg. In the absence of pulmonic stenosis, the right ventricular systolic pressure is equal to the pulmonary artery systolic pressure. Thus, by knowing the peak continuous-wave Doppler velocity of tricuspid regurgitation and the jugular venous pressure, it is possible to accurately estimate the pulmonary artery systolic pressure.

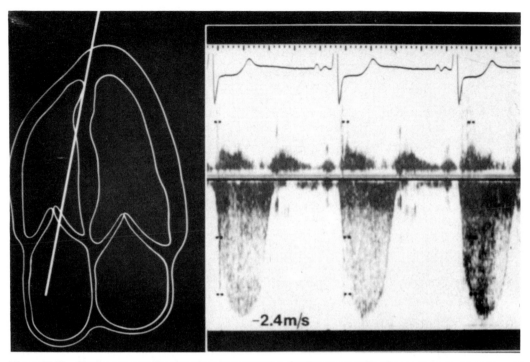

Figure 11.23. Continuous-wave Doppler: tricuspid regurgitation. Continuous-wave Doppler spectral recording of tricuspid regurgitation. The velocity scale is on the vertical axis, with each hash mark representing 1 m/sec. The peak velocity is measured at 2.4 m/sec.

Echocardiographic Predictors of Procedural Results

ECHO-SCORE

It is well recognized that certain echocardiographic features of mitral valve morphology can predict the likelihood of a successful surgical commissurotomy.[50] Recent experience with PMV has also confirmed that occurrence of severe degrees of mitral leaflet calcification, leaflet thickening, leaflet mobility, subvalvular thickening, and subvalvular calcification may identify patients in whom PMV is likely to be unsuccessful. In an effort to optimally select candidates for PMV, a number of investigators have developed "echo scores" based on these echocardiographic features.[51–54] The echo score is generated by either qualitatively or quantitatively grading the severity of these features. By correlating procedural results with retrospective analysis of these features, the echo score has been shown to have some predictive value in terms of identifying patients who are either likely or unlikely to derive hemodynamic benefit from PMV: the higher the echo score, the lower the likelihood of a successful

PMV, and conversely, the lower the echo score, the greater the likelihood of a successful PMV.

The scoring system of Wilkins et al. has been widely applied.[51] As shown in Table 11.1, valve mobility, subvalvular thickening, leaflet thickening, and leaflet calcification are each graded on a 0–4 scale. A maximum score of 16 is possible. While there was some overlap, in their initial studies, an echo score of ≥ 11 identified all patients with suboptimal results, whereas an echo score of ≤ 8 identified all patients with optimal results to PMV.[51] A more quantitative method for generating an echo score has been applied by Reid et al. to study echocardiographic features predictive of success with similar results.[53]

There are, however, a number of problems with the echo score. Among these are the fact that even patients with high echo scores obtain hemodynamic and symptomatic improvement after PMV.[20,55] Furthermore, not all studies are in agreement that either valve thickening,[20] subvalvular disease,[53] or the total echo score[54] are predictors of a successful procedure. There are few studies evaluating the utility of the echo score in a prospective manner.[54]

Table 11.1.
Grading of Mitral Valve Characteristics from the Echocardiographic Examination

Grade	Mobility	Subvalvular thickening	Leaflet Thickening	Calcification
1	Highly mobile valve with only leaflet tips restricted	Minimal thickening just below the mitral leaflets	Leaflets near normal in thickness (4–5 mm)	A single area of increased echo brightness
2	Leaflet mid and base portions have normal mobility	Thickening of chordal structures extending up to one-third of the chordal length	Mid-leaflets normal, considerable thickening of margins (5–8 mm)	Scattered areas of brightness confined to leaflet margins
3	Valve continues to move forward in diastole, mainly from the base	Thickening extending to the distal third of the chords	Thickening extending through the entire leaflet (5–8 mm)	Brightness extending into the mid-portion of the leaflets
4	No or minimal forward movement of the leaflets in diastole	Extensive thickening and shortening of all chordal structures extending down to the papillary muscles	Considerable thickening of all leaflet tissue (> 8 –10 mm)	Extensive brightness throughout much of the leaflet tissue

The total echocardiographic score was derived from an analysis of mitral leaflet mobility, valvular and subvalvular thickening, and calcification, which were graded from 0 to 4 according to the above criteria. This gave a total score of 0 to 16. Courtesy of Wilkins GT et al. *Br Heart J* 60:299–308, 1988.

Finally, as the technical aspects of PMV improve, more patients, especially those with higher echo scores may experience favorable results. It thus seems unreasonable to absolutely exclude patients for PMV purely on the basis of a high echo score.

BALLOON SIZE

Echocardiography may also be used to guide the selection of the most optimal balloon size for PMV. Because the mechanism of PMV involves commissural tearing along the natural commissures of the valve leaflets,[19,20,56,57] the balloon size that permits maximum extension of the commissures to the mitral anulus appears to be optimal.[54] Furthermore, selection of the appropriate balloon size is also important to protect against the development of excessive post-PMV mitral regurgitation.[54] A balloon size that is equivalent to, or slightly larger than, the mitral anular diameter measured from the apical four-chamber view during mid-diastole, when the mitral valve leaflets are at their maximal excursion, appears to result in the greatest likelihood of success.[35,54]

ECHO-DOPPLER EVALUATION FOLLOWING MITRAL VALVULOPLASTY
Hemodynamics

Both invasive and echo-Doppler measurements of mitral valve area and transmitral pressure gradients

may document post-PMV results. It has, however, recently been observed that post-PMV mitral valve areas determined by the Doppler pressure half-time method correlate less well with invasively obtained mitral valve areas than those pre-PMV.[19-23] In general, the Doppler mitral valve area overestimates the invasively derived mitral valve area immediately post-PMV. It has yet to be determined whether the discrepancy arises from inaccuracy with the invasive method, the Doppler method, or both. A number of factors may, however, play a role in the lowered correlation. Among these would include development of mitral regurgitation or intracardiac shunting through the development of an atrial septal defect, each of which may affect mitral valve area determinations by either invasive or Doppler methods. Furthermore, the dependence of the mitral valve area determined by the pressure half-time method on left atrial compliance and the initial transmitral pressure gradient has previously been noted.[23] Alterations in left atrial pressure, the transmitral gradient, transmitral flow, and left atrial and left ventricular dimensions and compliance all occur during PMV and so may affect mitral valve area determinations by the pressure half-time method and Gorlin formula in different ways.[21] Thomas et al. have recently shown that post-PMV the correlations of mitral valve area determinations by pressure half-time methods and the Gorlin formula may be improved when the pressure half-time determinations are corrected for left atrial compliance and the initial transmitral pressure gradient.[21] Whether left ventricular (LV) compliance is affected by the procedure is unsettled, though recently Harrison et al. found no evidence for LV diastolic dysfunction after the procedure.[58]

Correlations between Doppler and invasive measurements improve when determinations are made 24–48 hours after PMV, rather than immediately post-PMV.[21,22] Thus, beyond the initial, immediately post-PMV interval, echo-Doppler methods appear to be an accurate means to follow serial changes in mitral valve area after PMV and thus to detect mitral valve restenosis.

Mitral Regurgitation

While the degree of mitral regurgitation remains unchanged in most patients immediately after PMV, it may increase by one grade in 30–40% and by two grades in 5–15%.[36,59,60] Echo-Doppler examination is a convenient way to noninvasively follow the severity of mitral regurgitation after PMV. In late follow-up, most patients experience a decrease in the severity of mitral regurgitation, with less than 10% at six months after PMV having worse mitral regurgitation than was present before PMV.[60,61]

Atrial Septal Defect

Transseptal passage of balloon catheters results in the creation of transient and at times permanent atrial septal defects. The ability to detect these defects depends on the diagnostic techniques employed. While shunting by oximetry can be detected in 15–35% of patients immediately after PMV,[36,62] dye dilution methods can detect shunts in up to 75% of patients.[62] In most patients the severity of shunts is small, with a mean $Q_p:Q_s$ = 1.22, and only 2–15% have a $Q_p:Q_s$ >1.5.[36,62]

Echo-Doppler methods are more sensitive than either oximetry or dye dilution techniques. Immediately after PMV, atrial shunts are demonstrable in over 30% of patients assessed by chest wall contrast echocardiography,[57] over 50% using chest wall Doppler echocardiography,[63,64] and nearly 90% using transesophageal Doppler color flow mapping.[65]

Irrespective of which diagnostic method is used, the number of detectable shunts decreases with time. By 3–6 months after PMV, a detectable shunt is present in 20–25% of patients.[63,65] Creation and persistence of a significant left-to-right shunt, particularly in the presence of significant mitral regurgitation or mitral valve restenosis, which may exacerbate the left-to-right shunting, as well as with preexisting elevation in right-sided pressures, may cause hemodynamic deterioration.[41]

CONCLUSIONS

The echo-Doppler examination is an integral part of the PMV procedure. Not only does it offer a reliable way to diagnose mitral stenosis, but it may be used to both select candidates appropriate for PMV and identify those in whom PMV is contraindicated. While echo-Doppler is a convenient, noninvasive diagnostic method, it also provides unique and critical information necessary for the safe and successful performance of PMV. In many cases this information cannot be obtained from any other diagnostic modality, including cardiac catheterization.

REFERENCES

1. Edler I. Ultrasound cardiogram in mitral valve disease. *Acta Chir Scand* 11:230–231, 1956.
2. Edler I, Gustafson A. Ultrasonic cardiography in mitral stenosis. *Acta Med Scand* 159:85–90, 1952.
3. Nichol PM, Gilbert BW, Kisslo JA. Two-dimensional echocardiographic assessment of mitral stenosis. *Circulation* 55:120–128, 1977.
4. Gustafson A. Correlation between ultrasound cardiography, hemodynamics and surgical findings in mitral stenosis. *Am J Cardiol* 19:32–41, 1967.
5. Wharton CFP, Lopez-Bescos L. Mitral valve movement. A study using an ultrasound technique. *Br Heart J* 32:344–349, 1970.
6. DeMaria A, Miller R, Amsterdam E, Markson W, Mason D. Mitral valve early diastolic closing velocity in the echocardiogram: Relation to sequential diastolic flow and ventricular compliance. *Am J Cardiol* 37:693–700, 1976.
7. Quinones MA, Gaash WH, Waisser E, Alexander J. Reduction in the rate of diastolic descent of the mitral valve echocardiogram in patients with altered left ventricular diastolic pressure-volume relations. *Circulation* 49:246–254, 1974.
8. Henry WL, Griffith JM, Michaels LL, McIntosh CL, Morrow AG, Epstein SE. Measurement of mitral orifice area in patients with mitral valve disease by real-time two-dimensional echocardiography. *Circulation* 51:827–831, 1975.
9. Wann LS, Weyman A, Feigenbaum H, Dillon JC, Johnston KQW, Eggleton RC. Determination of mitral valve area by cross-sectional echocardiography. *Ann Intern Med* 88:337–341, 1978.
10. Hatle L, Grubakk A, Tromsdal A, Angelsen B. Noninvasive assessment of pressure drop in mitral

stenosis by Doppler ultrasound. *Br Heart J 40*: 131–140, 1978.

11. Holen J, Aaslind R, Lurdmark K, Simonsen S. Determination of pressure gradient in mitral stenosis with a noninvasive ultrasound Doppler technique. *Acta Med Scand 199*:455–460, 1976.

12. Libanoff AJ, Rodbard S. Atrioventricular pressure half-time: Measure of mitral valve orifice area. *Circulation 38*:144–150, 1968.

13. Hatle L. Angelsen B, Tromsdal A. Noninvasive assessment of atrioventricular pressure half-time by Doppler ultrasound. *Circulation 60*:1097–1104, 1979.

14. Pulsed and continuous wave Doppler in diagnosis and assessment of various heart lesions. In: *Doppler Ultrasound in Cardiology: Physical Principles and Clinical Applications*. ed by L. Hatle and B. Angelsen, Philadephia, Lea and Febiger, 1982, pp. 76–170.

15. Cannon SR, Richards KL, Crawford M. Hydraulic estimation of stenotic orifice area: A correction of the Gorlin formula. *Circulation 72*:1170–1178, 1985.

16. Segal J, Lerner DJ, Miller DC, et al. When should Doppler-determined valve area be better than the Gorlin formula?: Variation in hydraulic constants in low flow states. *J Am Coll Cardiol 9*:1294–1305, 1987.

17. Fredman CS, Pearson AC, Labovitz AJ, Kern MJ. Comparison of hemodynamic pressure half-time method and Gorlin formula with Doppler and echocardiographic determinations of mitral valve area in patients with combined mitral stenosis and regurgitation. *Am Heart J 119*:121–129, 1990.

18. Nakatani S, Masuyama T, Kodama K, Kitabatake A, Fujii K, Kamada T. Value and limitations of Doppler echocardiography in the quantification of stenotic mitral valve area: Comparison of the pressure half-time and the continuity equation methods. *Circulation 77*:78–85, 1988.

19. Reid CL, McKay CR, Chandraratna PAN, Kawanishi DT, Rahimtoola SH. Mechanisms of increase in mitral valve area and influence of anatomic features in double-balloon, catheter balloon valvuloplasty in adults with rheumatic mitral stenosis: A Doppler and two-dimensional echocardiographic study. *Circulation 76*:628–636, 1987.

20. Come PC, Riley MF, Diver DJ, Morgan JP, Safian RD, McKay RG. Noninvasive assessment of mitral stenosis before and after percutaneous balloon mitral valvuloplasty. *Am J Cardiol 61*:817–825, 1988.

21. Thomas JD, Wilkins GT, Choong CYP, et al. Inaccuracy of mitral pressure half-time immediately after percutaneous mitral valvotomy: Dependence on transmitral gradient and left atrial and ventricular compliance. *Circulation 78*:980–993, 1988.

22. Chen C, Wang Y, Guo B, Lin Y. Reliability of the Doppler pressure half-time method for assessing

effects of percutaneous mitral balloon valvuloplasty. *J Am Coll Cardiol 13*:1309–1313, 1989.

23. Thomas JD, Weyman AE. Doppler mitral pressure half-time: A clinical tool in search of theoretical justification. *J Am Coll Cardiol 10*:923–929, 1987.

24. Skjaerpe T, Hegrenaes L, Hatle L. Noninvasive estimation of valve area in patients with aortic stenosis by Doppler ultrasound and two-dimensional echocardiography. *Circulation 72*:810–818, 1985.

25. Zoghbi WA, Farmer KL, Soto JG, Nelson JG, Quinones MA. Accurate noninvasive quantification of stenotic aortic valve area by Doppler echocardiography. *Circulation 73*:452–459, 1986.

26. Omoto R, Yokote, Takamoto S, et al. The development of real-time two-dimensional Doppler echocardiography and its clinical significance in acquired valvular diseases with special reference to the evaluation of valvular regurgitation. *Jpn Heart J 25*:325–339, 1984.

27. Miyatake K, Izumi S, Okamoto M, et al. Semiquantitative grading of severity of mitral regurgitation by real-time two-dimensional Doppler color flow imaging technique. *J Am Coll Cardiol 6*:82–88, 1986.

28. Spain MG, Smith MD, Grayburn PA, et al. Quantitative assessment of mitral regurgitation by Doppler color flow imaging: Angiographic and hemodynamic correlations. *J Am Coll Cardiol 13*:580–590, 1989.

29. Sprecher DL, Adamic R, Adams D, Kisslo J. In vitro color flow, pulsed and continuous wave Doppler ultrasound masking of flow by prosthetic valves. *J Am Coll Cardiol 9*:1306–1310, 1987.

30. Sheikh KH, De Bruijn NP, Rankin JS, Clements FM, Stanley T, Wolfe WG, Kisslo J. The utility of transesophageal echocardiography and Doppler color flow imaging in patients undergoing cardiac valve surgery. *J Am Coll Cardiol 15*:363–372, 1990.

31. Schluter M, Langenstein BA, Hanrath P, Kremer P, Bleifeld W. Assessment of transesophageal pulsed Doppler echocardiography in the detection of mitral regurgitation. *Circulation 66*:784–789, 1982.

32. Shrestha NK, Moreno FL, Narciso FV, et al. Two-dimensional echocardiographic diagnosis of left atrial thrombus in rheumatic heart disease: A clinicopathologic study. *Circulation 67*:341–347, 1983.

33. Beppu S, Park Y, Sakakibara H, et al. Clinical features of intracardiac thrombosis based on echocardiographic observations. *Jpn Circ J 48*:75–82, 1984.

34. Shrestha NK, Moreno FL, Narciso FV, Torres L, Calleja HB. Two-dimensional echocardiographic diagnosis of left atrial thrombus in rheumatic heart disease. A clinicopathologic study. *Circulation 67*: 341–347, 1983.

35. McKay CR, Kawanishi DT, Rahimtoola SH. Catheter balloon valvuloplasty of the mitral valve in adults

using a double-balloon technique. *JAMA 257*: 1753–1761, 1987.

36. Ruiz CE, Allen JW, Lau FYK. Percutaneous double balloon valvotomy for severe rheumatic mitral stenosis. *Am J Cardiol 65*:473–477, 1990.

37. Kramer PH, Rowland AJ, Crouse LJ. Preoperative transesophageal echocardiography for candidates for balloon mitral valvuloplasty [Abstract]. *Circulation 80* (Suppl II): 71, 1989.

38. Matsumura M, Shah P, Kyo S, Omoto R. Advantages of transesophageal echo for correct diagnosis on small left atrial thrombi in mitral stenosis [Abstract]. *Circulation 80*(Suppl II): 678, 1989.

39. Dittmann H, Jacksch R, Voelker W, Karsch K-R, Seipel L. Accuracy of Doppler echocardiography in quantification of left to right shunts in adult patients with atrial septal defect. *J Am Coll Cardiol 11*: 338–342, 1988.

40. Bashi VV, Ravikumar E, Jairaj PS, Krishnaswami S, John S. Coexistent mitral valve disease with left-to-right shunt at the atrial level: Clinical profile, hemodynamics, and surgical considerations in 67 consecutive patients. *Am Heart J 114*:1406–1414, 1987.

41. Chen C-H, Lin S-L, Hsu T-L, Chen C-C, Wang S-P, Chang M-S. Iatrogenic Lutembacher's syndrome after percutaneous transluminal mitral valvotomy. *Am Heart J 119*:209–211, 1990.

42. Thiedemann KV, Ferrans VJ. Left atrial ultrastructure in mitral valvular disease. *Am J Pathol 89*: 575–604, 1977.

43. Unverferth DV, Fertel RH, Unverferth BJ, Leier CV. Atrial fibrillation in mitral stenosis: Histologic, hemodynamic and metabolic factors. *Int J Cardiol 5*: 143–152, 1984.

44. Sheikh KH, Davidson CJ, Skelton TN, Nesmith JW, Kisslo K, Bashore TM. Interatrial septal thickening preventing percutaneous mitral valve balloon valvuloplasty. *Am Heart J 117*:206–210, 1989.

45. Pandian NG, Isner JM, Hougen TJ, Desnoyers MR, McInerney K, Salem DN. Percutaneous balloon valvuloplasty of mitral stenosis aided by cardiac ultrasound. *Am J Cardiol 59*:380–381, 1987.

46. Berman AD, Weinstein JS, Safian RD, Diver DJ, Grossman W, McKay RG. Combined aortic and mitral balloon valvuloplasty in patients with critical aortic and mitral valve stenosis: Results in six cases. *J Am Coll Cardiol 11*:1213–1218, 1988.

47. Medina A, Bethencourt A, Coello I, et al. Combined percutaneous mitral and aortic balloon valvuloplasty. *Am J Cardiol 64*:620–624, 1989.

48. Bethencourt A, Medina A, Hernandez E, et al. Combined percutaneous balloon valvuloplasty of mitral and tricuspid valves. *Am Heart J 119*: 416–418, 1990.

49. Zitnik RA. The masking of aortic stenosis by mitral stenosis. *Am Heart J 69*:22–30, 1965.

50. Nanda NC, Gramiak R, Shah PM, DeWeese JA.

Mitral commissurotomy versus replacement. Preoperative evaluation by echocardiography. *Circulation 51*:263–267, 1975.

51. Wilkins GT, Weyman AE, Abascal VM, Block PC, Palacios IF. Percutaneous balloon dilatation of the mitral valve: An analysis of echocardiographic variables related to outcome and the mechanism of dilatation. *Br Heart J 60*:299–308, 1988.

52. Herrmann HC, Wilkins GT, Abascal VM, Weyman AE, Block PC, Palacios IF. Percutaneous balloon mitral valvotomy for patients with mitral stenosis. Analysis of factors influencing early results. *J Thorac Cardiovasc Surg 96*:33–38, 1988.

53. Reid CL, Chandraratna AN, Kawanishi DT, Kotlewski A, Rahimtoola SH. Influence of mitral valve morphology on double-balloon catheter balloon valvuloplasty in patients with mitral stenosis. *Circulation 80*:515–524, 1989.

54. Chen C, Wang X, Wang Y, Lan Y. Value of two-dimensional echocardiography in selecting patients and balloon sizes for percutaneous balloon mitral valvuloplasty. *J Am Coll Cardiol 14*:1651–1658, 1989.

55. Serra A, Bonan R, Lefevre T, Dyrda I. Balloon mitral valvuloplasty in patients with high echocardiographic score [Abstract]. *Circulation 80* (Suppl II): 71, 1989.

56. Block PC, Palacios IF, Jacobs ML, Fallon JT. Mechanism of percutaneous mitral valvotomy. *Am J Cardiol 59*:178–179, 1987.

57. McKay RG, Lock JE, Safian RD, et al. Balloon dilation of mitral stenosis in adult patients: Postmortem and percutaneous mitral valvuloplasty studies. *J Am Coll Cardiol 9*:723–731, 1987.

58. Harrison JK, Davidson CJ, Hanemann D, Harding MB, Bashore TM. Left ventricular diastolic performance and LV diastolic filling before and immediately after balloon mitral valvuloplasty. [Abstract] *Circulation 82* (Suppl III): III–501, 1990.

59. Abascal V, Wilkins GT, Choong CY, Block PC, Palacios IF, Weyman AE. Mitral regurgitation after percutaneous balloon mitral valvuloplasty in adults: Evaluation by pulsed Doppler echocardiography. *J Am Coll Cardiol 11*: 257–263, 1988.

60. Muller T, Petitclerc R, Lesperance J, et al. Mitral regurgitation assessed by echo-Doppler after percutaneous mitral valvuloplasty [Abstract]. *Circulation 80* (Suppl II):167, 1989.

61. Abascal VM, Wilkins GT, Choong CY, et al. Echocardiographic evaluation of mitral valve structure and function in patients followed for at least 6 months after percutaneous balloon mitral valvuloplasty. *J Am Coll Cardiol 12*:606–615, 1988.

62. Serra A, Bonan R, Cequier A, Crepeau J, Dyrda I. Atrial shunting after balloon mitral valvuloplasty: Prediction and follow-up [Abstract]. *Circulation 80* (Suppl II):72, 1989.

63. Bernard Y, Schiele F, Bassand J-P, Anguenot T,

Jacoulet P, Maurat J-P. Characteristics of flow through the atrial septal defect following percutaneous mitral valvuloplasty [Abstract]. *Circulation* *80*(Suppl II): 569, 1989.

64. Helmcke F, Parro A, Ballal RS, et al. Color Doppler assessment of iatrogenic atrial septal defect following percutaneous mitral valvuloplasty. *Circulation* *80*(Suppl II): 168, 1989.

65. Yoshida K, Yoshikawa J, Akasaka T. Assessment of left-to-right atrial shunting after percutaneous mitral valvuloplasty by transesophageal color Doppler flow-mapping. *Circulation* *80*:1521–1526, 1989.

12

Immediate Outcome of Percutaneous Mitral Balloon Valvotomy

IGOR F. PALACIOS, E. MURAT TUZCU, and PETER C. BLOCK

Since percutaneous mitral balloon valvotomy (PMV) was first performed in 1984,[1] the importance of patient selection in the immediate outcome of this procedure has become obvious.[1–8] PMV is not an easy technique, and operator experience and careful patient selection are necessary to achieve a good immediate outcome with minimal complications.

The criteria required for patients to be considered for PMV include

1. symptomatic mitral stenosis
2. no recent embolic event
3. less than 2 + of mitral regurgitation
4. no evidence of left atrial thrombus on 2-D echocardiography

Patients in atrial fibrillation and patients with previous embolic episodes should be anticoagulated with warfarin for 2 to 3 months before PMV. Patients with left atrial thrombus on 2-D echocardiography are excluded. A transesophageal echocardiogram should be performed if there is doubt of the presence of left atrial thrombus by transthoracic 2-D echocardiography or in patients with previous embolic events.

Percutaneous mitral balloon valvotomy results in immediate hemodynamic and clinical improvement in the great majority of patients with mitral stenosis.[2–8] Figure 12.1 shows the hemodynamic changes produced by PMV in a representative patient. In most series the mitral valve area increases from < 1.0 cm² to ≥ 2.0 cm². The mean changes in hemodynamics produced by PMV in 357 consecutive patients at the Massachusetts General Hospital are shown in Table 12.1; PMV

resulted in a significant decrease in mitral gradient and an increase in both cardiac output and mitral valve area. Mean pulmonary artery pressure, mean left atrial pressure, and calculated pulmonary vascular resistance decreased significantly following PMV. Pulmonary vascular resistance continues to decrease during the next 24 hours following PMV.[9]

A good hemodynamic outcome (defined as post-PMV mitral valve area ≥ 1.5 cm²) can be expected in 77% of the patients.[6] Although a suboptimal result (post-PMV mitral valve area < 1.5 cm²) occurred in 23% of the patients, a post-PMV mitral valve area ≤ 1.0 cm² (critical mitral valve area) was obtained in only 8% (Fig. 12.2).

Univariate and multiple stepwise regression analyses of multiple demographic, clinical, and hemodynamic variables of patients undergoing PMV at the Massachusetts General Hospital have demonstrated that the increase in mitral valve area with PMV is directly related to balloon size and inversely related to the echocardiographic score, presence of atrial fibrillation, presence of calcium under fluoroscopy, presence of mitral regurgitation before PMV, older age, lower cardiac output, New York Heart Association functional class before PMV, and a previous surgical mitral commissurotomy[3,6] (Tables 12.2, 12.3).

Experience with closed surgical mitral commissurotomy has shown that valve pliability, the degree of leaflet thickening, and the severity of subvalvular fibrosis and agglutination have an important impact on the immediate outcome of PMV. The most important predictor of the

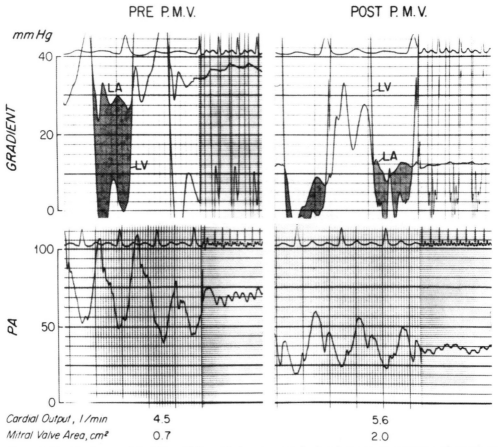

Figure 12.1. Simultaneous left atrial and left ventricular pressures (top), pulmonary artery pressure (bottom), cardiac output, and mitral valve area before (left) and after (right) successful PMV. (From Palacios IF, Block PC, Brandi S, et al. Percutaneous balloon valvotomy for patients with severe mitral stenosis. *Circulation* 75:778, 1987; with permission.)

Table 12.1.
Changes in Hemodynamic Variables Produced by PMV. (Massachusetts General Hospital. N = 357)

	Pre-PMV	Post-PMV
Mitral gradient (mm Hg)	15 ± 0.5	5 ± 0.2[a]
Cardiac output (liters/min)	3.9 ± 0.1	4.5 ± 0.1[a]
Mitral valve area (cm²)	0.9 ± 0.1	2.0 ± 0.1[a]
Mean PA pressure (mm Hg)	38 ± 1	29 ± 1[a]
Mean LA pressure (mm Hg)	25 ± 1	15 ± 1[a]
PAR (dynes-s-cm⁻⁵)	316 ± 15	268 ± 12[a]

[a]$p < 0.0001$
PA = pulmonary artery; LA = left atrium; PAR = pulmonary arteriolar resistance; PMV = percutaneous mitral balloon valvotomy.

Table 12.2.
Univariate Predictors of the Increase in MVA after PMV[a]

Directly related to:	
Balloon size	($p = .02$)
Inversely related to:	
Echo score	($p = .000000001$)
Older age	($p = .0001$)
Presence of AF	($p = .0003$)
NYHA FC pre-PMV	($p = .002$)
Mitral regurgitation	($p = .0004$)
Fluoroscopic calcium	($p = .0000009$)
Previous surgical commissurotomy	($p = .001$)

[a]Univariate analysis
AF = atrial fibrillation
FC = functional class

POST-PMV MITRAL VALVE AREA

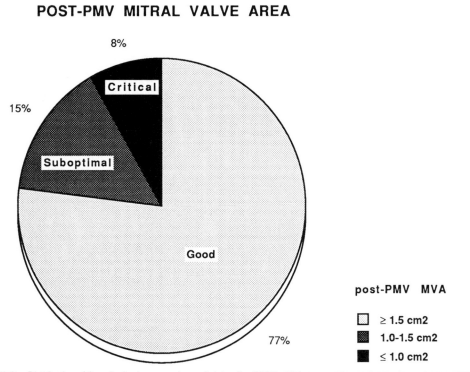

Figure 12.2. Distribution of the mitral valve areas immediately after PMV in 357 consecutive patients who underwent PMV at the Massachusetts General Hospital.

Table 12.3.
Independent Predictors of the Increase in MVA after PMV[a]

Directly related to:	
Balloon size	$(p = .02)$
Inversely related to:	
Echo score	$(p = .0001)$
Presence of AF	$(p = .009)$
Mitral regurgitation	$(p = .003)$

[a]Multiple stepwise regression analysis
AF = atrial fibrillation

immediate and long-term results of PMV is a morphologic echocardiographic score developed at the Massachusetts General Hospital.[10,11] The echocardiographic evaluation of the mitral valve is fundamental in the evaluation of patients for PMV. Since 2-D echocardiography shows the structure of the mitral valve apparatus, the severity of the stenotic lesion and chamber sizes, it provides information that may predict the likely outcome of PMV. In the echocardiographic score each of the following:—leaflet rigidity, leaflet thickening, val-

vular calcification, and subvalvular disease—are scored from 0 to 4.

Table 12.4 describes the scoring system. A higher score represents a heavily calcified and immobile valve with extensive thickening and agglutination of the subvalvular apparatus. Figure 12.3 shows the 2-D echocardiographic long axial view from two representative patients with mitral stenosis. One patient had an echocardiographic score of 4 (Fig. 12.3A) and the other an echocardiographic score of 11 (Fig. 12.3B). One would predict a poorer result in the patient with the higher echocardiographic score.

As can be seen in Figure 12.4, the best outcome with PMV occurs in patients with echocardiographic scores ≤ 8 (91% good results). The increase in mitral valve area is significantly greater in patients with an echocardiographic score ≤ 8 than in those with echocardiographic score > 8. An echocardiographic score ≤ 8 has a high sensitivity and specificity for predicting a good outcome (post-PMV mitral valve area ≥ 1.5 cm²).[12] Of the four components of the echocardiographic score, valve thickening correlates best with the absolute change in mitral valve area.[12]

Table 12.4.
The Echocardiographic Score

Grade	Mobility	Subvalvular Thickening	Valvular Thickening	Calcification
1	Highly mobile valve with only leaflet tips restricted	Minimal thickening just below the mitral leaflets	Leaflets near normal in thickness (4–5 mm)	A single area of increased echo brightness
2	Leaflet mid and base portions have normal mobility	Thickening of chordal structures extending up to one-third of the chordal length	Mid-leaflets normal, considerable thickening of margins	Scattered areas of brightness confined to leaflet margins
3	Valve continues to move forward in diastole, mainly from the base	Thickening extending to the distal third of the chords	Thickening extending through the entire leaflet (5–8 mm)	Brightness extending into the mid-portion of the leaflets
4	No or minimal forward movement of the leaflets in diastole	Extensive thickening and shortening of all chordal structures extending down to the papillary muscles	Considerable thickening of all leaflet tissue (> 8–10 mm)	Extensive brightness throughout much of the leaflet tissue

(From Wilkins GT, Weyman AE, Abascal VM, Block PC, Palacios IF. Percutaneous balloon dilatation of the mitral valve: An analysis of echocardiographic variables related to outcome and the mechanism of dilatation. *Br Heart J 60*:299, 1988; with permission.)

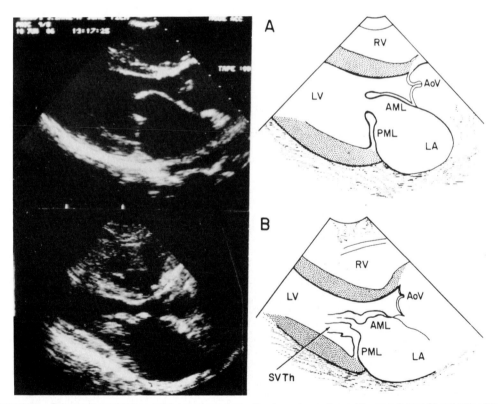

Figure 12.3.   Echocardiographic long axial view of a patient with a low echocardiographic score (panel **A**) and with a high echocardiographic score (panel **B**). (From Wilkins GT, Weyman AE, Abascal VM, Block PC, Palacios IF. Percutaneous balloon dilatation of the mitral valve: An analysis of echocardiographic variables related to outcome and the mechanism of dilatation. *Br Heart J 60*: 299, 1988; with permission.)

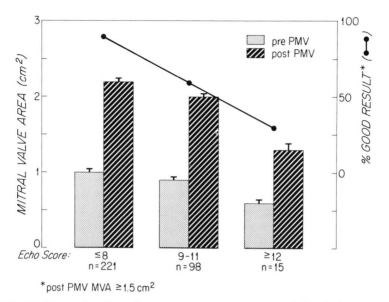

Figure 12.4. Relationship between the echocardiographic score (x axis), the increase in the mitral valve area produced by PMV (left axis), and the percentage of patients having a good result (post-PMV MVA $\geq$ 1.5 cm^2) (right axis).

Table 12.5.
Impact of the Effective Balloon Dilating Area (EBDA) on the Immediate Outcome of PMV

	MVA (cm^2)	
	pre-PMV	post-PMV
Single balloon (EBDA = 4.3 $\pm$ 0.2 cm^2) (N = 26)	0.8 $\pm$ 0.1	1.5 $\pm$ 0.1
Double Balloon (EBDA = 6.5 $\pm$ 0.03 cm^2) (N = 331)	0.9 $\pm$ 0.1	2.2 $\pm$ 0.1[a]

[a] $p < 0.0001$
EBDA = effective balloon dilating area; MVA = mitral valve area; PMV = percutaneous mitral balloon valvotomy.

Effective Balloon Dilating Area (cm^2)

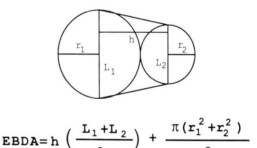

$$\text{EBDA} = h\left(\frac{L_1 + L_2}{2}\right) + \frac{\pi(r_1^2 + r_2^2)}{2}$$

Figure 12.5. Normogram used to calculate the effective balloon dilating area (EBDA) of any two balloon size combinations. (From Roth RB, Block PC, Palacios IF. Predictors of increased mitral regurgitation after percutaneous mitral balloon valvotomy. *Cathet Cardiovascular Diagn* 20:17, 1990; with permission.)

The increase of mitral valve area with PMV is also directly related to the inflated balloon size. The effect of balloon size was first evaluated in a subgroup of patients who underwent repeat PMV.[13] These patients had PMV with a single balloon resulting in a final mean mitral valve area of 1.2 $\pm$ 0.2 cm^2. They underwent repeat PMV using the double balloon technique, and this increased the effective balloon dilating area (EBDA), normalized by body surface area (EBDA:BSA) from 3.41 $\pm$ 0.2 to 4.51 $\pm$ 0.2 cm^2/m^2. The mean mitral valve area in this group after the repeat PMV was 1.8 cm^2 $\pm$ 0.2 cm^2. As can be seen in Table 12.5 the increase in mitral valve area in 331 patients who underwent PMV using the double balloon technique (EBDA of 6.5 $\pm$ 0.03 cm^2) was significantly greater than the increase in mitral valve area achieved in 26 patients who underwent PMV using the single balloon technique (EBDA of 4.33 $\pm$ 0.02 cm^2). The mean mitral valve area in patients who underwent PMV with the double balloon technique was 2.1 $\pm$ 0.1 cm^2; this value was greater than the valve area obtained in patients who underwent PMV with the single balloon

EFFECTIVE BALLOON DILATING AREA (cm²)

	0	15	18	20
15	1.77	4.02	4.89	5.55
18	2.54	4.89	5.78	6.46
20	3.14	5.55	6.46	7.14
23	4.15	6.57	7.55	8.27
25	4.91	7.46	8.41	9.11

Figure 12.6. Diagrammatic representation of the effective balloon dilating area (EBDA) for any two-balloon combination. (From Roth RB, Block PC, Palacios IF. Predictors of increased mitral regurgitation after percutaneous mitral balloon valvotomy. *Cathet Cardiovasc Diagn* 20:17, 1990; with permission.)

Table 12.6.
Effect of the Presence of Atrial Fibrillation on the Immediate Outcome of PMV

	MVA (cm²) pre-PMV	post-PMV
Normal sinus rhythm (N = 181)	1.0 ± 0.1	2.3 ± 0.1
Atrial fibrillation (N = 176)	0.9 ± 0.1	1.7 ± 0.1^a

[a]$p < 0.001$
MVA = mitral valve area; PMV = percutaneous mitral balloon valvotomy.

technique (1.5 ± 0.1 cm²). Care should be taken in the selection of dilating balloon catheters so as to obtain an adequate final mitral valve area without changing or minimally increasing mitral regurgitation. We have demonstrated that the ratio of the effective balloon dilating area to body surface area (EBDA:BSA) is the only predictor of increased mitral regurgitation after PMV.[14]

The EBDA is calculated using standard geometric formulas (Fig. 12.5). Using two balloons, the effective balloon dilating area can be derived from the chart in Figure 12.6. The incidence of mitral regurgitation is lower if balloon sizes are chosen so that EBDA:BSA is ≤ 4.0 cm²/m². The single balloon technique results in a lower incidence of mitral regurgitation but provides less relief of mitral stenosis than the double balloon technique. We think that this is due to the smaller EBDA:BSA of single balloon PMV. Thus, there is an optimal

Table 12.7.
Effect of Previous Surgical Commissurotomy on the Immediate Outcome of PMV

	MVA (cm²) pre-PMV	post-PMV
Previous surgical commissurotomy (N = 71)	0.9 ± 0.1	1.8 ± 0.1
No previous surgical commissurotomy (N = 286)	0.9 ± 0.1	2.1 ± 0.1^a

[a]$p < 0.01$
MVA = mitral valve area; PMV = percutaneous mitral balloon valvotomy.

balloon size between 3.1 and 4.0 cm²/m² that achieves a maximal mitral valve area with a minimal increase in mitral regurgitation.

The immediate outcome of patients undergoing PMV is also related to the severity of valvular calcification seen by fluoroscopy. Patients without fluoroscopic calcium have a greater increase in mitral valve area after PMV than patients with calcified valves. It is apparent that patients with either no or 1+ fluoroscopic calcium have a greater increase in mitral valve area after PMV than those patients with 2, 3, or 4+ of calcium (Fig. 12.7).

The increase in mitral valve area with PMV is inversely related to the presence of atrial fibrillation (Table 12.6); the post-PMV mitral valve area of 181 patients in normal sinus rhythm was 2.2 ± 0.1 cm², compared with a valve area of 1.8 ± 0.1 cm² of 176 patients in atrial fibrillation.

Although the increase in mitral valve area with PMV is also inversely related to the presence of previous surgical mitral commissurotomy (Table 12.7), PMV can produce a good outcome in this group of patients.[15] The mean mitral valve area in 71 patients with previous surgical commissurotomy was 1.8 ± 0.1 cm² (Table 12.7) compared with a valve area of 2.1 ± 0.1 cm² in patients without previous surgical commissurotomy. In this group of patients, an echocardiographic score ≤ 8 was again the most important predictor of a good immediate outcome.[15]

The immediate outcome of PMV is also directly related to the age of the patients. Elderly patients more frequently have atrial fibrillation, calcified valves, and higher echocardiographic scores (Fig. 12.8). Figure 12.9 shows the relationship between the age of the patients and the increase in mitral valve area produced by PMV. Figure 12.10 shows

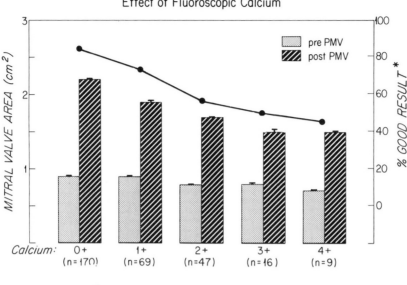

Figure 12.7. Relationship between the degree of calcium identified under fluoroscopy (x axis), the increase in mitral valve area produced by PMV (left axis), and the percentage of patients having a good result (post-PMV MVA ≥ 1.5 cm²) (right axis).

Effect of age on the determinants of immediate outcome of PMV

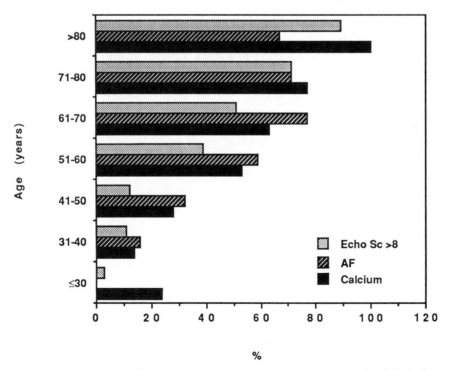

Figure 12.8. Relationship between patient's age (y axis) and the percentage of patients having an echocardiographic score > 8, presence of atrial fibrillation, and presence of calcium under fluoroscopy.

IMPACT OF AGE IN THE IMMEDIATE OUTCOME OF PMV

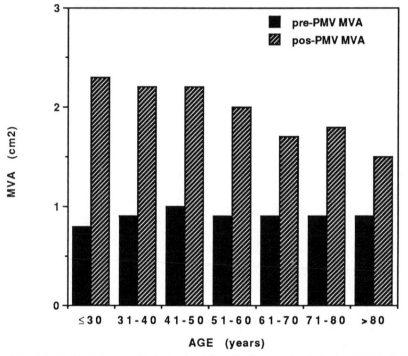

Figure 12.9.   Relationship between patient's age (x axis) and the increase in mitral valve area produced by PMV (y axis).

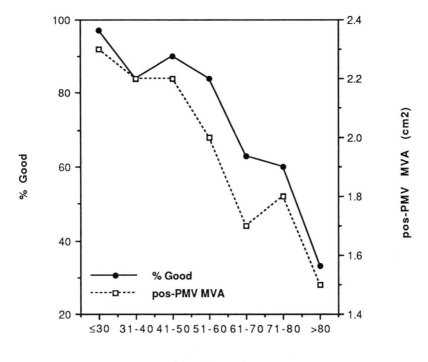

RELATIONSHIP BETWEEN AGE, post-PMV MVA AND % OF GOOD RESULTS

Figure 12.10.   Relationship between patient's age (y axis), the post-PMV mitral valve area (left axis), and the percentage of patients having a good result (post-PMV MVA $\geq$ 1.5 cm^2) (right axis).

the absolute post-PMV mitral valve area as well as the percentage of patients obtaining a good result with this procedure. A successful outcome from PMV (defined as post-PMV MVA ≥ 1.5 cm^2, < 2 grade increase in mitral regurgitation, and $\leq 1.5:1$ left-to-right shunt through the created interatrial communication) was obtained in only less than 50% of patients ≥ 65 years old. As can be seen in Figures 12.9 and 12.10, the increase in mitral valve area with PMV and the percentage of patients obtaining a good result with this technique decreases as age increases.

The presence and severity of mitral regurgitation before PMV is an independent predictor of unfavorable outcome of PMV. As can be seen in Figure 12.11, the increase in mitral valve area after PMV is inversely related to the severity of mitral regurgitation determined by angiography before the procedure. This negative relationship between presence of mitral regurgitation and immediate outcome is in part due to the fact that patients with mitral regurgitation are more frequently older. They more frequently have atrial fibrillation,

higher echocardiographic score, and evidence of calcified mitral valves under fluoroscopy (Fig. 12.12).

Complications. Mortality and morbidity with PMV is low and similar to surgical commissurotomy. In the series from the Massachusetts General Hospital[6] there is a less than 1% mortality. No death has occurred in the last 260 patients undergoing this procedure. There is a 1% incidence of thromboembolic episodes and stroke.

An increase in mitral regurgitation occurs in approximately 45% of patients.[3,6,11,14,16] However, in most patients this increase is only mild. Severe mitral regurgitation $(4+)$ occurred in only 0.9% of the patients. An undesirable increase in mitral regurgitation $(\geq 2+)$ occurs in 12.5% of patients[14] but is well tolerated in most. In more than half there is less mitral regurgitation at follow-up cardiac catheterization. The mechanism of undesirable severe mitral regurgitation is probably due to a tear of the posterior or anterior mitral leaflets in the paracommissural area. The role of mitral valve anatomy in the development of

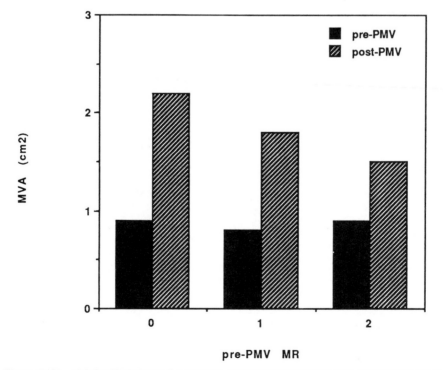

Figure 12.11.　Relationship between the presence of mitral regurgitation (x axis) and the increase in mitral valve area produced by PMV (y axis).

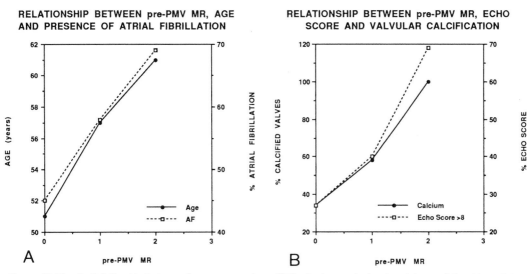

Figure 12.12. **A,** Relationship between the presence of pre-PMV mitral regurgitation (x axis), age (left axis), and the percentage of patients having atrial fibrillation (right axis). **B,** Relationship between the presence of pre-PMV mitral regurgitation (x axis), percentage of patients having calcified valves (left axis), and the percentage of patients having echocardiographic score > 8 (right axis).

significant post-PMV mitral regurgitation is controversial.[5,11] Nevertheless, unfavorable mitral valve anatomy (severe subvalvular fibrosis, calcification, and scarring) seems to be more likely associated with severe post-PMV mitral regurgitation.[5]

Transient heart block (< 24 hours' duration) occurred in 0.9% of the patients. Pericardial tamponade occurred in 0.9% of cases. PMV results in a 20% incidence of left-to-right shunt determined by oximetry immediately after the procedure.[6,17] The size of the defect is small (pulmonary to systemic flow ratio of < 2:1 in the majority of patients). A greater percentage of patients have a left-to-right shunt that can be detected with more sensitive techniques.[18] Transesophageal color flow Doppler echocardiography can demonstrate flow across the atrial septum in up to 87% of patients immediately after PMV.[18] Older age, fluoroscopic evidence of mitral valve calcification, higher echocardiographic score, a lower cardiac output pre-PMV, and a higher NYHA class are all factors that predispose patients to develop a left-to-right shunt post-PMV.[17] Clinical, echocardiographic, surgical, and hemodynamic follow-up of patients with a post-PMV left-to-right shunt demonstrates that the defect closed in 59% of the patients.[17] Any persistent left-to-right shunt is usually well tolerated.

Finally, the importance of operator experience and careful patient selection can not be overemphasized. In our recent experience, better patient selection with emphasis on echocardiographic scoring, proper sizing of balloon dilating catheters, and use of smaller balloons to dilate the atrial septum, coupled with increased operator experience, have resulted in a good outcome in the majority of cases, with fewer complications and no mortality.

REFERENCES

1. Inoue K, Owaki T, Nakamura T, Kitamura F, Miyamoto N. Clinical application of transvenous mitral commissurotomy by a new balloon catheter. *J Thorac Cardiovasc Surg 87*:394–402, 1984.
2. Lock JE, Kalilullah M, Shrivastava S, Bahl V, Keane JF. Percutaneous catheter commissurotomy in rheumatic mitral stenosis. *N Engl J Med 313*:1515–1518, 1985.
3. Palacios I, Block PC, Brandi S, Blanco P, Casal H, Pulido JI, Munoz S, D'Empaire G, Ortega MA, Jacobs M, Vlahakes G. Percutaneous balloon valvotomy for patients with severe mitral stenosis. *Circulation 75*:778–784, 1987.
4. Al Zaibag M, Ribeiro PA, Al Kassab SA, Al Fagig MR. Percutaneous double balloon mitral valvotomy for rheumatic mitral stenosis. *Lancet 1*:757–761, 1986.
5. Vahanian A, Michel PL, Cormier B, Vitoux B, Michel X, Enriquez M, Sarano L, Slama M, Trabelsi S, Ben Ismail M, Ascar J. Results of percutaneous mitral commissurotomy in 200 patients. *Am J Cardiol 63*:847–852, 1989.
6. Palacios IF, Block PC, Wilkins GT, Weyman AE.

Follow-up of patients undergoing percutaneous mitral balloon valvotomy: Analysis of factors determining restenosis. *Circulation 79*:573–579, 1989.

7. McKay RG, Lock JE, Safian RD, Come PC, Diver DJ, Baim DS, Berman AD, Warren SE, Mandell VE, Rotal HD, Grossman W. Balloon dilatation of mitral stenosis in adult patients: Postmortem and percutaneous mitral valvuloplasty studies. *J Am Coll Cardiol 9*:723–731, 1987.

8. McKay CR, Kawanishi DT, Rahimtoola SH. Catheter balloon valvuloplasty of the mitral valve in adults using a double balloon technique. Early hemodynamic results. *JAMA 257*:1753–1761, 1987.

9. Block PC, Palacios IF. Pulmonary vascular dynamics after percutaneous mitral valvotomy. *J Thorac Cardiovasc Surg 96*:39–43, 1988.

10. Wilkins GT, Weyman AE, Abascal VM, Block PC, Palacios IF. Percutaneous mitral valvotomy: An analysis of echocardiographic variables related to outcome and the mechanism of dilatation. *Brit Heart J 60*:299–308, 1988.

11. Abascal VM, Wilkins GT, Choong CY, Block PC, Palacios IF, Weyman AE. Mitral regurgitation after percutaneous mitral valvuloplasty in adults: Evaluation by pulsed Doppler echocardiography. *J Am Coll Cardiol 2*:257–263, 1988.

12. Abascal VM, O'Shea JP, Wilkins GT, Palacios IF, Thomas JD, Rosas E, Newell JB, Block PC, Weyman AE. Prediction of successful outcome in 130 patients undergoing percutaneous balloon mitral valvotomy. *Circulation 82*:448–456, 1990.

13. Herrman HC, Wilkins GT, Abascal VM, Weyman AE, Block PC, Palacios IF. Percutaneous balloon mitral valvotomy for patients with mitral stenosis: Analysis of factors influencing early results. *J Thorac Cardiovasc Surg. 96*:33–38, 1988.

14. Roth RB, Block PC, Palacios IF. Predictors of increased mitral regurgitation after percutaneous mitral balloon valvotomy. *Cathet Cardiovasc Diagn 20*:17–21, 1990.

15. Rediker DE, Block PC, Abascal VM, Palacios IF. Mitral balloon valvuloplasty for mitral restenosis after surgical commissurotomy. *J Am Coll Cardiol 2*:252–256, 1988.

16. Abascal VM, Wilkins GT, Choong CY, Palacios IF, Block PC, Weyman AE. Echocardiographic evaluation of mitral valve structure and function in patients followed for at least 6 months after percutaneous balloon mitral valvuloplasty. *J Am Coll Cardiol 12*:606–615, 1988.

17. Casale P, Block PC, O'Shea JP, Palacios IF. Atrial septal defect after percutaneous mitral balloon valvuloplasty: Immediate results and follow-up. *J Am Coll Cardiol 15*:1300–1304, 1990.

18. Yoshida K, Yoshikawa J, Yamaura Y, Shakudo M, Hozumi T, Fukaya T. Assessment of left to right shunting after percutaneous mitral valvuloplasty by transesophageal color Doppler flow mapping. *Circulation 80*:1521–1526, 1989.

13

Techniques and Complications
Related to Mitral Balloon Valvotomy

CHARLES R. MCKAY

Progressive scarring and distortion of the mitral valve continues for decades after an acute episode of rheumatic fever has resolved. Typical morphologic findings from mitral valves of symptomatic patients include commissural fusion. leaflet thickening, and calcification, with fusion and shortening of the chordae tendinae. Commissural fusion is present in a majority of the patients and is the major cause of restricted leaflet opening.[1] Experience with closed surgical commissurotomy has shown that fused commissures are amenable to simple mechanical separation.[2–4] This separation of the commissures relieves transvalvular gradients and reduces patients' symptoms for years.[5] Transluminal balloon catheter treatment of intracardiac lesions and pulmonary and aortic valvuloplasty procedures were first performed by pediatric cardiologists.[6,7] The early reports of the relief of rheumatic mitral valve stenosis by mitral balloon valvuloplasty demonstrated remarkable changes in hemodynamics.[8] The valve gradients are typically reduced from 15–30 mm Hg to 0–6 mm Hg, and valve areas are increased to 1.5–3.0 cm².

Although the term "valvuloplasty" has been used to refer to the mitral balloon technique, there is a growing trend to refer to the procedure as "mitral balloon commissurotomy or valvotomy"[22,24] because (1) the mechanism by which the mitral orifice is widened is well understood to result from splitting of the commissures or "commissurotomy",[11,2] not a plastic surgical repair or "valvuloplasty"; and (2) the term "mitral valvuloplasty" can be mistaken for surgical mitral valvuloplasty.[12,13] This can lead to confusion in the medical literature, in educational conferences, and

in hospital discharge records. Surgical mitral valvuloplasty is a true plastic repair of the mitral valve, which restructures regurgitant and stenotic valves and is becoming more commonly practiced by many cardiac surgeons.[14,15] The terms "percutaneous transluminal balloon valvuloplasty," "catheter balloon valvuloplasty," and "catheter balloon commissurotomy" are redundant since balloons are always introduced on a catheter using a percutaneous transluminal approach.

Although the use of the balloon device is still investigational, there is the general acceptance of the efficacy and safety of the mitral balloon valvotomy procedure. In experienced centers, where there is a high success rate and low morbidity, mitral balloon valvotomy is a treatment of choice for selected patients with severe, symptomatic mitral valve stenosis. At the same time, surgical mitral valvuloplasty is an increasingly preferred and successful treatment for mitral valve regurgitation instead of mitral valve replacement. The identity of these two successful new procedures should not be confused.

This chapter will outline the technical aspects of performing mitral balloon valvotomy and will focus on the transseptal catheterization technique, on the balloon valvotomy equipment, and on the balloon technique. Certain aspects of patients' anatomy and the clinical settings that are likely to favor or complicate the mitral balloon valvotomy procedure in a given patient will be discussed. The variations in the technique of performing mitral balloon valvotomy will be reviewed. The complications of the procedure, considering how one might anticipate and avoid these complications, will then be discussed.

199

THE TECHNIQUE OF TRANSSEPTAL CATHETERIZATION

The success of mitral balloon valvotomy depends on performing successful transseptal catheterization. Today, younger invasive cardiologists who train in centers without a high prevalence of patients with valvular heart disease may not obtain extensive practice with transseptal heart catheterization. Therefore, a review of patient anatomy and the technique of transseptal catheterization is warranted here.

Morphologic Relationships in Transseptal Catheterization

Several anatomic relationships of the left atrium, right atrium, and mitral valve are of key importance in performing successful transseptal catheterization. Figure 13.1 demonstrates right atrial anatomy of a cadaver heart in a cutaway anteroposterior view. The inferior vena cava (IVC) and superior vena cava (SVC) are both posterior structures, and the opening of the SVC into the right atrium at the crista terminalis is below the roof of the right atrium. The posterior right atrial wall is covered by pericardium. The interatrial septum runs from the right posterior atrial wall anterior to the tricuspid valve anulus. The key anatomic structure to be identified is the limbic ledge. This crescentic muscular ridge is located in the posterior central portion of the interatrial septum. It is located just below the level of the aortic valve and is just posterior to the coronary sinus. In approximately 10% of patients, the thin membranous septum of the fossa ovalis is incomplete or "probe patent," which facilitates catheter entry into the left atrium with the gentle pressure of a blunt transseptal dilator. In contrast, after open-heart surgery, this membranous septum may be fibrosed and thickened, and in some patients the fossa ovalis bulges into the right atrium due to the high left atrial pressure. In these patients, the limbic ledge may not be easily engaged or the muscle easily crossed even with firm pressure on the transseptal needle. If the limbic ledge is high or posterior, the transseptal catheter may pass posteriorly as it crosses into the left atrium. This has little consequence for diagnostic left atrial catheterization; however, it can make positioning the catheters for mitral balloon valvotomy much more difficult. In this situation one should avoid a high and posterior left atrial entry during transseptal catheterization.

Transseptal Catheter Equipment

Before the transseptal equipment enters the body, it is important to assemble all of the equipment on the table and be sure that the pieces fit together

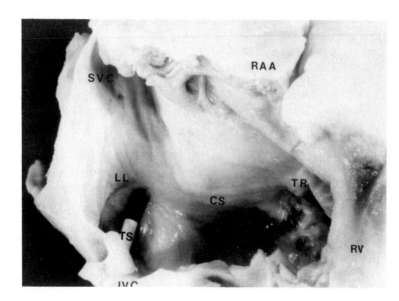

Figure 13.1. Right atrial anatomic relationships.
Photograph of the right atrium, PA cutaway view, with transseptal sheath and dilator placed across fossa ovalis into left atrium.
RAA = right atrial appendage; SVC = superior vena cava; LL = limbic ledge; TS = transseptal sheath; TR = tricuspid valve; CS = coronary sinus; RV = right ventricle; IVC = inferior vena cava.

properly. Transseptal equipment has changed somewhat over the years.[16] The original Ross needle with an 18-gauge tip has been replaced by the Brockenbrough needle (Fig. 13.2A) with a 21-gauge tip. The Brockenbrough catheter (Fig. 13.2B) with Criley tip occluder (Fig. 13.2C) and Harris adapter (Fig. 13.2C) is used to perform angiography. The more recently introduced Mullins sheath system (Fig. 13.2D) with a curved 65-cm sheath[17] is made with a sidearm adapter and can be used with a 7-French end-hole balloon catheter (Fig. 13.2E) for mitral balloon valvotomy procedures.

It is important to make two measurements on the equipment before it enters the patient (Fig. 13.3). First, with the tip of the dilator at the distal end of the Mullins sheath, measure the length of the dilator that is protruding proximally out of the sheath. This measurement can be taken directly with the millimeter markers on the proximal end of the dilator and usually ranges from 35 to 45 mm. This is the distance to advance the sheath over the dilator to be sure the sheath is in the left atrium before the needle and dilator are removed from the sheath. For the second measurement, with the dilator advanced distally all the way out of the sheath, the Brockenbrough needle tip (without the Bing stylet) is placed just inside the tip of the dilator. Proximally, measure the length of needle protruding from the proximal end of the dilator back to the arrowhead-shaped crosspiece on the Brockenbrough needle. The arrowhead on this crosspiece points in the direction of the curvature of the distal end of the needle. Various methods to measure or mark this distance are used by different operators. A steel millimeter ruler, the operator's left index finger, a "mosquito" clamp, or positioning screws at this point can be used to firmly maintain the relative distance between the needle and the hub of the dilator. In this manner the sheath, dilator, and needle can be manipulated as a unit without the needle protruding from the catheter tip.

When selecting transseptal equipment for mitral balloon valvotomy procedures, some details of equipment design are important. The older Ross needle has an 18-gauge curved tip and easily obtains left atrial pressures, but it can also puncture the right atrial or left atrial posterior walls, leaving larger holes with inadvertent perforation. It therefore may carry increased risks of hemodynamic compromise, even after "needle only" perforations. The 21-gauge tip on the Brockenbrough needle requires meticulous flushing to directly measure atrial pressure but may lead to less atrial wall trauma from "needle only" perforations.

During mitral balloon valvotomy procedures, the Mullins sheath technique is used to achieve entry into the left atrium and into the left ventricle. The 8.2-French Mullins sheath with a sidearm and hemostatic valve easily accommodates a 7-French end-hole balloon-tipped catheter (Fig. 13.4B), allowing for safe entry into the left atrium and left ventricle. One disadvantage of the sheath tech-

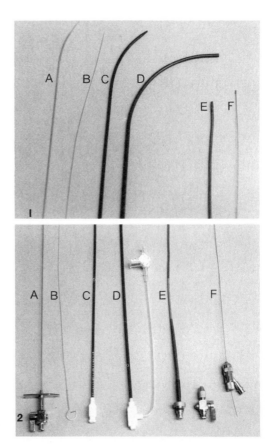

Figure 13.2.   Transseptal equipment. **1** = distal ends, **2** = proximal ends. From left to right: **A,** Brockenbrough needle with 21-gauge curved tip and crosspiece proximally. Arrow at proximal end points in direction of needle curvature. **B,** Bing stylet used during needle insertion into catheters to avoid needle tip or catheter lumen damage. **C,** Curved dilator for 7-French Mullins sheath with proximal millimeter marks. **D,** Mullins sheath (65-cm length), curved distally, 8-French, with sidearm adapter and hemostatic valve. **E,** Brockenbrough 7-French catheter, woven Dacron with both end-holes and side-holes. When Kifa catheter material was used, it was flanged proximally to accept removable metal luerlock adapter (shown separately). **F,** Criley tip occluder converts end- and side-hole Brockenbrough catheter to side-hole catheter for angiography. **G,** Harris adapter is shown with shaft of tip occluder loaded through rubber gasket. Sidearm with luerlock is used for injection and pressure monitoring.

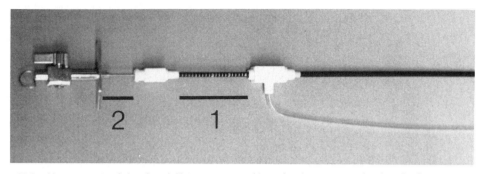

Figure 13.3. Measurements of sheath and dilator system used in performing transseptal catheterization. Measurement 1. Distally the dilator is just inside the distal end of the sheath. Proximally the distance that the dilator protrudes from the end of the sheath is measured using the millimeter markers provided on the proximal dilator shaft.
Measurement 2. The distal end of the Brockenbrough needle is just inside the distal end of the dilator. Proximally the distance from the end of the dilator to the arrowhead crosspiece on the needle is measured using a sterile metal ruler or bent pipe cleaner. Alternatively a removable screw clamp can be placed to maintain this relationship, then removed to protrude the needle distally.

nique, however, is that neither the tip nor the body of the sheath is radiopaque, and it is difficult to see on fluoroscopy without either a catheter or some contrast in its lumen. Previously, the Brockenbrough catheters with precurved distal tips of various diameters were used with curved guidewires to enter the left atrium and ventricle in diagnostic cases. Various "j curves," preset to diameters of 2.5 to 3.5 cm were selected to facilitate passage from smaller or larger left atria across the stenotic mitral valve into the left ventricle. Although this technique can still be used for diagnostic cases, it is not easily adapted to the mitral balloon valvotomy technique. In addition, the Mullins sheath and end-hole catheter are safer, and the unit can be used to measure transmitral valve gradients in patients with coexisting aortic stenosis or an aortic valve prosthesis that cannot be crossed retrograde.

Dilator and Sheath Technique for Transseptal Catheterization

The original technique for performing transseptal catheterization has been well described.[16,18] To perform the transseptal catheterization with the dilator-sheath system, the 0.032″ j-wire is placed from the right femoral vein up to the SVC.[17] The Mullins sheath and dilator are advanced to the SVC. The j-wire is exchanged for the curved Brockenbrough needle. Care is taken to (1) align the curves of the needle and the sheath in the same direction and (2) not extend the needle tip beyond the end of the dilator (second measurement described previously). The SVC or right atrial pressure is then monitored through the tip of

the needle. Holding the needle just inside the dilator at the premeasured distance (second measurement) and holding the curves of the needle and sheath as a unit at the 12 o'clock (upward or anterior) position, the operator slowly withdraws the equipment from the SVC to the right atrium while turning the curve of the needle and sheath from the 12 o'clock to the 4 o'clock position. While being withdrawn, the catheter will abruptly move medially (rightward) as it descends into the right atrium (Fig. 13.6). The first abrupt rightward movement is encountered as the dilator tip passes from the SVC over the aortic root into the right atrium. The second abrupt rightward movement is encountered as the dilator tip passes over the limbic ledge into the fossa ovalis, which is usually anterior to the spine in the PA view (Fig. 13.1). The catheter can then also be viewed from the RAO position. The tip of the dilator should be down just below the level of the aortic valve and posterior to it. The curve of the sheath and needle should face slightly anteriorly. The level of the aortic valve anulus is marked by (1) a pigtail catheter resting in the sinus of Valsalva, (2) a calcified native valve or prosthetic valve seen on fluoroscopy, or (3) counting 2.5 vertebral bodies below the carina. The dilator and needle can now be held firmly together and advanced. The dilator will engage the septum and stop on the limbic ledge. Gentle steady pressure on the dilator may allow one to advance the Mullins dilator tip into the left atrium without advancing the needle out of the dilator. Alternatively, the Brockenbrough needle can be sharply advanced out of the dilator and across the septum, holding the dilator rigidly in place. In either case the needle tip entry into the left

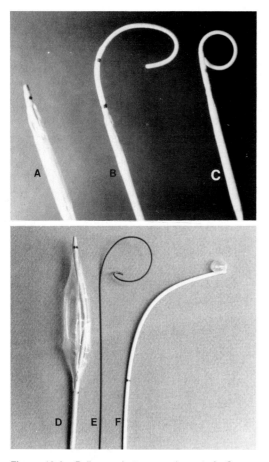

Figure 13.4. Balloon valvotomy equipment. **A,** Owens balloon, 20-mm diameter, 3-cm working length (14-French). **B,** Cribier-Letac aortic valvuloplasty balloon (10-French). **C,** Triad balloon 20-mm diameter, 4-cm working length, with pigtail end (10-French). **D,** Owens 25-mm balloon inflated. **E,** Curved j-exchange wire. **F,** End-hole 7-French balloon catheter.

atrium is confirmed by (1) feeling a "give" during pressure on the needle, (2) seeing a sudden increase in the atrial pressure, (3) noting the typical large left atrial A and V waveforms, (4) drawing a left atrial oxygen saturation, or (5) hand injection of 1–3 cc of contrast material through the needle tip. The latter maneuver produces a fine "jet" of contrast in the left atrial cavity demonstrating that the needle is free in the chamber and not near the roof or side walls of the left atrium. Once the needle tip is confirmed to be in the left atrial chamber, the needle and sheath are advanced as a unit under fluoroscopic guidance 3–5 mm while the operator observes continuous undamped waveforms on the pressure monitor. This is particularly important in postoperative thickened

atrial septa. Then the needle is held still while the sheath and dilator are advanced an additional 2–3 cm over the needle into the left atrium. Monitoring the left atrial pressure and the catheter position on fluoroscopy during these maneuvers reassures the operator of the correct placement of the equipment. The sheath is then advanced 35–45 mm into the left atrium (measurement 1 previously). The sheath is held firmly while the dilator and needle are slowly withdrawn. During dilator and needle withdrawal, the sheath will bend downward into the left atrium. Slight counterclockwise torque on the sheath will move it off the posterior wall, left pulmonary vein, or left atrial appendage and allow it to fall onto the base of the atrium or mitral valve anulus. Gentle removal of the needle and dilator is warranted as the patient may experience some back discomfort as the curved needle is withdrawn.

The lumen of the 7-French balloon catheter is initially flushed. The balloon is then filled with carbon dioxide gas or air and the catheter is advanced into the left atrium. But turning the sheath counterclockwise and advancing the inflated balloon, one can avoid the posterior atrial wall, the pulmonary vein, and the left atrial appendage. Moving the catheter forward into the mitral inflow tract with the balloon inflated allows the mitral diastolic flow to propel the balloon catheter into the left ventricle. With posterior transseptal punctures in larger left atria, the balloon may tend to move into the pulmonary veins (best seen in the LAO view) or superiorly into the left atrial appendage (best seen in the RAO view). Advancing the sheath forward along the catheter shaft toward the inflated balloon will change the angle of curvature of the sheath-catheter system and will allow the operator to place the inflated balloon at the mitral valve orifice. In cases with very tight valve stenosis or with valves with calcific spicules in the mitral orifice, the balloon may have to be partially deflated in order to advance the catheter across the mitral valve into the left ventricle. It is important, however, to leave the balloon inflated as much as possible as it crosses the mitral valve to avoid entangling the balloon and subsequently the long guidewires and larger catheters in the chordae tendinae. With the distal end of the sheath in the left atrium and the end-hole catheter in the left ventricle, a transmitral valve gradient can be obtained. Alternatively, the transmitral valve gradient can be obtained earlier while the balloon catheter and sheath are in the left atrium and a pigtail catheter is advanced retrograde from the aorta into the left ventricle.

MITRAL BALLOON VALVOTOMY EQUIPMENT

Standard equipment for mitral balloon valvotomy has improved rapidly over the last four years. Figure 13.4 shows the standard Owens balloon catheter, which has been used for several years for aortic, pulmonary, tricuspid, and mitral valve procedures. Investigators have evolved individual preferences for different balloon widths and lengths, each of which has strengths and weaknesses. The balloons with 3-cm working lengths will "fit into" smaller left ventricles with less chance of dilating the atrial septum or traumatizing the ventricle during inflation but may be more difficult to hold still across pliable mitral valves during balloon inflation. The balloons with 5.5-cm working lengths have less movement during balloon inflation but have significantly longer inflation and deflation times and may press against the left ventricular apex or the interatrial septum. Standard inflated balloon diameters are 15, 18, 20, 23, and 25 mm. Mitral balloon valvotomy using a single 25-mm diameter balloon has the technical advantage that only a single balloon and guidewire need to be placed across the mitral valve. However, these balloons are more "globular" as they inflate and are difficult to hold in place in the valve plane during balloon inflations. Their larger volumes require longer inflation and deflation times. Also, after they have been inflated across the mitral valve, they have very large "profiles"; therefore, they can enlarge the holes in the atrial septum and femoral vein as they are pulled out of the patient. The guidewires used are 0.038″, 260-cm length, exchange j-wires (Fig. 13.4B). Standard stiffness wires are used when the wires are placed out the aorta, and the extra-stiff wires are used when the wires are curled and placed into the left ventricular apex. The double lumen catheter is used to place two wires into the heart without twisting or binding them together, as they are advanced to the LV apex or out the aorta. An 8-mm diameter balloon catheter is used to dilate the interatrial septum. Newer equipment includes the Mansfield Triad balloon with three lumens. Two lumens are used to inflate and deflate the balloon rapidly. The third lumen extends to the distal catheter tip and is used for the guidewire. The smaller shaft and thinner polyethylene balloon material result in a 9-French profile, which is much improved from the 14-French profile of the Owens balloon. The pigtail tip tracks the curved guidewire to the left ventricular apex and greatly diminishes the ten-

dency for left ventricular myocardial trauma or perforation with these balloons (Fig. 13.4A). The larger 4-cm working length is a compromise between the 3- and 5.5-cm lengths.

The single balloon developed by Dr. Inoue (Fig. 13.5) has an 8-French profile and a curved shaft, which helps the operator cross the mitral valve without a guidewire.[19] This balloon is made of a latex material that can expand up to 32 mm in diameter, depending on the balloon inflation pressure used by the operator. The balloon has the unique ability of allowing distal inflation initially, then proximal expansion (Fig. 13.5). Once the catheter is manipulated into the LV, the distal inflation is performed. The balloon is then pulled back into the mitral orifice and the proximal inflation results in the opening of the valvular orifice. The novel design of the catheter allows for much greater tip control.

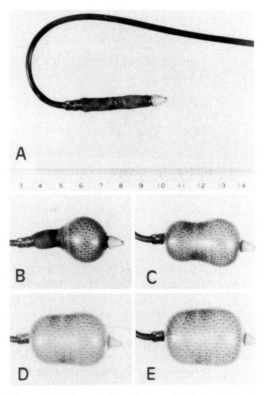

Figure 13.5. Inoue balloon. **A,** Curved catheter shaft and hard plastic tip to dilate and cross interatrial septum (8-French). **B–E,** Inflation of latex balloon. With progressive increase in pressure, first the distal end and then the proximal end of the balloon inflate and apply force to the mitral valve commissures. (From Inoue K, et al. *J Thorac Cardiovasc Surg* 87:394, 1984. Used with permission.)

TECHNIQUE OF MITRAL BALLOON VALVOTOMY

The first reports of mitral balloon valvotomy used a 32-mm latex balloon in 6 patients[19] or a single 25-mm polyethylene balloon in 8 adolescent and young adult patients[8] introduced by a transseptal approach and placed over a wire into the left ventricular apex. Since the early reports, it has become clear that larger openings in the mitral valve are needed in adult patients.[20,21] The double balloon technique in its early reports[22,23] and in recent reports[24,25] has continued to yield larger mitral valve areas and has become the standard approach to the treatment of adult patients in many centers.[26] A standard double balloon technique[23] is diagrammed in Figure 13.6. After the transseptal catheterization is performed and the left atrium to left ventricular gradient is measured, the direct Fick and/or thermodilution cardiac outputs are obtained.

Now, two approaches can be taken. A 0.038″, 260-cm length extra-stiff j-guidewire can be pre-curled (Fig. 13.4B) and placed into the apex of the left ventricle (Fig. 13.6). As a second alternative, a wire of normal stiffness can be placed out the ascending aorta (Fig. 13.7). The distal 10–12 cm of wire is curled with a larger circle or j, which presents a curved portion of the wire to the apex of the left ventricular endocardium and helps avoid balloon trauma to the ventricular wall. The 30″

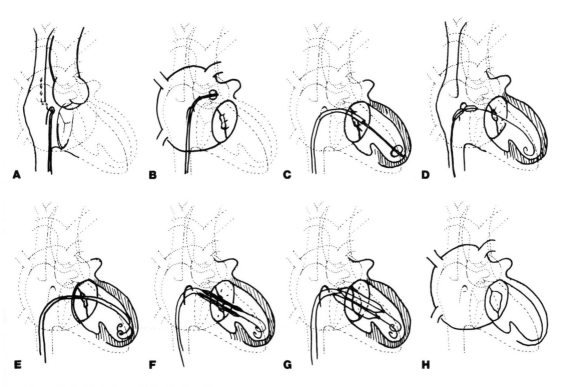

Figure 13.6. Technique of Mitral Balloon Valvotomy.
A, Transseptal catheterization. Cardiac chambers are outlined by fine dotted lines. Transseptal catheter is shown in fossa ovalis as in Figure 13.1. Right atrium and aorta outlined in solid lines. Path of transseptal catheter from SVC to RA to fossa ovalis shown in double shafted arrows. **B,** Passage of end-hole balloon catheter through sheath into left atrium. Mitral valve anulus and stenotic valve leaflets shown. **C,** Passage of end-hole balloon catheter and sheath anteriorly through mitral valve into left ventricle. **D,** Dilation of interatrial septum by 8-mm balloon catheter. This catheter can then be advanced through the mitral valve and into the left ventricular apex to confirm that the wire is not caught through chordae tendinae. **E,** Two stiff 260-cm j-guidewires with formed curved distal ends resting across the mitral valve in the left ventricle. A block double lumen catheter is useful for placing the second wire and for making hemodynamic measurements. **F,** Two 20-mm diameter balloon catheters placed across the stenotic mitral valve. The cylindrical working area of the balloons should be centered anterior to the A-V groove in the left ventricle to engage the mitral valve orifice. The wire curves should rest gently against the left ventricular endocardium. **G,** Two balloon catheters inflated, opening the fused mitral commissures. **H,** Opened mitral valve commissures improve orifice area in diastole; shown with equipment removed.

RAO view is best for observing placement of the guidewire and subsequent balloon valvotomy equipment (Fig. 13.6). With the j-wire looped into the left ventricular apex, the Mullins sheath and 7-French end-hole balloon catheter are removed. A 9-French dilator is used to dilate the femoral vein. An 8-mm balloon angioplasty catheter is then advanced to the left atrial and is inflated in order to dilate the atrial septum. A "waist" can be seen on fluoroscopy when the balloon is correctly placed and inflated across the atrial septal muscle. The inflated 8-mm balloon catheter can also be advanced across the mitral valve anulus, through the mitral valve inflow tract, and into the left ventricle to be sure that the guidewire is not wedged into a calcified commissure or entangled in the mitral valve chordae. The 8-mm balloon is then deflated and removed. The double lumen catheter is then advanced from the femoral vein to inferior vena cava, and across the atrial septum and mitral valve into the left ventricle. A second 260 cm long curved j-guidewire is then placed into the left ventricular cavity using the double lumen sheath. Again, the large loop of guidewire should be presented to the left ventricular endocardium. Ectopy is usually encountered as the wires exit the catheters and curve into the LV chamber. In smaller ventricles, wires with smaller or tighter curls or loops may be needed to achieve a quiet position. The double lumen catheter is removed and the two large balloon valvotomy catheters to be used for the valve dilation are sequentially placed across the atrial septum and mitral valve into the left venticular apex. The two catheters should be placed such that the proximal and distal balloon markers are aligned in the RAO view. This alignment should optimize lateral force on the mitral valve and avoid having one balloon slip back into the left atrium during balloon inflation. There should be slight forward pressure on the catheter shafts, and the wires should be positioned in the left ventricle so that the curled wire ends are positioned down into the apex. Wires that are "pushed" into the apex may force the balloons back into the left atrium during an inflation or may cause perforation of the left ventricular apex.

Inflation of both balloons simultaneously, observed on fluoroscopy, will demonstrate a "waist" in the balloons. If the balloons remain in position without slipping back proximally, full inflation should be continued for a total of 10–15 sec. Heavy hand pressure on the 30-cc luerlock syringes can generate the 3 to 3.5 atmospheres of pressure that are needed to put sufficient lateral force on the valve commissures. The total inflation and deflation times may be 20–40 sec for larger diameter balloons. As this usually stops mitral inflow during the first inflation, the arterial pressure may transiently drop to 60–80 mm Hg of systolic pressure in some patients. As the balloons are deflated, the arterial pressure should return to near normal levels. If at least one commissure is open, the increase in systolic pressure is rapid.

The goal of simultaneous balloon inflations is to put lateral pressure on the two fused mitral valve commissures and separate the scar tissue that is tethering the commissures. With commissural splitting, the mitral valve orifice is larger, and the deflated balloons can be seen on fluoroscopy to have increased mobility during systole. If the commissures have not been opened during the balloon inflation, then the deflated balloons, which now have a larger profile than when they were first introduced into the heart, may continue to significantly obstruct the mitral valve inflow tract. In this situation, lower arterial pressures can persist.

Since one is at this point "committed" to the placement of the balloon catheters across the interatrial septum and valve, a judgment is needed as to the stability of the catheters and the patient. If the judgment is that the patient is stable, then repositioning the balloon catheters across the interatrial septum and valve; and repeating the balloon inflation can further open the mitral valve commissures. The improved forward flow is associated with increased arterial pressure. Some patients do not tolerate the hypotension, especially older patients, volume depleted patients, patients with concomitant aortic valve disease, or patients with severe left ventricular dysfunction. Elderly patients who have lower pressures with the equipment across the valve may need to be temporarily supported with intravenous fluids and low-dose dopamine in order to complete the procedure. In severe stenosis, sequentially inflating the balloons can partially open one commissure and allow both balloons to be placed across the valve plane. With both balloons stable, they can then be inflated simultaneously, opening both commissures. Usually only 2–4 inflations are needed to achieve an optimal result. When the commissures are opened, subsequent inflations show no "waist," less hypotension, and the deflated balloons have increased mobility in systole when viewed on fluoroscopy.

The balloons can then be removed sequentially across the atrial septum to the right atrium or back into the inferior vena cava. The mitral valve gradient is remeasured by (1) placing the double lumen catheter over a wire into the left atrium and a pigtail catheter in the left ventricle; or (2) placing the Mullins sheath, preloaded with the 7-French end-hole balloon catheter, across the mitral valve and removing the guidewire. If the mitral valve gradient is acceptable, then the final gradient should be obtained with no equipment across the mitral valve. Cardiac outputs are again obtained by thermodilution and/or direct Fick methods. A full right-sided oximetric saturation run is obtained. Left ventricular angiography is repeated to check left ventricular function and to document any changes in the mitral regurgitation.

The advantages of placing the wires in the left ventricular apex rather than out the aorta are (1) minimal extra fluoroscopy time to position the wire and (2) direct alignment of the balloons in the mitral inflow track with the long axis of the left ventricle. The disadvantages of placing wires in the left ventricular apex are (1) in patients with small left ventricles and large left atria, where the balloons may push back into the atrium during the first or second balloon inflation (this effect can be countered by carefully checking that there is no excessive forward pressure on the wires curled in the apex); (2) elderly hypoxic patients tend to have more ventricular ectopy; and (3) with the older Owens catheters there is some tendency for myocardial trauma or ventricular perforation. Recent data suggest that this tendency is much reduced using the newer pigtail-tiped catheters.[32]

The alternative standard approach to mitral balloon valvotomy, placing the long guidewires of normal stiffness through the left ventricular outflow tract into the descending aorta,[24] is also commonly practiced (Fig. 13.7). The 7-French end-hole catheter is looped in the left ventricular apex using a curved 0.035″ guidewire (Fig. 13.7A). With the balloon inflated and the 0.035″ guidewire fixed in the left ventricle, the catheter is advanced through the left ventricular outflow tract to the descending aorta (Fig. 13.7B). A 260-cm exchange j-wire is placed down into the distal aorta being careful to maintain the loop of wire and catheter in the left ventricular apex (Fig. 13.7C).

The procedure then can be performed over the two wires as outlined previously. The advantage of this technique is that the two balloons, once placed across the mitral valve, may have less tendency to "squeeze" back into the left atrium during balloon inflation. The disadvantages of this technique are (1) extra fluoroscopy time is needed to place the 7-French end-hole catheter and the long guidewire out the aorta; (2) elderly patients also experience ectopy with protracted wire manipulations; (3) there is a significant danger of "losing" the loop of wire in the left ventricle (Fig. 13.7D), which will cause the wires or balloons to straighten out and put direct traction on the anterior mitral valve leaflet. This can cause acute mitral regurgitation or may tear the mitral valve chordae or leaflets while one is trying to manipulate or merely remove the equipment; and (4) in patients with aortic valve stenosis or mechanical aortic prosthetic valves this approach is technically complex or not possible.

There are several alternative techniques that are also successfully used to perform mitral balloon valvotomy. The Inoue "self-guiding" single balloon has enjoyed extensive experience in Asia[19] and is currently being investigated in the United States and Europe (Fig. 13.5). Several clever features of this balloon design include (1) the low profile of the catheter and shaft; (2) the ability of the balloon to differentially inflate first distally then proximally with increasing pressures. The distal end of the balloon opening at the lower pressures allows the operator to "lock" the balloon against the mitral valve during inflation; and (3) the preformed curved shaft and curved wire within the shaft help direct the balloon across the mitral valve and into the left ventricle. The disadvantages of this balloon catheter may be its inability (1) to achieve widths of 38–42 mm during inflation, which is the usual mitral valve diameter in larger patients or (2) to exert lateral pressure on calcified valves. An explicit algorithm to size the balloon for each patient has been developed and should be followed to avoid inducing significant mitral regurgitation.

Other investigators have placed the two balloon catheters across the mitral valve through separate transseptal punctures. Both adults and pediatric patients have been treated with this technique.[7,22] The advantages of this technique are (1) better control over homeostasis and (2) possibly smaller atrial septal defects. The disadvantage is the need to perform two transseptal punctures and to manipulate two sets of equipment separately across the mitral valve.

In a somewhat more complicated technique, a "snare" device is placed through the transseptal sheath to the left ventricle and out the aorta.[27] A long guidewire is placed transarterially into the aorta, snared and pulled back through the aorta, the left ventricle, and down through the left and right atria and the inferior vena cava to exit

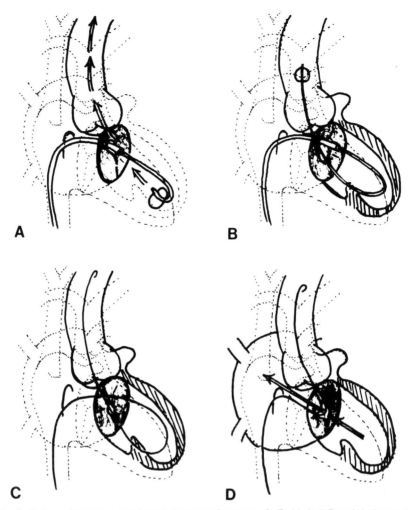

Figure 13.7. Technique of placing guidewire out the ascending aorta. **A,** End-hole 7-French balloon catheter through transseptal sheath at left ventricular apex. Reverse curve at tip of catheter is formed over 0.035″ wire. Wire is precurved and advanced to catheter tip. Catheter is turned to face backwards up the left ventricular outflow tract (double shafted arrows). **B,** Holding 0.035″ wire fixed in left ventricular apex, the balloon catheter is advanced with the balloon inflated with CO_2 to float the catheter out the left ventricular outflow tract. **C,** A long 260-cm j-wire is placed out the aorta and into the descending aorta. The balloon catheter and sheath are removed carefully to maintain a large loop of the exchange wire in the left ventricular apex. A second wire can be placed parallel to this wire using an 8-French double lumen catheter. **D,** If, while manipulating the wires or balloons, the wire loop in the left ventricle is lost, pulling the wire will place direct traction on the anterior mitral valve leaflet causing mitral regurgitation or leaflet damage. If the loop cannot be maintained, the entire procedure should be repeated before balloon valvotomy catheters are introduced.

through the right femoral vein. If the double balloon technique is used, the two balloons are placed through separate arterial sheaths in this way. Each 18–20-mm diameter balloon is placed into the patient transarterially and manipulated across the stenotic mitral valve. Simultaneous balloon inflations are performed. Advantages of this technique include reduced trauma to the femoral vein and atrial septum and fewer iatrogenic atrial septal defects. Disadvantages of the technique include (1) excessive use of fluoroscopy time, (2) possibility of bilateral femoral arterial trauma, (3) inability to readily withdraw and replace balloons across the mitral anulus, and (4) a complex and technically demanding technique.

The present generation of equipment has substantially reduced the risks and difficulty of all these techniques. Further design changes in the next generation of equipment will not be immediately available. The present devices are currently being reviewed for FDA approval, and a broader clinical experience with current techniques is needed.

Expected equipment advances include (1) very low profile catheters; (2) a "bifoil" balloon placed on a single catheter shaft; and (3) modified Inoue-type balloons, which can be precisely sized to each patient's valve anulus.

MORPHOLOGIC FACTORS THAT INFLUENCE THE SUCCESS OF THE PROCEDURE

In choosing to perform mitral balloon valvotomy in a given patient, it is important to consider anatomic factors of the patient that may decrease or increase the chances of achieving a successful, complete mitral balloon valvotomy procedure (Table 13.1). These patient-related factors have

been identified from operators' clinical experience over the last few years.[28] Responsible industry-sponsored registries, which have reported early hemodynamic results and complications at open scientific meetings, have been very helpful in this regard.

Several anatomic features of the patient are important. In smaller patients the smaller mitral valve anulus and left ventricle require smaller length and diameter balloons. Because we routinely see patients from 1.3 to 2.2 m² body surface area, we measure the mitral anulus diameter and size the balloons accordingly. For most younger patients, between 1.7 and 2.0 m², two 18- or 20-mm diameter balloons are used.

Table 13.1.
Morphologic Factors Contributing to Technical Difficulties during Mitral Balloon Valvotomy Procedures

Morphologic Factors	Potential Technical Problems	Possible Solutions
Inferior vena cava occlusion, Chiari network	Difficult transseptal	TEE or TC echo guidance
Large right atrium	Difficult transseptal	TEE or TC echo guidance
Small left atrium	Double balloons produce ASD	Smaller (3-cm length) balloons
Very large left atrium with small left ventricle	Balloon instability during inflation	Larger (5.5-cm length) balloons
Thickened interatrial septum	Difficult transseptal	New needle, echo guidance
Left atrial thrombus	Embolus	Verify with TEE, CT, or MRI; reconsider MBV
Mitral regurgitation	Falsely elevated PA wedge	Directly measure LA pressure
	Catheter instability with ↑ MR	Longer balloons
		Careful sizing diameter of balloons to anulus
Calcified mitral valve anulus	Posterior anulus tear	Undersize balloon diameters
Calcified mitral valve commissure	Potential leaflet tear	Undersize balloon or abandon MBV
Narrowed or "pointed" left ventricular apex	Catheter instability with inflation	Undersize balloon diameters
Native aortic valve stenosis	Hemodynamic instability	Consider combined aortic and mitral dilation or surgery
Mechanical aortic valve prosthesis	Hard to measure MV gradient	Mullins sheath in LA and balloon catheter in LV
	Difficult LV angio	Use balloon catheter through Mullins sheath
Decreased left ventricular function	Low blood pressure	Low-dose dobutamine infusion
	Excessive ectopy	Antiarrhythmics
Coronary artery stenosis	Low blood pressure with ischemia	Consider PTCA with MBV
		Abandon MBV, refer to Surgery
Tricuspid valve disease	Inaccurate thermodilution output	Direct Fick cardiac output
	Increased pulm. hypertension or right heart failure with iatrogenic ASD	Avoid ASD: Short balloon length, use echo, and fluoro, guided balloon inflations

TEE = transesophageal echo; TC = transcutaneous echo; CT = X-ray cine computed tomography; MRI = magnetic resonance imaging; ASD = atrial septal defect; MV = mitral valve; MR = mitral regurgitation; LV = left ventricle; LA = left atrium; MBV = mitral balloon valvotomy.

The transseptal puncture in patients with a larger right atrium or right ventricle may be more difficult. The atrial septum after open-heart surgery may be stiff and fibrotic, making needle puncture more difficult.

The combination of a very large left atrium and a very small left ventricle and a calcified mitral valve is often seen in elderly patients. In those cases it may be difficult to float the 7-French end-hole balloon catheter across the mitral valve into the left ventricle and to maintain balloon and wire position across the mitral valve during double balloon inflations. Undersizing the balloons and inflating the balloons sequentially before they are inflated simultaneously can be helpful in this situation. When the left ventricular cavity, seen in the RAO view, is a more "globular" shape, it is easier to place the curled guidewire in the left ventricular apex. Conversely, when the left ventricle is more "triangular" shaped, the sharply angled left ventricular apex can make it more difficult to maintain the j-guidewire position in the left ventricular apex and more difficult to inflate the balloons without having them push back during systole into the left atrium. Slightly undersizing balloon diameter in these ventricles is also helpful. In patients with smaller left atria, using the shorter 3-cm length balloons may avoid atrial tears, atrial septal defects, and trauma to the left ventricular endocardium which may be produced by the longer 5.5 cm balloons (Fig. 13.8 & 13.9).

The presence of mitral regurgitation can complicate the procedure in several ways. First, in selecting patients for balloon valvotomy, it is important to be clear that large "V-waves" do not falsely elevate the mitral gradient and lead to overestimation of the degree of stenosis. It is therefore important to directly measure left atrial pressures in patients with mixed mitral stenosis and regurgitation in order to obtain accurate mitral valve gradients. If a large gradient exists, patients with mixed stenosis and regurgitation can still benefit substantially from balloon valvotomy treatment. Second, some patients can have increased regurgitation after a "successful" balloon valvotomy. It is therefore important that the regurgitation be evaluated before and after the procedure by angiography and Doppler echocardiography. Follow-up has shown that the increased mitral regurgitation noted immediately after the procedure can decrease over 3–6 months in many of these patients.[28,29] Third, in patients with calcified mitral valves, it is important to be sure that heavy nodules of calcium are not binding the commissures (Fig.

13.10). In these cases transverse leaflet tears may markedly increase the mitral regurgitation. Fourth, in patients with concomitant aortic valve disease or disease of multiple valves, it is important for the operator to be convinced that there is a large mitral valve gradient, which, if it is reduced, will significantly improve the patient's hemodynamic status. Merely relieving a small mitral valve gradient in a patient with complex valvular heart disease will yield minimal clinical improvement.

The presence of a left atrial thrombus seen on two-dimensional echo is a contraindication to mitral balloon valvotomy. In most laboratories attempts at detecting left atrial thrombus have relied on transthoracic echocardiography. Currently transesophageal echocardiography, magnetic resonance imaging (MRI) scanning, and cine computed tomography (CT) scanning are being evaluated and may be more sensitive techniques. Transesophageal echocardiography is likely the most sensitive of these newer technologies.

Various other factors may add to the difficulty or risk of performing mitral balloon valvotomy procedures. In patients with severe pulmonary hypertension, that is, systolic pulmonary pressures greater than two-thirds of systemic levels, vasovagal reactions or ventricular arrhythmias can precipitate prolonged hypotension and hemodynamic instability. Patients with pulmonary hypertension, tricuspid regurgitation and right ventricular dysfunction may not tolerate the volume overload if a moderate or large atrial septal defect is produced after balloon valvotomy. Elderly patients with significant lung disease or poor left ventricular function may have prolonged hypotension or prolonged ventricular ectopy when the two large balloon dilation catheters are placed across the mitral valve. Patients with neurological, pulmonary, or orthopaedic impairment who have been referred because of increased operative risks may have trouble lying flat on the cardiac catheterization table for the longer periods of time needed to complete the procedure. Patients who refuse potential blood transfusions also remain a problem. Although the need for transfusions in patients undergoing mitral balloon valvotomy procedures is now very small, the possibility of cardiac trauma and the need for open-heart surgery remain possible outcomes. One cannot guarantee that a transfusion would not be needed during a particular procedure.

Finally, there are factors in dealing with the patient as an individual that must be assessed before mitral balloon valvotomy can be advocated

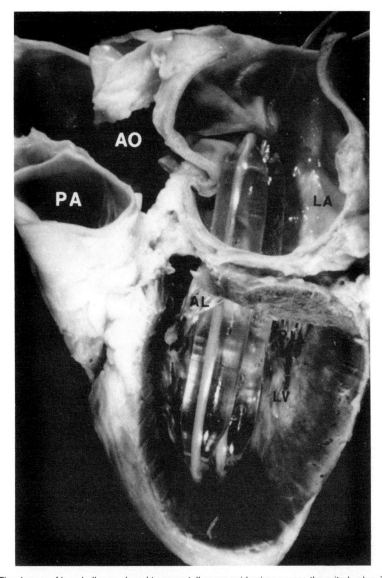

Figure 13.8. The danger of long balloons placed transseptally over guidewires across the mitral valve. The left ventricle (LV) and left atrium (LA) are shown in a cutaway LAO view. Two 18-mm diameter, 5.5-cm length balloons are placed transseptally across the mitral valve and 0.038″ j-guidewires are placed in the aortic outflow tract (AO). During inflation, the longer balloons may push the guidewires forward into the myocardium. Alternatively, the catheter shafts just proximal to the balloons are of necessity separated by 18 mm during inflation. The proximal ends of the balloons are near the atrial muscle. During inflation, the two shafts will push back and separate, spreading open the entry hole in the membranous atrial septal tissue.

instead of the surgical procedure. The patient's preferences and family preference for the balloon technique should be of primary concern. Therefore both the alternative treatments of surgical versus balloon valvotomy should be discussed at length with the family and the patient. Because the patients are receiving most of their continuing care with the referring physician and are usually living at some distance from the tertiary care hospital, referring physicians' preferences are also of importance. Referring physicians should have all of the patient's hemodynamic and echo-Doppler results after the procedure and be confident that further consultative and referral care remain available to them and their patients after these procedures.

It is important to assess the expectations of the

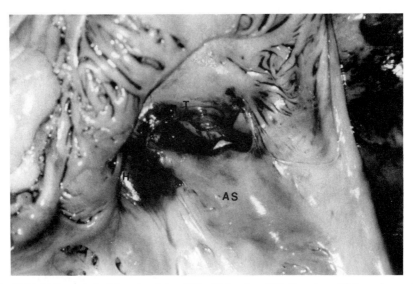

Figure 13.9.   Right atrial aspect of a 1.8-cm length tear (T) in atrial septum (AS). Hematoma (H) formed around torn muscle is shown.

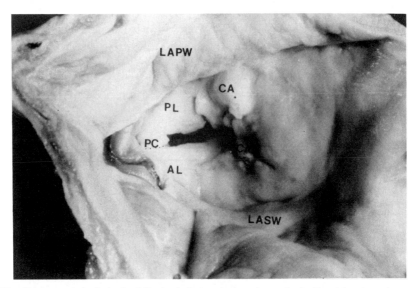

Figure 13.10.   Atrial aspect of mitral valve following balloon valvotomy in a patient with calcium-bound commissures. Left atrial posterior wall (LAPW) and septal wall (LASW) are seen. The anterior leaflet (AL) of the mitral valve is seen inferiorly. The posterior leaflet (PL) contains a 1-cm diameter localized calcified nodule (CA). While the posterior commissure (PC) is free of calcium, the dark area of anterior commissure has heavy verrucous calcifications, which "bind" the two leaflets together. Dilation with two balloons (15- and 18-mm diameter) resulted in 1.1-cm opening of the posterior commissure and a 1.2-cm tear transverse to the mitral orifice in the posterior leaflet just to the left of the calcified nodule.

referring physician, the patient, and the family for the functional recovery of the patient after the procedure. In young patients with only mitral stenosis as their medical problem, one should anticipate full recovery and return to a very active life-style with family and work. In the elderly patients, however, other medical conditions may severely limit the overall functional ability, and merely improving symptoms of pulmonary congestion, regardless of other medical problems, may be the goal of a successful procedure. The clinical expectations should be clearly discussed with the patient, the family, and the referring physician. The expected results of surgical commissurotomy or mitral valve replacement should also be discussed along with those of mitral balloon valvotomy. Mitral balloon valvotomy remains, at this writing, an investigational procedure. It is routinely practiced under investigational protocols, and many tertiary care centers have considerable experience with the technique. With continued technique and equipment improvements there has been reduced morbidity and mortality. The accumulating long-term follow-up is showing that symptomatic improvement persists in many patients. These experiences have supported and increased our enthusiasm for this treatment. However, the procedure still has associated complications that should be noted and understood by both practitioners and patients.

COMPLICATIONS OF MITRAL BALLOON VALVOTOMY

Table 13.2 lists the procedure-related risks of mitral balloon valvotomy. The procedure-related mortality ranges from 0 to 3%. It may not be possible to complete the procedure in up to 8% of patients due to a variety of untoward events or patient inability to tolerate lying on the catheteriza-tion table for 60–120 min. "Suboptimal results" are variously defined, but recent studies have noted that spontaneous variability in valve measurements range around ± 15%.[30] Optimal results have been defined as increases in mitral valve area to at least 1.5 cm^2 or by 25% increase in area.[28] Left ventricular perforation or trauma, although more commonly seen with the older Owens balloons, also remains a possible risk. Increased mitral regurgitation by greater than one angiographic grade may be seen in up to 30% of the patients immediately after the procedure.

Perioperative emboli or stroke may occur in 0 to 2%. Patients in these studies did not have a history of recent embolic events and were screened by transthoracic echocardiography. Hypotension due to arrhythmias, volume depletion, or vasovagal reactions can be easily treated. Hypotension during balloon inflation is now less of a problem with the newer low-profile balloons. Iatrogenic atrial septal defects can be documented by oximetry in 5–33% of the patients. By color Doppler studies, up to 53% of patients will have some atrial septal defect flow. In many cases, this will decrease or disappear over 6–12-month follow-up. Because authors use various criteria for a "significant

Table 13.2.
Immediate Complications of Mitral Balloon Valvotomy

Complication	Incidence (%)	References
Procedure-related mortality	0–3	21,25,27,28,29
Unable to complete procedure	0–8	10,21,25,27,29
Suboptimal increase in MV area	35	28
Increased mitral regurgitation	5–30	21,25,27,28,29
With surgical repair/placement	1–4	21,26
Cardiac perforation	0–2	25,28
With tamponade	0–2	25,26
With surgical correction	0–3	25,26
Embolization		
CVA	0–2	25,26,27
Systemic	0–2	24,25
Blood transfusion	0–3	22,23
Atrial septal defect (by oximetry)	5–33	20,21,25,27,28
Arrhythmias		
AV block	0–2	24,28
Balloon rupture		
With sequelae	0–5	25,30
Vascular complication		
With surgical repair	0–2	25,26,27,28,29

CVA = cerebrovascular accident, AV = atrioventricular

step-up" by oximetry, the reported incidence of atrial septal defect is quite variable in the literature. Transverse balloon rupture has been well described in balloon dilation of coarctation of the aorta but is rarely seen in mitral balloon valvotomy.[31] The mechanism of transverse rupture may be quite similar in these cases. Balloon expansion against a stenotic pliable valve or a valve with calcific spicules will create radial stress in a very small "ring" around the balloon, causing local stress and radial tears. Vascular complications are unusual with femoral venous entry and may be more serious with the arterial entry of larger balloons.

Mechanisms of Complications of Mitral Balloon Valvotomy

In centers with greater experience, it has become clear that certain constellations of factors may predispose a patient to complications. Early recognition of these situations may cause the operators to alter technique or abandon the procedure before they encounter a major complication (Table 13.2).

Potential complications related to the transseptal catheterization have been reviewed. Most large series document a 2–5% major complication rate and 0.5–1% mortality related to transseptal catheterization. These statistics would also pertain to patients undergoing mitral balloon valvotomy. The importance of avoiding a very high, posterior transseptal needle and sheath placement has been discussed. In performing a lower transseptal catheterization, or two transseptal catheterizations, operators may encounter difficulty engaging the thin-walled fossa ovalis and elect to cross the thicker atrial wall muscle. If they engage the base of the septum or the coronary sinus and place a large sheath into the left atrium, they may not have a complication during a procedure but may encounter progressive hypotension after the procedure when the sheaths are pulled back, leaving open tears in the inferior atrial wall. Delayed tamponade 1–6 hours after otherwise successful balloon valvotomy can be encountered due to this problem. Difficulty in placing the balloons across the calcified mitral valve may lead the operator to "accept" nonoptimal balloon positions for a "first inflation." During these inflations, excessive forward balloon movement may produce perforation of the left ventricular apex, while excessive backward movement may force the balloon shafts, which are separated by the inflated balloons, back into the atrial septum enlarging the atrial septal defect.

In the small left atria and left ventricles, the larger 5.5-cm balloons may also push the catheter tip into the apex or the proximal catheter shafts into the atrial septum during systole (Fig. 13.8). Checking the balloon position in both the RAO and angulated LAO views by fluoroscopy is useful in these circumstances. In addition, we have found that two-dimensional echocardiography performed at the time the balloons are placed across the mitral valve can reassure the operator that the shafts at the proximal ends of the balloons are not dilating the interatrial septum during balloon inflation. Simply advancing the proximal ends of the shorter balloons farther into the left atrium can reduce this problem. Echocardiography is also useful in monitoring patients with persistent hypotension to rule out impending tamponade in the cardiac catheterization laboratory.

Trauma to the femoral vein was thought to be a considerable risk with transvenous entry of two large catheters through a single site. However, extensive experience has shown that venous entry site complications are uncommon and minimized by (1) placing both of the catheters through a single hole, (2) carefully dilating the skin and fascia with a 9-French dilator before the balloon catheters are introduced, (3) not using large venous sheaths, (4) removing all catheters and wires soon after the procedure in the laboratory, and (5) placing direct local pressure for 20 to 30 min on the femoral vein. Often there is no hematoma and very little groin tenderness after 24 hours. On the other hand, in obese patients, or in elderly patients with a tendency to move excessively in bed, persistent local pressure and observation may be necessary.

In some elderly patients with coexisting lung disease and hypoxia, we have encountered excessive ectopy during catheter placement. We have abandoned the procedure in some of these cases because we could not find a balloon and wire position either in the left ventricle or out the aorta that did not induce persistent ectopy with hemodynamic compromise. The Inoue balloon technique may have an advantage in these patients. These elderly or very ill patients often have associated right heart failure, hypoxia, and chronic lung disease and are therefore also very high risk surgical patients.

When using the technique where the long guidewires are placed out the left ventricle and stabilized in the descending aorta, it is mandatory that the loop of the guidewire be maintained in the left ventricular apex. Several cases of direct trauma to the mitral valve resulting in acute mitral regurgitation and need for emergent surgery have been encountered. In small ventricles or triangular-shaped left ventricular chambers seen on RAO angiography, it can be very difficult to maintain this loop of wire in the apex.

Perforation of the left ventricular apex has been reported by several investigators during otherwise successful mitral balloon valvotomy. There are several factors that may contribute to this risk: (1) using longer 5.5-cm balloons in a smaller ventricle (Fig. 13.8), (2) placing the old Owens catheters in the left ventricular apex without adequate coils on the long exchange guidewire, and (3) using relatively oversized diameter balloons, which tend to "lock" the catheters in the mitral valve anulus and therefore force stiffer catheters and catheter tips down onto the contracting left ventricular myocardium during systole. Fortunately, if one uses the newer pigtail catheters and sizes the balloon according to each patient's anulus diameter, these complications may be avoided. The mitral anulus diameter is best measured by echocardiography in the apical four-chamber view.[23]

There are also several mechanisms of producing interatrial septal defects after an otherwise successful mitral balloon valvotomy. The older balloons with thicker polyethylene balloon material tended to form "wings" as they were deflated. They therefore presented a large "deflated profile" to the atrial septum and the femoral vein as they were retracted out of the body. Although with newer balloons, this complication is diminished, atrial septal defects are still encountered. This can be related to the use of longer balloons in the smaller left atria or forcing the catheter shafts, just proximal to the balloons, back into the septum during balloon inflations.

Interatrial openings through the septal muscle persist long after a successfully completed procedure. This has been observed at the time of operation in the occasional patient who has gone on to have mitral valve replacement several months after the balloon valvotomy procedure. The interatrial septum does not heal by forming a clot in the defect. Rather, interstitial edema and a hematoma form locally around the 0.5- to 1.0-cm split in the muscle. This tissue tends to stiffen and fibrose over time forming a "baffle." As long as the mitral valve remains open and the left atrial pressure is low, there is no driving pressure to open the slit. However, if there is mitral valve restenosis, there is also a possibility of observing a recurrent left-to-right shunt that was once closed. Fortunately, this must be rare and has yet to be documented in vivo.

Avoiding procedure-related complications can be achieved first by becoming experienced with the transseptal technique. In those cases where some difficulty is anticipated, patient referral to an experienced center may be indicated. Where specific technical difficulties are encountered in balloon or wire placement, it may be best to abandon the technique and refer the patient to surgery or to stabilize the patient and reattempt the procedure after some period of recovery time. A repeated attempt may then prove successful after discussion with other operators.

Diagnosis and Avoidance of Procedure-Related Complications

The serious procedure-related complications usually begin in the catheterization laboratory (Table 13.2) and are obvious during the case. The most difficult situations are encountered from (1) persistent ectopy, (2) inability to stabilize the balloons during inflation, (3) persistent hypotension, (4) mitral regurgitation, and (5) tamponade. Persistent ventricular or supraventricular ectopy can occur despite careful and proper wire and balloon placement across the mitral valve. Avoiding excessive forward pressure of the balloons on left ventricular apex can usually control this problem. Intravenous beta-blockers or other antiarrythmics have been helpful to control ventricular ectopy in some patients. The inability to stabilize the balloon across the mitral valve during inflation may occur especially in younger patients with pliable valves and hyperdynamic hearts. The use of longer length balloons or sequential inflation of the balloons prior to simultaneous inflations are useful maneuvers.

Persistent hypotension during successive balloon inflations can be very difficult to control. Patients may be volume depleted, have vasovagal reactions, have poor RV or LV function, have obstruction of the mitral valve by the balloon catheters, or have excessive ectopy, which results in hypotension. These conditions are usually controlled by fluids, atropine, dopamine, or expeditious balloon manipulation.

Acute mitral regurgitation may be induced by catheter or wire position or by valve trauma. When the guidewires are placed out the left ventricle to the aorta and the large left ventricular "loop" is lost, there is direct pressure and traction on the anterior mitral valve leaflet (Fig. 13.7). Although restoring a partially lost loop in the left ventricle can be accomplished by advancing the guidewire into the LV apex, once the loop is completely lost it pulls directly from the aortic to the mitral valve and is almost impossible to restore. On the other hand, continuing to pull a guidewire without a loop back to the left atrium may create a "band saw" effect and tear into the anterior mitral leaflet or the chordae. If gentle traction does not remove such wires, they may be removed through a pigtail or stiffer double lumen catheter.

Cases of acute mitral regurgitation due to rupture of chordae or transverse tears of the leaflets have been encountered. Valves with heavy fibrosis and calcification on echo and fluoroscopy may be prone to this problem. Using large balloon combinations that stretch the mitral anulus can produce posterior anulus tears into the left atrial myocardium or pericardium. Smaller valves with mitral annular calcification in the elderly may be prone to these tears.[32]

Cardiac tamponade due to difficulties with the transseptal catheterization has been discussed. Posterior anulus tears that reach the pericardium can also present as tamponade. Left ventricular apical perforation is probably the most devastating hemodynamic complication. The use of longer balloons in patients with small left ventricles and atria and the inability to maintain the curled guidewires in the left ventricular apex may predispose to perforation. Left ventricular perforation has also occurred when the guidewires were placed out the aorta. Immediate recognition of clinical signs of tamponade and marked increase in right atrial pressure on a monitoring right heart catheter can lead to early treatment by pericardial tap and pericardial catheter placement while arranging for emergency surgical repair.

STATE OF THE ART OF MITRAL BALLOON VALVOTOMY TECHNIQUE

The procedure and equipment have improved rapidly over the last four years.[33] This may have contributed to a reduced procedure-related morbidity and mortality. Mitral balloon valvotomy is an important new treatment for patients with symptomatic rheumatic mitral stenosis. It can effect immediate major improvements in hemodynamics, and patients notice obvious improvements in symptoms over minutes or hours. Long-term follow-up studies are of the greatest importance in establishing the persistent effectiveness of this new treatment modality.

Acknowledgments

The author has benefitted greatly from clinical collaboration with Dr. David Kawanishi and from extensive and continuing collaboration with Dr. Bruce F. Waller.

REFERENCES

1. Rasted IE, Scheifly CH, and Edwards JE. Studies of the mitral valve II. Certain anatomic features of the mitral valve and associated structures in mitral stenosis. *Circulation 14*:398, 1956.
2. Bailey CP. The surgical treatment of mitral stenosis (mitral commissurotomy). *Dis Chest 15*:377, 1949.
3. Harken DE, Ellis LB, Ware PF, et al. The surgical treatment of mitral stenosis. I. Valvuloplasty. *N Engl J Med 239*:801, 1948.
4. Logan A, Turner R. Surgical treatment of mitral stenosis with particular reference to the transventricular approach with a mechanical dilator. *Lancet 2*: 874, 1959.
5. John S, Bashi VV, Jairaj PS, et al. Closed mitral valvotomy: Early results and long-term follow-up of 3724 consecutive patients. *Circulation 68*:891, 1983.
6. Kan J, White RI, Mitchell SE, et al. Percutaneous balloon valvuloplasty: A new method for treating congenital pulmonary valve stenosis. *N Engl J Med 307*:540, 1982.
7. Mullins CE, Nihill MR, Vick GW, et al. Double balloon technique for dilation of valvular or vessel stenosis in congenital and acquired heart disease. *J Am Coll Cardiol 10*:107, 1987.
8. Lock JE, Khalilullah M, Shrivastava S, et al. Percutaneous catheter commissurotomy in rheumatic mitral stenosis. *N Engl J Med 313*:1515, 1985.
9. McKay CR, Otto C, Block P, et al. Immediate results of mitral balloon commissurotomy in 737 patients. *Circulation 82*:(Suppl III), III-545, 1990.
10. Dean LS, Davis K, Feit F, et al. Complications and mortality of percutaneous mitral balloon commissurotomy. *Circulation 82*:(Suppl III), III-545, 1990.
11. Waller BF, McKay CR, Lewon RF, et al. Morphologic analysis of 23 operatively excised and intact stenotic cardiac valves from patients undergoing prior clinical catheter balloon valvuloplasty. *Circulation 78*:II-592, 1988.
12. Carpentier A, Deloche A, Dauptain J, et al. A new reconstructive operation for correction of mitral and tricuspid insufficiency. *J Thorac Cardiovasc Surg 61*: 1–13, 1971.
13. Antanes MJ, Colsen PR, Kinsley RH. Mitral valvuloplasty: A learning curve. *Circulation 68*: II-70, 1983.
14. Cheitlin MD. Mitral valve repair: Procedure of choice for mitral regurgitation. *Council on Clinical Cardiology Newsletter*, Winter 1990, p. 3.

15. Cosgrove DM. Mitral valvuloplasty. *Curr Probl Cardiol 14*:354, 1989.

16. Braunwald E. A new technique for left ventricular angiography and transseptal left heart catheterization. *Am J Cardiol 6*:1062, 1960.

17. Lasley WK, et al. Transseptal left heart catheterization; use of a sheath technique. *Cathet Cardiovasc Diagn 8*:535, 1982.

18. Ross J Jr. Considerations regarding the technique for transseptal left heart catheterization. *Circulation 34*:391, 1966.

19. Inoue K, Owaki T, Nakamura T, et al. Clinical application of transvenous mitral commissurotomy by a new balloon catheter. *J Thorac Cardiovasc Surg 87*:394, 1984.

20. McKay RG, Lock JE, Keane JF, et al. Percutaneous mitral valvuloplasty in an adult patient with calcific mitral stenosis. *J Am Coll Cardiol 7*:1410, 1986.

21. Chen C, Wang Y, Qing D, et al. Percutaneous mitral balloon dilatation by a new sequential single- and double-balloon technique. *Am Heart J 116*:1161, 1988.

22. Al Zaibag MA, Kasab SA, Ribeiro PA, et al. Percutaneous double-balloon mitral valvotomy for rheumatic mitral-valve stenosis. *Lancet 1*:757, 1986.

23. McKay CR, Kawanishi DT, Rahimtoola SH. Catheter balloon valvuloplasty of the mitral valve in adults using a double-balloon technique. *JAMA 257*:1753, 1987.

24. Palacios I, Block P, and Brandi S. Percutaneous balloon valvotomy for patients with severe mitral stenosis. *Circulation 75*:778, 1987.

25. Vahanian A, Michel PL, Cormier B, et al. Results of percutaneous mitral commissurotomy in 200 patients. *Am J Cardiol 63*:847, 1989.

26. Block PC. Early results of mitral balloon valvuloplasty (MBV) for mitral stenosis: Report from the NHLBI registry. *Circulation 78*:II489, 1988.

27. Babic UU, Dorros G, Pijcic P, et al. Percutaneous mitral valvuloplasty: Retrograde transarterial double balloon technique utilizing the transseptal approach. *Cathet Cardiovasc Diagn 14*:229, 1988.

28. Abscal VM, Wilkins GT, O'Shea JP, et al. Prediction of successful outcome in 130 patients undergoing percutaneous balloon mitral valvotomy. *Circulation 82*:448, 1990.

29. McKay CR, Kawanishi DT, Kotlewski A, et al. Improvement in exercise capacity and exercise hemodynamics three months after double-balloon, catheter balloon valvuloplasty treatment of patients with symptomatic mitral disease. *Circulation 77*:1013, 1988.

30. Kawanishi DT, McKay CR, Reid CL. Spontaneous variation and exercise induced changes in measurement of mitral valve areas using the Gorlin Formula: Implications for evaluation of changes following catheter balloon valvuloplasty for mitral stenosis. *J Am Coll Cardiol 11*:234A, 1988.

31. Dev V, Shrivastava S. Transverse balloon tear in valvuloplasty (letter). *Am Heart J 117*:1397, 1989.

32. Waller BF, VanTassel JW, McKay CR. Anatomic basis for the morphologic results from catheter balloon valvuloplasty of stenotic mitral valves. *Clin Cardiol 13*:655, 1990.

33. Berland J. Gamva H, Rocha P, et al. Mitral valvuloplasty: Improvement in safety and efficacy by using two new pigtail balloons. *Circulation 78*:II-490, 1988.

14

Follow-up Studies:
Effect of Balloon Mitral Valvotomy
on Symptoms, Outcome, and Hemodynamics

RAOUL BONAN, ANTONIO SERRA, and THIERRY LEFÈVRE

Percutaneous mitral balloon valvotomy (PMV) is now a well-established alternative to surgical mitral commissurotomy for patients with symptomatic mitral stenosis.[1–8] Immediate hemodynamic results are excellent in patients with a mobile, pliable, noncalcified, and nonthickened valve, which occurs more frequently in young patients. More recently it has been shown that PMV is also feasible in older patients with more extensive valvular disease.[9–13] However, the resultant mitral valve area obtained after PMV is strongly dependent on mitral valve morphology.[8,14–16]

In vivo[17] and postmortem in vitro studies[13,18–21] have shown that successful PMV enlarges valve area through separation of fused commissures, similar to surgical commissurotomy, and by fracture of calcified nodular deposits. Therefore, the expected mid- and long-term follow-up of patients after successful PMV should be comparable to surgery. The small series published to date have confirmed this hypothesis.[8,20–23] Using our data, we will document the initial follow-up of this percutaneous therapeutic procedure.

METHODS
Patient Selection

In our first 113 cases, all patients with symptomatic mitral stenosis were considered candidates for PMV. Patients with mitral regurgitation $> 2+/4+$ according to Sellers criteria,[24] those with a contraindication for transseptal catheterization,

with a recent history of systemic emboli ($<$ 3 months), or with left atrial thrombus documented by transthoracic echocardiography were excluded from PMV. Recently, transesophageal echocardiography has been used to detect atrial thrombus and has demonstrated a much greater sensitivity and specificity than transthoracic echocardiography. There was no prospective contraindication regarding mitral valve morphology or left atrial size. Patients with intractable pulmonary edema during pregnancy were not excluded, because the expected fetal risk from surgery is higher than that from x-ray exposure.

We have shown[13] that the outcome of PMV is related to the morphology of the mitral apparatus quantified by the echocardiographic score described by Wilkins et al.[14] and discussed in Chapters 11 and 12. For this reason, we now exclude patients for PMV who have severe alteration of the mitral valve morphology as assessed by an echocardiographic score $\geq$ 11 and who have no contraindication for surgery.

Patient Characteristics

Percutaneous mitral balloon valvotomy was performed from March 1987 to April 1989 in 113 consecutive patients (Tables 14.1 and 14.2). The majority were female; 25% had previous surgical open or closed commissurotomy, 15% a prior history of emboli, 47% calcification on x-ray and 68% were in NYHA functional class III or IV. Eighteen percent had a left atrial diameter $\geq$ 60 mm

Table 14.1.
Patient Characteristics ($N = 113$)

Age (years)	53 ± 14 (27 to 81)
Sex (F:M)	101:12
Previous commissurotomy	27 (25%)
Previous embolism	17 (15%)
Atrial fibrillation	40 (36%)
Anticoagulation	46 (42%)
Calcification (on X-ray)	52 (47%)
NYHA CHF Class 4	13 (12%)
3	62 (56%)
2	35 (32%)

Table 14.2.
Echocardiographic Characteristics

Left atrial diameter (mm)	52 ± 8
≥ 60 mm	20 (18%)
Mitral valve thickness > 2*	15 (13%)
calcification > 2*	33 (29%)
mobility > 2*	32 (28%)
Subvalvular fibrosis > 2*	25 (22%)
Mean echo score*	8.4 ± 1.6
Echo score > 8*	50 (44%)

*Numbers represent echo score[14]

and 44% an echocardiographic score > 8. Some patients with severe alteration of the mitral valve morphology (echo score ≥ 10) were selected for PMV because the expected risk of surgery was prohibitive (> 10–20%). Six patients had moderate to severe tricuspid regurgitation, two moderate aortic insufficiency, one severe aortic stenosis, two significant coronary artery disease, and two severe obstructive pulmonary disease (FEV_1 < 1000 cc/min).

Procedure and Hemodynamic Measurements

Before PMV the right and left heart pressures, an oximetric run, and the arteriovenous and the venovenous indicator dilution curves (indocyanine green) were obtained using a left femoral artery (7-French pigtail) and left femoral venous approach (8-French Goodale-Lubin). Cardiac output was determined by the Fick method. Oxygen consumption was measured directly with a metabolic rate meter (Waters Instrument, Harrow, UK). Left atrial transseptal catheterization was performed by the right femoral venous approach with a standard Brockenbrough needle using an 8-French Mullins transseptal long sheath and dilator (USCI, Billerica, MA). Correct needle position in the left atrium was confirmed by pressure measurement. The sheath and dilator were then advanced, and the needle was removed. After achieving left atrial access, 4000 units of heparin were given intravenously. The mitral valve area was calculated using the Gorlin formula. Mean transmitral pressure gradient was measured by planimetry from the simultaneous left atrial and left ventricular pressure recordings, averaging 3 consecutive beats if the patient was in sinus rhythm and 10 if atrial fibrillation was present. Left ventriculography in the 30° RAO projection was done, and mitral regurgitation was quantified

according to the criteria of Sellers.[24] After pre-PMV measurements, the dilator was removed and a 7-French balloon-tipped end-hole catheter was advanced though the sheath into the left ventricle in order to facilitate crossing the mitral valve and to avoid accidental passage of the guidewire between chordae. The long sheath was then advanced to the left ventricle and a 0.038-inch, 260-cm long "extra stiff" Teflon-coated guidewire was positioned at the apex of the left ventricle. The J-tip of the guidewire was manually precurved in order to create a loop in the apex and prevent left ventricular damage. The 7-French balloon catheter and the sheath were removed, and a 7-French, 6-mm angioplasty catheter balloon (Cook Inc., Bloomington, IN) was passed over the guidewire to the level of the interatrial septum, and the septum was dilated. After removal of this catheter, a 12-French catheter with two balloons in a single shaft (Bifoil, Schneider, Zurich, Switzerland) or two 9-French separated balloon catheters were positioned across the mitral valve. When a second catheter balloon was used, a second long exchange guidewire was placed in the left ventricle apex using the long double-lumen sheath catheter. Two to five inflations by hand were performed until the waist in the balloons caused by the mitral stenosis disappeared. The first inflation was performed at low pressure in order to remove air from the balloon catheter. Two separate balloons were used in 53% of cases, one bifoil catheter balloon in 44%, and one single balloon in 3%. The most frequent balloon diameter combination was 19 + 19 mm (67%). To prevent additional damage of the interatrial septum, the dilation catheters were removed by first performing several aspirations under negative pressure in order to obtain the thinnest profile and then by rotating the catheter on its long axis during the pull-back across the septum.

Immediately after PMV, hemodynamic measurements, left ventriculography, an oximetric run, and dye dilution curves were repeated.

IMMEDIATE OUTCOME
Completed PMV

As shown in Figure 14.1, PMV was completed in 103 of 113 (91%) patients. Complete success, defined as a final mitral valve area ≥ 1.5 cm^2 and an increase in mitral valve area $\geq 25\%$ was obtained in 82 (80%) patients. In 12 (11%) patients the result was an incomplete success defined as a 25% increase in mitral valve area but a final mitral valve area between 1 and 1.5 cm^2. Nine (9%) patients were considered hemodynamic failures with a final mitral valve area < 1 cm^2 and a gain $< 25\%$.

As shown in Table 14.3, a substantial decrease in left atrial and mean pulmonary artery pressure, mitral valve gradient, and pulmonary arteriolar resistance was obtained after PMV, with a dramatic increase observed in mitral valve area.

Multivariate analysis and stepwise logistic regression identified independent predictive factors of success (vs. failure or incomplete success): cardiac index (2.6 ± 0.7 vs. 1.9 ± 0.7 liters/min/m^2, $p = 0.0001$), NYHA class < 3 (39% vs. 7%, $p = 0.002$), left atrial diameter (50 ± 8 vs. 56 ± 8 mm, $p = 0.05$), and echo score ≤ 8 (60% vs. 36%, $p = 0.01$). Lower cardiac output and higher functional class have also been associated with less favorable short- and long-term results of closed mitral commissurotomy.[25–27]

The quality of the leaflets and the subvalvular apparatus appears to be a major determinant of outcome in mitral valve balloon dilation, thus corroborating previous experience with surgical commissurotomy.[27–29] The mechanism of PMV has been shown to be similar to surgical commissurotomy.[17–19] Therefore use of two-dimensional echocardiography to detect the mitral anatomy should be useful in the evaluation of candidates for PMV. Using the scoring system to describe mitral valve morphology outlined by Wilkins et al.[14] it was found that a lower echocardiographic score was associated with a higher rate of optimal hemodynamic outcome. In a recent study, Palacios et al.[20] found that a good hemodynamic result (post-PMV mitral valve area ≥ 1.5 cm^2) was obtained in 88% of patients with echo scores of 8 or less and in 44% of patients with echo scores of more than 8. In our series, success rate was also related to echo score as shown in Figure 14.2. The same relationship was observed between the percentage increase in mitral valve area and echocardiographic score (Fig. 14.3).

Other studies, using a different grading system of the mitral valve anatomy,[7,8,16] have found the same negative correlations between deterioration of the mitral valve apparatus and PMV effectiveness.

Uncompleted PMV

Percutaneous mitral balloon valvotomy was not completed in 10 patients. Five technical failures

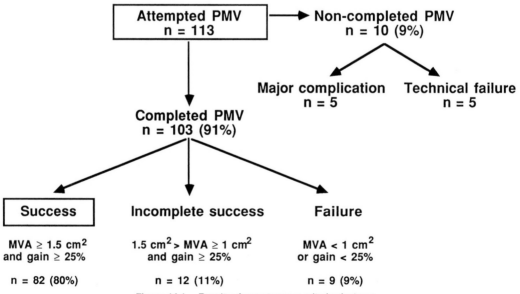

Figure 14.1. Results of percutaneous mitral valvotomy.

Table 14.3.
Immediate Hemodynamic Results

	Pre-PMV	Post-PMV	p value
Cardiac output (liters/min)	3.8 ± 1.2	4.2 ± 1.3	< 0.001
Mean pressures (mm Hg)			
Pulmonary artery	37 ± 13	26 ± 10	< 0.0001
Left atrium	26 ± 6	14 ± 5	< 0.0001
Right atrium	7 ± 4	6 ± 3	< 0.05
Mitral gradient (mm Hg)	16 ± 5	6 ± 3	< 0.0001
Mitral valve area (cm^2)	1.1 ± 0.4	2.1 ± 0.8	< 0.0001
Pulmonary resistance			
Arteriolar (dynes $\cdot$ sec^{-1} $\cdot$ cm^{-5})	300 ± 350	225 ± 190	< 0.001
Total (dynes $\cdot$ sec^{-1} $\cdot$ cm^{-5})	880 ± 570	465 ± 285	< 0.0001

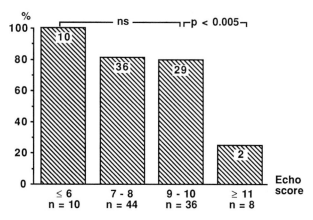

Rate of success

Figure 14.2. Relationship between percutaneous mitral valvotomy success rate and echocardiographic score.

occurred. In one case the transseptal catheterization could not be performed. In the remaining four patients, the balloon catheter could not be placed properly across the mitral valve. The left atrial diameter of these patients was 70, 61, 60, 72, and 55 mm respectively.

Major complications occurred in five cases. Acute mitral regurgitation occurred in two and was caused by mitral leaflet tear. Both required urgent or delayed surgery without further complications. There were two left ventricular perforations. One occurred in a 73-year-old patient who had urgent surgery (including mitral valve replacement) due to acute tamponade and died 48 hours later. The other patient developed a pseudoaneurysm in the left ventricular apex and was not operated on because the surgical risk was considered excessive. Another patient had a left atrial perforation with acute tamponade treated by emergency surgery without further complication. Technical failure and left heart perforation seem to

decrease with experience since most occurred in our first 50 patients.

Acute mitral regurgitation due to mitral leaflet rupture has also been reported in patients undergoing surgical commissurotomy.[25,26] In one patient, following unsatisfactory increase of the mitral valve area after conventional double balloon technique, a 15-mm balloon was used in conjunction with a bifoil (19 + 19 mm). The effective balloon area:mitral anulus area ratio was 9.45:10.8 cm^2. The echocardiographic score was 10 of 16 with subvalvular fibrosis of 2 of 4. Mitral regurgitation increased from 1 to 4 of 4. In the second case, two single balloons (18 + 20 mm) were used. The balloon area:mitral anulus area ratio was 6.47:10.8. The echocardiographic score was 5 of 10 with subvalvular fibrosis of 1 of 4. Mitral regurgitation increased from 0 to 4 of 4.

Severe mitral regurgitation has been reported to occur after PMV in 4 to 5% of patients[7,8] and is especially a concern in patients with extensive

Figure 14.3. Relationship between increase in mitral valve area obtained by percutaneous mitral valvotomy and echocardiographic score.

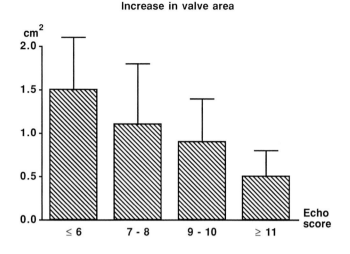

valvular and subvalvular disease. This may be related to a high ratio of effective balloon:mitral anulus area as occurred in our first case. However, other mechanisms have to be evoked to explain why severe mitral regurgitation would occur in patients with a low echocardiographic score[19] and a low effective balloon:mitral anulus area ratio as in our second case. The spatial orientation of the balloon within the valve at the beginning of inflation and the relative fragility of noncalcified valves compared to the thickened fibrosis of the commissures in some patients may play an important role in these cases.

PMV in Candidates for Closed Commissurotomy

As early as 1953, Sellers et al.[28] suggested that the type of mitral stenosis influenced the rate of success of closed surgical commissurotomy. Subsequent studies have confirmed that the mobility of the valve leaflets,[25] the degree of fibrosis,[29] the amount of calcification,[27] and the severity of mitral regurgitation[27] were the major determinants of the success of closed mitral commissurotomy.

In the 1970s, closed commissurotomy was recommended for significant mitral stenosis with mobile, nonthickened, and noncalcified valves without moderate or severe mitral regurgitation or need for an associated procedure during surgery.[28–30]

Among our 113 patients, 49 were considered ideal candidates for closed commissurotomy because there was minimal calcification of the mitral valve ($\leq$ 2 of 4), minimal subvalvular fibrosis ($\leq$ 2 of 4), mild mitral regurgitation ($\leq$ 2 of 4), and no

need for an associated procedure. Three of 49 PMV procedures were not completed: 1 technical failure, 1 left ventricular perforation, and 1 acute mitral regurgitation. Hemodynamic failure occurred in 3 of 49 patients. The 43 (88%) remaining patients had a complete or incomplete hemodynamic success. In comparison to nonideal candidates, these "ideal" patients were younger (47 $\pm$ 11 vs. 57 $\pm$ 14 years, $p < 0.01$), had a higher cardiac output (4.3 $\pm$ 1.1 vs. 3.4 $\pm$ 1.2 liters/min, $p < 0.001$), a smaller left atrium (50 $\pm$ 7 vs. 54 $\pm$ 9 mm, $p < 0.01$), and a lower echocardiographic score (7.1 $\pm$ 1.0 vs. 9.4 $\pm$ 1.3, $p < 0.004$).

PMV After Previous Commissurotomy

Recurrent mitral valve stenosis following surgical commissurotomy is a recognized event that occurs over varying periods of time.[31–33] This problem is becoming more frequent than "primary" mitral stenosis in Western countries. PMV in this setting has been proposed as a suitable alternative to surgery,[6,34] essentially because reoperation in this context is associated with a higher risk of morbidity and mortality[35,36] and also requires valve replacement in most cases.[37]

Twenty-seven of our 113 (24%) patients had a previous surgical commissurotomy and were dilated at 14 $\pm$ 5 years following surgery. PMV was not completed in 2 patients (1 technical failure and 1 complication), whereas hemodynamic failure occurred in 4 patients (one had a massive cerebrovascular accident and subsequent death). A complete or incomplete hemodynamic success was obtained in 21 (78%) patients. In comparison to the risk of mitral valve replacement,[35] PMV can be offered to post-commissurotomy patients with an echocardiographic score under 11.

PMV in High Surgical Risk Patients

Thirty-one of our patients were considered high risk for surgery due to: age > 70 years, NYHA functional class = 4, severe pulmonary hypertension, need for an associated procedure during surgery, or severe obstructive pulmonary disease. The expected perioperative risk of surgery (mitral valve replacement) in the majority of cases was > 20% according to the surgeon's evaluation. Five PMV procedures were not completed (2 technical failures and 3 complications), and 5 patients had a hemodynamic failure; PMV was successful in the remaining 21 (68%) patients. This lower rate of success must be compared to the need of mitral valve replacement and its high rate of morbidity and mortality in this subset of patients. For this reason, PMV can be performed in high surgical risk patients, especially if the echocardiographic score is ≤ 10.

Management of Unsuccessful PMV

Technical failure, major complications, and hemodynamic failure occurred in 19 of 113 (18%) patients. Five patients had a technical failure. Three had elective surgery including 2 perioperative deaths. One patient died 48 hours after PMV from multisystemic failure. In the remaining patient, elective surgery was declined due to a prohibitive perioperative risk. Two of the 3 patients who died were in the high surgical risk group.

Among 5 patients with major complications, 4 had emergency surgery with 1 immediate postoperative death. This patient was also classified as a high-risk patient for surgery. The remaining patient had a successful repeated PMV.

In the 9 patients considered a hemodynamic failure, 1 patient died 48 hours after PMV from the massive cerebral embolism that occurred during PMV. Three patients had elective mitral valve replacement without further complications. Mitral valve replacement was not offered to the remaining 3 patients because of their high perioperative risk. One of them died at 6 months from cardiac heart failure. These 2 deaths also occurred in the high surgical risk group.

CLINICAL FOLLOW-UP
Mortality

The cumulative Kaplan Meier survival curve of the 113 patients is illustrated in Figure 14.4 showing 92% survival at both 18 months and 24 months. The majority of deaths occurred within 3 months, 6 of 8 after unsuccessful PMV. The in-hospital mortality after PMV was 4 of 113 (3.5%) (Table 14.4). Three patients were in the high-risk group (in-hospital mortality of high-risk patients = 9.7%) and 1 had previous commissurotomy (in-hospital mortality = 3.7%).

After discharge, 4 patients died during follow-up. Two patients had an unsuccessful PMV (10.5%) and 2 patients a successful PMV (2.1%). One of the 12 patients with an incomplete hemodynamic success died from pneumonia 1 month after PMV. One of the 82 patients with

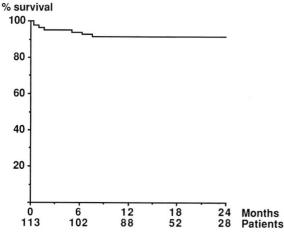

% survival

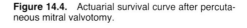

Figure 14.4. Actuarial survival curve after percutaneous mitral valvotomy.

Table 14.4.
Mortality

	In-hospital mortality	Long-term cumulative mortality
All patients	4/113 (3.5%)	8/113 (7.0%)
Ideal candidates	0/49	0/49
Post-commissurotomy	1/27 (3.7%)	1/27 (3.7%)
High risk	4/31 (13%)	6/31 (19%)

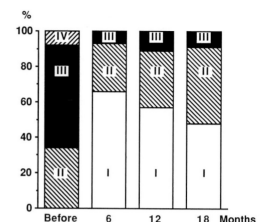

Figure 14.5. New York Heart Association functional class of patients undergoing percutaneous mitral valvotomy.

hemodynamic success died at the 6-month follow-up from unknown causes.

Similar results were observed by Palacios et al.[20] who found a 7% mortality after PMV at a mean follow-up of 13 ± 1 months. They also demonstrated that no death occurred in patients with an echo score of 8 or less, whereas 7 of 43 (16%) deaths occurred in patients with an echo score of more than 8. Similarly no death occurred in our 49 ideal candidates for closed commissurotomy, whereas 8 of 64 (13%) patients who were not ideal candidates died.

Elective Mitral Valve Replacement or Repeat PMV

Among the 94 patients with successful PMV, 3 patients with immediate complete hemodynamic success had recurrence of symptoms during the follow-up period. Two patients had restenosis documented by invasive hemodynamics, and a repeat successful PMV was done. One patient had grade 3 mitral regurgitation noted at 6 months and required mitral valve replacement.

This suggests a "clinical restenosis" rate of 2% at a mean follow-up interval of 16 months. This is similar to previously reported studies after closed commissurotomy.[25,27,30]

Functional Improvement After Successful PMV

Six-month clinical follow-up was obtained after 83 successful PMV procedures. Patients were improved by at least one functional class in 72 of 83 (87%). The functional class was sustained in 48 of 56 (86%) patients who had a clinical evaluation at one year and increased only by one grade in the remaining patients. Only 3 patients returned to their pre-PMV functional class at one-year follow-up. The functional class remained unchanged from 12 to 18 months' follow-up in 21 of 23 (91%) patients. As shown in Figure 14.5, whereas 66% of patients were in functional class 3 or 4 before

PMV, 89% were in functional class 1 or 2 at any time of follow-up.

Similar results were obtained in other North American studies.[20,21,23] In the study of Palacios et al.,[20] 80% of patients were improved by at least one functional class at follow-up. In the subgroup of patients with an echocardiographic score > 8, only 27 of 43 (63%) patients were clinically improved. PMV candidates in North America are older, with more severe mitral valve disease, as reflected by higher echocardiographic scores, than European patients. These differences may explain the better rate of clinical improvement observed in European and North African series.[7,22] The mean age of patients in the study of Al Zaibag et al. was 26 ± 9 years. At one-year follow-up, 90% were improved by at least one functional class. In the study of Vahanian et al.,[7] patients were 43 ± 16 years old (10 years younger than in our series). At a mean follow-up of 9 ± 3 months, 96% were improved by at least one functional class.

Six-month clinical follow-up was obtained in 42 of 43 ideal candidates for closed commissurotomy who underwent successful PMV. Thirty-six (86%) patients were improved by at least one functional class. The 6 patients who were not improved were already in functional class 2 before PMV. Clinical status remained unchanged from 6- to 12-month follow-up in 32 of 35 (91%) patients.

In patients with successful PMV after previous commissurotomy, 17 had clinical evaluation at 6-month follow-up. All but 2 (88%) were improved by at least one functional class. Symptomatic improvement remained unchanged in 10 of 11 (91%) patients at 12-month follow-up.

Eighteen of the 21 successful PMV procedures performed in high surgical risk patients were available for 6-month follow-up. Sixteen (89%) were improved by at least one functional class. This improvement was maintained at 12-month follow-up in 11 of 13 (85%) patients.

Mid-term clinical results are very encouraging not only in patients with favorable anatomy but even in poor surgical candidates and patients with previous commissurotomy. Clinical improvement after PMV appears comparable to that obtained after surgical commissurotomy.

ECHOCARDIOGRAPHIC FOLLOW-UP

Mitral Valve Area

As shown in Table 14.5, similar increases in mitral valve area were observed by hemodynamic and echocardiographic (pressure half-time) measurements. Mitral valve area decreased slightly at follow-up from 2.0 ± 0.6 post-PMV to 1.8 ± 0.4 cm^2 at 12 months. Echocardiographic restenosis, defined as a mitral valve area under 1.5 cm^2 and loss of 50% of the gain, was found in 5 of the 27 patients (19%) followed at 12 months. This is consistent with the 16% rate of restenosis found by Palacios et al.[20] at a mean follow-up of 11 ± 3 months. In fact, only 2 of these 5 patients returned to pre-PMV clinical status. At 12 months, no predictive factor for restenosis was found, probably due to the small number of patients. Four restenosis patients had an echocardiographic score of 8 and one had a score of 9.

Correlations Between Hemodynamic and Echocardiographic Measurements of the Mitral Valve Area

Pressure half-time is widely used as an independent measure of mitral valve area in patients undergoing PMV. However, pressure half-time is dependent on chamber compliance and early peak transmitral gradient.[38] These factors may render pressure half-time inaccurate under several clinical settings such as immediately post-PMV or in chronic aortic regurgitation.[39,40]

Mitral valve area was measured by echocardiography and invasive hemodynamics along with measurement of chamber compliance and filling pressure in 2 patients at 6-month follow-up. Mitral valve area assessed by pressure half-time ($T_{1/2}$) is similar to mitral valve area calculated by the Gorlin formula (1.88 ± 0.42 vs. 1.86 ± 73, p = NS) but correlation is poor ($r = 0.45$, $p = 0.03$). This is partly related to the absence of simultaneous measurements by the two methods. Thomas et al.[38] developed a mathematical formulation for mitral valve area using mean net chamber compliance (cn) and the square root of the early gradient (ΔP_o): $MVA = \dfrac{11.6\ cn\sqrt{\Delta P_o}/cc}{T_{1/2}}$ where cc is the coefficient of orifice contraction. By analogy with the Hatle formula,[41] $MVA = K/T_{1/2}$ where K was empirically = 220, we calculated a new constant $K = 11.6\ cn\sqrt{\Delta P_o}/cc$ and found better correlations with this new constant ($r = 0.85$, $p = 0.00001$). Although these results do not have practical applications in the assessment of mitral valve area by echocardiography, they demonstrate the potential inadequacy of the empirical constant of 220.

For these reasons, we retrospectively analyzed correlations between Doppler and hemodynamically derived measurements of mitral valve area in patients without significant aortic stenosis, aortic insufficiency > grade 1 or left atrial enlargement > 55 mm. Correlations were strongly improved in this subgroup ($r = 65$, $p = 0.003$).

These results demonstrate the potential lack of accuracy of pressure half-time in several clinical settings even 6 months after PMV, particularly in patients with aortic valve disease or left atrial

Table 14.5.
Mitral Valve Area at Follow-up. Hemodynamic and Echocardiographic Evaluation

	Before PMV	After PMV	3 months	6 months	12 months
MVA (Gorlin) cm^2	1.1 ± 0.4	2.1 ± 0.8		1.8 ± 0.7	
Number of pts	113	103		50	
MVA (PHT) cm^2	1.2 ± 0.8	2.0 ± 0.6	1.9 ± 0.6	1.9 ± 0.5	1.8 ± 0.4
Number of pts	108	99	42	54	27

MVA = mitral valve area; PHT = pressure half-time (echocardiographic); Gorlin = MVA using invasive data.

enlargement. The continuity equation method might be more accurate than pressure half-time in patients with moderate to severe aortic regurgitation,[40] however. Color Doppler flow imaging of the mitral valve is now under evaluation, and preliminary results are encouraging. Kawahana et al.[42] found a correlation of $r = .93$ between MVA measured by color Doppler and by catheterization.

Atrial Shunting

Atrial shunting was detected by transthoracic color flow mapping in 65% of patients after PMV. This incidence decreased to 40% and 21% at 6- and 12-month follow-up, respectively. Others have found left-to-right atrial shunts to be present in up to 80% of cases immediately after PMV[43] and to disappear in the majority of cases, with a rate of 21% at 12-month follow-up.[44] Color Doppler imaging is important for the serial assessment of atrial shunting after PMV.

Mitral Regurgitation

As shown in Figure 14.6, mitral regurgitation increased by one grade or more in 43% of patients after PMV. This is consistent with the 45% reported rate of previous studies.[45,46]

Besides two episodes of acute mitral regurgitation ($4+$) requiring surgery, two other patients had grade 3 mitral regurgitation after PMV. One of them had a functional class decrease from 4 to 1 and remained in functional class 1 at the 12-month follow-up. The other was not clinically improved and had mitral valve replacement at 6 months. Severe mitral regurgitation is rare and can be caused by tearing of one of the mitral leaflets,[47] or rupture of chordae or papillary muscle.[48] The influence of valvular anatomy on increases in mitral regurgitation after PMV is controversial. Abascal et al.[45] found no relation between valve anatomy and mitral regurgitation increase.

Moderate mitral regurgitation after PMV tends to decrease with time. Mitral regurgitation decreased by one or two grades in 8 of 48 (17%) patients at 6-month follow-up. From 6 to 12 months, mitral regurgitation decreased by one or two grades in 4 of 20 (20%) patients and increased in 8% and 10% of patients at 6- and 12-month follow-up, respectively. This overall decrease in the severity of mitral regurgitation has also been demonstrated by Palacios et al.[20] The mechanism is unclear, although three possible mechanisms are suggested: (1) reversible mitral valve stretching, (2) healing of an excessively split commissure to the mitral anulus, and (3) reversible papillary muscle dysfunction caused by balloon trauma at the time of PMV.

Echocardiography not only provides data predictive of immediate outcome after PMV but also should permit objective follow-up. Repeated evaluations of valve area, mitral regurgitation, and atrial shunting confirm the long-term symptomatic improvement with stable, mild regurgitation and further a decrease or disappearance of the left-to-right atrial shunt.

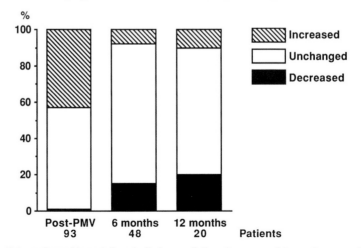

Figure 14.6.   Echocardiographic evolution of mitral regurgitation after successful percutaneous mitral valvotomy.

HEMODYNAMIC FOLLOW-UP

Of the first 85 patients with completed PMV, 50 patients (59%) underwent prospective recatheterization 6 ± 1 months after PMV. Hemodynamic measurements and assessment of atrial shunting and mitral regurgitation were repeated. Baseline characteristics of this population, which were not substantially different from the entire population, are listed in Table 14.6. Twelve patients had had prior surgical commissurotomy 14 ± 6 years before; 11 patients were at high risk for surgery, and 32 patients were considered as ideal candidates for closed commissurotomy. As no selective criteria were used for hemodynamic follow-up, 41 of 82 patients (50%) from the success group of PMV and 9 of 21 patients (43%) from the incomplete success or failure groups (Fig. 14.2) were recatheterized.

Patients with Incomplete Success or Failure of PMV

Of these 9 patients, 6 were not considered for surgical commissurotomy because of heavily calcified valves or severe submitral disease. Four were considered at increased risk for surgery. Four had prior surgical commissurotomy. After PMV, mitral valve area insignificantly increased from 1.0 ± 0.6 to 1.3 ± 0.4 cm² (p = NS) (Table 14.7). Nevertheless, a significant decrease in left atrial pressure, mean mitral gradient, and total pulmonary vascular resistance was obtained. At 6 months, hemodynamic measurements remained unchanged. However, 6 patients were clinically improved at follow-up.

Patients with Initially Successful PMV

Of these patients, 29 (71%) were considered as ideal candidates for commissurotomy; 7 (17%) were at high risk for surgery, and 8 (19%) had a prior surgical commissurotomy. As shown in Table 14.8, PMV produced an immediate improvement in right heart pressures, left atrial pressure, transmitral gradient, pulmonary vascular resistances, and a marked increase in mitral valve area. At 6 months, heart rate was lowered significantly, and there was an increase in left atrial pressure. Cardiac output and mean mitral gradient were not significantly different from immediate post-PMV values. However, the overall hemodynamic changes produced a significant decrease in the calculated mitral valve area from 2.5 ± 0.8 post-PMV to 2.0 ± 0.7 cm² at 6 months (p <

Table 14.6.
Hemodynamic Follow-up: Population Data

Pre-PMV characteristics of the population (N = 50)	
Age (years)	50 ± 13 (27 to 75)
Female sex	46 (92%)
NYHA CHF Class ≥ 3	30 (60%)
Prior commissurotomy	12 (24%)
Prior systemic embolism	7 (14%)
Atrial fibrillation	10 (20%)
Anticoagulant therapy	20 (40%)
Valve calcification (x-ray)	24 (48%)
Mean echo score	8.0 ± 1.4
Echo score > 8	17 (34%)
Mitral valve thickness > 2*	4 (8%)
calcification > 2*	10 (20%)
mobility > 2*	11 (22%)
Subvalvular thickening > 2*	5 (10%)
Left atrial diameter (mm)	50 ± 8
Left atrial diameter ≥ 60 mm	4 (8%)

*Echo scores

0.001). Other studies[7,20] have also shown a significant decrease of mitral valve area at follow-up, suggesting either overestimation of mitral valve area immediately after successful PMV or some degree of mitral restenosis.

Levine et al.[49] found a progressive regression of pulmonary hypertension 7 ± 4 months after PMV. In our study, no further improvement was observed in pulmonary vascular resistances at 6 months, even in patients with pulmonary hypertension before PMV. Clinical follow-up at 6 months showed functional improvement in 36 of 41 patients (88%). Four of the 5 patients who returned to pre-PMV functional status had objective recurrent mitral stenosis at recatheterization.

Mitral Valve Restenosis

After closed surgical mitral commissurotomy, the rate of recurrent mitral stenosis has been determined to be between 10 and 30% at 5 years[33,50,51] and as high as 60% at 10–15 years.[52] However, the actual restenosis rate is largely unknown because of the lack of prospective hemodynamic follow-up studies after surgical commissurotomy. In our 6-month hemodynamic follow-up study, patients were prospectively recatheterized regardless of symptoms. The criteria employed to define restenosis after PMV are arbitrary and vary from one series to another[7,20,53] (loss of > 2 standard deviation of the interobserver variability; loss of ≥ 50% of the gain in valve area obtained after PMV; loss of > 25% of the gain; and valve area at

Table 14.7.
Hemodynamic Follow-up with Failure or Success of PMV

	Pts with incomplete success or failure of PMV (N = 9)			Pts with successful PMV (N = 41)		
	Pre-PMV	Post-PMV	6 months	Pre-PMV	Post-PMV	6 months
Heart rate	71 ± 11	77 ± 8	77 ± 23	80 ± 13	85 ± 17	74 ± 11†††
Cardiac ouput (liters/min)	2.6 ± 1.2	2.7 ± 0.6	2.8 ± 0.8	4.4 ± 1.1	4.7 ± 1.2	4.4 ± 1.1
Mean pressures (mm Hg)						
Right atrium	10 ± 5	9 ± 3	8 ± 5	6 ± 3	5 ± 3**	6 ± 4
Pulmonary artery	39 ± 16	32 ± 12	30 ± 5	35 ± 11	22 ± 8****	22 ± 8
Left atrium	25 ± 7	15 ± 3**	16 ± 5	25 ± 5	11 ± 5****	14 ± 6††
Aorta	92 ± 13	90 ± 15	98 ± 11	92 ± 11	90 ± 12	92 ± 15
Mitral gradient (mm Hg)	13 ± 4	5 ± 2***	6 ± 3	16 ± 5	5 ± 2****	6 ± 3
Mitral valve area (cm²)	1.0 ± 0.6	1.3 ± 0.4	1.2 ± 0.4	1.2 ± 0.3	2.5 ± 0.8****	2.0 ± 0.7†††
Pulm. vasc. resist.[a]						
Arteriolar	655 ± 780	431 ± 390	390 ± 265	230 ± 235	170 ± 120*	160 ± 120
Total	1575 ± 1260	805 ± 515*	835 ± 465	705 ± 355	340 ± 150****	400 ± 195

$*p < 0.05$; $**p < 0.01$; $***p < 0.001$; $****p < 0.0001$ between pre- and post-PMV.
$†p < 0.05$; $††p < 0.01$; $†††p < 0.001$ between post-PMV and 6 months.
[a]in dynes · sec^{-1} · cm^{-5}
All other comparisons are not statistically significant.

follow-up < 1.5 cm^2). We defined hemodynamic restenosis as a loss of $> 50\%$ of the gain in valve area along with a drop in mitral valve area to below 1.5 cm^2 among our 41 patients with initially successful PMV. Patients with incomplete success or hemodynamic failure after PMV were excluded from the analysis of the restenosis data.

Using these criteria, hemodynamic restenosis was found in 11 patients (27%). To assess which factors could be associated with restenosis, univariate analysis of 52 pre- and post-PMV variables was performed between patients with recurrent mitral stenosis and those without (Table 14.8). Patients with hemodynamic restenosis were older, had a smaller mitral valve area, had more severe valvular abnormalities evidenced by a higher echocardiographic score or a higher frequency of valve calcification, and had a poorer result from PMV than patients without restenosis. Multiple stepwise logistic regression analysis identified the post-PMV mitral valve area (1.94 ± 0.35 vs. 2.76 ± 0.78, $p < 0.0001$) as the only independent predictor of recurrent mitral stenosis 6 months after PMV. A similar restenosis rate of 22% after

successful PMV was reported by Palacios et al.[20] in a hemodynamic study involving 37 patients at a mean follow-up of 9 months. They observed recurrent stenosis in 70% of patients with echocardiographic scores > 8 as opposed to 4% in patients with scores ≤ 8. Recurrent mitral stenosis after closed surgical commissurotomy has also been more frequently observed in patients with calcified valves.[51] In addition to the echocardiographic score, Abascal et al.[53] also found mitral valve area after PMV to be an independent predictor of recurrent stenosis. However, important differences in the incidence of restenosis have been reported in echocardiographic follow-up studies,[7,22] (Table 14.9) in our hemodynamic follow-up results, and in those reported by Palacios et al.[20] After successful PMV, Zaibag et al.[22] did not find recurrent stenosis at one year in a series involving young patients. Vahanian et al.[7] found 4% mitral restenosis at 9 months in a series of patients with a mean age of 43 years. However, the incidence of restenosis by echocardiography was 20% in the study of Abascal et al.[53] The mean age of those patients was similar to ours but was 9 and 26 years

Table 14.8.
Predictive Factors of Restenosis

	Restenosis (N = 11)	No restenosis (N = 30)	p
Age (years)	55 ± 14	44 ± 10	< 0.02
Pre-PMV valve area (cm^2)	0.96 ± 0.30	1.25 ± 0.30	< 0.01
Post-PMV cardiac output (liters/min)	4.0 ± 1.0	4.9 ± 1.1	< 0.05
Post-PMV valve area (cm^2)	1.94 ± 0.35	2.76 ± 0.78	< 0.0001
Calcification (x-ray)	7 (64%)	9 (30%)	< 0.05
Mean echo score	8.5 ± 1.4	7.4 ± 1.2	< 0.02
Echo score > 8	6 (55%)	5 (17%)	< 0.04
Leaflet mobility score > 2	5 (45%)	1 (3%)	< 0.006

Table 14.9.
Echocardiographic Follow-up Studies

Author (Ref)	N	Age	Months follow-up	Restenosis rate %	Mitral valve area (cm^2)			
					Pre-PMV	Post-PMV	Follow-up	p
Al Zaibag (22)	41	26	12	0	0.8 ± 0.2	1.6 ± 0.3	1.7 ± 0.3	NS
Vahanian (7)	91	43	9	4	1.0 ± 0.4	1.9 ± 0.3	1.8 ± 0.4	*
Abascal (53)	20	52	7.5	20	0.9 ± 0.3	1.8 ± 0.4	1.6 ± 0.5	**

*$p < 0.05$; **$p < 0.001$ between post-PMV and follow-up.

older than the two other echocardiographic series, respectively. These results illustrate the importance of age and the more severe morphologic alterations of the mitral apparatus found in patients with long-standing mitral stenosis. A suboptimal result of PMV is more likely to be obtained in those patients.

In our study, 17% of restenosis was found in patients with echocardiographic scores ≤ 8, but restenosis increased to 55% among those with scores > 8 ($p < 0.04$). Patients considered as ideal candidates for closed commissurotomy had a restenosis rate of 14%, significantly lower than the 50% observed in the rest of the population ($p < 0.03$). As for surgical commissurotomy, the morphological characteristics of the mitral valve not only adversely affected the immediate outcome of PMV[14] but also its mid-term and probably long-term results.

Atrial Shunting

No atrial shunting was detected before PMV. Venovenous dye dilution curve (Fig. 14.7) identified left-to-right atrial shunting after PMV in 35 patients (70%). This incidence is higher than the 8–24% rate reported in the literature[7,20,54] and is due to the sensitivity of the indicator dilution method. Transesophageal color Doppler flow-mapping, a new echocardiographic technique more sensitive than the traditional transthoracic approach, also detected a higher incidence of atrial shunting after PMV,[55] in accordance with our results.

The oximetric method employed in other studies lacks sensitivity[56,57] and does not consistently detect left-to-right shunts of less than 15–20% of the pulmonary blood flow. In our study, oximetry detected atrial shunting in only 18 of 50 patients (36%) after PMV. Shunts detected by oximetry were always identified by venovenous indicator dilution curves. Mean post-valvuloplasty $Q_p{:}Q_s$ of the 50 patients was 1.23 ± 0.24. In 15 patients the $Q_p{:}Q_s$ was 1, in 17 patients 1.1, in 3 patients 1.3, in 5 patients 1.4, and in 10 patients > 1.5. No patient had a severe shunt with $Q_p{:}Q_s$ > 2. In a previous study,[58] we found that the use of a bifoil balloon catheter ($p < 0.005$), a smaller left atrium ($p < 0.01$), and the presence of mitral valve calcification ($p < 0.003$) were independent predictors for the development of atrial shunting after PMV. Palacios et al.[59] also correlated atrial shunting detected by oximetry after PMV with mitral valve calcification. However, we did not find any predictive factor that satisfactorily explained the occurrence of shunts of significant ($Q_p{:}Q_s$ >1.5) severity after mitral valvuloplasty. At follow-up, atrial shunting had disappeared in 13 of the 35 patients (37%) who had a shunt immediately after PMV, had decreased in magnitude in 9 patients (26%), and had persisted unchanged or even increased in 13 patients (37%). In 2 patients, shunts not detected immediately after PMV were recognized at 6 months, but only by venovenous dilution curve. The incidence of shunts detected by indicator dilution curves decreased from 70% post-PMV to 48% at 6 months ($p < 0.01$); those detected by the oximetric method, from 36% to 18% ($p < 0.04$). Mean $Q_p{:}Q_s$ decreased from 1.23 ± 0.27 to 1.13 ± 0.24 ($p < 0.01$). At 6 months, the $Q_p{:}Q_s$ was 1 in 26 patients, in 15 patients was 1.1, in 1 patient was 1.2, in 2 patients was 1.3, and in 1 patient was 1.4. A moderate shunt with $Q_p{:}Q_s$

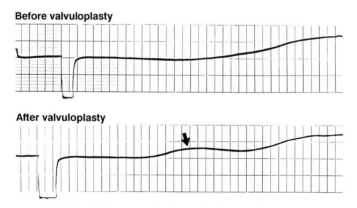

Before valvuloplasty

After valvuloplasty

Figure 14.7. Venovenous indication dilution curves before and after percutaneous mitral valvotomy. These main pulmonary artery–right ventricle curves detect early appearance of indication after PMV (arrow) compared to before PMV.

Hemodynamic follow-up

Evolution of mitral regurgitation

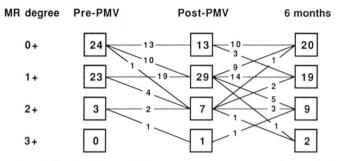

Figure 14.8.   Hemodynamic evolution of mitral regurgitation after percutaneous mitral valvotomy in the 50 recatheterized patients (MR degree: 0 to 4 +).

> 1.5 persisted in only 5 patients. Of these, 3 patients had recurrent mitral stenosis, and 1 patient was considered as a hemodynamic failure from PMV.

No differences in the incidence, magnitude, or evolution of the post-PMV atrial shunting were discovered in our subgroups of patients.

Mitral Regurgitation

Figure 14.8 shows the evolution of mitral regurgitation before and after PMV and at 6-month follow-up in the 50 patients who underwent repeat cardiac catheterization. In 16 patients (32%), PMV resulted in an increase in the degree of mitral insufficiency compared with pre-PMV status. Data from our entire population showed an accentuation of mitral regurgitation after PMV in 36% of the patients. In 15 patients, the severity of mitral regurgitation increased by 1 + according to Sellers criteria,[24] and only 1 patient progressed by 2 + . As mentioned in the echocardiographic follow-up section, no relation was found between morphologic features of mitral apparatus and mitral regurgitation after PMV. In a recent echocardiographic study involving 38 patients, Chen et al.[60] reported that the severity of subvalvular disease and the sum of balloon diameters to mitral anulus diameter ratio were independent predictors of an increase in mitral regurgitation after valvuloplasty. In 72 patients with left ventriculography, the effective balloon:mitral anulus area ratio was evaluated. We observed a higher incidence of mitral regurgitation after PMV when this ratio was >0.7 (60% vs. 25% p <0.02). At follow-up ventriculography, the severity of mitral regurgita-

tion decreased in 13 patients (25%) but increased in 10 patients (20%). No specific pattern was recognized in the variation in mitral regurgitation at 6-month follow-up. However, only two patients had 3 + mitral regurgitation.

Statistical analysis failed to reveal any relation between morphologic aspects of the mitral apparatus or procedural variables and the further changes observed in mitral regurgitation at follow-up. Variations in mitral regurgitation could be related not only to changes in hemodynamic conditions or in left atrium size at 6 months, but also to the inaccuracy of the semiquantitative method of mitral regurgitation quantification.

Thus, the efficacy of PMV is hemodynamically confirmed at 6 months. Two elements will need further long-term evaluation: the rate of restenosis and the course of atrial shunting. Restenosis after PMV appears similar to that seen after surgical mitral commissurotomy. It appears related to both anatomy and the evolution of the disease process. When present, atrial shunting, although small and generally decreasing with time, will be the only scar from the procedure.

CONCLUSION

Interventional cardiology, already rich with coronary angioplasty, now adds another exciting effective procedure: "balloon mitral valvotomy."

Percutaneous mitral valvotomy provides excellent long-term symptomatic relief from mitral stenosis comparable to surgical mitral commissurotomy in patients with favorable anatomy. The clinical benefits obtained in patients with previous commissurotomy and in high-risk surgical candidates widen its indications. Restenosis, a reality, not only is the result of an inadequate valvotomy but also is a fraction of the magnitude of the disease of the mitral apparatus. The adverse sequelae from the procedure appear acceptable, one, mild mitral regurgitation, already is found after surgical commissurotomy, the other, atrial shunting, small in magnitude and decreasing with time, represents the "price to pay" for a nonsurgical procedure. As for mitral commissurotomy, percutaneous mitral valvotomy is still a palliative procedure, and progression of the disease must be expected in the decade without the "trauma and morbidity" of surgery.

Acknowledgments

We with to acknowledge the contribution of Monique Brouillette, R.N., Jacques Crépeau, M.D., Ihor Dyrda, M.D., and Robert Petitclerc, M.D., for their participation to the PMV and the collection of the follow-up data, and Luce Bégin for her secretarial assistance.

REFERENCES

1. Inoue K, Owaki T, Nakamura T, Kitamura F, Miyomoto N. Clinical application of transvenous mitral commissurotomy by a new balloon catheter. *J Thorac Cardiovasc Surg 87*:394–402, 1984.
2. Lock JE, Khalilullah M, Shrivastava S, Bahl V, Keane JF. Percutaneous catheter commissurotomy in rheumatic mitral stenosis. *N Engl J Med 313*: 1515–1518, 1985.
3. McKay RG, Lock JE, Safian RD, et al. Balloon dilatation of mitral stenosis in adult patients: Postmortem and percutaneous mitral valvuloplasty studies. *J Am Coll Cardiol 9*:723–731, 1987.
4. Al Zaibag M, Ribeiro PA, Al Kasab S, Al Fagih MR. Percutaneous balloon mitral valvotomy for rheumatic mitral valve stenosis. *Lancet 1*:757–761, 1986.
5. McKay CR, Kawanishi DT, Rahimtoola SH. Catheter balloon valvuloplasty of the mitral valve in adults using a double balloon technique: Early hemodynamic results. *JAMA 257*:1753–1761, 1987.
6. Rediker DE, Block PC, Abascal VM, Palacios IF. Mitral balloon valvuloplasty for mitral restenosis after surgical commissurotomy. *J Am Coll Cardiol 11*:252–256, 1988.
7. Vahanian A, Michel PL, Cormier B, et al. Results of percutaneous mitral commissurotomy in 200 patients. *Am J Cardiol 63*:847–852, 1989.
8. Nobuyoshi M, Hawasaki N, Kimura T, et al. Indications, complications, and short-term clinical outcome of percutaneous transvenous mitral commissurotomy. *Circulation 80*:782–792, 1989.
9. Babic UU, Pejcic P, Djurisic Z, Vucinic M, Grujicic SM. Percutaneous transarterial balloon valvuloplasty

for mitral valve stenosis. *Am J Cardiol 57*:1101–1104, 1986.
10. Palacios IF, Lock JE, Keane JF, Block PC. Percutaneous transvenous balloon valvotomy in a patient with severe calcific mitral stenosis. *J Am Coll Cardiol 7*:1416–1419, 1986.
11. Ubago JLM, De Prada JA, Bardaji JC, et al. Percutaneous balloon valvulotomy for calcific rheumatic mitral stenosis. *Am J Cardiol 59*:1007–1008, 1987.
12. Palacios IF, Block PC, Brandi S, et al. Percutaneous balloon valvotomy for patients with severe mitral stenosis. *Circulation 75*:778–784, 1987.
13. Serra A, Bonan R, Lefèvre T, Dyrda I. Balloon mitral valvuloplasty in patients with high echocardiographic score (Abstract). *Circulation 80*(Suppl II):II–71, 1989.
14. Wilkins GT, Weyman AE, Abascal VM, Block PC, Palacios IF. Percutaneous mitral valvotomy: An analysis of echocardiographic variables related to outcome and the mechanism of dilatation. *Br Heart J 60*:299–308, 1988.
15. Reid CL, McKay CR, Chandranatra PAN, Kawanishi DT, Rahimtoola SH. Mechanisms of increase in mitral valve area and influence of anatomic features in double balloon catheter balloon valvuloplasty in adults with rheumatic mitral stenosis — A Doppler and two dimensional echocardiographic study. *Circulation 76*:628–636, 1987.
16. Reid CL, Chandranatra AN, Kawanishi DT, Kotlewski A, Rahimtoola SH. Influence of mitral valve morphology on double-balloon catheter balloon valvuloplasty in patients with mitral stenosis. Analysis of factors predicting immediate and 3 month results. *Circulation 80*:515–524, 1989.
17. Block PC, Palacios JF, Jacobs ML, Fallon JT. Mechanism of percutaneous mitral valvotomy. *Am J Cardiol 59*:178–179, 1987.
18. Kaplan JD, Isner JN, Karas RH, et al. In vitro analysis of mechanisms of balloon valvuloplasty of stenotic mitral valves. *Am J Cardiol 59*:318–323, 1987.
19. Ribeiro PA, Al Zaibag M, Rajendran U, et al. Mechanism of mitral valve area increased by in vitro single and double balloon mitral valvotomy. *Am J Cardiol 62*:264–269, 1988.
20. Palacios IF, Block PC, Wilkins GT, Weyman AE. Follow-up of patients undergoing percutaneous mitral balloon valvotomy. Analysis of factors determining restenosis. *Circulation 79*:573–579, 1989.
21. McKay C, Kawanishi D, Kotlewski A, Gonzalez A, Parise K, Rahimtoola S. Long-term improvement in rest and exercise hemodynamics and in treadmill performance after mitral catheter balloon valvuloplasty (Abstract). *J Am Coll Cardiol 11*(Suppl II):15A, 1988.
22. Al Zaibag A, Ribeiro P, Al Kasab S, et al. One year follow-up results after percutaneous double balloon mitral valvotomy. *Am J Cardiol 1*:126–127, 1989.

23. Cunningham MJ, Diver DJ, Berman AD, et al. Acute hemodynamic results and clinical follow-up in patients undergoing balloon mitral valvuloplasty (Abstract). *J Am Coll Cardiol 11*(Suppl II):15A, 1988.

24. Sellers RD, Levy MJ, Amplatz J, Lillehei CW. Left retrograde cardioangiography in acquired cardiac disease. Technic indication and interpretations in 700 cases. *Am J Cardiol 14*:437–447, 1964.

25. Hockjema TD, Wallace RB, Kirklin JW. Closed mitral commissurotomy recent results in 291 cases. *Am J Cardiol 17*:825–828, 1966.

26. Smith WM, Netuze JM, Baratt-Boyes BG, Lowe JB. Open mitral valvotomy—effect of preoperative factors on results. *J Thorac Cardiovasc Surg 82*:738–751, 1981.

27. Grantham RN, Daggett WM, Cosimi AB, et al. Transventricular mitral valvulotomy: Analysis of factors influencing operative and late results. *Circulation 49* (Suppl II): 200–212, 1974.

28. Sellers TH, Bedford DE, Somerville W. Valvotomy in the treatment of mitral stenosis. *Br Med J ii*:1059–1067, 1953.

29. Morrow, AG, DuPlessis LA, Wilcox BR. Hemodynamic studies after mitral commissurotomy. *Surgery 54*:463–470, 1963.

30. Ellis LB, Benson H, Harken DE. The effect of age and other factors on the early and late results following closed mitral valvuloplasty. *Am Heart J 74*:743–751, 1968.

31. Logan A, Lowther CP, Turner RW. Reoperation for mitral stenosis. *Lancet 1*:443–449, 1962.

32. Belcher JR. Restenosis of the mitral valve. An account of fifty second operations. *Lancet 1*:181–184, 1960.

33. Heger JJ, Werr LS, Weyman AE, Dillon JC, Feigenbaum H. Long-term changes in mitral valve area after successful mitral commissurotomy. *Circulation 59*:443–447, 1979.

34. Acar J, Vahanian A, Michel PL, et al. Percutaneous balloon valvotomy in patients with previous surgical mitral commissurotomy (Abstract). *Eur Heart J 9*(Suppl 1):240, 1988.

35. Fraser K, Sugden BA. Second closed mitral valvotomy for recurrent mitral stenosis. *Thorax 32*:759–761, 1977.

36. Peper WA, Lytle BW, Cosgrove DM, Goormastic M, Loop FD. Repeat mitral commissurotomy: Long-term results. *Circulation 76*(Suppl III):97–101, 1987.

37. Rutledge R, McIntosh CL, Morrow AG, et al. Mitral valve replacement after closed mitral commissurotomy. *Circulation 66*(Suppl I):162–166, 1982.

38. Thomas JD, Weyman AE. Doppler mitral half-time: A clinical tool in search of theoretical justification. *J Am Coll Cardiol 10*:923–929, 1987.

39. Moro E, Nicolosi L, Zanuttini D, Cervesato E, Roelandt J. Influence of aortic regurgitation on the assessment of the pressure half-time and derived mitral valve area in patients with mitral stenosis. *Eur Heart J 9*:1010–1017, 1988.

40. Nakatani S, Mosuyama T, Kodama K, Kitabataka A, Fujii K, Kamado T. Value and limitations of Doppler echocardiography in the quantification of stenotic mitral valve area: Comparison of the pressure half-time and the continuity equation methods. *Circulation 77*:78–85, 1988.

41. Hatle J, Angelsen B. *Doppler ultrasound in cardiology: Physical principles and clinical applications.* Philadelphia, Lea & Febiger, 1982 pp. 110–124.

42. Kawahana T, Tamai J, Mihari M, Seo H, Yamagishi M, Miyataka K. A new method for determination of mitral valve area in mitral stenosis by color Doppler flow imaging technique (Abstract). *Circulation 4*:2659, 1989.

43. Bernard Y, Schiele F, Jacoulet P, Anguenot T, Maurat JP, Bassand JP. Assessment with color flow mapping of mitral regurgitation and left to right atrial shunting after percutaneous mitral valvuloplasty (Abstract). *Circulation 78*(Suppl II):II–1, 1988.

44. O'Shea JP, Abascal VM, Marshall JE, Wilkins GT, Thomas JD. Long-term persistence of atrial septal defect following percutaneous mitral valvuloplasty: A Doppler-echocardiographic follow-up study (Abstract). *Circulation 78*(Suppl II):II–1, 1988.

45. Abascal VM, Wilkins GT, Choong GY, Block PC, Palacios IF, Weyman AE. Mitral regurgitation after percutaneous mitral valvuloplasty in adults: Evaluation by pulsed Doppler echocardiography. *J Am Coll Cardiol 11*:257–263, 1988.

46. Roth RB, Block PC, Palacios IF. Mitral regurgitation after percutaneous mitral valvuloplasty: Predictors and follow-up (Abstract). *Circulation 78*(Suppl II):II–488, 1988.

47. Cequier A, Bonan R, Crépeau J, Dethy M, Dyrda I, Waters D. Massive mitral regurgitation caused by tearing of the anterior leaflet during percutaneous mitral balloon valvuloplasty. *Am J Med 85*:100–103, 1988.

48. O'Shea JP, Abascal VM, Wilkins GT, et al. Unusual sequelae of percutaneous mitral valvuloplasty: A Doppler-echocardiographic study (Abstract). *Circulation 78*(Suppl II):II–32, 1988.

49. Levine MJ, Weinstein JS, Diver DJ, et al. Progressive improvement in pulmonary vascular resistance after percutaneous mitral valvuloplasty. *Circulation 79*:1061–1067, 1989.

50. Higgs LM, Glancy DL, O'Brien KP, Epstein JE, Morrow AG. Mitral restenosis: An uncommon cause of recurrent symptoms following mitral commissurotomy. *Am J Cardiol 26*:34–37, 1970.

51. Eskilsson J. Mitral stenosis after closed commissurotomy. A clinical and echocardiographic long-term follow-up study. *Acta Med Scand 664*(Suppl): 1–116, 1982.

52. Lyons WS, Tompkins RG, Kirklin JW, Wood

EH. Early and late hemodynamic effects of mitral commissurotomy. *J Lab Clin Med 53*:499–516, 1959.

53. Abascal VM, Wilkins GT, Choong CY, et al. Echocardiographic evaluation of mitral valve structure and function in patients followed for at least 6 months after percutaneous balloon mitral valvuloplasty. *J Am Coll Cardiol 12*:606–615, 1988.

54. Come PC, Riley MF, Diver DJ, Morgan JP, Safian RD, McKay RG. Noninvasive assessment of mitral stenosis before and after percutaneous balloon mitral valvuloplastly. *Am J Cardiol 61*:817–825, 1988.

55. Yoshida K, Yoshikawa J, Akasaka T, et al. Assessment of left-to-right atrial shunting after percutaneous mitral valvuloplasty by transesophageal color Doppler flow-mapping. *Circulation 80*:1521–1526, 1989.

56. Wood, EH. Diagnostic applications of indicator-dilution techniques in congenital heart disease. *Circ Res 10*:531–569, 1962.

57. Yang SS, Bentivoglio LG, Maranhao V, Goldberg H. *From cardiac catheterization data to hemodynamic parameters.* Philadelphia, F. A. Davis Company, 1988; pp. 166–188.

58. Serra A, Bonan R, Cequier A, Crépeau J, Dyrda I. Atrial shunting after balloon mitral valvuloplasty: Prediction and follow-up (Abstract). *Circulation 80*(Suppl II):II–72, 1989.

59. Palacios IF, Block PC. Atrial septal defect during percutaneous mitral valvotomy: Immediate results and follow-up (Abstract). *Circulation 78*(Suppl II):II–529, 1988.

60. Chen C, Wang X, Wang Y, Lan Y. Value of two-dimensional echocardiography in selecting patients and balloon sizes for percutaneous balloon mitral valvuloplasty. *J Am Coll Cardiol 14*:1651–1658, 1989.

15

Balloon Mitral Valvotomy: A Surgical Perspective

PETER Van TRIGT

The relief of mitral stenosis has traditionally been the role of the cardiac surgeon, as mitral commissurotomy was the first successful cardiac operation of the modern era beginning with Bailey's report of closed commissurotomy in 1949. Since the original report of Inoue and associates in 1984,[1] mitral balloon valvotomy has been performed in many centers. This technique has extended the applicability of percutaneous catheter technology for stenotic valvular lesions and has provided an alternative to surgical procedures for patients who are high-risk candidates or refuse operation.[2,3] The ultimate role of balloon valvotomy remains to be determined and will depend on its efficacy, durability, complication rate, and cost. Technically, it is analogous to surgical mitral commissurotomy, which was initially performed in a closed approach over 40 years ago, then extended to the direct open approach on cardiopulmonary bypass, which has been used routinely and preferentially since 1960.[4] The lessons learned from the previous and well-documented surgical experience with mitral commissurotomy should be a foundation of useful information for all cardiologists initiating the use of the percutaneous balloon catheter for the relief of mitral stenosis. Cardiac surgeons have developed well-recognized indications and contraindications for mitral commissurotomy, and the natural history and long-term outcome of the mitral valve following the procedure has been well documented in several large surgical series. The potential benefits of the procedure as well as its limitations should be recognized by invasive cardiologists in order to prevent repeating mistakes of the past by applying the technique inappropriately. Successful mitral commissurotomy and repair, as surgeons have come to understand, require great care, understanding of the exact pathology of the stenotic valve, precise intervention, and gentle technique.

MITRAL STENOSIS—ANATOMIC AND PATHOLOGIC FEATURES

Although the mitral valve is quadricuspid during embryogenesis, the commissural cusps regress and two leaflets are present at birth—the large sail-like anterior leaflet and the smaller posterior, or mural, leaflet. The two commissures do not divide the leaflet tissue completely to the valve anulus. The anterior leaflet has a greater base to margin length, but because the posterior leaflet has a greater amount of annular attachment, the surface area of each leaflet is nearly equal. The leaflets are trapezoidal and are attached by chordae tendineae to the papillary muscles, which arise from the endocardial surface of the ventricular chamber. Each leaflet is attached to both the anterior and posterior papillary muscles by the thin fibrous chordae, which fan out along the leaflet margin, as well as along the ventricular surface of the leaflets. Approximately three times as many chordae attach to the leaflets as to the papillary muscles.

Functionally, the mitral valve allows free flow of blood from the left atria to the left ventricle during ventricular diastole and prevents regurgitation of blood into the atria during systole. This is achieved through a coordinated contraction pattern of myocardium and papillary muscles during the cardiac cycle. Early transmitral flow is the result of a pressure gradient across the mitral valve as well as active forces related to myocardial relaxation. The major orifice of the valve is between the leaflets, but much blood passes between the interchordal spaces, and chordal fusion can narrow the mitral inlet. During ventricular systole after closure of the mitral valve, competence is aided by active motion of the valve anulus and papillary muscles. Regardless of the presence of intact normal leaflets, competence of the mitral valve is lost in the presence of annular dilation, chordal disruption, or papillary muscle dysfunction.

The predominant cause of mitral stenosis is rheumatic fever, and isolated mitral stenosis occurs in approximately 40% of all patients with rheumatic valvular heart disease. Congenital mitral stenosis is rare, with other uncommon causes of mitral stenosis including malignant carcinoid, systemic lupus erythematosus, and endomyocardial fibrosis. Fusion of the valve leaflets at the commissures is the most common result of rheumatic inflammation, occurring alone in 30% of involved valves.[5] The endocardial surface ulcerates where the two leaflets normally coapt in systole. The valve leaflets become thickened, calcified, and rigid, with the ingrowth of fibrous tissue. Concomitantly, the chordae tendineae may become thickened, retracted, and fused, with displacement of the valve into the left ventricular chamber. These combined processes result in the end-stage in a rigid, narrowed mitral valve that is funnel-shaped and with an orifice frequently described as "fish-mouth" (Fig. 15.1). The amount of calcium in the leaflets of the stenotic mitral valve varies considerably. Generally calcium is more frequent and in larger quantity in men than women, in older than younger patients, and in patients with higher transvalvular gradients.[5] Previous surgical experience has documented that if commissural fusion alone is present, excellent results can be obtained by commissurotomy.[6–8] More commonly, extensive fibrosis and calcification of the leaflets with leaflet retraction and fusion of the chordae require mitral valve replacement.[9]

INDICATIONS FOR INTERVENTION

Justification for an aggressive approach to mitral stenosis is based on the natural history of the disease. It appears that after a relatively asymptomatic latent period of 10–20 years following an episode of rheumatic fever, the condition of most patients will progress from a functional class of I–II to total disability in 5–10 years. This deterioration occurs rapidly in up to half of the affected patients, commonly as the result of the onset of atrial fibrillation. It has been shown clearly that operation or intervention should not be delayed until Class IV symptoms develop.[4] In patients with

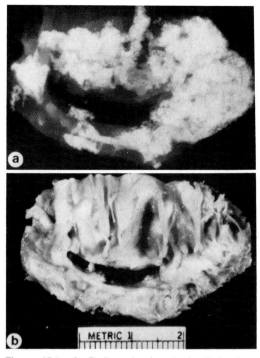

Figure 15.1. A, Radiograph of excised mitral valve showing extensive calcification of leaflets and commissures. **B,** View of whole valve from ventricular surface showing narrowed orifice in the characteristic "fish-mouth" configuration.

less severe symptoms (Class II), cardiac catheterization should be performed and valve cross-sectional area calculated. If mitral orifice size is less than $1.0 \text{ cm}^2/\text{m}^2$ of body surface area, intervention should generally be recommended. Available data support early application of valve dilation, commissurotomy, or valve replacement to patients with mitral stenosis. Roberts has concluded that the national history of mitral stenosis ranks second only to aortic stenosis in terms of mortality from all forms of valvular heart disease.[5]

MITRAL COMMISSUROTOMY

The vast majority of cardiac surgeons currently favor open direct vision commissurotomy for mitral stenosis over the more historical closed commissurotomy.[10,11] Most surgical series report that operative mortality is equivalently low with the open approach and that the quality of the procedure is enhanced in terms of both hemodynamic improvement and incidence of operative complications.[12] The chances of embolizing a left atrial thrombus or creating serious regurgitation are lessened by direct visualization during commissurotomy. An open commissurotomy has been shown to be more effective in relieving obstruction, especially when mild calcification or subvalvular stenosis is present (Fig. 15.2). The open approach allows access for a maximal safe commissurotomy as well as exposure to the chordae tendineae, which may be released by an incision to separate areas of fusion. With further retraction of the chordae to the level of papillary muscle, the papillary muscle may also be incised to correct foreshortening of the chordae (Fig. 15.3).

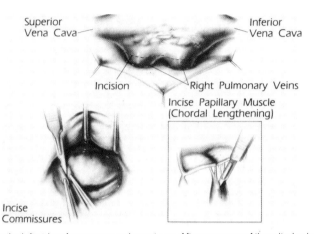

Figure 15.2. Approach to the left atrium for open commissurotomy. After exposure of the mitral valve, a scalpel is used to accurately incise the anterior commissure. The chordae tendineae and papillary muscles may be lengthened if necessary (inset).

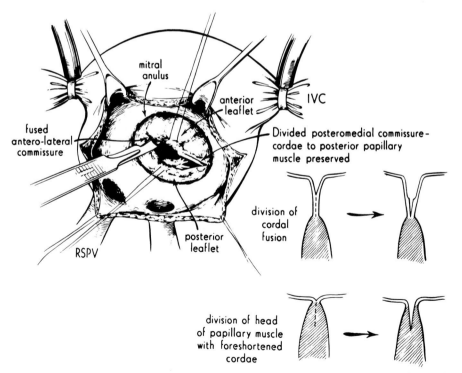

Figure 15.3. Demonstration of commissural incision for open commissurotomy. When the chordae are found and foreshortened, a subvalvular release is required to provide adequate relief from obstruction.

The indications for open commissurotomy include those patients with pure or predominant rheumatic mitral stenosis who have evidence of leaflet pliability, minimal or no calcification, and insignificant regurgitation.[11] The operation is performed through a median sternotomy on cardiopulmonary bypass. Cold cardioplegic arrest is used to protect the ventricular myocardium and the aorta is cross-clamped. The left atrium is opened through the interatrial groove, and exposure is facilitated by mobilizing the superior and inferior vena cavae. The left atrium is examined for thrombotic material, and the valve is inspected. In severe mitral stenosis, the commissures can be fused to the point that leaflets cannot be delineated (Fig. 15.4). Chordal fusion and foreshortening can further obscure the normal anatomy. Gentle traction on the chordae of the anterior leaflet creates a folding of the leaflet at the commissure allowing an incision to be performed through the endocardial layer. Usually a combination of sharp and blunt techniques is required to complete an effective commissurotomy. The scalpel is used to initiate the commissurotomy at the point of leaflet fusion.

Placement of the Tubb's dilator into the anulus is effective in further developing the commissures, which usually split precisely along anatomic lines. The commissural incisions are made to within 3 mm of the anulus and not extended to the annular tissue since normal leaflet is contiguous at the anulus. Minor amounts of calcium can be debrided; however, significant calcification is associated with a poor long-term result and should indicate valve replacement. Next, attention is turned to the subvalvular apparatus. If subvalvular fusion is evident, the chordae are carefully sharply divided, taking care to avoid injury of the chordal attachments to the leaflets. If the chordae are severely shortened, the papillary muscle heads are essentially inserted into the leaflets, creating further subvalvular obstruction. In this situation, the papillary muscle heads are sharply incised to open up the mitral inflow (Fig. 15.3). After the commissurotomy is completed, valve competence is assessed by injection of saline into the ventricle or by induction of aortic insufficiency after removal of the aortic cross-clamp. If significant regurgitation is present, consideration is given to

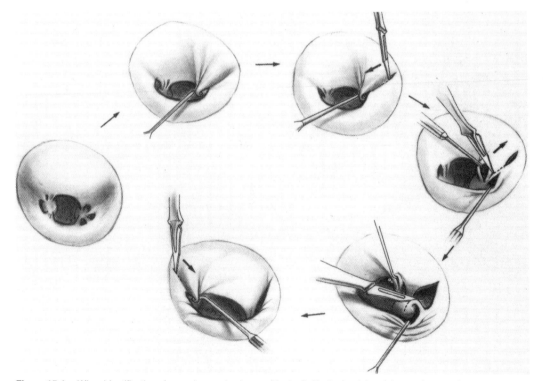

Figure 15.4.   When identification of commissures is obscured by leaflet fusion and chordal retraction, gentle traction on the chordae produces a folding along the natural commissural line, which is sharply incised.

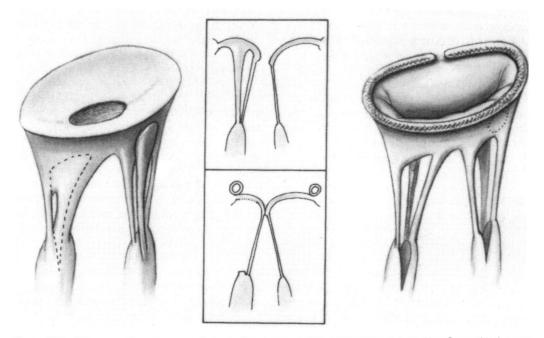

Figure 15.5. When commissurotomy results in significant regurgitation, annular remodeling with a Carpentier ring can restore competency.

valve replacement or annular remodeling[13] with a prosthetic Carpentier ring (Fig. 15.5). The air is vented from the left atrium and ventricle as the atriotomy is closed. After discontinuing cardiopulmonary bypass, assessment of residual mitral stenosis or the appearance of mitral regurgitation can be accurately assessed with transesophageal color-flow Doppler echocardiography. Most patients should have an uncomplicated postoperative course after commissurotomy with a surgical mortality of 1–4% being reported by most series.[14]

RESULTS OF MITRAL COMMISSUROTOMY

Mitral commissurotomy is not a curative procedure as the underlying inflammatory rheumatic process or continuing valvular injury from turbulence will eventually cause recurrent valvular obstruction. Immediate improvement in symptoms is seen with reduction of the transvalvular gradient by commissurotomy usually to less than 5 mm Hg. In a series of patients undergoing open commissurotomy for mitral stenosis,[14] two-thirds of 85 patients were in Class III or IV congestive heart failure preoperatively, while 95% reverted to functional Class I or II following open commis-

surotomy. In this series the operative mortality was under 2%, and the long-term follow-up to five years was excellent with only one patient requiring a second open commissurotomy and two patients requiring valvular replacement for progressive mitral insufficiency.

The NYU experience with open radical mitral commissurotomy was reviewed by Gross et al.,[11] documenting the experience with 200 patients undergoing the procedure. The operative mortality was 1.7%, and 77% of the patients were in functional Class III or IV preoperatively. At follow-up 90% were in functional Class I or II, and the long-term complication-free survival rate in the group was 87% in those patients in whom neither residual transmitral gradient nor regurgitation was present at the end of the procedure. A postoperative mitral gradient greater than 3 mm Hg or postoperative mitral regurgitation was significantly correlated to the need for valve replacement by multivariant analysis. The 10-year complication-free survival in these patients was 70% (complications included increasing congestive heart failure, worsening of functional cardiac classification, need for reoperation, and thromboembolic complications). The authors strongly recommend the advantages of open commissurotomy over closed commissurotomy, as the open technique offers the opportunity for debridement of calcium, precise splitting of fused chordae tendineae and papillary muscles, and evaluation for mitral regurgitation after repair. The significance of left atrial thrombus was also emphasized by the authors as 20% of the patients in the series were found to have significant atrial thrombus at operation, and this was safely removed during the open commissurotomy. The actuarial survival at 10 years was 92%, and significant postoperative complications were noted to be rare.

Open commissurotomy has also proven to be extremely beneficial in reduction of the postoperative incidence of systemic embolization and infective endocarditis. In a report of 100 patients undergoing open commissurotomy,[10] 13 had preoperative emboli and only 2 had postoperative emboli. Risk of emboli was higher in patients with atrial fibrillation (21%); however, no correlation between the incidence of embolism and the presence of left atrial thrombus at operation was found. The low incidence of systemic emboli following commissurotomy was also documented by the other surgical series,[14] with an incidence of postoperative emboli of 2–4%. Long-term anticoagulation is usually restricted to older patients with atrial fibrillation. Surgical experience with open commissurotomy for mitral stenosis has also documented that patients experiencing atrial fibrillation for less than one year have an excellent chance of reverting to sinus rhythm following commissurotomy and standard medical therapy.[15]

The development of pulmonary hypertension in patients with mitral stenosis has been shown to be an important indication for commissurotomy, and elevated pulmonary vascular resistance has been shown to significantly decrease after successful commissurotomy or valve replacement.[9] Patients with end-stage valvular disease, emphysema, or chronic pulmonary emboli may have persistent pulmonary hypertension following commissurotomy, however. This can cause incomplete resolution of symptoms and persistent right ventricular failure.

The incidence of restenosis following commissurotomy varies among surgical series,[14,16] with the best series following 100 patients operated on between 1960 and 1976 with 16 of 99 survivors requiring reoperation. The median time to significant recurrent symptoms or reoperation in the series was 8–10 years.[16] A distinct relationship was found in the study between leaflet deformity (mobility, thickening, calcification) and the need for reoperation. Of 77 patients with fair or poor leaflet anatomy, which correlates with poor mobility, significant thickening, and at least moderate calcification, 23% had undergone reoperation at the time of study, whereas none of 10 patients with good leaflet anatomy had done so (Fig. 15.6).

Close medical follow-up is required following open commissurotomy to assess for evidence of recurrent symptoms. When significant symptoms reappear or significant restenosis is found, operation should be considered early with mitral valve replacement generally being required at the second procedure.[17,18] Late occurrence of mitral regurgitation is uncommon following the procedure as this will usually become immediately apparent following the procedure and should be optimally determined prior to completion of the operation so that either reparative techniques or mitral valve replacement can be applied. Generally, 20% of patients with mitral stenosis undergoing planned commissurotomy will instead require mitral valve replacement due to underestimated severity of the valve disease, with significant involvement of the subvalvular mechanism or heavy leaflet calcification being the most common features necessitating mitral valve replacement.

MITRAL VALVE REPLACEMENT

Mitral valve replacement uses the same techniques of cardiopulmonary bypass, myocardial protection, and left atrial exposure as those discussed for mitral commissurotomy. The mitral valve is visualized and the pathology carefully assessed (Fig. 15.7). When the decision to replace the valve is made, the valve is excised, first removing the anterior leaflet leaving a 2 mm rim of cusp tissue attached to the anulus for the annular sutures. Care is taken not to cut through the anulus, especially in the area of the posterior leaflet, as a dissecting hematoma and atrioventricular rupture can result. The chordae are divided at their origin of the papillary muscles (Fig. 15.8), and it is important not to divide or otherwise damage the papillary muscles, which can also cause later myocardial rupture. Although recent authors have recommended leaving the posterior leaflet intact when performing mitral valve replacement (as a means of preserving left ventricular function), in general this is not always possible in the setting of mitral stenosis due to extreme thickening and subvalvular fusion. Calcium in the anulus is carefully removed by gently crushing the deposits with rongeurs and debriding the calcium, taking care not to extend the dissection through the anulus or the heart wall.

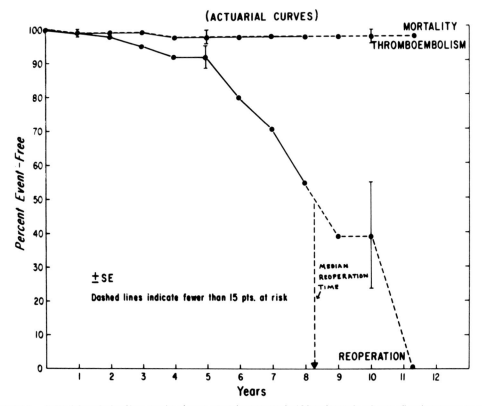

Figure 15.6. Actuarial analysis of late results of open commissurotomy in 100 patients showing median time to reoperation being 8.2 years. Mortality and thromboembolism curves are superimposed. (Reproduced with permission, Mosby-Year Book, Inc.)

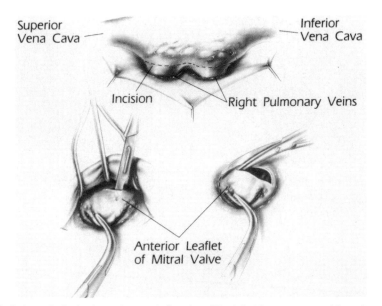

Figure 15.7. Technique of mitral valve replacement. Opening of the left atrium, exposure of the valve, and excision of anterior leaflet.

After the annular circumference has been adequately debrided and prepared, the anulus is sized for the appropriate valve. Valve sutures are then placed using horizontal pledgeted mattress sutures (Fig. 15.9), placing the sutures precisely into the annular tissue but not into the ventricular myocardium so as to avoid the circumflex coronary artery, the aortic valve, and the conduction system. The sutures are then passed through the valve sewing ring, and the valve is seated and the sutures tied. After completion, the annular tissue becomes sandwiched between the Teflon felt suture pledgets and the valve sewing ring (Fig. 15.10). Clinical experience using this technique with horizontal pledgets has demonstrated a negligible incidence of perivalvular leak and dehiscence.

Excellent long-term survival has also been reported in a current series with both bioprosthetic

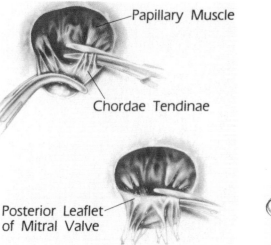

Figure 15.8. Mitral valve replacement. Division of chordae tendineae at junction with papillary muscle.

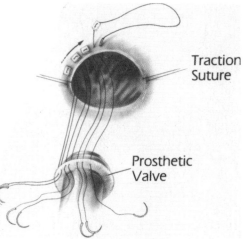

Figure 15.9. Mitral valve replacement. Interrupted horizontal mattress sutures are placed around the anulus then through the sewing ring of the valve.

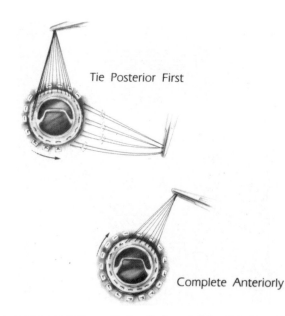

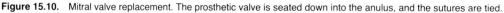

Figure 15.10. Mitral valve replacement. The prosthetic valve is seated down into the anulus, and the sutures are tied.

and mechanical valve replacement for mitral valve disease. Carpentier recently reported[19] three groups of 100 patients each who had undergone mitral valve replacement using the porcine, Starr-Edwards, or Bjork-Shiley prostheses. The series included predominantly mitral regurgitation or mixed mitral regurgitation and mitral stenosis as the underlying etiology of valve disease, with ischemia being present in 25% of the patients. Operative mortality was 12% in all three groups. The long-term actuarial survival curves are shown in Figure 15.11 with approximately 80% of patients in each group being free of valve-related death at 12 years. The most common cause of valve-related death in the bioprosthetic group was peri-prosthetic leak and valvular dysfunction. The most common cause of valve-related death in the Starr-Edwards and Bjork-Shiley groups was thromboembolism. To assess long-term performance of the porcine versus mechanical valve, actuarial representation of valve failure–free patients is shown in Figure 15.12. This shows a 70% incidence of freedom from valve failure in the mechanical mitral valve replacement patients and a 56% incidence of freedom from valve failure in the tissue valve group due to the natural degeneration of the tissue valves over time.

ROLE OF MITRAL BALLOON VALVOTOMY

The utility of balloon valvotomy for treatment of mitral stenosis depends greatly on the morphologic features of the stenotic valve. It has been shown that the mechanism by which the procedure works is through commissural splitting[20,21] along the natural planes of the anterior and posterior commissures. Only those patients with obstruction at the leaflet level due to commissural fusion and not at the subvalvular apparatus have demonstrated benefits from the procedure. The mobility and flexibility of the leaflets, determined by the amount of fibrosis and calcification within the tissue, have been shown to be important factors in determining the safety and efficacy of the procedure.[22,23] In patients with highly calcified and fibrotic valves, the risks are increased and the results are inferior to surgical management.[24-26] This was clearly demonstrated in an experimental study of mitral valves excised at the time of surgery that were found to be unsuitable for commissurotomy according to standard surgical criteria.[21] When these fibrotic and calcified valves were mounted in a specially designed chamber and dilated using current valvotomy techniques, the results were suboptimal with either incomplete

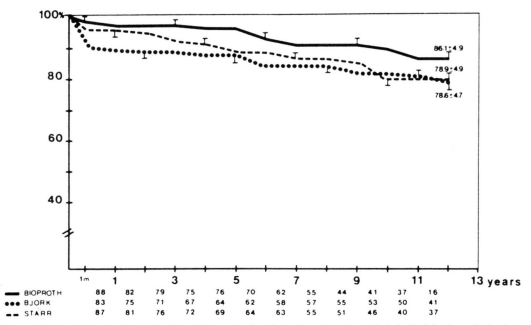

Figure 15.11. Survival after MVR. Actuarial curves of patients free of valve-related death following mitral valve replacement. Numbers of patients at each anniversary are shown below. (Reproduced with permission, Futura Publishing Company, Inc.[19])

commissural splitting or leaflet rupture occurring in the majority of valves. The residual mitral stenosis was graded as moderate to severe following the experimental dilation as the maximal area achieved was only 2.2 cm². The authors conclude that in severely fibrotic valves, dilation with the percutaneous balloon can result in stretching of the anulus rather than splitting the commissures. This results in only a transient improvement in mitral valve area and may explain the restenosis phenomenon seen in some patients after balloon valvotomy.

In the presence of a mobile, noncalcified valve without subvalvular fusion, the results reported for balloon dilation have been acceptable,[27] resulting in mitral valve area greater than 2 cm² and transvalvular gradients in the range of 5–10 mm Hg (Fig. 15.13). Two-dimensional echocardiography has had a significant impact on the application

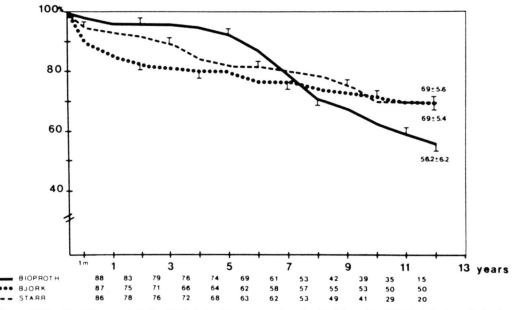

Figure 15.12. Event-free survival after MVR. Actuarial representation of valve failure–free patients following mitral valve replacement. (Reproduced with permission, Futura Publishing Company, Inc.[19])

HEMODYNAMIC RESULTS OF MITRAL BALLOON VALVULOPLASTY

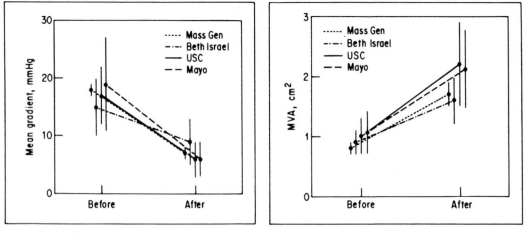

Figure 15.13. Results of percutaneous mitral balloon valvuloplasty. **A,** Acute decrease in mean transvalvular gradient is shown in four series. **B,** Acute increase in mitral valve area (MVA) is shown in four series. (Reproduced with permission, Mayo Clinic Proceedings.[27])

of balloon valvotomy, and an echocardiographic score has been developed[27] to quantitate the degree of leaflet mobility, thickening, calcification, and subvalvular obstruction (Table 15.1). Patients with scores less than 8 have had excellent results after mitral balloon valvotomy. Patients with echo scores greater than 10 have demonstrated a higher incidence of complications and suboptimal results.

Review of the literature examining residual gradients following balloon mitral valvotomy reveals that residual gradients in the order of 5–10 mm Hg are commonly measured following this procedure.[3,23,25] This residual gradient is higher than those reported by the NYU surgical series of open commissurotomy.[11] In this surgical review of 200 patients undergoing open mitral commissurotomy, a postoperative gradient of greater than 3 mm Hg significantly correlated to the subsequent need for reoperation and subsequent valve replacement. From these surgical data, it would be predicted that a significant number of patients treated with balloon valvotomy would redevelop significant gradients and re-present with symptoms of congestive heart failure.

Review of the reported complications of balloon mitral valvotomy relative to the morbidity and mortality of surgical commissurotomy is important in assessing the current role of balloon valvotomy. Kirklin reported in 1986 that open commissurotomy can be performed with extremely low operative mortality—only one death in a series of 259 open commissurotomies done over several years.[28] The incidence of perioperative cerebrovascular accident is also extremely low for this procedure, as direct exposure is afforded of the left atrial chamber and any thrombi can be carefully removed by the surgeon prior to commissurotomy.

The risks associated with mitral valve dilation are listed in Table 15.2. The most threatening complication is ventricular perforation with tamponade, usually resulting from the guidewire or the actual balloons rupturing the left ventricular myocardial wall. The left ventricle in mitral stenosis is not subjected to pressure or volume overload and is usually small and thin, making it susceptible to perforation. This has been reported in several cases, some of which resulted in fatality.[29,30] Bleeding from left ventricular perforation is generated from a high pressure chamber, and the risk of tamponade is significant. Although the incidence of this devastating complication is low and formal OR standby is not generally required for routine balloon valvotomy, the cardiac surgical and anesthesiology services should be able to mobilize and transfer a patient to the operating room for immediate intervention within 20–30 min as appropriate support for balloon mitral valvotomy.

Acute severe mitral insufficiency rarely occurs following mitral balloon valvotomy, although up to 30% of patients will increase the severity of preexisting mitral regurgitation by one or two grades following the dilation.[31] Severe mitral regurgitation may occur in 3% of patients and appears to be related to the use of the double balloon technique.[2] The mechanism of severe

Table 15.1.
Mitral Valve Echocardiography Score— Morphologic Features

Grade	Definition
	Mobility
1.	Highly mobile valve with only leaflet tips restricted
2.	Normal mobility of leaflet midportion
3.	Valve moves forward in diastole mainly from base
4.	No or minimal forward movement of leaflets in diastole
	Leaflet thickening
1.	Leaflets nearly normal in thickness (4–5 mm)
2.	Midportion of leaflets normal but marked thickening of margins (5–8 mm)
3.	Thickening extending to distal third of chords
4.	Extensive thickening and shortening of all chordal structures extending to papillary muscles
	Calcification
1.	Single areas of increased echo brightness
2.	Scattered areas of brightness confined to leaflet margins
3.	Brightness extending to midportion of leaflets
4.	Extensive brightness throughout leaflet tissue

Table 15.2.
Reported Complications of Mitral Valvuloplasty

Complication	McKay (N = 63) No.	%	NHLBI (N = 72) No.	%	Babic (N = 76) No.	%
CVA	2	3.2	3	4.2	3	3.9
Tamponade	0	0	4	5.6	—	—
Death	1	1.6	1	1.4	1	1.3
Mitral regurgitation	0	0	2	2.8	2	2.6
ASD	13	20.6	—	—	—	—

CVA = cerebrovascular accident; ASD = atrial septal defect.

mitral regurgitation following balloon dilation has been attributed to anterior leaflet tear, paracommissural tear, and rupture of the papillary muscle.[30] These reports reinforce the fact that patients with heavily calcified, rigid leaflets are not candidates for the dilation procedure, which will result in tearing of the leaflets rather than separation of the commissures.

Embolization with a resulting cerebrovascular accident has occurred in 3–4% of patients in reported series and remains one of the largest concerns of the procedure. Two-dimensional echocardiography will not identify all patients with left atrial thrombus. The presence of left atrial thrombus should definitely indicate that the procedure be deferred to surgical intervention. Embolization of calcific debri from the valve during the dilation has also been implicated in the embolic complications of the procedure. The risks of embolization parallel that risk associated with a closed mitral commissurotomy, due to the nondirect exposure of the mitral valve for the procedure.

Creation of a left-to-right atrial shunt following balloon mitral valvotomy is not rare[32] due to the transseptal puncture necessitated by the procedure. These are usually modest shunts without clinical consequence (shunt fraction less than 1.5). Occassionally large atrial septal defects have been reported following mitral balloon valvotomy, most likely due to unintentional inflation of a valvotomy balloon across the fossa ovalis of the interatrial septum. Routinely, a small balloon dilation or a large introducer is used to create a path through the septum to introduce the valvotomy balloons. This alone can result in a residual defect.

RECOMMENDATIONS— CONCLUSION

It is clear that long-term follow-up is essential to determine the role of balloon mitral valvotomy in the treatment of mitral stenosis. In its early application, the procedure should be limited to patients who are relatively ideal candidates for closed commissurotomy, which balloon dilation closely parallels in mechanism of action and potential complications. Unless the patient has noncalcified pliable leaflets with stenosis due to commissural fusion, no evidence of left atrial thrombus, and nonsignificant mitral regurgitation, percutaneous dilation should be deferred to a standard, open, surgical approach.[33] Open commissurotomy can provide better relief of obstruc-

tion and at a lower risk of complication than balloon dilation in the majority of patients. The initial data in valvotomy series indicate that the relief of obstruction is less and the incidence of complications (significant mitral regurgitation) is higher in those patients with preexisting calcification, fibrosis, and subvalvular fusion. A similar experience was reported during the development of surgical commissurotomy, and predictably there will be many parallels in patient selection and outcome between these two procedures, introduced over three decades apart. Balloon valvotomy should not be regarded as a means of temporizing valve replacement, as delay in mitral valve replacement of a severely diseased valve with mixed mitral stenosis–mitral insufficiency will only limit the functional recovery of the patient.

REFERENCES

1. Inoue K, Owaki T, Nakamura T, Kitamura F, Miyamoto N. Clinical application of transvenous mitral commissurotomy by a new balloon catheter. *J Thorac Cardiovasc Surg 87*:394–402, 1984.
2. Nobuyoshi M, Hamasaki N, Kimura T, et al. Indications, complications, and short-term clinical outcome of percutaneous transvenous mitral commissurotomy. *Circulation 80*:782–792, 1989.
3. Lock JE, Khalilullah M, Shrivastava S, Bahl V, Keane JF. Percutaneous catheter commissurotomy in rheumatic mitral stenosis. *N Eng J Med 313*:1515–1518, 1985.
4. Sealy WC, Young WG. Acquired mitral stenosis: An inquiry into its progressive and recurrent nature and the influence of preventive measures and surgery on its natural history. *Ann Thorac Surg 1*:244–258, 1965.
5. Roberts WC. Mophologic features of the normal and abnormal mitral valve. *Am J Cardiol 51*:1005–1028, 1983.
6. John S. Bashi VV, Jairaj PS, et al. Closed mitral valvotomy: Early results and long-term follow-up of 3724 consecutive patients. *Circulation 68*:891–896, 1983.
7. Cohn LH, Allred EN, Cohn LA, Disesa VJ, Shemin RJ, Collins JJ. Long-term results of open mitral valve reconstruction for mitral stenosis. *Am J Cardiol 55*:731–734, 1985.
8. Breyer RH, Mills SA, Hudspeth AS, et al. Open mitral commissurotomy: Long-term results with echocardiographic correlation. *J Cardiovasc Surg 26*:46–52, 1985.
9. Foltz BD, Hessel EA, Ivey TD. The early course of pulmonary artery hypertension in patients undergoing mitral valve replacement. *J Thorac Cardiovasc Surg 88*:238–244, 1984.
10. Bocheck LI. Current status of mitral commis-

surotomy: Indications, techniques, and results. *Am J Cardiol* 52:411–415, 1982.

11. Gross RI, Cunningham JN, Snively SL, et al. Long-term results of open radical mitral commissurotomy: Ten year follow-up study of 202 patients. *Am J Cardiol* 47:821–825, 1981.

12. Schoevaerdts JC, Jaumin P, Kremer R, Ponlot R, Chalant ChH. Surgical treatment of mitral stenosis. *J Cardiovasc Surg* 22:109–112, 1981.

13. Carpentier A. Cardiac valve surgery—the "French correction." *J Thorac Cardiovasc Surg* 86:323–337, 1983.

14. Montoya A. Mulet J, Pifarre R, Moran JM, Sullivan HJ. The advantages of open mitral commissurotomy for mitral stenosis. *Chest* 75:131–135, 1979.

15. Hansen JF, Anderson ED, Olsen ES, et al. DC cardioversion of atrial fibrillation after mitral valve operation. *Scand J Thorac Cardiovasc Surg* 13:267–275, 1979.

16. Housman LB, Bonchek L, Lambert L, Grunkemeier G, Starr A. Prognosis of patients after open mitral commissurotomy: Actuarial analysis of late results in 100 patients. *J Thorac Cardiovasc Surg* 73:742–745, 1977.

17. Higgs LM, Glancy DL, O'Brien KP, Epstein SE, Morrow AG. Mitral restenosis: An uncommon cause of recurrent symptoms following mitral commissurotomy. *Am J Cardiol* 26:34–37, 1970.

18. John S, Perianayagam WJ, Abraham KA, et al. Restenosis of the mitral valve: Surgical considerations and results of operation. *Ann Thorac Surg* 25:316–321, 1978.

19. Perier PP, Deloche A, Chauvaud S, et al. Clinical comparison of mitral valve replacement using porcine, Starr, and Bjork valves. *J Cardiac Surg* 3:359–368, 1988.

20. Reid CL, McKay CR, Chandraratna PAN, Kawanishi DT, Rahimtoola SH. Mechanisms of increase in mitral valve area and influence of anatomic features in double-balloon, catheter balloon valvuloplasty in adults with rheumatic mitral stenosis: A Doppler and two-dimensional echocardiographic study. *Circulation* 76:628–636, 1987.

21. Reifart N, Nowak B, Baykut D, Satter P, Bussmann WD, Kaltenbach M. Experimental balloon valvulo-plasty of fibrotic and calcific mitral valves. *Circulation* 81:1005–1011, 1990.

22. Babic UU, Pejcic P, Djurisic Z, Vucinic M, Grujicic SM. Percutaneous transarterial balloon valvuloplasty for mitral valve stenosis. *Am J Cardiol* 57:1101–1104, 1986.

23. McKay CR, Kawanishi DT, Rahimtoola SH. Catheter balloon valvuloplasty of the mitral valve in adults using a double-balloon technique: Early hemodynamic results. *JAMA* 257:1753–1761, 1987.

24. Palacios I, Block PC, Brandi S, et al. Percutaneous balloon valvotomy for patients with severe mitral stenosis. *Circulation* 75:778–784, 1987.

25. Palacios IF, Lock JE, Keane JF, Block PC. Percutaneous transvenous balloon valvotomy in a patient with severe calcific mitral stenosis. *J Am Coll Cardiol* 7:1416–1419, 1986.

26. McKay RG, Lock JE, Keane JF, Safian RD, Aroesty JM, Grossman W. Percutaneous mitral valvuloplasty in an adult patient with calcific rheumatic mitral stenosis. *J Am Coll Cardiol* 7:1410–1415, 1986.

27. Nishimura A, Holmes DR, Reeden GS. Percutaneous balloon valvuloplasty. *Mayo Clin Proc* 65:198–220, 1990.

28. Kirklin JW, Barrett-Boyes BG. *Cardiac Surgery*. New York, John Wiley and Sons, 1986.

29. Roberston JM, de Virgilio C, French W, Ruiz C, Nelson RJ. Fatal left ventricular perforation during mitral balloon valvoplasty. *Ann Thorac Surg* 49:819–821, 1990.

30. Acar C, Deloch A, Tibi PR, et al. Operative findings after percutaneous mitral dilatation. *Ann Thorac Surg* 49:959–963, 1990.

31. Abascal VM, Wilkins GT, Choong CY, et al. Mitral regurgitation after percutaneous balloon mitral valvuloplasty in adults: Evaluation by pulsed Doppler echocardiograpy. *J Am Coll Cardiol* 11:257–263.

32. Bernard Y, Schiele F, Bassard JP, et al. Characteristics of flow through the atrial septal defect following percutaneous mitral valvuloplasty. *Eur Heart J* 10:96–104, 1989.

33. Roberts WC, Perloff JK. Mitral valvular disease. A clinicopathologic survey of the conditions causing the mitral valve to function abnormally. *Ann Intern Med* 77:939–975, 1972.

CATHETER INTERVENTIONAL PROCEDURES
IN NEONATES AND CHILDREN

16

Percutaneous Balloon Valvotomy/Angioplasty in Congenital Heart Disease

P. SYAMASUNDAR RAO

Rubio and Limon Lason[1] in 1954 described a technique by which pulmonic and tricuspid valve stenoses could be relieved via a catheter; they used a ureteral catheter with a wire. Twenty-five years later, Semb and his associates[2] used a Berman balloon angiographic catheter to produce rupture of the pulmonary valve (commissures); they withdrew an inflated balloon from the main pulmonary artery to the right ventricle and reduced the pulmonary valve gradient. More recently, Kan and her associates[3] used a static dilation technique (similar to that used by Dotter and Judkins[4] and Gruntzig and his associates[5,6] in which they introduced a deflated balloon across the pulmonic valve and inflated the balloon; the radial forces of balloon inflation produced relief of pulmonary valve obstruction. This static dilation technique is what is currently used. The purpose of this chapter is to present the role of percutaneous balloon dilation in the treatment of congenital heart disease, utilizing our personal experience with balloon dilation in approximately 200 children. Our previously reported material and that reported in the literature will be used as supportive material.

TECHNIQUE

The diagnosis and assessment of the obstructive lesions of the heart are made by the usual clinical, roentgenographic, electrocardiographic, and echo-Doppler data. Once a moderate to severe obstruction is diagnosed, cardiac catheterization and cineangiography are performed percutaneously to confirm the clinical impression and to consider for balloon dilation of the stenotic lesion. The indica-

tions for catheter intervention (described later for each lesion) are usually those prescribed for surgical intervention. Once balloon dilation is decided on, (1) a 5- to 7-F end-hold (or multi-A-2) catheter is introduced percutaneously into either the femoral vein or artery and advanced across the stenotic lesion, (2) a 0.014- to 0.035-inch guidewire is passed through the catheter into the vessel or cardiac chamber beyond the stenotic lesion, (3) a 4- to 9-F balloon dilation catheter is advanced over the guidewire and the balloon is positioned across the stenotic lesion, (4) the balloon is inflated with diluted contrast media to approximately 3 to 5 atmospheres of pressure, and (5) measurement of pressure gradients across the obstructive region and angiographic demonstration of the relief of obstruction are recorded. The recommended duration of inflation is 5 sec. Usually a total of three to four balloon inflations are performed, 5 min apart. We use a double balloon technique (two balloons simultaneously inflated across the stenotic region) when the valve anulus or the vessel diameter is too large to dilate with a commercially available single balloon. Recordings of heart rate, systemic pressure, and cardiac index prior to and after balloon dilation are made to assure that change in pressure gradient is not related to change in cardiac index but is indeed related to the procedure.

PULMONIC STENOSIS

Valvular pulmonary stenosis constitutes 7.5 to 9.0% of all congenital heart defects.[7,8] Children with pulmonic stenosis usually present with asymptomatic murmurs, although they can present with signs of congestive heart failure due to severe right ventricular dysfunction or cyanosis because of a right-to-left shunt across the atrial septum. Clinical findings of an ejection systolic click, an ejection systolic murmur at the left upper sternal border, right ventricular hypertrophy on an electrocardiogram, a prominent main pulmonary artery segment on a chest roentogenogram, and an increased Doppler flow velocity in the main pulmonary artery are characteristic for this anomaly. When the pulmonary valvular obstruction is moderate to severe, relief of the obstruction is recommended to treat symptoms, or to prevent right ventricular fibrosis and dysfunction. Until recently, surgical valvotomy was the only treatment available, but at the present time, relief of pulmonary valve obstruction can be accomplished by balloon valvuloplasty.

Indications

By and large, the indications for balloon dilation of pulmonic stenosis are essentially the same as those used for surgical intervention. The indications for surgical pulmonary valvotomy are reasonably clear: patients with moderate to severe degree of stenosis irrespective of the symptoms are candidates for surgical relief of the obstruction.[9,10] The indications for balloon valvuloplasty appear less clear and are rarely defined.[11] Careful examination of all the available studies reveals that many patients with what may be considered mild pulmonic stenosis (natural history study definition[10]: gradient < 25 mm Hg = trivial, 25 to 49 mm Hg = mild, 50 to 79 mm Hg = moderate, and ≥ 80 mm Hg = severe) undergo balloon valvuloplasty.[3,11–20] Review of the results of balloon valvuloplasty in these patients with mild stenosis reveals that residual right ventricular peak systolic pressures at follow-up are 75 ± 18% of pre-valvuloplasty values.[21] Furthermore, natural history studies of pulmonic stenosis[10,22,23] indicate that mild pulmonary stenosis remains mild on follow-up. Therefore, the advisability of balloon valvuloplasty for mild obstruction can be questioned. My recommendations are to consider the indications for balloon valvuloplasty to be the same as those used for surgical valvuloplasty and that balloon dilation should not be performed in patients with peak-to-peak gradients less than 50 mm Hg. Because noninvasive Doppler estimates of pulmonary valve gradients are reasonably accurate,[24,25] patients with mild stenosis can be followed periodically. Once the Doppler estimate of

the pulmonic valvular gradient is in excess of 50 mm Hg, they should be considered candidates for balloon valvuloplasty. Some investigators consider dysplastic pulmonary valves as a relative contraindication for balloon valvuloplasty,[26,27] but based on results of others[18,28] and our own data,[29] balloon valvuloplasty is the initial treatment of choice; though larger balloons to produce a balloon:anulus ratio of 1.4 to 1.5 should be used.[29] In conclusion, moderate to severe valvular pulmonic stenosis (gradient ≥ 50 mm Hg), irrespective of previous surgical intervention and pulmonary valve dysplasia, is an indication for percutaneous balloon pulmonary valvuloplasty.

Technical Issues

The general technique of balloon valvuloplasty is as described in the beginning of the chapter. Some specific aspects of importance will be mentioned here.

A. *Passing an end-hold catheter across the pulmonic valve.* This may be difficult in some patients, particularly in young children and neonates. In such occasions we employ several maneuvers: (1) the use of an end-hole catheter (usually a multi-A2), positioning it just underneath the pulmonary valve and advancing the floppy end of a straight guidewire through the tip of the catheter into the main pulmonary artery; (2) use of a balloon-wedge catheter, positioning it just beneath the pulmonic valve and quickly deflating the balloon and advancing the catheter into the main pulmonary artery. Failing this, use a guidewire as described earlier; (3) use of flexible, steerable coronary guidewire through an end-hole catheter. We have encountered one child in whom we could not advance any catheter across the right ventricular infundibulum because of severe infundibular constriction. In this child administration of propranolol (0.1 mg/kg i.v., slowly) made it possible to pass a catheter across the pulmonary valve and eventually perform balloon pulmonary valvuloplasty.[30]

B. *Choice of size of balloon dilation catheter.* The current recommendations are to use a balloon that is 1.2 to 1.4 times the size of the pulmonary valve anulus. These recommendations are formulated on the basis of immediate[17] and follow-up results.[31–33] For further discussion of reasoning behind such recommendations, the reader is referred to these publications.[31–34] Balloons larger than the 1.5 times the size of the pulmonary valve anulus are not recommended because of potential damage to the right ventricular outflow tract caused by use of large balloons.[35] However it may be advisable to use large balloons to achieve a balloon anulus ratio of 1.5 when pulmonary valve dysplasia is present.[29]

When the pulmonary valve anulus is too large to dilate with a single balloon, valvuloplasty with simultaneous inflation of two balloons across the pulmonary valve anulus should be performed. When two balloons are used, the following formula is used to calculate the effective balloon size[31]:

$$\frac{D_1 + D_2 + \pi \left(\dfrac{D_1}{2} + \dfrac{D_2}{2} \right)}{\pi}$$

where D_1 and D_2 are diameters of the balloons used.

Although we do not believe that the double balloon technique is superior to the single balloon technique,[32,36,37] it does reduce injury to the femoral veins because smaller-sized catheters can be used.

On occasion, it may be difficult to advance the balloon angioplasty catheter across the pulmonic valve. It is important to avoid kinking or looping of the guidewire to prevent such a problem. Replacement of the guidewire with an extra-stiff Amplatz guidewire may circumvent the problem.

Acute Results

Several groups,[11–18,38–43] including our group,[33,34,44–47] have reported excellent immediate relief of pulmonic valve obstruction following balloon valvuloplasty. From our group, 66 infants and children, aged 2 days to 20 years (median 6 years), underwent balloon dilation of valvular pulmonic stenosis during a 6-year period ending September 1989. Following valvuloplasty, the peak systolic pressure in the right ventricle decreased (108 ± 44 [mean $\pm$ SD] vs. 55 ± 20 mm Hg, $p < 0.001$) as did the peak systolic gradient across the pulmonic valve (92 ± 43 vs. 29 ± 20 mm Hg, $p < 0.001$). The cardiac index did not change ($p = 0.1$). Width of the jet of the contrast media through the pulmonary valve as visualized in the lateral view of the cineangiogram (Fig. 16.1) increased. Less doming and much more "free" movement of the pulmonary valve leaflets occurred following the valvuloplasty in each case. Surgical intervention was avoided in all cases. Most patients were discharged home within 24 to 48 hours following the procedure.

Follow-up Results

Several authors[11–16,18,38,40,41] have obtained follow-up catheterization data in 6 to 44 patients, one

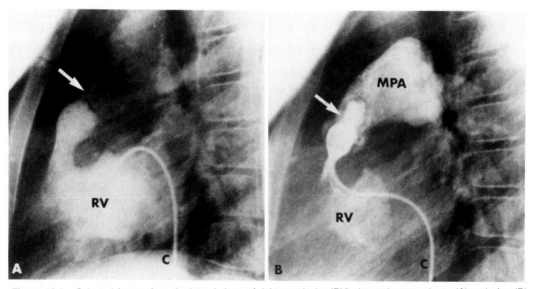

Figure 16.1. Selected frames from the lateral views of right ventricular (RV) cineangiogram prior to (**A**) and after (**B**) balloon pulmonary valvulplasty. Note extremely thin jet prior to balloon dilation (**A**), which increased to a much wider jet (arrow) after valvuloplasty (**B**), opacifiying the main pulmonary artery (MPA). C = catheter. (Reproduced with permission from Rao PS. *Current Problems in Cardiology* 14(8):417–500, 1989.)

week to 17 months following balloon valvuloplasty and have reported 14 to 33% recurrence of the gradient (Table 16.1). Our own catheterization experience in 40 children, 6 to 34 months (mean, 11.0 months) after balloon valvuloplasty,[37] reveals the peak systolic pressure gradient across the pulmonic valve (93 ± 45 vs. 31 ± 24 mm Hg, $p < 0.001$) and the peak systolic pressure in the right ventricle (110 ± 43 vs. 57 ± 22 mg Hg, $p < 0.001$) are decreased, and the pulmonary artery pressure (17 ± 5 vs. 24 ± 6 mm Hg, $p < 0.001$) is increased immediately after balloon dilation. The cardiac index (3.3 ± 0.9 vs. 3.2 ± 0.7 liters/min/ m^2, $p > 0.1$) remains unchanged. Upon follow-up approximately 11 months later, systolic pressure gradient across the pulmonic valve (29 ± 34 mm Hg, $p < 0.001$) and right ventricular peak systolic pressure (55 ± 32 mm Hg, $p > 0.001$) remain improved when compared to predilation values. The cardiac index (3.5 ± 0.8 liters/min/m²) does not significantly ($p > 0.1$) change.

Despite improvement as a group, several children developed restenosis of the pulmonary valve (Fig. 16.2). Seven of 40 (17.5%) had pulmonary valve gradients in excess of 30 mm Hg. Five of these children underwent repeat balloon valvuloplasty with larger balloon diameters (Fig. 16.2) and the pulmonary valvular gradients were reduced from 102 ± 40 to 38 ± 12 mm Hg ($p < 0.01$). The other two children with residual gradients of 45 and 60 mm Hg are being followed clinically. A restenosis rate of 17.5% in our group is comparable to the 14 to 33% reported by other workers.[11–16,18,38,40,41] Electrocardiographic and echo-Doppler follow-up studies also reflect the pressure gradient reduction.[48,49]

Applicability to All Ages

Although balloon pulmonary valvuloplasty is used most frequently in childhood, it has also been used in neonates[18,50–52] and in adults.[53–57] The experi-

Table 16.1.
Intermediate-Term Follow-up Catheterization Results of Balloon Pulmonary Valvuloplasty (BPV) from the Literature

Author & Year	Number of patients undergoing BPV	Number of patients with follow-up	Duration of follow-up, mean (range), months	Poor result[a] on follow-up No. (%)	Comments
Kan et al. 1983	20	11	7(2–12)	2(18)	The failure was in patients with dysplastic valve or after previous valvotomy
Tynan et al. 1985	27	6	—(2–6)	2(33)	Both patients underwent surgery
Kveselis et al. 1985	19	7	12(9–13)	7(100)[b]	Repeat BPV in one patient with 52 mm Hg gradient with reduction to 34 mm Hg
Miller, 1985	16	7	4(3–6)	1(14)	Two patients with gradients of 24 and 22 mm Hg at follow-up underwent repeat BPV with excellent results
Sullivan et al. 1985	23	12	5.5 (0.25–6)	6(50)	Repeat valvuloplasty in 4 patients with good results
Khan et al. 1986	32	14	10(6–14)	2(14)	—
Srivastava et al. 1987	32	21	(3–18)	9(43)	—
Rey et al. 1988	51	23	—(1–17)	5(22)	Repeat BPV in 5 patients with satisfactory results.
Fontes et al. 1988	100	44	12(3–14)	10(23)	Repeat BPV in 6 patients with success. Two with dysplastic valves underwent surgery
Rao, 1990	66	40	11(6–34)	7(18)	Repeat BPV in 5 patients with good results

[a]Poor result is defined as pulmonary valve gradient in excess of 30 mm Hg at follow-up.
[b]The pulmonary valve gradient ranged between 31 and 52 mm Hg with a mean of 38 mm Hg.
Modified from Rao PS. *Current Problems in Cardiology* 14(8):417–500, 1989.

FOLLOW-UP RESULTS OF
BALLOON PULMONARY VALVULOPLASTY

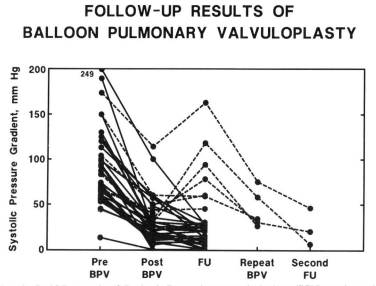

Figure 16.2. Longitudinal follow-up data following balloon pulmonary valvuloplasty (BPV) are shown. In 33 patients (solid lines) the peak systolic pressure gradient across the pulmonic valve improved or remained unchanged at follow-up (FU) when compared to the immediate post-BPV gradient. In seven children (interrupted lines), the gradient remained high or increased at FU. Five of these children underwent repeat valvuloplasty with larger balloons and subsequent improvement in pulmonary valvular gradients. A second FU study in three patients shows further fall in the gradient in each patient. (Modified from Rao PS. *Clin Cardiol 12*:55–74, 1989.)

ence with pulmonary valvuloplasty in the neonate with critical pulmonary stenosis will be discussed in Chapter 18 and will not be dealt with further here. Relief of pulmonary stenosis in adult patients has also been accomplished by balloon valvuloplasty.[53–57] Because of the physical size of the pulmonary valve ring, many adults may require balloon valvuloplasty using two balloons.[55,56] However, as pointed out elsewhere,[32,36] the double balloon technique is comparable to, but not superior to the single balloon technique when equivalent balloon:anulus ratios are compared.

Based on our own experience with teenage children[47,58] and that of others in adults,[53,55,57] infundibular obstruction following balloon valvuloplasty appears to be more common in older than in young patients. The reason for this is probably related to long-standing right ventricular hypertension and consequent right ventricular hypertrophy in older patients.

Comparison with Surgical Results

Over the years, the risk from surgical correction of congenital cardiac defects has diminished markedly. Despite this, there are many negative aspects to the surgical repair of cardiac defects including prolonged hospitalization, frightening postopera-

tive appearance (especially to the parents), residual scars, possible psychologic trauma to the child, and quite an expense. For these reasons, there is an advantage to treating cardiac defects by catheter techniques, provided morbidity and mortality figures and recurrence rates are better than, or at least comparable to, those of surgical therapy. However, comparison of immediate and follow-up results of surgical versus balloon therapy is fraught with problems because of (1) the small number of balloon valvuloplasty patients available for follow-up; (2) the shorter duration of balloon follow-up; and (3) the possible inaccuracy of comparing "older" surgical studies with "current" balloon dilation.

Surgical treatment for valvular pulmonic stenosis has been available for 40 years since the first description by Brock.[59] Six representative surgical pulmonary valvuloplasty papers[10,60–64] can be used for comparison with balloon valvuloplasty results. These authors followed 50 to 234 patients for "months" to 30 years after surgical relief of pulmonary valve obstruction. Operative mortality varied between 3 to 14%; a cooperative study involving several institutions had only 3% mortality in 304 patients presented.[10] Poor results at follow-up were noted in 0 to 8%, with the cooperative study having 4% poor results (defined as a pulmonary valvular gradient in excess of 50 mm Hg) at follow-up. Pulmonary valve insufficiency was reported in all studies. Follow-up catheterization studies after balloon valvuloplasty,[11–16,18,37,38,40,41,47] including the current study, involved recatheterization in from 6 to 44 patients at one week to 34 months after valvuloplasty (Table 16.1). Restenosis was reported in 14 to 33%. No significant mortality has been reported following balloon valvuloplasty.[65] The mortality figures and morbidity appear higher following surgery; however, the recurrence rate appears higher following the balloon procedure. With refinement of balloon techniques,[32,33,66] the restenosis rate may be able to be brought down to extremely low levels; of the 32 patients in whom dilation with balloons larger than 1.2 times of the pulmonary valve anulus diameter was performed, none required repeat valvuloplasty and none had pressure gradients in excess of 30 mm Hg at follow-up (Table 16.2). Based on the available information, it is evident that both immediate and follow-up results after balloon valvuloplasty are comparable or superior to surgical pulmonary valvuloplasty. Such a categoric statement will be able to be substantiated when 5- and 10-year follow-up studies of balloon valvuloplasty confirm the current intermediate-term follow-up results.

AORTIC STENOSIS

Valvular aortic stenosis accounts for approximately 5% of all congenital heart defects.[7,8] Children with aortic stenosis usually come to the attention of physicians because of a cardiac murmur alone. Rarely children with aortic stenosis present with symptoms of heart failure, syncope, chest pain, or even sudden death. Findings on examination include a systolic ejection click at the apex and at the right upper sternal border, a systolic ejection murmur best heard at the right upper sternal border with radiation into the carotid vessels, and a prominent left ventricular impulse on palpation. The electrocardiogram may or may not show evidence for left ventricular hypertrophy or abnormal ST-T wave changes. Exercise electrocardiography may be useful in detecting severe stenosis by demonstrating reduced cardiac reserve. Quantitation of the degree of obstruction can be made by Doppler flow velocity analysis. Surgical aortic valvotomy is usually recommended for moderate to severe aortic stenosis to prevent myocardial decompensation and to prevent sudden death.

Indications

By and large, the indications for balloon dilation of stenotic aortic valve are essentially similar to those used for surgical correction.[67–70] A peak-to-peak systolic pressure gradient in excess of 80 mm Hg, irrespective of the symptoms, or a peak-to-peak gradient $\geq$ 50 mm Hg with a normal stroke volume and either symptoms or electrocardiographic ST-T wave changes are generally considered as indicators for catheter intervention. Since the aortic valvular gradient after balloon valvuloplasty appears to decrease to only approximately 50 to 60% of prevalvuloplasty values (Table 16.3), and because

Table 16.2.
Prevalence of Repeat Valvuloplasty and Significant Residual Gradients at Follow-up in Various Groups

	Number of patients needing repeat valvuloplasty	p value[a]	Number of patients with pulmonary valve gradient > 30 mm Hg	p value[a]
B:A ratio ≤ 1.0 N = 7	4		5	
		0.002		0.001
B:A ratio > 1.0 N = 33	1		2	
B:A ratio ≤ 1.2 N = 21	5		7	
		0.05		0.002
B:A ratio > 1.2 N = 19	0		0	

B:A, Balloon:Anulus
N = number of patients with intermediate-term follow-up catheterization.
[a]Fisher's exact test
Modified from Rao PS. *Am Heart J 116*:577–580, 1988.

Table 16.3.
Acute Results of Balloon Aortic Valvuloplasty in Children[a]

Authors, year	Number of patients undergoing BAV	Age, yrs. mean ± SD (range)	Pre-BAV gradient[b] (mm Hg)	Gradient[b] immediately after BAV (mm Hg)	Percentage reduction of gradient mean ± SD (range)	Comments
Lababidi et al. 1984	23	9 ± 5 (2–27)	113 ± 48	32 ± 15	71 ± 1 (51–89)	two patients required surgery
Walls et al.[c] 1984	27	9 ± 5 (1.7–17)	108 ± 46	32 ± 16	—	
Choy et al. 1987	8	7 ± 5 (0.25–12)	74 ± 25	38 ± 14	47 ± 16 (29–67)	—
Helgason et al.[d] 1987	14	9 ± 5 (0.2–15)	85 ± 23	27 ± 14	68 ± 15 (49–94)	—
Wren et al. 1987	54	0.6 ± 0.3 (0.2–0.9)	80 ± 18	25 ± 30	69 ± 38 (29–94)	one death
Mullins et al. 1987	14	—	68	24	65	only double balloon BAV
Beekman et al.[e] 1988	16	8 ± 2 (0.25–17)	2 ± 24	46 ± 16	43	only single balloon BAV
	11	10 ± 2 (0.25–21)	76 ± 16	22 ± 13	67	only double balloon BAV
Sholler et al.[f] 1988	68	11 ± 9 (0.2–39)	9 ± 23	34 ± 19	55 ± 21 (0–94)	three patients required surgery
Rao et al. 1989	17	7 ± 5 (0.6–16)	74 ± 21	29 ± 13	60 ± 17 (35–92)	—

[a]Excludes neonates and literature reports containing less than 3 patients.
[b]Gradient is peak to peak systolic pressure gradient across the aortic valve obtained at cardiac catheterization.
[c]Includes the patients previously reported by Lababidi et al. 1984
[d]Neonates in these series were excluded.
[e]Includes the patients previously reported by Choy et al. 1987
[f]Includes the patients previously reported by Helgason et al. 1987
BAV = Balloon aortic valvuloplasty.

of the lack of long-term follow-up results documenting its effectiveness, one may question the routine use of balloon aortic valvuloplasty. However, based on reasonably good intermediate-term results[71–73] and significant early and late surgical mortality and need for reoperation following surgical aortic valvotomy,[67,70,74–78] I would recommend balloon aortic valvuloplasty as the initial treatment option in children with moderate to severe valvular aortic stenosis. Previous surgical valvotomy does not affect the result unfavorably. Critical aortic stenosis in the neonate and young infant is a particularly good indication for balloon therapy because of the high morbidity and mortality associated with surgical intervention.

Presence of significant (greater than 2 + angiographically) aortic insufficiency is considered a contraindication for balloon valvuloplasty for fear of increasing the degree of aortic insufficiency. A stenotic porcine heterograft in aortic position is probably poorly treated by balloon catheter techniques.

Technical Issues

The basic technique was described earlier in the chapter. Some important additional technical aspects of percutaneous aortic valvuloplasty are (1) 100 units/kg body weight of intravenous heparin (maximum 2500 units) are administered prior to balloon valvuloplasty, (2) the size of the balloon chosen is within 1 to 2 mm of the size of the aortic valve anulus, and (3) when the size of the aortic valve anulus is too large to dilate with a commercially available single balloon, or when a single balloon cannot be safely passed from the femoral artery, a double balloon technique with two balloons simultaneously inflated across the stenotic aortic valve is used. Effective balloon size is calculated as described for the therapy of pulmonary stenosis. Over the last two years we have used the 5.5-cm long, low-profile balloons, which have made it easier to maintain the position of the balloon(s) across the aortic valve during valvuloplasty.

Acute Results

Balloon aortic valvuloplasty has been performed in children by several groups of workers, and the results, though acceptable, are not as good as those following pulmonary valvuloplasty. Generally the valvular gradient is acutely reduced by about 60% of prevalvuloplasty values. The reported results are shown in Table 16.3.[20,71,73,79–83] No significant increase in aortic insufficiency has been reported. Our own experience with this lesion[73,84] is not as extensive as in the other lesions; we have performed balloon aortic valvuloplasty in only 20 children, aged 7 months to 16 years (7.6 ± 5.1 years). The peak systolic pressure gradient across the aortic valve has been reduced from 73 ± 22 to 25 ± 14 mm Hg ($p < 0.001$) in this group. The percentage reduction of aortic valvular gradient has ranged between 35 and 99% (65 ± 18%) with the left ventricular end-diastolic pressure decreasing from 13.9 ± 4.5 to 9.4 ± 6.1 mm Hg ($p < 0.01$). There was no significant change in the cardiac index observed. No evidence for increase in aortic insufficiency was seen, and no patient required immediate surgical intervention.

Follow-up Results

Although the acute results of balloon aortic valvuloplasty and the clinical follow-up are available from many studies, hemodynamic follow-up results have not been extensively documented.[71–73,79,82] Walls et al.[82] reported 3- to 13-month follow-up catheterization data in 14 patients and found residual gradients of 37 ± 22 mm Hg. However, the number of patients with moderate to severe stenosis has not been mentioned. Sholler et al.[72] reported recatheterization results in 16 patients from 1 to 25 months after valvuloplasty and found that significant residual aortic valve gradients (45 ± 28 mm Hg) were present at follow-up. They also performed Doppler evaluation of the gradient in a total of 29 patients followed for 1 to 24 months after dilation and found a peak instantaneous gradient of 40 ± 22 mm Hg was present. However, it is not clear how many patients had residual gradients in excess of 50 mm Hg at follow-up. The follow-up results in our study[73,84] are from 18 children evaluated at 3 to 32 months (mean 12 months) after valvuloplasty. The residual gradient in these patients was 38 ± 24 mm Hg. These values were lower ($p < 0.001$) than those observed prior to valvuloplasty and were not significantly different ($p > 0.1$) from the immediate post-valvuloplasty gradients. However when individual values were examined, 4 of 18 (22%), had follow-up gradients in excess of 50 mm Hg. Two of these four children had repeat balloon valvuloplasty and two surgical valvotomy, all with good results.

Although balloon aortic valvuloplasty was first utilized in children,[85] it has now been successfully performed in both neonates and adults. The issues related to neonates and adults are discussed in other chapters in this book and therefore will not be discussed further here.

Comparison with Surgical Results

Since the first description of surgical aortic valvotomy in the mid-1950s,[86,87] surgery has been extensively used to relieve aortic valve obstruction in children. Nine representative papers[67–70,74–78] investigating the long-term follow-up can be examined to assess the results. These authors collectively followed 41 to 179 patients for 0.3 to 26 years following surgical aortic valvotomy. Operative mortality varied between 0 to 4% when neonates and young infants were excluded; the cooperative study[75] had a 1.2% operative mortality in 162 children undergoing open aortic valvotomy. Late mortality varied between 4 to 22%[67–70,74,76–78], in the cooperative study[75] it was only 1.9%. Restenosis of the aortic valve was noted in 16 to 78% of patients, while significant insufficiency at follow-up developed in 6 to 65% of patients. Reoperation either to relieve residual aortic obstruction or to correct aortic insufficiency was required in 16 to 36% of patients. Thus, the significant incidence of early and late mortality, the development of aortic valve restenosis and insufficiency at follow-up, and the need for reoperation with surgical aortic valvotomy[67–70,74–78] make balloon aortic valvuloplasty an attractive alternative to surgical valvotomy.

MITRAL VALVE STENOSIS

Since the first description in 1984,[88] several workers have utilized the technique of balloon valvuloplasty for relief of rheumatic mitral valvular stenosis. This procedure consists of initial transseptal catheterization of the left atrium, dilation of the interatrial septum, positioning of the balloon dilation catheter across the mitral valve, and inflating the balloon within the mitral valve orifice. A reduction of the diastolic gradient across the mitral valve and an increase in the cardiac output have been noted in most studies. There has been minimal, if any, increase in mitral insufficiency noted. Our limited experience in two patients is consistent with the reported results. Balloon dilation of congenital mitral valvular obstruction has also been attempted in a limited number of patients[89–91] with an immediate reduction in the mitral valve gradient and an increase in valve area reported. Few follow-up studies are available, but restenosis has been noted.[89] This technique might be useful in selected cases of congenital mitral stenosis, though the data are incomplete at this time.

COARCTATION OF THE AORTA

Five to 8% of congenital heart defects are accounted for by aortic coarctation.[7,8] These patients may present with signs of congestive heart failure in the neonatal period or during infancy, or they may be detected during evaluation for a cardiac murmur, hypertension, or an absent femoral pulse during childhood. Decreased or absent femoral pulses, higher arm blood pressure than lower limb blood pressure, and a nonspecific ejection murmur are usually found. Other findings depend on the nature of associated cardiac defects. Clinical findings are characteristic, and the diagnosis of coarctation can be confirmed by echo-Doppler studies and/or catheterization and angiography. Relief of coarctation is recommended to relieve signs of heart failure and to potentially reduce or prevent hypertension.

Indications

The indications for balloon coarctation angioplasty include the presence of systemic failure.[45,92,93] These indications are similar to those used to recommend surgery. Although there is some concern with regard to the development of aneurysms[94–99] following balloon angioplasty of native coarctations and evidence for postoperative recurrent coarctations, a general consensus is emerging that native coarctations should be treated with balloon dilation.[45,92,93,97,98,100] This is particularly true in the neonate and small infant because of the high morbidity and mortality as well as the high recurrence rate with surgery.[101–115] Balloon dilation of coarctation of the aorta appears to offer a

relatively safe and effective alternative to surgical repair in the neonates and young infants. With angioplasty, operative intervention may be avoided entirely or at least be postponed until the patient is older and larger in size, since surgical results are better with regard to operative mortality and recoarctation in older children. Should recurrence occur following angioplasty, or should aneurysm form at the site of dilation, the infant could undergo surgical resection at a later date when not as acutely ill.

With regard to the older child with native coarctation, because of concern for developing an aneurysm at the dilation site, this procedure should probably be performed only at selected centers with expertise in this lesion; its general use in other sites should await longer follow-up results from a larger number of patients.[116,117] Balloon dilation of postoperative recoarctations has also been recommended[65,118] as the therapy of choice for restenosis. Such a recommendation, though, has been made prior to the availability of data on immediate results in a significant number of patients and prior to the availability of any follow-up results. This type of recommendation is based in part on the speculation that the scar tissue in recoarctation may prevent the development of aneurysms or their progression once they develop. Based on recent data,[99,118–122] the immediate results of balloon angioplasty in recoarctation are excellent with a significant reduction in gradient across the coarctation demonstrable. However, the follow-up data are scanty and inconclusive at this time.

Technical Issues

The technique of the percutaneous balloon coarctation angioplasty is similar to that described for balloon valvuloplasty. It will not be detailed here, except to point out some important technical aspects of the procedure, namely: (1) 100 units/kg of heparin (maximum of 2500 units) are administered immediately after the introduction of the arterial catheter. The heparin effect is neither reversed nor continued after balloon angioplasty; (2) the size of the balloon chosen for angioplasty should be two times (or more) the size of the coarcted segment, but no larger than the size of the descending aorta at the level of diaphragm as measured from a frozen frame of the video recording; (3) at no time should a catheter or guidewire be manipulated back over the area of freshly dilated coarctation of the aorta since intimal damage may be accentuated or perforation induced; and (4) although most coarctation balloon dilations are performed by the retrograde arterial approach, a transvenous approach can also be applied in certain patients. With the transvenous method, the catheter is advanced antegrade from the ascending to the descending aorta after the catheter is positioned in the ascending aorta either directly from the right ventricle (when transposition of the great arteries is present) or via a ventricular septal defect.

Acute Results

For the purpose of this discussion, aortic coarctation will be divided into 3 groups: (1) native coarctation in the neonate and infants ≤ 1 year, usually associated with other cardiac defects; (2) native coarctation in children; and (3) postoperative recoarctation.

NEONATES AND INFANTS (≤ 1 YEAR)

Despite initial reports of marginal to poor results,[118,123] subsequent experience with dilating the native neonatal and infant aortic coarctation[92,97,100,124–128] appears encouraging. Review of the literature (excluding our reports) reveals that 37 neonates and infants (≤ 1 year) have undergone balloon angioplasty; these data are derived from nine reports.[97,100,118,123–128] Balloon angioplasty reduced the peak systolic pressure gradient across the aortic coarctation from 64 ± 32 to 23 ± 26 mm Hg ($p < 0.001$) in 25 infants in whom pressure data were available. Only 2 of these 37 infants required surgical intervention. In our cases, including those reported previously,[45,92,93,129,130] 18 infants, aged 4 days to 12 months (median 2.7 months), have undergone balloon angioplasty with a resultant reduction in peak systolic pressure gradient across the coarctation from 40 ± 12 to 11 ± 8 mm Hg ($p < 0.001$). All children have improved symptomatically and none have required surgical intervention. The infants who were in heart failure benefitted equally well as those with systemic hypertension. The femoral pulses, which had been either absent or markedly reduced or delayed, became palpable with an increased pulse pressure following angioplasty. Most patients were discharged within 24 to 48 hours following the procedure.

CHILDREN WITH NATIVE COARCTATION

Although not as extensively documented as pulmonic stenosis, several reports,[95–98,100,119,128,131–]

[133] including our own studies,[45,93,129,130] suggest good immediate results. There have been 99 children reported in nine studies.[95–97,100,119,128,131–133] In these studies, the pressure gradient across the coarctation fell from 52 ± 16 to 12 ± 11 mm Hg ($p < 0.001$) in 43 of the children in whom adequate pre- and post-angioplasty pressure data were available for review. From our study of 28 children, aged 14 months to 13 years (median 6.5 years) undergoing balloon angioplasty of unoperated aortic coarctation, the resultant reduction in peak systolic pressure gradient across the aortic coarctation was from 49 ± 23 to 10 ± 9 mm Hg ($p < 0.001$). No patient required immediate surgical intervention. As in the neonate, the femoral pulses became palpable with an increased pulse volume following angioplasty and the hypertension improved. All patients were discharged home within 24 hours following the procedure.

RECOARCTATION FOLLOWING PREVIOUS SURGERY

There are a few reports of balloon angioplasty for recoarctation,[99,117,119–122,134] each reporting good immediate results. Our own experience with recurrent coarctation is limited to nine patients. These children developed recoarctation 6 months to 7 years (26 ± 25 months) following surgical repair. Previous surgery included end-to-end anastomosis after resection of the coarctation in four, patch angioplasty in four (Dacron, 2; subclavian flap, 2), and repair of interrupted aortic arch in one. At the time of balloon angioplasty these children were 6 months to 7 years old (median 22 months). The peak systolic pressure gradient across the coarctation was reduced from 52 ± 20 to 16 ± 8 mm Hg by the procedure. Systemic hypertension improved with a fall in peak systolic pressure from 144 ± 30 to 121 ± 16 mm Hg. All patients improved angiographically.

Follow-up Results

NEONATES AND INFANTS (≤ 1 YEAR)

Follow-up catheterization and angiographic data are available in 8 neonates and infants[91,100,127] from among the 37 infants reported in the literature that have undergone balloon angioplasty. These data were obtained 11 ± 4 months after the procedure. Residual gradients of 22 ± 10 mm Hg are present, and this is significantly improved when compared to the preangioplasty gradients of 50 ± 31 mm Hg. From our group of 18 neonates and infants, follow-up catheterization and angiography were performed in 14 infants, 12 ± 4 months after angioplasty. A mean residual gradient of 18 ± 16 mm Hg was observed, and this was significantly improved compared to the preangioplasty mean gradient of 45 ± 12 mm Hg ($p < 0.001$). Three of these patients developed recoarctation with gradients ≥ 30 mm Hg[130]; two of these patients underwent surgical repair of residual coarctation, and the remaining infant underwent repeat balloon angioplasty, all with good results.

CHILDREN WITH NATIVE COARCTATION

Several groups of workers[96–98,100,199,128,131,133] restudied 7 to 19 children, 1 to 31 months following angioplasty and reported a 14 to 31% rate of recoarctation. From our study group, 16 children underwent repeat catheterization 11 ± 6 months following angioplasty with a residual gradient of 15 ± 12 mm Hg observed. The preangioplasty gradient in these 16 patients was 59 ± 22 mm Hg ($p < 0.001$). Repeat balloon angioplasty was required in two children (12.5%), both with good results. The remaining children are asymptomatic with a reduction in systemic blood pressure (138 ± 27 vs. 110 ± 15 mm Hg, $p < 0.01$) on follow-up.

RECOARCTATION FOLLOWING PREVIOUS SURGERY

Follow-up catheterization and angiographic studies in patients who have had balloon angioplasty for restenosis after surgical repair have been performed by only a few workers.[99,122] Saul and his associates[99] restudied five patients; one patient developed recoarctation, and two patients developed local aortic aneurysms. Cooper et al.[122] recatheterized 21 patients 12 ± 8 months after angioplasty; the residual gradient across the coarctation was 12 ± 9 mm Hg. This had previously been decreased by angioplasty from 37 ± 16 to 14 ± 11 mm Hg. Three of these 21 patients required repeat balloon angioplasty. Two patients developed aneurysms at follow-up, while an aneurysm that developed immediately after angioplasty persisted at follow-up. From our own series, 4 patients underwent follow-up catheterization, and the remaining patients were followed with upper and lower limb blood pressure measurements. The follow-up duration was 3 to 23 months with mean of 11 months. The residual gradient was 6 ± 6 mm Hg with a range of 0–18 mm Hg in those recatheterized. These gradients had been 52 ± 20 mm Hg prior to angioplasty and

16 ± 8 mm Hg immediately following the procedure. No aneurysms were noted.

Applicability to Adult Patients

Although balloon angioplasty of aortic coarctation has most frequently been applied to neonates, infants, and children, it can be used in adults as well.[100,135–137] Although the experience with this procedure in adults is limited, results so far[137] are encouraging. Follow-up studies are required prior to recommending angioplasty as an alternative to surgical therapy in adult patients.

Comparison with Surgical Results

Surgical treatment of coarctation has been available since its initial description by Crafoord[138] and Gross.[139] Fifteen representative studies published since 1980[101–115] are available to assess the results of coarctation surgery. These authors reported follow-up of 25 of 317 patients operated during variable periods of time from 1960 to 1985. Surgical mortality ranges from 0 to 43%, while the late mortality ranges between 4 and 32%. Recoarctation rates also vary between 3 and 25%. The younger the infant in whom one operates, the higher the operative mortality reported and the greater the rate of recurrence. Associated cardiac defects increase both initial and late mortality. Finally, many surgical studies suggest a similar mortality rate and incidence of recoarctation. The balloon angioplasty results, with mortality and recurrence rates (14 to 31%) being similar to those after surgery, appear attractive. Aneurysms following balloon angioplasty,[94,95,97,98] though of concern, have also been seen following surgical correction of coarctation.[140–146] Based on these data, balloon coarctation angioplasty appears to have some advantages over surgery.

Other Issues

REMODELING OF THE AORTA AFTER ANGIOPLASTY

We have examined the data to see if remodeling of the aorta takes place following successful balloon angioplasty of aortic coarctation.[147] The data from the same group of children in whom we examined the causes of recoarctation[130] were utilized for this purpose; group A (13 patients) had good results (peak gradient ≤ 20 mm Hg and no recoarctation on angiography), and group B (7 patients) had fair and poor results (peak gradient > 20 mm Hg with or without recoarctation on angiography). Measurements of the aortic diameter at five sites, namely ascending aorta (immediately proximal to right innominate artery), isthmus, coarctation segment, and descending aorta distal to coarctation and at the level of diaphram, were made in two angiographic views, corrected for magnification, and averaged. A standardized diameter of the aorta at the five locations measured was calculated (Fig. 16.3) for each case pre-angioplasty and at follow-up. The variance (variance is the sum of the squared differences of each measure divided by the degrees of freedom) from norm or unity was determined for each patient before angioplasty and at follow-up. The variance of standardized aortic measures (0.233 vs. 0.287) was similar ($p > 0.05$) in both groups prior to angioplasty, while at follow-up (0.057 vs. 0.129), they were different ($p = 0.01$). There was a greater percentage improvement at follow-up (0.233 vs. 0.057) in group A with good results ($p = 0.002$) than in group B (0.287 vs. 0.129, $p = 0.04$) with fair and poor results. Cluster analysis and visual inspection of aortic shapes (Fig. 16.4) were also indicative of remodeling of the aorta in the group with good results. These data indicate a greater remodeling and normalization of the aorta following successful

balloon angioplasty of aortic coarctation, suggesting that normalized flow across the dilated coarctation allows optimal growth of the aortic segments.[147] A quantitative analysis of angiographic data by Suarez de Lezo[128] suggests a tendency to realignment as determined by a change in configuration angle between proximal and distal aortic segments at follow-up, and these data are supportive of remodeling of the aorta that we observed. The data of Beekman,[97] showing improvement toward unity of the ratio of coarctation site to isthmus diameter, are also indicative of anatomic remodeling after balloon angioplasty.

An 8 to 55% incidence of aneurysms at the site of balloon dilation of aortic coarctation has been reported with native[94,95,97,98] and postoperative[99,122] coarctation. None of these patients with aneurysm required therapy nor did any aneurysm rupture, although elective resection and repair has been advocated by some workers.[95,133] We restudied 30 infants and children 6 to 30 months following dilation of native coarctations and 4 children 6 to 22 months following dilation of recoarctation; one child developed a small aneu-

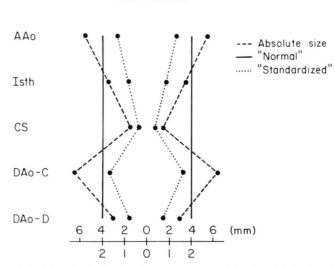

Figure 16.3. Method of obtaining standardized aortic measures. Absolute sizes (dashed line) at all five locations measured are shown. These were then averaged and are represented by the solid lines. The standardized (or normalized) aortic diameter at each site is then calculated by dividing the absolute size by the average (mean) of all the five measurements. The dotted lines represent the final, standardized (or normalized) aortic shape and can be compared to that of other patients or to the same patient after an intervention. AAo, ascending aorta; Isth, aortic isthmus; CS, coarcted segment; DAo-C, descending aorta immediately distal to coarctation; DAo-D, descending aorta at diaphragm. (Reproduced with permission from Rao PS and Carey P. *J Am Coll Cardiol* 14:1312–1317, 1989.)

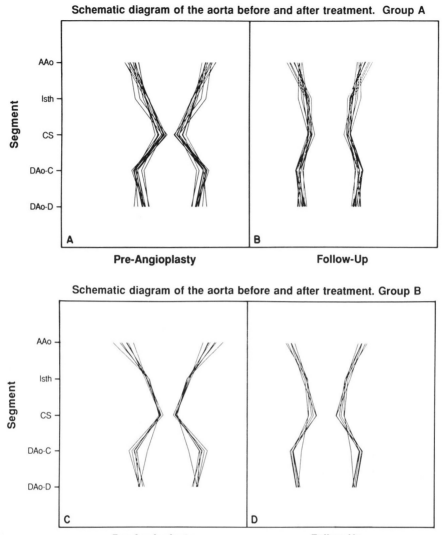

Figure 16.4. Line drawings of the standardized aortic measurements in group A (top panel) and group B (bottom panel). Each pair of lines represent a single patient. Group A patients noted a good hemodynamic result as opposed to group B. Note that aortic shapes are similar in both groups (**A** and **C**) pre-angioplasty. The shape of the aorta improved markedly in group A (**B**), but not in group B. Baseline shape does not appear to play a role in the results from the procedure. Abbreviations as in Figure 16.3 (Reproduced with permission from Rao PS and Carey P. *J Am Coll Cardiol 14*:1312–1317, 1989.)

rysm.[148] We postulate use of large balloons, inadvertent manipulation of catheters/guidewires in the region of freshly dilated aortic coarctation, and misinterpretation or over interpretation of the presence of an aneurysm as possible causes for the aneurysms observed.[93] The observations of Isner et al.[149] of severe depletion and disarray of elastic tissue (so-called cystic medial necrosis) in two-thirds of resected aortic coarctation segments may provide a pathologic basis for this phenomenon.

Further studies to identify factors causing aneurysms following balloon coarctation angioplasty are warranted.

CYANOTIC CONGENITAL HEART DEFECTS

Cyanotic heart defects as a group contribute up to 20 to 25% of all congenital heart defects.[8] In many of these patients, pulmonic stenosis is an integral part of a cardiac malformation that includes a right-to-left shunt. These patients usually present with symptoms in the neonatal period or early infancy. The degree of cyanosis and the level of hypoxemia determine the symptomatology. Physical findings and laboratory data depend on the defect complex and are reasonably characteristic for each defect complex. Total surgical correction and, if that is not feasible, palliation by some type of systemic-to-pulmonary artery anastomosis to augment pulmonary blood flow and to improve oxygenation are usually recommended. With the availability of transluminal balloon dilation, we and others have used this technique to augment pulmonary flow instead relying on the initial or repeat systemic-to-pulmonary shunts. This has been accomplished by use of balloon pulmonary valvuloplasty or by dilating previously created but narrowed Blalock-Taussig (BT) shunts.

INDICATIONS

The indication for balloon pulmonary valvuloplasty in this setting[51] is the presence of cardiac defects not amenable to surgical correction at the time of presentation, while, at the same time, palliation for pulmonary oligemia is required.

Symptoms related to hypoxemia and progressive polycythemia are indications for intervention. The presence of two or more sites of obstruction to pulmonary blood flow (Fig. 16.5) has been considered a prerequisite when employing balloon pulmonary valvuloplasty. If valvular stenosis is the sole obstruction, relief of such an obstruction may result in a marked increase in pulmonary blood flow and elevation of pulmonary artery pressure.

The indications for dilating narrowed BT shunts are similar: cyanotic heart defects not amenable to total surgical correction either because of the age and size of the patient or because of anatomic complexity, while at the same time requiring palliation of pulmonary oligemia.[150] The majority of these patients have associated pulmonary atresia or have a pulmonary artery that cannot be catheterized either because of the severity of obstruction or because of an abnormal or atypical position.

Technical Issues

BALLOON PULMONARY VALVULOPLASTY

The technique of balloon valvuloplasty in patients with complex cyanotic heart defects is similar to that described in the beginning of the chapter and in the

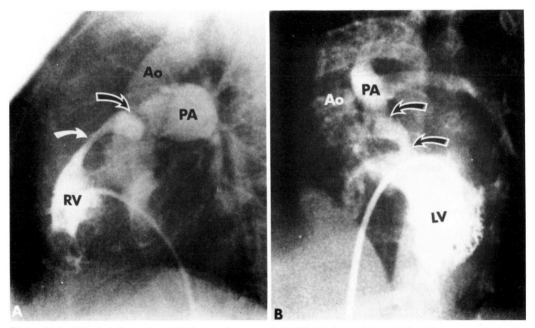

Figure 16.5. Selected cineangiographic frames from a patient with tetralogy of Fallot (**A**) and from a patient with transposition of the great arteries (**B**) demonstrating two sites of pulmonary outflow obstruction (two arrows) in each situation. When the pulmonary valvular obstruction is relieved by balloon valvuloplasty, the subvalvular obstruction remains and prevents flooding of lungs. Ao, aorta; LV, left ventricle; PA, pulmonary artery; RV, right ventricle. (Reproduced with permission from Rao PS. *Current Problems in Cardiology* 26:417–500, 1989.)

section dealing with pulmonic valvular stenosis. At times it may be more difficult to accomplish balloon valvuloplasty in this group compared to patients with simple pulmonary stenosis. We use a balloon maximal diameter that is 1.2 to 1.4 times the pulmonary valve anulus.

BALLOON DILATION OF NARROWED BT SHUNTS

Entry of BT shunts is slightly tricky. We have used custom-made 5-F right coronary catheters to enter the subclavian artery. When it is difficult to advance the catheter across the narrowed shunts, use of 0.014-inch flexible, steerable guidewires and balloon on a wire (USCI) type of devices has been found successful in entering the pulmonary artery through the BT shunt.[150] Progressive dilation with balloons having a diameter equivalent to the diameter of the subclavian artery may be necessary to provide an adequate increase in the pulmonary blood flow.

Acute Results

BALLOON PULMONARY VALVULOPLASTY

Balloon pulmonary valvuloplasty for infants with cyanotic heart defects and pulmonary oligemia has been used by us[51] and others[39,151,152] to augment pulmonary blood flow. Boucek et al.[151] performed balloon pulmonary valvuloplasty in seven children and improved their oxygen saturations from $72 \pm 5\%$ to $83 \pm 5\%$ ($p < 0.005$). The pulmonary arterial pressure and pulmonary blood flow also increased. Qureshi et al.[152] reported their observations after balloon dilation of the pulmonary valve in 15 patients with tetralogy of Fallot and the systemic arterial saturation increased in the majority of patients. In four of the children either no significant change or a deterioration in oxygen saturation occurred. Six children did not require further intervention and four children received a systemic to pulmonary artery shunt at a mean of 1.6 months (0 to 3 months) after the procedure. The authors conclude that balloon dilation may be useful in the management of infants with severe tetralogy of Fallot, and that it should be considered as initial palliative treatment.

Our experience with this procedure, including that reported previously,[51] has been in 12 infants with congenital cyanotic heart defects, aged 3 days to 24 months, weighing 2.9 to 12.0 kg. Percutaneous balloon pulmonary valvuloplasty was performed as a palliative procedure to improve pulmonary oligemia. The diagnoses in these cases included tetralogy of Fallot in five; transposition of

the great arteries (S, D, D) with ventricular septal defect and both valvular and subvalvular pulmonic stenosis in three; critical pulmonary stenosis with intact ventricular septum and hypoplastic right ventricle in three; and ventricular inversion, ventricular septal defect, and both valvular and subvalvular pulmonic stenosis in the final case. Following balloon valvuloplasty, there was an increase of the arterial oxygen saturation ($65.9 \pm 9.7\%$ to $78.4 \pm 13.6\%$, $p < 0.05$), pulmonary blood flow index (1.83 ± 0.55 to 3.14 ± 0.6 liters/min/m^2, $p < 0.05$), pulmonary-to-system flow ratio (0.62 ± 0.35 to 1.2 ± 0.6, $p < 0.05$), and pulmonary artery pressure (16.8 ± 7.2 to 29.2 ± 11.1 mm Hg, $p < 0.02$). Immediate surgical intervention was avoided in all 12 patients.

BALLOON DILATION OF NARROWED BT SHUNTS

Balloon angioplasty of a narrowed BT shunt was initially reported by Fischer and associates[153] and subsequently employed by others.[150,154] Fischer[153] dilated a narrowed BT shunt in a 4-year-old and increased the systemic arterial saturation from 68% to 80%. Marx[154] successfully performed this procedure in five of six patients in whom they attempted the dilation. Two of the five patients benefited markedly and one moderately. In the remaining patients no benefit was shown. We[150] performed this procedure in six children with an increase in arterial oxygen saturations from $71 \pm 8\%$ to $81 \pm 6\%$ ($p < 0.05$). Five children improved markedly, but there was no improvement in the remaining child. This latter child eventually underwent another BT shunt procedure with good results.

Follow-up Results

BALLOON PULMONARY VALVULOPLASTY

There is a limited amount of follow-up data. Boucek et al.[151] reported 0.5- to 2.8-year follow-up results in 7 patients. Four tetralogy of Fallot patients eventually underwent surgical correction, one patient undergoing a systemic-to-pulmonary shunt. The other two did not require surgical intervention. Qureshi[152] reported follow-up observations after balloon angioplasty in 15 tetralogy of Fallot patients. Seven children did not require further palliation during a mean follow-up period of 12.9 months (3.5 to 26 months). Four children required systemic-to-pulmonary artery shunt operation at 0 to 3 months (mean 1.6 months) after balloon valvuloplasty. The final four patients had a corrective operation at 6 to 10 months (mean 8 months) after the procedure.

From our group of patients, with follow-up at 4 to 26 months after the balloon valvuloplasty, all infants are thriving well with decreased hypoxemia and polycythemia. Follow-up catheterization data are available in 10 patients, 3 to 15 months following valvuloplasty, and in all, the immediate post-balloon valvuloplasty improvement has persisted or has shown further improvement. None of the patients had significant elevation of pulmonary arterial systolic pressure at follow-up (23.1 ± 5.8 mm Hg, range 12–28 mm Hg). Two infants with tetralogy of Fallot underwent successful total surgical correction at 6 and 12 months respectively following balloon valvuloplasty. Two infants with transposition of the great arteries showed evidence for an increase in the size of their pulmonary arteries, but because of persistence of hypoxemia, Blalock-Taussig shunts were performed 6 months and 2 years, respectively, following initial balloon valvuloplasty. The other six infants are doing well clinically with continued palliation of pulmonary oligemia. In two of these children, significant improvement in the size of the pulmonary artery has been noted, making it feasible for a safer eventual surgical correction. These data suggest that pulmonary valvuloplasty offers excellent palliation of pulmonary oligemia in cyanotic heart defects, thus avoiding the risks of immediate surgical palliation and paving the way for a better result from eventual total surgical correction. We also suggest that multiple obstructions in series are a necessary prerequisite (Fig. 16.5) for performing balloon valvuloplasty because, if valvular stenosis is the sole obstruction, relief of such an obstruction may result in a marked increase in pulmonary flow, elevation of pulmonary artery pressure, and the development of pulmonary vascular obstructive disease.

BALLOON DILATION OF NARROWED BT SHUNTS

Follow-up data after balloon angioplasty of narrowed BT shunts are scanty. Fischer[153] stated that a dilated shunt was patent two months after angioplasty. Marx[154] stated that on short-term follow-up, three patients (out of five) improved and two did not benefit. Of the six patients from our group, one was a failure. The remaining five children were followed for 3 to 12 months (mean 6 months). Previously symptomatic children had abatement of their symptoms. Hemoglobin levels decreased (19.0 ± 2.7 vs. 17.1 ± 1.9 gm%). Aterial oxygen saturation for the group as a whole remained unchanged from the immediate post-angioplasty values (81 ± 4 vs. 78 ± 10%). One child decreased the oxygen saturation markedly and required further palliation with a contralateral BT shunt. The remaining four children are stable at last follow-up visit without need for further palliation.

VALVULOPLASTY/ANGIOPLASTY FOR OTHER LESIONS

Balloon dilation techniques have been applied to other congenital, acquired, and postoperative stenotic lesions, namely, tricuspid valve stenosis,[155,156] discrete subaortic membranous stenosis,[157–160] pulmonary vein stenosis,[161,162] patent ductus arteriosus (to improve systemic perfusion in patients with interrupted aortic arch,[163] hypoplastic left heart syndrome,[164] and aortic coarctation,[165] respectively), vena caval[166,167] or interatrial baffle[168] obstruction following Mustard or Senning operation for transposition of the great arteries, supravalvular pulmonic stenosis[37] following arterial switch procedure for transposition of the great arteries, bioprosthetic valve stenosis in pulmonary,[169–172] aortic,[173] mitral,[174] and tricuspid[175] positions, and branch pulmonary artery stenosis.[176–178] However, the success of balloon angioplasty/valvuloplasty has varied depending on the lesion dilated and the technique of dilation used. Discussion of these details is beyond the scope of this chapter.

COMPLICATIONS
Immediate

Complications during and immediately after balloon valvuloplasty have been remarkably minimal. Transient bradycardia, premature beats, and a fall in systemic pressure during balloon inflation have been uniformly noted by all workers, particularly with valvular dilations. These return rapidly to normal following balloon deflation. Blood loss requiring transfusion has been reported in many studies. Complete right bundle branch block, transient left bundle branch block,[69] and other transient electrocardiographic abnormalities,[179] transient or permanent heart block,[11,180] ventricular fibrillation (particularly with aortic valvuloplasty[73,179]), cerebrovascular accident,[52,97] loss of consciousness,[11] cardiac arrest,[179] convulsion,[11] transmural tears with vessel wall perforation,[98,179,181–183] balloon rupture at high inflation pressures,[12,40,42,44,184] tricuspid valve papillary muscle rupture,[185] severe infundibular obstruction (following pulmonary valvuloplasty) requiring propranolol administration[18,30,40,47,58] and/or surgical intervention,[40,186] aortic insufficiency or mitral valve tears (following aortic valvuloplasty[179]), hypertension with a *forme fruste* post-coarctectomy syndrome,[45,119,135] and unilateral pulmonary edema,[187,188] though rare, have been reported. Femoral artery thrombosis requiring heparin, streptokinase, or thrombectomy occurred in 39% (12 of 31) of patients undergoing balloon dilation of aortic coarctation or stenosis while such a complication occurred in only 2.2% of arterial catheterizations not involving balloon dilation.[189] Deaths associated with balloon dilation have been reported after angioplasty of peripheral pulmonary artery stenosis,[178,179] of coarctation of the aorta,[120,123,126] and of aortic stenosis[181]; these were either related to vessel wall rupture,[123,178,179,181] occlusion of extremely critical obstruction,[179] or ventricular fibrillation.[120,126]

Fellows and his associates[179] carefully analyzed complications of catheter therapy over a three-year period and reported a 12% incidence of acute complications. Six percent of these were considered major and 6% were considered minor. The mortality rate was 0.7%. The complication rate appears to be related to age of the patient and type of lesion dilated. Patients younger than 6 months of age had a higher rate of complication than older children. Dilation of recurrent coarctations appeared to have the lowest rate of complications (4%), while aortic valvuloplasty has the highest complication rate (40%). Some of these complications may be unavoidable. However, meticulous attention to the details of the technique, use of the appropriate length of the balloon, avoiding extremely high inflation pressures, and short inflation/deflation cycles may help to prevent or reduce complications.

Holter monitoring for 24 hours following balloon valvuloplasty[14] revealed premature ventricular contractions (grade 1, Lown criteria) in one-third of the patients studied. It was not clear[14] whether the premature beats were present prior to valvuloplasty and for how long after valvuloplasty the premature beats persisted. Transient prolongation of the QTc interval following balloon angioplasty/valvuloplasty[190,191] may be a potential hazard for developing R-on-T phenomenon in children with ventricular ectopy. The Holter findings[14] of premature beats following valvuloplasty may have a significance in the light of prolongation of QTc interval.[146] However, no patients from our series or many other studies have been known to develop ventricular arrhythmias. Two cases of sudden death from ventricular

fibrillation shortly after balloon angioplasty of aortic coarctation[120,126] have been reported though. Whether these arrhythmias are related to QTc prolongation is not known. However, patient monitoring following balloon valvuloplasty/angioplasty seems warranted.

Complications at Follow-up

With regard to complications at intermediate-term follow-up, femoral vessel occlusion, aneurysms at the coarctation dilation site, pulmonary valve insufficiency, and the recurrence of obstruction have been noted.

VESSEL OCCLUSION

Between 10 to 29%[14,18,40] of femoral veins through which balloon valvuloplasty hardware has been inserted have been noted to be occluded at follow-up. In the present series, 3 out of 40 patients (8%) that we restudied following pulmonary valvuloplasty have had an occluded femoral vein. It is the general consensus that femoral venous occlusion is more common in small infants.[14,18]

Data with regard to the incidence of femoral artery occlusion at follow-up are not readily available from the literature. Of the 34 infants and children that underwent follow-up catheterization after balloon coarctation angioplasty from our study, three femoral arteries were found to be obstructed (complete in two and partial in one). All of the arteries had good collateral flow.

ANEURYSMS

Aneurysms at the site of balloon dilation of aortic coarctation have been discussed in an earlier section of this chapter.

PULMONARY INSUFFICIENCY

Doppler evidence for pulmonary insufficiency appears sensitive but has been studied by only a few investigators.[14,18,19,192] Rocchini and Beekman[192] reported pulmonary insufficiency in 31 of 37 (84%) patients, while Robertson et al.[19] found mild pulmonary insufficiency in all 29 patients studied. In our group, 34 out of 43 (79%) patients had Doppler evidence for pulmonary insufficiency. However, the pulmonary insufficiency is likely minimal as evidenced by lack of right ventricular volume overloading (normal-sized right ventricle and no paradoxical septal motion) in this group of patients. Similar conclusions have been reported by Tynan using equilibrium-gated radionuclide angiograms.[11] Although long-term follow-up studies for progressive right ventricular volume overloading are not available, the current data suggest that the pulmonary insufficiency produced by balloon valvuloplasty is unlikely to be problematic.

Restenosis

Few studies report intermediate- or long-term results and fewer have investigated causes of recurrence following balloon dilation. The available information[193] with regard to pulmonic stenosis, aortic coarctation, and aortic stenosis will be reviewed.

PULMONIC STENOSIS

Recurrence of valve stenosis following balloon pulmonary valvuloplasty has been reported,[11,13–18] but the reasons for the restenosis at intermediate-term follow-up have been studied only to a limited degree.[11,13–18,31] We have systematically investigated the cause of recurrence of pulmonic stenosis following balloon valvuloplasty.[37,66] On the basis of results of 6- to 34-month follow-up catheterization data in 40 children, two groups were identified: group I with good results (pulmonary valve gradient of 30 mm Hg or less), 33 patients; group II with poor results (gradient greater than 30 mm Hg), 7 patients. Fourteen biographic, anatomic, physiologic, and technical factors were examined by multivariate logistic regression analysis to identify factors associated with restenosis. The identified risk factors were (1) residual pulmonary valve gradient in excess of 30 mm Hg immediately following balloon valvuloplasty and (2) balloon to pulmonary valve anulus ratio less than 1.2. Dysplastic pulmonary valves did not seem to play a role in recurrence, and this may have been due to use of large balloons in patients with dysplastic valves. The data suggest that a balloon:anulus ratio of less than 1.2 is associated with pulmonary valve restenosis at intermediate-term follow-up, and such recurrences can be predicted by noting an immediate post-valvuloplasty pulmonary valve gradient in excess of 30 mm Hg. We suggest use of progressively larger balloons to reduce the valve gradient to less than 30 mm Hg acutely.[66,193]

AORTIC COARCTATION

Recoarctation following balloon angioplasty has been reported by several groups,[92,94,96–98,100,117]

but the reason for recurrence at intermediate-term follow-up has been studied only to a limited degree.[97] We investigated causes of recoarctation following balloon angioplasty of aortic coarctation.[130] On the basis of results of 6 to 30 months' follow-up catheterization data in 20 children, groups were divided based on hemodynamic outcomes: group I, with good results (gradient ≤ 20 mm Hg and no recoarctation on angiograms), 13 patients; group II with fair and poor results (gradients > 20 mm Hg with or without recoarctation on angiography), 7 patients. None developed angiographic aneurysms. Thirty biographic, anatomic, physiologic, and technical variables were examined by multivariate logistic regression analysis, and four factors were identified as risk factors associated with recoarctation: (1) age less than 12 months, (2) an aortic isthmus less than half the size of the ascending aorta, (3) a coarcted aortic segment smaller than 3.5 mm prior to dilation, and (4) a coarcted aortic segment less then 6 mm after angioplasty. A predilation systolic pressure gradient across the aortic coarctation in excess of 50 mm Hg, previously implicated as a risk factor for recurrence by some authors,[97] and the ratios of balloon diameter to both coarcted aortic segment or descending aortic diameter were carefully scrutinized, but neither seemed to influence the presence of recoarctation. The identification of risk factors should help in the selection of patients for balloon angioplasty. Avoiding or minimizing those risk factors should help reduce the rate of recoarctation following angioplasty.[130,193]

AORTIC STENOSIS

Although acute results of balloon aortic valvuloplasty are well-described, only a few studies[71,72,79,82] have reported follow-up results and restenosis rates. To our knowledge, the causes for recurrence of aortic valve stenosis at follow-up have not been studied by others. On the basis of 3- to 32-month (mean 12 months) follow-up results in 18 children, two groups were identified: group I with good results (gradient ≤ 49 mm Hg), 14 patients; and group II with poor results (gradient ≥ 50 mm Hg), 4 patients. All four patients in group II required repeat balloon valvuloplasty or surgical valvotomy; none from group I required surgical procedures. Seventeen biographic, anatomic, physiologic, and technical variables were examined by a multivariate logistic regression analysis to identify factors associated with restenosis. Restenosis was most common in the following situations: (1) age $\leq$ 3 years and (2) an immediate post-valvuloplasty aortic valvular gradient $\geq$ 30 mm Hg.[73–193] Aortic valve morphology[72] and balloon to anulus ratio may also play a significant role in the recurrence of aortic stenosis, but due to the small number of patients evaluated and the narrow range of variability found in our study,[73,193] these factors could not be verified. Identification of risk factors for restenosis should help in patient selection. Because an immediate post-valvuloplasty aortic valvular gradient in excess of 30 mm Hg is a potentially alterable and significant risk factor for restenosis, one might consider using progressively larger balloons in order to reduce the gradient to less than 30 mm Hg.

With regard to other lesions, the data either from the reports in the literature or from our own experience are not adequate for analysis.

MECHANISM OF VALVULOPLASTY AND ANGIOPLASTY

Inflation of a balloon placed across an obstructive lesion exerts radial forces on the stenotic lesion without any axial component.[194] Several physical principles of the "dilating force" are important in the mechanism of action and should be understood for successful application of the balloon dilation technique[194]: (1) for the same pressure, there is a greater dilating force with a larger diameter balloon than with a small diameter balloon; (2) for the same pressure, longer balloons have greater dilating force than shorter balloons; (3) for the same size balloon, the higher the inflation pressure, the greater is the dilating force—these are related in a linear fashion; (4) for the same pressure, a tighter stenotic area will receive a greater dilating force than a less tight stenosis; (5) for the same pressure, a more stenotic area will receive a higher dilating force compared to a less stenotic area; and (6) high inflation pressures will not significantly increase the diameter of the balloon, because the balloon material (especially the treated polyethylene in most pediatric dilation balloons) does not overexpand. The balloon material "yield strength" (the force at which permanent deformation of the material occurs) and "ultimate tensile strength" (the force necessary to break the material) are very close to each other.

Based on these principles and our experience with balloon dilations in children, we now routinely perform sequential balloon inflations every 5 minutes with 3, 4, and 5 atmospheres of pressure

using 5 sec duration each time. If the waist in the balloon cannot be abolished, then we sequentially increase the pressure of inflation to 6, 7, and 8 atmospheres of pressure. This has been required on only two occasions (both native coarctations) out of a total experience of 200 balloon dilations in children.

The mechanism of congenital aortic and pulmonic valvuloplasty has been assessed by Walls and his associates by direct vision at surgery.[82] They found tearing of valve raphae, tearing of the valve leaflets themselves, and avulsion of the valve leaflets. Direct visual observations by others,[11–13,51] though limited in numbers, and echocardiographic observations[19] also indicate similar mechanisms. The circumferential dilating force exerted by balloon inflation is likely to rupture (tear) the weakest part of the valve mechanism. It is likely that the fused commissures are the weakest links that can be broken with balloon dilation. However, in a given patient, when the fused commissures are strong and cannot be torn, tears in the valve cups or avulsion of the valve leaflets[82] can occur. The latter events may cause severe semilunar valve insufficiency.

Lock and his associates[195,196] created aortic coarctations and branch pulmonary artery stenoses in newborn lambs and balloon-dilated the stenotic lesions in order to examine the mechanism of balloon angioplasty. Linear intimal tears were observed in both types of lesions located at or near the area of maximal narrowing in branch pulmonary artery stenotic lesions and in the nonoperated aortic wall in aortic coarctations. The intimal tears were noted to extend into the media with intramedial hemorrhage. No evidence for adventitial rupture was observed.[195,196] These mechanisms of relief may be similar in postoperative recoarctations but may not be applicable to native, previously unoperated stenotic lesions. The presence of intimal and medial tears following dilation of human aortic coarctation in both in vivo[119,120,123] and in excised coarctation segments[197] and branch pulmonary arteries[198] has also been reported by several workers, although these observations have been in a small number of cases. Thus the mechanism of relief of arterial obstruction is likely by tearing the intima and media.

CONCLUSIONS AND FUTURE DIRECTIONS

The technique of balloon dilation of stenotic lesions of the heart and great vessels in infants and children has been available since 1982. This technique has been used extensively in isolated valvular pulmonic stenosis with excellent immediate and reasonably good intermediate-term follow-up results. Refinements in the technique may further decrease the restenosis rate. *Balloon pulmonary valvuloplasty* is now the procedure of choice in the treatment of moderate to severe valvular pulmonic stenosis. *Balloon dilation of aortic valve stenosis* produces reasonable immediate results, but long-term studies are needed prior to making definitive recommendations. However, the aortic valvuloplasty technique is attractive in neonates with critical aortic obstruction. Although good immediate and intermediate-term follow-up results of *balloon angioplasty of coarctation of the aorta* have been reported, recommendations for use of this technique as the treatment of choice have been clouded by the reports of aneurysms at the site of coarctation dilation. We interpret the available data as supportive for the recommendation of balloon angioplasty as the treatment of choice in neonates and infants with aortic coarctations. General use of this technique in children should perhaps await longer follow-up results in a larger number of children. *Balloon valvuloplasty of pulmonary stenosis in association with other congenital heart defects* and *dilation of the narrowed BT shunt*, though reported by only a few groups, has been associated with good immediate and follow-up results and appears to be an effective alternative to surgical aorta-to-pulmonary artery anastomosis. Despite good results in many other lesions, there is very little experience in children with other defects to make a definitive recommendation at this time.

The indications for balloon dilation of stenotic lesions of the heart and great vessels are essentially the same as those used for surgical therapy. The technique of balloon angioplasty/valvuloplasty should now be added to the therapeutic armamentarium available to the pediatric cardiologist in the management of infants and children with heart disease.

Thus far only one- to two-year follow-up results are available. Five- to 10-year follow-up results to document long-term effectiveness of balloon dilation are needed for all stenotic lesions.

Miniaturization of currently bulky dilating catheter systems and improvement in the inflation/deflation time for these balloons are necessary for increasing the safety and effectiveness of this technique in infants and children. Meticulous attention to the details of the technique and further refinement of the procedure will likely further reduce the complication rate. Transcatheter laser techniques to relieve stenotic lesions and visualization of these lesions while relieving the obstruction by dual fiberoptic catheters have been used in postmortem stenotic lesions and animal models. Further development and refinement of these latter techniques in animal models followed by clinical trials may result in their application to infants and children with obstructive lesions in the heart and great vessels.

The transcatheter techniques offer promise as excellent alternatives to open or closed heart surgery in the treatment of several congenital heart defects.

Acknowledgment

The author wishes to acknowledge the contribution to this material made by past and present pediatric cardiology and cardiovascular surgery staff at the King Faisal Specialist Hospital and Research Center, Riyadh, Saudi Arabia, and University of Wisconsin Medical School/Children's Hospital, Madison, Wisconsin, including Dr. J. Al Halees, M. Brais, P. S. Chopra, M. E. Fawzy, O. Galal, F. Kutayli, J. M. Levy, M. K. Mardini, H. N. Najjar, L. Solymar, M. K. Thapar, and A. D. Wilson. The author also thanks Mr. P. Carey and Mrs. M. Kraak for their help, in the statistical analysis and manuscript preparation, respectively.

REFERENCES

1. Rubio V, Limon Lason R. Treatment of pulmonary valvular stenosis and tricuspid stenosis using a modified catheter. Second World Congress on Cardiology, Washington, DC, 1954, Program Abstracts II, p. 205.
2. Semb BKH, Tijonneland S, Stake G, Aabyholm G. Balloon valvulotomy of congenital pulmonary valve stenosis with tricuspid valve insufficiency. *Carciovasc Radiol 2*:239–241. 1979.
3. Kan JS, White RI Jr., Mitchell SE, Gardner TJ. Percutaneous balloon valvuloplasty: A new method for treating congenital pulmonary valve stenosis. *N Engl J Med 307*:540–542, 1982.
4. Dotter CT, Judkins MP. Transluminal treatment of arteriosclerotic obstuction: Description of a new technique and a preliminary report of its application. *Circulation 30*:654–670, 1964.
5. Zeitler E, Gruntzig A, Schoop W. *Percutaneous vascular recanalization: Technique, application, clinical results.* Berlin, Springer-Verlag, 1978.
6. Grunzig AR, Senning A, Siegothaler WE. Nonoperative dilatation of coronary artery stenosis: Percutaneous transluminal coronary angioplasty. *N Engl J Med 301*:61–68, 1979.

7. Nadas AS, Fyler DC. *Pediatric Cardiology*, 3rd ed., Philadelphia, W.B. Saunders, 1972, p. 683.

8. Keith JD, Rowe RD, Vlad P. *Heart Disease in Infancy and Childhood*, 3rd ed, New York, The MacMillan Co., 1978, pp. 4–6.

9. Nadas AS. Pulmonary stenosis: Indications for surgery in children and adults. *New Engl J Med* 287:1196–1197, 1972.

10. Nugent EW, Freedom RM, Nora JJ, Ellison RC, Rowe RD, Nadas AS. Clinical course of pulmonic stenosis. *Circulation* 56(Suppl I):1-18–1-47, 1977.

11. Tynan M, Baker EJ, Rohmer J, et al. Percutaneous balloon pulmonary valvuloplasty. *Br Heart J* 53:520–524, 1985.

12. Lababidi Z, Wu JR. Percutaneous balloon pulmonary valvuloplasty. *Am J Cardiol* 52:560–562, 1983.

13. Kan JS, White RI Jr, Mitchel SE, Anderson JH, Gardner TJ. Percutaneous transluminal balloon valvuloplasty for pulmonary valve stenosis. *Circulation* 69:554–560, 1984.

14. Kveselis DA, Rocchini AP, Snider AP, Rosenthal A, Crowley DC, Dick M. Results of balloon valvuloplasty in the treatment of congenital valvar pulmonary stenosis in children. *Am J Cardiol* 56:527–532, 1985.

15. Miller GAH. Balloon valvuloplasty and angioplasty in congenital heart disease. *Br Heart J* 54:285–289, 1986.

16. Sullivan ID, Robinson PJ, Macartney FJ, et al. Percutaneous balloon valvuloplasty for pulmonary stenosis in infants and children. *Br Heart J* 54:435–441, 1986.

17. Radtke W, Keane JF, Fellows KE, Lang P, Lock JE. Percutanous balloon valvotomy of congenital pulmonary stenosis using oversized balloons. *J Am Coll Cardiol* 8:909–915, 1986.

18. Rey C, Marche P, Francart C, Dupuis C. Percutaneous transluminal balloon valvuloplasty of congenital pulmonary valve stenosis, with a special report on infants and neonates. *J Am Coll Cardiol* 11:815–820, 1988.

19. Robertson M, Benson LN, Smallhorn JF, Musewe N, Freedom RM, Moes CAF, Burrows P, Johnston AE, Burrows FA, Rowe RD. The morphology of the right ventricular outflow tract after percutaneous pulmonary valvotomy: Long term follow-up *Br Heart J* 58:239–244, 1987.

20. Mullins CE, Nihill MR, Vick WG III, Ludomirsky A, O'Laughlin MP, Bricker JT, Judd VE. Double balloon technique for dilatation of valvar or vessel stenosis in congenital and acquired heart disease. *J Am Coll Cardiol* 10:107–114, 1987.

21. Rao PS. Indications for balloon pulmonary valvuloplasty (Editorial). *Am Heart J* 116:1661–1662, 1989.

22. Engle MA, Ito T, Goldbery HP. The fate of the patient with pulmonic stenosis. *Circulation* 30:554–561, 1964.

23. Mody MR. The natural history of uncomplicated valvar pulmonic stenosis. *Am Heart J* 90:317–321, 1975.

24. Stevenson JG, Kawabori I. Noninvasive determination of pressure gradients in children: Two methods employing pulsed Doppler echocardiography. *J Am Coll Cardiol* 3:179–192, 1984.

25. Rao PS. Doppler ultrasound in the prediction of transvalvar pressure gradients in patients with valvar pulmonic stenosis. *Internat J Cardiol* 15:195–203, 1987.

26. Musewe NN, Roberston MA, Benson LN, Smallhorn JR, Burrows PE, Freedom RM, Moes CAF, Rowe RD. The dysplastic pulmonary valve: Echocardiographic features and results of balloon dilatation. *Br Heart J* 57:364–370, 1987.

27. DiSessa TG, Alpert BS, Chase NA, Birnbaum SE, Watson DG. Balloon valvuloplasty in children with dysplastic pulmonary valves. *Am J Cardiol* 66:405–407, 1987.

28. Marantz PM, Huhta JC, Mullins CE, Murphy DM Jr., Nihill MR, Ludomirsky A, Yoon GY. Results of balloon valvuloplasty in typical and dysplastic pulmonary valve stenosis: Doppler echocardiographic follow-up. *J Am Coll Cardiol* 12:476–479, 1988.

29. Rao PS. Balloon dilatation in infants and children with dysplastic pulmonary valves: Short-term and intermediate-term results. *Am Heart J* 116:1168–1176, 1988.

30. Thapar MK, Rao PS. Use of propranolol for severe dynamic infundibular obstruction prior to balloon pulmonary valvuloplasty. *Cathet Cardiovasc Diagn* 19:240–241, 1990.

31. Rao PS. Influence of balloon size on the short-term and long-term results of pulmonary valvuloplasty. *Texas Heart Institute J* 14:57–61, 1987.

32. Rao PS. How big a balloon and how many balloons for pulmonary valvuloplasty? (Editorial). *Am Heart J* 116:577–580, 1989.

33. Rao PS. Further observations on the role of balloon size on the short-term and intermediate-term results of balloon pulmonary valvuloplasty. *Br Heart J* 60:507–511, 1988.

34. Rao PS. Balloon pulmonary valvuloplasty: A review. *Clin Cardiol* 12:55–74, 1989.

35. Ring JC, Kulik TJ, Burke BA. Morphologic changes induced by dilatation of pulmonary valve annulus with over-large balloons in normal newborn lamb. *Am J Cardiol* 55:210–214, 1986.

36. Rao PS, Fawzy ME. Double balloon technique for percutaneous balloon pulmonary valvuloplasty: Comparison with single balloon technique. *J Interventional Cardiol* 1:257–262, 1988.

37. Rao PS. Balloon angioplasty and valvuloplasty in infants, children, and adolescents. *Current Problems in Cardiol* 14(8):417–500, 1989.

38. Srivastava S, Sundar AS, Muhkopadyaya S, Rajani M. Percutaneous transluminal balloon pulmonary

valvuloplasty: Long-term results. *Internat J Cardiol* 17:303–314, 1987.

39. McCredie RM, Lee CL, Swinburn MJ, Warner G. Balloon dilatation pulmonary valvuloplasty in pulmonary stenosis. *Aust NZ J Med* 16:20–23, 1986.

40. Ali Khan MA, Al Yousef S, Mullins CE. Percutaneous transluminal balloon pulmonary valvuloplasty for the relief of pulmonary valve stenosis with special reference to double-balloon technique. *Am Heart J* 112:158–166, 1986.

41. Fontes VF, Sousa JEMR, Esteves CA, Silva MVD, Cano MN, Maldonado G. Pulmonary valvuloplasty—Experience of 100 cases. *Internat J Cardiol* 21:335–342, 1988.

42. Mullins CE, Ludomirsky A, O'Laughlin MP, et al. Balloon valvuloplasty for pulmonic valve stenosis: Two year follow-up hemodynamic and Doppler evaluation. *Cathet Cardiovasc Diagn* 14:76–81, 1988.

43. Ali Khan MA, Al-Yousef S, Huhta JC, Bricker JT, Mullins CE, Sawyer W. Critical pulmonary valve stenosis in patients less than 1 year of age: Treatment with percutaneous gradational balloon pulmonary valvuloplasty. *Am Heart J* 117:1008–1014, 1989.

44. Rao PS, Mardini MK. Pulmonary valvotomy without thoracotomy: The experience with percutaneous balloon pulmonary valvuloplasty. *Ann Saudi Med* 5:149–155, 1985.

45. Rao PS. Transcatheter treatment of pulmonic stenosis and coarctation of the aorta: The experience with percutaneous balloon dilatation. *Br. Heart J* 56:250–258, 1986.

46. Rao PS. Transcatheter management of heart disease in infants and children. *Pediat Rev Comm* 1:1–18, 1987.

47. Rao PS, Fawzy ME, Solymar L, Mardini MK. Longterm results of balloon pulmonary valvuloplasty. *Am Heart J* 115:1291–1296, 1988.

48. Rao PS, Solymar L. Electrocardiographic changes following balloon dilatation of valvar pulmonic stenosis. *J Interventional Cardiol* 1:189–197, 1988.

49. Rao PS. Value of echo-Doppler studies in the evaluation of the results of balloon pulmonary valvuloplasty. *J Cardiovasc Ultrasonography* 5:309–312, 1986.

50. Tynan M, Jones O, Joseph MC, Deverall PB, Yates AK. Relief of pulmonary valve stenosis in the first week of life by percutaneous balloon valvuloplasty (letter). *Lancet* 1:123, 1984.

51. Rao PS, Brais M. Balloon pulmonary valvuloplasty for congenital cyanotic heart defects. *Am Heart J* 115:1105–1113, 1988.

52. Zeevi B, Keane JF, Fellows KE, Lock JE. Balloon dilatation of critical pulmonary stenosis in the first week of life. *J Am Coll Cardiol* 11:821–824, 1988.

53. Pepine CJ, Gessner IH, Feldman RL. Percutaneous balloon valvuloplasty for pulmonic valve stenosis in the adult. *Am J Cardiol* 50:1442–1445, 1983.

54. Gibbs, JL, Stanley CP, Dickenson D. Pulmonary balloon valvuloplasty in late adult life. *Internat J Cardiol* 11:237–239, 1986.

55. Al Kasab S, Riberio P, Al Zaibag M. Use of double balloon technique for percutaneous balloon pulmonary valvotomy in adults. *Br Heart J* 58:136–141, 1987.

56. Fawzy ME, Mercer EN, Dunn B. Late results of pulmonary balloon valvuloplasty in adults using double balloon technique. *J Interventional Cardiol* 1:35–42, 1988.

57. Al Kasab S, Ribeiro PA, Al Zaibag M, Halim M, Haggab MA, Shahid M. Percutaneous double balloon pulmonary valvotomy in adults: One- to two-year follow-up. *Am J Cardiol* 62:822–825, 1988.

58. Thapar MK, Rao PS. Significance of infundibular obstruction following balloon valvuloplasty for valvar pulmonic stenosis. *Am Heart J* 118:99–103, 1989.

59. Brock RC. Pulmonary valvotomy for relief of congenital pulmonary stenosis: Report of three cases. *Brit Med J* 1:1121–1126, 1948.

60. Campbell M, Brock R. The results of valvotomy for simple pulmonary stenosis. *Br Heart J* 17:229–246, 1954.

61. Engle MA, Ito T, Goldberg HP. The fate of the patient with pulmonic stenosis. *Circulation* 30:554–561, 1964.

62. Reid JM, Coleman EN, Stevenson JG, Inall JA, Doig WG. Longterm results of surgical treatment for pulmonary valve stenosis. *Arch Dis Child* 51:79–81, 1976.

63. McNamara DG, Latson LA. Longterm follow-up of patients with malformations for which definitive surgical repair has been available for 25 years or more. *Am J Cardiol* 50:560–568, 1982.

64. Kopecky SL, Gersh BJ, McGoon MD, et al. Longterm outcome of patients undergoing surgical repair of isolated pulmonary valve stenosis: Follow-up at 20-30 years. *Circulation* 78:1150–1156, 1988.

65. Lock JE, Keane JE, Fellows KE. The use of catheter intervention procedures for congenital heart disease (Editorial). *J Am Coll Cardiol* 6:1420–1423, 1986.

66. Rao PS, Thapar MK, Kutayli F. Causes of restenosis following balloon valvuloplasty for valvar pulmonic stenosis. *Am J Cardiol* 62:979–982, 1988.

67. Jones M, Barnhart GR, Morrow AG. Late results after operations for left ventricular outflow tract obstruction. *Am J Cardiol* 50:569–579, 1982.

68. Ankeney JL, Tzeng TS, Liebman J. Surgical therapy for congenital aortic valvular stenosis: A 23-year experience. *J Thorac Cardiovasc Surg* 85:41–48, 1983.

69. Hsieh KS, Keane JF, Nadas AS, Bernhard WF, Castaneda AR. Longterm follow-up of valvotomy

before 1968 for congenital aortic stenosis. *Am J Cardiol* 58:338–341, 1986.

70. Jack WD II, Kelly DT. Long-term follow-up of valvulotomy for congenital aortic stenosis. *Am J Cardiol* 38:231–234, 1976.

71. Lababidi Z, Wu J, Walls JT. Percutaneous balloon aortic valvuloplasty: Results in 23 patients. *Am J Cardiol* 53:194–197, 1984.

72. Sholler GF, Keane JF, Perry SB, Sanders SP, Lock JE. Balloon dilatation of congenital aortic valve stenosis: Results and influence of technical and morphologic features on outcome. *Circulation* 78:351–360, 1988.

73. Rao PS, Thapar MK, Wilson AD, Levy JM, Chopra PS. Intermediate-term follow-up results of balloon aortic valvuloplasty in infants and children with special reference to causes of restenosis. *Am J Cardiol* 64:1356–1360, 1989.

74. Sandor GGS, Olley PM, Trussler GA, Williams WG, Rowe RD, Morch JE. Long-term follow-up of patients after valvotomy for congenital valvar aortic stenosis in children. *J Thorac Cardiovasc Surg* 80:171–176, 1980.

75. Wagner HR, Ellison RC, Kenae JF, Humphries JO, Nadas AS. Clinical course in aortic stenosis. *Circulation* 56(Suppl I):147–156, 1977.

76. Lawson RM, Bonchik LI, Menashe V, Starr A. Late results of surgery for left ventricular outflow tract obstruction in children. *J Thorac Cardiovasc Surg* 71:334–342, 1976.

77. Dobell ARC, Bloss RS, Gibbons JE, Colins GF. Congenital valvular aortic stenosis: Surgical management and long-term results. *J Thorac Cardiovasc Surg* 81:916–920, 1981.

78. Presbitero P, Somerville J, Revel-chion R, Ross D. Open aortic valvotomy for congenital aortic stenosis: Late results. *Br Heart J* 42:26–34, 1982.

79. Helgason H, Keane JF, Fellows KE, Kulik TJ, Lock JE. Balloon dilatation of aortic valve: Studies in normal lambs and in children with aortic stenosis. *J Am Coll Cardiol* 9:916–920, 1987.

80. Choy M, Beekman RH, Rocchini AP, Crowley DC, et al. Percutaneous balloon valvuloplasty for valvar aortic stenosis in infants and children. *Am J Cardiol* 59:1010–1013, 1987.

81. Wren C, Sullivan I, Bull C, Deanfield J. Percutaneous balloon dilatation of aortic valve stenosis in neonates and infants. *Br Heart J* 58:608–612, 1987.

82. Walls JT, Lababidi Z, Curtis JJ, Silver D. Assessment of percutaneous balloon pulmonary and aortic valvuloplasty. *J Thorac Cardiovasc Surg* 88:352–356, 1984.

83. Beekman RH, Rocchini AP, Crowley DC, Snider AR, Serwery GA, Dick M II, Rosenthal A. Comparison of single and double balloon valvuloplasty in children with aortic stenosis. *J Am Coll Cardiol* 12:480–485, 1988.

84. Rao PS. Balloon aortic valvuloplasty in children: A review. *Clin Cardiol* 13:458–466, 1990.

85. Lababidi Z. Aortic balloon valvuloplasty. *Am Heart J* 106:751–752, 1983.

86. Swan H, Korz A. Direct vision trans-aortic approach to the aortic valve during hypothermia: Experimental observations and report of a successful clinical case. *Ann Surg* 144:205–214, 1956.

87. Lewis FJ, Shumway NE, Niazi SA, Benjamin RB. Aortic valvotomy under direct vision during hypothermia. *J Thorac Surg* 32:481–499, 1956.

88. Inoue K, Owaki T, Nakamura T, et al. Clinical applications of transvenous mitral commissurotomy by a new balloon catheter. *J Thorac Cardiovasc Surg* 87:394–402, 1984.

89. Kvesellis DA, Rocchini AP, Beekman R, Snider AR, Crowley DN, Dick M, Rosenthal A. Balloon angioplasty for congenital and rheumatic mitral stenosis. *Am J Cardiol* 57:348–350, 1986.

90. Alday LE, Juaneda E. Percutaneous balloon dilation in congenital mitral stenosis. *Br Heart J* 57:479–482, 1987.

91. Perry SB, Zeevi B, Keane JF, Lock JE. Interventional catheterization of left-heart lesions, including aortic and mitral valve stenosis and coarctation of the aorta. *Cardiol Clinics* 7(2):341–349, 1989.

92. Rao PS. Balloon angioplasty for coarctation of the aorta in infancy. *J Pediatr* 110:713–718, 1987.

93. Rao PS, Najjar HN, Mardini MK, Solymar L, Thapar MK. Balloon angioplasty for coarctation of the aorta: Immediate and long-term results. *Am Heart J* 115:657–664, 1988.

94. Marvin WJ, Mahoney LT, Rose EF. Pathological sequelae of balloon dilation angioplasty for unoperated coarctation of the aorta in children (Abstract). *J Am Coll Cardiol* 7:117A, 1986.

95. Cooper RS, Ritter SB, Rothe WB, Chen CK, Griepp R, Golinko RJ. Angioplasty for coarctation of the aorta: Long-term results. *Circulation* 75:600–604, 1987.

96. Wren C, Peart I, Bain H, Hunter S. Balloon dilatation of unoperated aortic coarctation: Immediate results and one year follow-up. *Br Heart J* 58:369–373, 1987.

97. Beekman RH, Rocchini AP, Dick M II, Snider AR, Crowley DC, Serwer GA, Spicer RL, Rosenthal A. Percutaneous balloon angioplasty for native coarctation of the aorta. *J Am Coll Cardiol* 10:1078–1084, 1987.

98. Morrow WR, Vick GW III, Nihill MR, Rokey R, Johnston DL, Hedrick TD, Mullins CE. Balloon dilatation of unoperated coarctation of the aorta: Short- and intermediate-term results. *J Am Coll Cardiol* 11:133–138, 1988.

99. Saul JP, Keane JF, Fellows KE, Lock JE. Balloon dilatation angioplasty of postoperative aortic obstructions. *Am J Cardiol* 59:943–948, 1987.

100. Lababidi ZA, Daskalopoulos DA, Stoeckle H Jr.

Transluminal balloon coarctation angioplasty: Experience with 27 patients. *Am J Cardiol 54*:1288–1291, 1984.

101. Coganoglu A, Teply JF, Grunkemeier GL, Sunderland CO, Starr A. Coarctation of the aorta in patients younger than three months: A critique of the subclavian flap operation. *J Thorac Cardiovasc Surg 89*:128–135, 1985.

102. Kopf GS, Hellenbrand W, Kleinman C. Lister G, Talner N, Laks H. Repair of aortic coarctation in the first three months of life: Immediate and long-term results. *Ann Thorac Surg 41*:425–430, 1986.

103. Goldman S, Hernandez J, Pappas G. Results of surgical treatment of coarctation of the aorta in the critically ill neonate: Including the influence of pulmonary artery banding. *J Thorac Cardiovasc Surg 91*:732–737, 1986.

104. Sanchez GR, Balara RK, Dunn JM, Mehta AV, O'Riordan AC. Recurrent obstruction after subclavian flap repair of coarctation of the aorta in infants. Can it be predicted or prevented? *J Thorac Cardiovasc Surg 91*:738–746, 1986.

105. Beekman RH, Rocchini AP, Behrendt DM, et al. Long-term outcome after repair of coarctation in infancy: Subclavian angioplasty does not reduce the need for reoperation. *J Am Coll Cardiol 8*:1406–1411, 1986.

106. Metzdorff MT, Cobanoglu A, Grunkemeier GL, Sunderland CO, Starr A. Influence of age at operation on late results with subclavian flap aortoplasty. *J Thorac Cardiovasc Surg 89*:235–241, 1985.

107. Lerberg DB, Hardesty RL, Siewers RD, Zuberbuhler JR, Bahnson HT. Coarctation of the aorta in infants and children; 25 years of experience. *Ann Thorac Surg 33*:159–170, 1982.

108. Fyler DC, Buckley LP, Hellenbrand WE, et al. Report of the New England Regional Infant Cardiac Program. *Pediatrics 65*(Suppl.):375–461, 1980.

109. Kamau P, Miles V, Toews W, et al. Surgical repair of coarctation of the aorta in infants less than six months of age. *J Thorac Cardiovasc Surg 82*:171–179, 1981.

110. Hesslein PS, McNamara DG, Morris MJH, Hallman GL, Cooley DA. Comparison of resection versus patch aortoplasty for repair of coarctation in infants and children. *Circulation 64*:164–168, 1981.

111. Ziemer G, Jonas RA, Perry SB, Freed MD, Casteneda AR. Surgery for coarctation of the aorta in the neonate. *Circulation 74*:I-25–I-31, 1986.

112. Yee ES, Soifer SJ, Turley K, Verrier ED, Fishman NH, Ebert PA. Infant coarctation: A spectrum in clinical presentation and treatment. *Ann Thorac Surg 42*:488–493, 1986.

113. Fenchel G, Steil E, Seybold-Epting W, Seboldt H, Apitz J, Hoffmeister H. Repair of symptomatic aortic coarctation in the first three months of life: Early and late results after resection and end-to-end anastomosis and subclavian flap angioplasty. *J Cardiovasc Surg 29*:257–263, 1988.

114. Koller M, Rothlin M, Senning A. Coarctation of the aorta: Review of 362 operated patients. Long-term follow-up and assessment of prognostic variables. *Eur Heart J 8*:670–679, 1987.

115. Vouhe PR, Trinquet F, Lecompte Y, Verhant F, Roux P, Touati G, Pome G, Leca F, Weveux J. Aortic coarctation with hypoplastic aortic arch: Results of extended end-to-end aortic arch anastomosis. *J Thorac Cardiovasc Surg 96*:557–563, 1988.

116. Rao PS. Balloon dilatation in infants and children with cardiac defects. *Cathet Cardiovasc Diagn 18*:136–149, 1989.

117. Rao PS. Which aortic coarctations should we balloon-dilate? (editorial) *Am Heart J 117*:987–989, 1989.

118. Lock JE, Bass JL, Amplatz K, Fuhrman BP, Castaneda-Zuniga W. Balloon dilatation angioplasty of aortic coarctations in infants and children. *Circulation 68*:109–116, 1983.

119. Allen HD, Marx GR, Ovitt TW, Goldberg SJ. Balloon dilatation angioplasty for coarctation of the aorta. *Am J Cardiol 57*:828–832, 1986.

120. Kan JS, White RI Jr, Mitchell SE, Farmiett EJ, Danahoo JS, Gardner TJ. Treatment of restenosis of coarctation by percutaneous transluminal angioplasty. *Circulation 68*:1087–1094, 1983.

121. Hess J, Mooyaart EL, Busch HJ, Bergstra A, Landsman MI. Percutaneous transluminal balloon angioplasty in restenosis of coarctation of the aorta. *Br Heart J 55*:459–461, 1986.

122. Cooper SG, Sullivan ID, Wren C. Treatment of recoarctation: Balloon dilatation angioplasty. *J Am Coll Cardiol 14*:413–419, 1989.

123. Finley JP, Beaulieu RG, Nanton MA, Roy DL. Balloon catheter dilatation of coarctation of the aorta in young infants. *Br Heart J 50*:411–415, 1983.

124. Lababidi Z. Neonatal transluminal balloon coarctation angioplasty. *Am Heart J 106*:752–753, 1983.

125. Sperling DR, Dorsey TJ, Rowen M, Gazzaniga AB. Percutaneous transluminal angioplasty of congenital coarctation of the aorta. *Am J Cardiol 51*:562–564, 1983.

126. Suarez de Lezo J, Fernandez R, Sancho M, et al. Percutaneous transluminal angioplasty for aortic isthemic coarctation in infancy. *Am J Cardiol 54*:1147–1149, 1984.

127. Alyousef S, Khan A, Nihill M, Lababidi Z, Mullins C. Perutane transvenose antegrade balloon angioplastie bei Aortenisthmusstenose. *Herz 13*:36–40, 1988.

128. Suarez de Lezo J, Sancho M, Pan M, Romero M, Olivera C, Liques M. Antiographic follow-up after balloon angioplasty for coarctation of the aorta. *J Am Coll Cardiol 13*:689–695, 1989.

129. Rao PS, Mardini MK, Najjar HN. Relief of coarctation of the aorta without thoracotomy: The experience with percutaneous balloon angioplasty. *Ann Saudi Med* 6:193–203, 1986.

130. Rao PS, Thapar MK, Kutayli F, Carey P. Causes of recoarctation following balloon angioplasty of unoperated aortic coarctations. *J Am Coll Cardiol* 13:109–115, 1989.

131. Cooper RS, Ritter SB, Golinko RJ. Balloon dilatation angioplasty: Nonsurgical management of coarctation of the aorta. *Circulation* 70:903–907, 1984.

132. Brodsky SJ. Percutaneous balloon angioplasty: Treatment for congenital coarctation of the aorta and congenital valval pulmonic stenosis. *Am J Dis Child* 138:851–854, 1984.

133. Brandt B III, Marvin WJ Jr., Rose EF, Mahoney LT. Surgical treatment of coarctation of the aorta after balloon angioplasty. *J Thorac Cardiovasc Surg* 94:715–719, 1987.

134. Lorber A, Ettedgui JA, Baker EJ, Jones ODH, Reidy J, Tynan M. Balloon angioplasty for recoarctation following the subclavian flap operation. *Internat J Cardiol* 10:57–63, 1986.

135. Lababidi Z, Madigan N, Wu J, Murphy TJ. Balloon coarctation angioplasty in an adult. *Am J Cardiol* 53:350–351, 1984.

136. Tegtmeyer CJ, Wellons HA, Thompson RN. Balloon dilatation of the abdominal aorta. *J Am Med Assoc* 23:2636–2637, 1980.

137. Attia IM, Lababidi ZA. Early results of balloon angiography of native aortic coarctation in young adults. *Am J Cardiol* 61:930–931, 1988.

138. Crafoord D, Nylin G. Congenital coarctation of the aorta and its surgical treatment. *J Thorac Cardiovasc Surg* 14:347–361, 1945.

139. Gross RE, Hufnagel CA. Coarctation of the aorta. Experimental studies regarding its surgical correction. *N Engl J Med* 237:287–293, 1945.

140. Olsson P, Soderland S, Dabiel WT, Ovenfors CO. Patch grafts or tubular grafts in repair of coarctation of the aorta. *Scand J Thorac Cardiovasc Surg* 10:139–143, 1976.

141. Rheuban K, Gutgesel HP, Carpenter MA, et al. Aortic aneurysms after patch angioplasty for aortic isthmic coarctation in childhood. *Am J Cardiol* 58:178–180, 1986.

142. Hehrlein FW, Mulch J, Rautenburg HW, Schlepper M, Scheld HH. Incidence and pathogenesis of late aneurysms after patch graft aortoplasty for coarctation. *J Thorac Cardiovac Surg* 92:226–230, 1986.

143. Kirsh MM, Perry B, Spooner E. Management of pseudoaneurysm following patch grafting for coarctation of the aorta. *J Thorac Cardiovasc Surg* 74:636, 1977.

144. Bergdahl L, Ljunqvist A. Long-term results after repair of coarctation of the aorta by patch grafting. *J Thorac Cardiovasc Surg* 80:177–181, 1980.

145. Clarkson PM, Brandt PWT, Barratt-Boyer BG, et al. Prosthetic repair of coarctation of the aorta with particular reference to Dacron onlay patch grafts and late aneurysm formation. *Am J Cardiol* 56:342–346, 1985.

146. del Nido J, Williams WG, Wilson GJ, et al. Synthetic patch angioplasty for repair of coarctation of the aorta: Experience with aneurysm formation. *Circulation* 74:I-32–I-36, 1986.

147. Rao PS, Carey P. Remodeling of the aorta following successful balloon coarctation angioplasty. *J Am Coll Cardiol* 14:1312–1317, 1989.

148. Rao PS. Should balloon angioplasty be used instead of surgery for native coarctations? *Circulation* (In Press)

149. Isner JM, Donaldson RF, Fulton D, Bhan I, Payne DD, Cleveland RJ. Cystic medial necrosis in coarctation of the aorta: A potential factor contributing to adverse consequences observed after percutaneous balloon angioplasty of coarctation sites. *Circulation* 75:689–695, 1987.

150. Rao PS, Levy JM, Chopra PS. Balloon angioplasty of stenosed Blalock-Taussig anastomosis: Role of balloon on a wire in dilating occluded shunts. *Am Heart J* 120:1173–1178, 1990.

151. Boucek MM, Webster HE, Orsmond GS, Ruttenberg HD. Balloon pulmonary valvuloplasty: Palliation for cyanotic heart disease. *Am Heart J* 115:318–322, 1988.

152. Qureshi SA, Kirk CR, Lamb R, Arnold R, Wilkinson JL. Balloon dilatation of the pulmonary valve in the first year of life in patients with tetralogy of Fallot: A preliminary study. *Br Heart J* 60:232–235, 1988.

153. Fischer DR, Park SC, Neches WH, Beerman LB, Fricker FJ, Mathews RA, Zuberbuhler JR, Wedemeyer AL. Successful dilatation of stenotic Blalock-Taussig anastomosis by percutaneous transluminal balloon angioplasty. *Am J Cardiol* 55:861–862, 1985.

154. Marx GR, Allen HD, Ovitt TW, Hanson W, Keiter-Marek J. Balloon dilatation angioplasty of Blalock-Taussig shunts. *Am J Cardiol* 62:834–837, 1988.

155. Al Zaibag M, Ribeiro PA, Al Kasab S. Percutaneous balloon valvotomy in tricuspid stenosis. *Br Heart J* 57:51–53, 1987.

156. Riberio PA, Al Zaibag M, Al Kasab S, et al. Percutaneous double balloon valvotomy for rheumatic tricuspid stenosis. *Am J Cardiol* 61:660–662, 1988.

157. Suarez de Lezo J, Pan M, Sancho M, Herrera N, Arizon J, Franco M, Conche M, Valles F, Romanos A. Percutaneous transluminal balloon dilatation of discrete subaortic stenosis. *Am J Cardiol* 58:619–621, 1986.

158. Lababidi Z, Weinhaus L, Stoeckle H, Walls JT. Transluminal balloon dilatation for discrete subaortic stenosis. *Am J Cardiol* 59:423–425, 1987.

159. Arora R, Goel PK, Lochan R, Mohan JC, Khalilullah M. Percutaneous transluminal balloon dilatation in discrete subaortic stenosis. *Am Heart J* 116:1041–1042, 1988.

160. Rao PS, Wilson AD, Chopra PS. Balloon dilatation for discrete subaortic stenosis: Immediate and intermediate-term results. *J Invasive Cardiol* 2:65–71, 1990.

161. Massumi A, Woods L, Mullins CE, et al. Pulmonary venous dilatation in pulmonary veno-occlusive disease. *Am J Cardiol* 48:585–589, 1981.

162. Driscoll DJ, Hesslein PS, Mullins CE. Congenital stenosis of individual pulmonary veins: Clinical spectrum and unsuccessful treatment of transvenous balloon dilatation. *Am J Cardiol* 49:1767–1772, 1982.

163. Corwin RD, Singh AK, Karson KE. Balloon dilatation of ductus arteriosus in a newborn with interrupted aortic arch with ventricular septal defect. *Am Heart J* 102:446–447, 1981.

164. Suarez de Lezo J, Lopez-Rubio F, Guzman J, Galan A. Percutaneous transluminal angioplasty of stenotic ductus arteriosus. *Cathet Cardiovasc Diagn* 11:493–500, 1985.

165. Rao PS, Solymar L. Transductal balloon angioplasty for coarctation of the aorta in the neonate: Preliminary observations. *Am Heart J* 116:1558–1562, 1988.

166. Rocchini AP, Cho KJ, Byrum C, et al. Transluminal angioplasty of superior vena cava obstruction in a 15-month-old child. *Chest* 82:506–508, 1981.

167. Benson LN, Yeatman L, Lako H. Balloon dilatation for superior vena caval obstruction after Senning procedure. *Cathet Cardiovasc Diagn* 11:63–68, 1985.

168. Waldman JD, Waldman J, Jones MC. Failure of balloon dilatation in mid-cavity obstruction of the systemic venous atrium after the Mustard operation. *Pediatr Cardiol* 4:151–154, 1983.

169. Waldman JD. Schoen FJ, Kirkpatrik SE, et al. Balloon dilatation of porcine bioprosthetic valve in the pulmonary position. *Circulation* 76:109–114, 1987.

170. Lloyd TR, Marvin WJ Jr, Mahoney LT, Lauer RM. Balloon dilatation valvuloplasty of bioprosthetic valves in extracardiac conduits. *Am Heart J* 114:268–274, 1987.

171. Ensing GJ, Hagler DJ, Seward JB, Julsrud PR, Mair DD. Caveats of balloon dilatation of conduits and conduit valves: *J Am Coll Cardiol* 14:397–400, 1989.

172. Zeevi B, Keane JF, Perry SB, Lock JE. Balloon dilatation of postoperative right ventricular outflow obstructions. *J Am Coll Cardiol* 14:401–408, 1989.

173. McKay CR, Waller BF, Hong R, Rubin N, Reid CL, Rahimthoola SH. Problems encountered with catheter balloon valvuloplasty of bioprosthetic aortic valves. *Am Heart J* 115:463–465, 1988.

174. Calvo OL, Sobrino N, Gamallo C, Oliver J, Dominquez F, Iglesias A. Balloon percutaneous valvuloplasty for stenotic bioprosthetic valves in mitral position. *Am J Cardiol* 60:736–739, 1987.

175. Feit F, Stecy PJ, Nachamie MS. Percutaneous balloon valvuloplasty for stenosis of a porcine bioprosthesis in the tricuspid valve position. *Am J Cardiol* 58:363–364, 1986.

176. Lock JE, Castaneda-Zuniga WR, Fuhrman BP, et al. Balloon dilatation angioplasty of hypoplastic and stenotic pulmonary arteries. *Circulation* 67:962–967, 1983.

177. Rocchini AP, Kveselis D, Dick M, Crowley D, Snider AP, Rosenthal A. Use of balloon angioplasty to treat peripheral pulmonary stenosis. *Am J Cardiol* 54:1069–1073, 1984.

178. Ring JC, Bass JL, Marvin W, Fuhrman BP, Kulik TJ, Foker JE, Lock JE. Management of congenital stenosis of branch pulmonary artery with balloon dilatation angioplasty. *J Thorac Cardiovasc Surg* 90:35–44, 1988.

179. Fellows KE, Radtke W, Keane JF, Lock JE. Acute complications of catheter therapy for congenital heart disease. *Am J Cardiol* 60:679–683, 1987.

180. Lo RNS, Lau KC, Leung MP. Complete heart block after balloon dilatation of congenital pulmonary stenosis. *Br Heart J* 59:384–386, 1988.

181. Waller BF, Girod DA, Dillon JC. Transverse aortic wall tears in infants after balloon angioplasty for aortic valve stenosis: Relation of aortic valve damage to diameter of inflated angioplasty balloon and aortic lumen in seven necropsy cases. *J Am Coll Cardiol* 4:1235–1241, 1984.

182. Burrows PE, Benson LN, Moes F, Freedom RM. Pulmonary artery tears following balloon valvotomy for pulmonic stenosis. *Cardiovasc Interventional Radiol* 12:38–42, 1989.

183. Krabill KA, Bass JL, Lucas RV Jr, Edwards JE. Dissecting transverse aortic arch aneurysm after percutaneous transluminal balloon dilatation angioplasty of an aortic coarctation. *Pediat Cardiol* 8:39–42, 1987.

184. Weinhaus L, Lababidi Z. Catheter rupture during balloon valvuloplasty. *Am Heart J* 113:1035–1036, 1987.

185. Attia I, Weinhaus L, Walls JT, Lababidi Z. Rupture of tricuspid valve papillary muscle during balloon pulmonary valvuloplasty. *Am Heart J* 113:1233–1234, 1987.

186. Ben-Shachar G, Cohen MH, Sivakoff MC, Portman MA, Riemenschneider TR, Van Heekeran DW. Development of infundibular obstruction after percutaneous pulmonary balloon valvuloplasty. *J Am Coll Cardiol* 5:754–756, 1985.

187. Arnold LW, Keane JF, Kan JS, Fellows KE, Lock JE. Transient unilateral pulmonary edema after successful balloon dilatation of peripheral pulmonary artery stenosis. *Am J Cardiol* 26:326–330, 1988.

188. Gibbs JL, Wilson W, deCosta P. Balloon dilatation of a Waterston aorto-pulmonary anastomosis. *Br Heart J* 59:596–597, 1988.
189. Wessel DL, Keane JF, Fellows KE, Robicharud H, Lock JE. Fibrinolytic therapy for femoral arterial thrombosis after cardiac catheterization in infants and children. *Am J Cardiol* 58:347–351, 1986.
190. Martin GR, Stanger P. Transient prolongation of the QTc interval after balloon valvuloplasty and angioplasty in children. *Am J Cardiol 58*:1233–1235, 1986.
191. Levine JH, Guarmieri T, Kadish AH, Shie RI, Calkins H, Kan JS. Changes in myocardial repolarization in patients undergoing balloon valvuloplasty for congenital pulmonary stenosis: Evidence for contraction excitation on feedback in humans. *Circulation 77*:70–77, 1988.
192. Rocchini AP, Beekman MA. Balloon angioplasty in the treatment of pulmonary valve stenosis and coarctation of the aorta. *Texas Heart Inst J 13*:377–382, 1987.
193. Rao PS. Causes of restenosis following balloon angioplasty/valvuloplasty: A review. *Pediat Rev Comm 4*:157–172, 1990.
194. Abels JE. Balloon catheters and transluminal dilatation: Technical considerations. *Am J Roentgen 135*:901–906, 1980.
195. Lock JE, Niemi T, Einzig S, Amplatz K, Burke B, Bass JL. Transvenous angioplasty of experimental branch pulmonary artery stenosis in newborn lambs. *Circulation 64*:880–893, 1981.
196. Lock JE, Niemi T, Burke BA, Einzig S, Castaneda-Zuniga WR. Transcutaneous angioplasty of experimental aortic coarctation. *Circulation 66*:1280–1286, 1982.
197. Ho SY, Somerville J, Yip WCL, Anderson RH. Transluminal balloon dilation of resected coarcted segments of thoracic aorta: Histologic study and clinical implications. *Internat J Cardiol 19*:99–105, 1988.
198. Edwards BS, Lucas RV Jr, Lock JE, Edwards JE. Morphologic changes in the pulmonary arteries after percutaneous balloon angioplasty for pulmonary artery stenosis. *Circulation 71*:195–202, 1985.

17

Acute Interventional Procedures in the Neonate

STANTON B. PERRY and RONALD J. KANTER

The first widely used transvascular intervention was balloon atrial septostomy for critically ill newborns with transposition of the great arteries. In the last several years, a wide range of transcatheter techniques have been developed, including ablation of obstructions with balloons and closure of intra- and extracardiac defects with devices. Many of these techniques are now being applied to the infant less than one month of age. For example, neonates with critical pulmonary or aortic valve stenosis and some with coarctation of the aorta are now considered suitable candidates for nonsurgical treatment. Rapid and accurate diagnostic methods such as Doppler echocardiography and expedient initial management through rapid regional transport and pharmacologic and respiratory support are permitting neonates to enter the catheterization laboratory in better condition than in the past, thus, reducing the overall risk from the procedure.

This chapter addresses current applications of balloon and blade atrial septostomy and balloon valvuloplasty and angioplasty in the neonate: clinical indications, methodologies, results, and complications.

BALLOON ATRIAL SEPTOSTOMY

Certain congenital heart lesions are incompatible with long-term postnatal survival unless an adequate interatrial communication exists. These include d-transposition of the great arteries (d-TGA), total anomalous pulmonary venous return (TAPVR), pulmonary atresia with intact ventricular septum, atresia or severe stenosis of either atrioventricular valve, and double outlet ventricle with an inadequate ventricular septal defect. The commonest of these is d-TGA (approximately one in 4000 live births[1]), which if untreated carries a

one-year mortality rate of greater than 90%.[2,3] The need to palliate these patients until surgical correction can be undertaken provides the impetus for development of an alternative to surgical septectomy.[4-8] In 1965, Rashkind and Miller reported the use of a balloon catheter to create an atrial septal defect, which permitted immediate increase in arterial oxygen saturation, decompression of left atrial hypertension, and improvement in the clinical status in three infants with d-TGA.[9] This section will focus on the clinical role of balloon atrial septostomy (BAS) for congenital heart defects in the context of current surgical management.

d-Transposition of the Great Arteries

In infants with d-TGA with an intact ventricular septum and a closed ductus arteriosus, successful septostomy usually results in better oxygenation of venous return with relief of systemic arterial hypoxemia. Following septostomy, shunting across the defect is right-to-left during ventricular diastole and left-to-right at the onset of systole.[10] The arterial oxygen saturation can be expected to increase by 13 to 26%,[4,11-15] and some equalization of atrial mean pressures also occurs. The left atrial mean pressure usually exceeds the right by less than 4 mm Hg following the procedure.[8,13,16] The drop in pulmonary venous pressure following septostomy may be important in patients with a ventricular septal defect or patent ductus arteriosus by reducing pulmonary arterial pressure.

Successful BAS results in improved arterial oxygenation and reduction in signs of congestive heart failure. Failure of BAS to improve the clinical condition may be due to hypovolemia, pulmonary hypertension, or, occasionally, by a prohibitively small fossa ovalis. Late failure of BAS is defined as recurrence of cyanosis with or without signs of heart failure. Powell et al. demonstrated higher left and right atrial pressures, higher pulmonary artery pressures, and lower arterial oxygen saturations during follow-up catheterizations in infants who were in need of further palliation.[12] The infants had smaller atrial septal defects (less than 10 mm in diameter by sizing with balloon catheters) than did those babies not requiring additional palliation. The change in arterial oxygen saturation during initial BAS did not predict subsequent failure in this investigation or in those by Hawker et al.[17] or Baker et al.[8] The initial equalization of atrial pressures has likewise not been a strong predictor of eventual successful palliation.[8,13,17] Baker et al.[8] demonstrated during follow-up catheterizations inadequate atrial septal defects (less than 12 mm in diameter) in cyanotic infants who had initially responded to BAS with an adequate decrease in left atrial pressure and a reduction in cyanosis.[8] Reversibly stretching the foramen ovale without tearing the fossa ovalis may account for this phenomenon in some instances. It is currently believed that the initial pullback of the balloon should be at maximum desired volume, rather than performing sequential pullbacks with increasing balloon volumes from 1.5 to 4.0 milliliters.[4,6,18] Most currently available balloons maintain a turgid configuration with a diameter of nearly 15 mm at a volume of 2.0 milliliters. There are a small number of infants whose septostomy size is limited by an undersized fossa ovalis, as proven at surgery or postmortem examination.[19] Conversely, some infants have been found at follow-up catheterization or in surgery to have an adequate atrial septal defect, despite becoming increasingly or intermittently cyanotic. Their cyanosis is due to evolving pulmonary hypertension or to the development of dynamic or fixed left ventricular outflow tract obstruction.[20,21] Fortunately, late failure of BAS is becoming less of an issue with the contemporary trend toward the arterial switch operation in the first week of life.

The mortality rate of BAS in neonates with d-TGA (0 to 11%[4,6–8,12–14,16–18,22–24]) is much lower than that of the Blalock-Hanlon atrial septectomy.[4–8] Most deaths have been related to the moribund status of some newborns prior to BAS. This is less frequent with the advent of echocardiography and earlier diagnosis, the use of prostaglandins, and the expeditious transport of critically ill infants to regional facilities.

Infants with d-TGA have a higher mortality rate in the months following BAS if there is a coexistent patent ductus arteriosus,[11,12] a large ventricular septal defect,[11] or coarctation of the aorta.[7,11,25] Having undergone BAS at an older age or having incurred a thrombotic event (especially stroke) also adversely influences survival rate.[11] The left and right atrial pressures prior to BAS appear not to predict survival rate, whereas a low pulmonary artery pressure (with or without left ventricular outflow tract obstruction), elevated hemoglobin concentration, and an elevated arterial oxygen content at follow-up catheterization all predict improved survival.[11] Even after an initially successful BAS, 15 to 40% of unoperated infants with d-TGA will die during the first six months without surgery.[1,11] This has prompted a movement toward earlier reparative procedures, such as the Mustard and Senning operations, even into the neonatal period.[26] The current trend toward an anatomic correction obviates concerns over many of these issues.

Total Anomalous Pulmonary Venous Return

In children with TAPVR, an intact ventricular septum, and a closed ductus arteriosus, the entire systemic cardiac output must pass across the atrial septal defect. A restrictive atrial septum results in systemic and pulmonary venous congestion and low systemic output. Some investigators have found that despite minimal pressure difference between the atria,[27] BAS results in rapid clinical improvement, with diminution of pulmonary artery and right atrial pressures.[15,24,27–29] However, many centers now proceed directly to surgical correction without BAS or catheterization.

If surgical intervention is not feasible and BAS is necessary, several caveats exist. The performance of a septostomy in an infant with TAPVR is more difficult than in those with d-TGA, owing to the small size of the left atrium, the absence of left-sided pulmonary veins to serve as landmarks, and the large—often numerous—orifices entering the right atrium. The procedure must be performed expeditiously, as the entire left-sided output is obstructed when the balloon is maximally inflated. Older reports recommend the use of double-lumen septostomy catheters so that left atrial pressure and oxygen saturation sampling may confirm catheter position.[27,29] The current availability of echocardiographic guidance has obviated that need. Echocardiographic proof of defect adequacy is also desirable, in that the interatrial pressure gradient may[27] or may not[28] be large prior to BAS, and gradient reduction may be by less than 2 mm Hg,[28] thus, serving little notice that a successful septostomy has been performed.

Right-Sided Atrioventricular Valve Atresia

In infants with right-sided atrioventricular valve atresia, an adequate atrial septal defect is necessary to prevent systemic venous congestion and low cardiac output. Most infants with tricuspid atresia never require enlargement of their atrial septal defect. If the atrial septal defect is obstructive, the right atrium hypertrophies, and a balloon catheter may not be capable of tearing the atrial septum. Nevertheless, improvement following BAS for tricuspid atresia is well known; 29 of the 36 infants reported in two large series were under four months old at the time of septostomy.[15,24]

During catheterization, the interatrial pressure gradient is a useful guide to the adequacy of the septostomy. There are reports of mean pressure gradients falling from greater than 10 mm Hg to 3 mm Hg[30,31] and of even more impressive equalization of the atrial A wave amplitudes following BAS. Defect size is probably better reflected in the A wave differences than is the mean pressure gradient.[24] Immediately following BAS, improvement in systemic output may "outstrip" pulmonary blood flow, and the infant may become more cyanotic, necessitating an aortopulmonary shunt.[15,24]

Pulmonary Atresia with Intact Ventricular Septum

Children having this lesion also require an atrial level right-to-left shunt until the right ventricle and outflow tract grow to a size adequate to support the entire systemic venous return. In the most severe form, this growth may never occur. Nevertheless, BAS is rarely required for this lesion. In fact, it can be argued that performance of a septostomy in an infant who is to undergo a right ventricular outflow tract patch may discourage forward flow through the right ventricle. The clinical success rates after BAS in infants with pulmonary atresia with intact ventricular septum also reflect the wide range of severity of this lesion, including the presence of right ventricle to coronary artery fistulae in 0[15] to 77%.[32] Routine BAS in children with this lesion is not recommended; only in the rare neonate with a diminutive right ventricle who is not a candidate for an outflow

tract patch and in whom there is systemic venous obstruction should it be considered.

Left-Sided Atrioventricular Valve Atresia

An inadequate atrial septal defect in patients with left-sided atrioventricular valve atresia or stenosis results in pulmonary venous hypertension with pulmonary edema. Atrial septostomy can reduce the left atrial pressure. This category of lesions includes the hypoplastic left heart syndrome, severe mitral atresia or stenosis with a ventricular septal defect or double outlet right ventricle, and single ventricle (usually morphologically left) with atresia or severe stenosis of the left atrioventricular valve. In this group, BAS rarely provides long-term palliation,[15,24,29,33] and, therefore, close follow-up is required even after initial reduction in interatrial pressure gradient.

Technique

The neonate requiring balloon atrial septostomy is in a high-risk group. During transport from intensive care facilities to the catheterization laboratory, meticulous attention to the airway, to arterial and venous infusion lines, and to portable electrocardiographic and pressure monitors is necessary. Once in the laboratory, frequent appraisal of body temperature, acid-base balance, serum glucose concentration, and oxygenation and ventilation will prevent many complications. With the help of echocardiography, the option of performing the BAS in the intensive care unit may avoid many of these potential complications.[34]

Many cardiologists favor the percutaneous femoral venous approach. Although gradual dilation of the vein to accept up to an 8-French (F) catheter is possible in infants as small as 2.0 kg, availability of lower profile balloon catheters with smaller sheaths makes this unnecessary; the risk of femoral vein thrombosis may also be reduced by using the smaller sheaths. Percutaneous cannulation may be associated with less bleeding or less risk of local infection compared with saphenous vein cutdown,[35] but the procedural time may not be much different. Successful transumbilical septostomies using umbilical veins have been reported since 1974.[36,37] Operators have successfully passed up to 6-F single lumen septostomy catheters through the ductus venosus,[36-38] although ductal patency is greatly reduced after 72 hours of age. When using this approach, care should be taken to withdraw the catheter's introducer sheath an appropriate distance back into the inferior vena cava so that the balloon catheter can be freely jerked back to the low right atrium. The practical advantages of this approach must be weighed against the reported risks of omphalitis, portal vein thrombosis, and hepatic necrosis.[36]

Catheter selection is based on the desired balloon size and the requisite for simultaneous pressure monitoring or blood sampling. The 5.5-F double-lumen Rashkind catheter requires an 8-F sheath but will permit blood sampling. The tiny sampling port requires frequent flushing. The 5-F Edwards Miller catheter requires a 7-F sheath, has only one lumen, but, like the double-lumen Rashkind, will accept a volume of over 4 milliliters to give a diameter of 18 mm. These catheters have particular application to older infants and children as part of a blade septostomy procedure, although normal-sized term newborns whose left atrium is of average size will also tolerate a balloon inflated to 3.0 to 3.5 milliliters. The USCI 6-F septostomy catheter fits into a 6-F sheath, allowing the procedure to be performed on smaller infants. Its maximum volume of 1.8 milliliters gives a diameter of 13 mm, and overdistension to 3.0 milliliters will increase the diameter to 15 mm. This size is especially safe for newborns with small left atria, such as those with mitral atresia or TAPVR, although we routinely create adequate defects in term babies with d-TGA using this catheter.

The balloon should always be tested prior to entering the patient. All catheter models have a distal bend that permits ready negotiation of the foramen ovale using fluoroscopy or two-dimensional echocardiography. Echocardiographic assistance using the subxyphoid short-axis view (long axis of the cavae) will allow visualization of the inferior vena cava, right atrium, and atrial septum in the approximate plane of the foramen ovale.[39] Once the catheter is across the atrial septum, the long-axis subxyphoid view (four-chamber) will demonstrate the balloon position.[40,41] A leftward, slightly posterior position of the catheter tip as viewed radiographically will also prove that it is not in the right ventricular outflow tract. Entry into a left pulmonary vein or sampling of well-oxygenated blood provides further confirmation. Rarely, levoposition of the right atrial appendage may not permit radiographic discrimination from the left atrium, unless pressure or oxygen saturation measurement is available.[42] The balloon may be inflated with dilute contrast (33%) if viewed radiographically and saline if visualized echographically. Once inflated, balloon distortion or absence of free movement suggests entrapment in the mitral valve, the left atrial appendage, a pulmonary vein, or a small left atrium. Once properly positioned, the inflated balloon is briskly jerked across the atrial septum under constant visualization and readvanced into the body of the right atrium prior to entry into the mouth of the inferior vena cava (Fig. 17.1). Most operators repeat the maneuver once or twice to ensure free passage of the balloon, but multiple pullbacks using gradually larger volumes are not recommended. Availability of echocardiography confers one final advantage: prompt visualization and measurement of the new defect (Fig. 17.2). One expects to see disruption of the central portion of the fossa ovalis, with flailed elements of the septum primum fluttering between the atria.[43]

Complications

Complications of the procedure include right or left atrial or right ventricular perforation,[8,16,23,43–46] tricuspid or mitral valve rupture,[8,25,46] failure of the balloon to deflate,[8,47,48] arrhythmia,[4,16] and intraabdominal hemorrhage.[49] Not all chamber perforations result in death; volume replacement and rapid surgical intervention sometimes prove lifesaving.[43,44] Inability to deflate a balloon may occur when it is wedged into the proximal inferior vena cava, and the proximal binding of the balloon to the catheter detaches and slips distally. The balloon can be ruptured by passing a stiff wire through a sheath up to the caval-atrial junction. The balloon is then pulled down onto the exposed wire tip.[48] Finally, iliac vein thrombosis has been reported in 7% of children who had undergone BAS as infants, an incidence higher than in any other group examined.[49]

Contemporary Role of Balloon Atrial Septostomy

The role of this intervention in children with congenital heart disease is changing with the remarkable strides in corrective heart surgery in neonates. In most centers, babies with d-TGA continue to undergo BAS at the initial catheterization prior to an arterial switch procedure in the first week of life or an atrial switch procedure somewhat later. Infants with TAPVR can expect to undergo complete cardiac repair in the neonatal period or early infancy. Indeed, an inadequate atrial septal defect and congestive heart failure is an

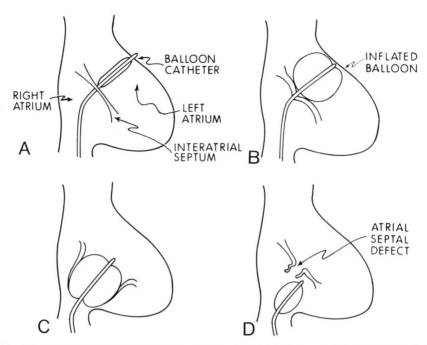

Figure 17.1. Diagrammatic representation of balloon atrial septostomy as it appears in an anteroposterior projection. **A,** Balloon is deflated in left atrium; **B,** inflated balloon prior to pullback: **C,** beginning of pullback as atrial septum stretches; **D,** following pullback with balloon in right atrium and new septal defect.

indication for complete correction rather than for enlargement of the septal defect. Children with two atria, but with an outlet from only one, must have an adequate atrial septal defect until a Fontan operation can be performed—usually at one to four years of age.

BLADE ATRIAL SEPTOSTOMY

In 1975, Park introduced a technique for enlarging or creating an atrial septal defect using a catheter with a retractable blade. The technique is useful for the child in whom the atrial septum is too thick or tough for balloon septostomy. The original blade measured 12 mm in length and successfully created defects 8.5 to 11.0 mm in three experimental newborn lambs.[50]

A collaborative effort describing the initial experience with this technique included 52 patients, most beyond the neonatal period.[51] Thirty-one children had d-TGA, 10 had mitral atresia, 5 tricuspid atresia, 2 double-outlet right ventricle with an inadequate ventricular septal defect, 2 pulmonary atresia with intact ventricular septum, 1 TAPVR, and 1 Taussig-Bing anomaly with inadequate venous admixture. According to their prees-

tablished criteria, 79% improved following the procedure, and five patients (10%) had significant complications, including one death. During follow-up of four months to two years, the septal defect remained large in 84%. This procedure has also been used in children with primary pulmonary hypertension and life-threatening syncope, as a means of improving systemic, albeit desaturated, blood flow.

Technique

The blade septostomy catheter has a distal bend similar to that of balloon septostomy catheters, a distal metal tube that houses the blade, a central guidewire that controls the blade, a proximal gasket through which the wire passes and which prevents back-bleeding, a sidearm for continuous pressure monitoring or contrast injection, and an adjustable locking device/wire holder located at the operator's end of the wire (Fig. 17.3). Three blade lengths are available, 9.4, 13.4, and 20.0 mm; the two smaller blades are on 5.7-F catheters, and the larger is on a 7.3-F catheter.

The procedure requires adequate sedation, and biplane fluoroscopy is optimal. The device should be tested outside the patient first. It is passed into the left atrium through an existent atrial septal defect or a long sheath following transseptal puncture. The transseptal sheath should then be pulled back into the inferior vena cava. Confirmation of its location in the left atrium may be by the methods described for balloon septostomy catheter placement. The angle subtended by the distal angulation of the catheter should point inferior, leftward, and anterior and will correspond to the direction of the sidearm, which is in view of the operator (Fig. 17.4). The locking device is loosened and pulled back over the wire by the distance that the blade will be extruded and is then retightened. The blade is extruded by pushing the locking device forward against the gasket, and the entire apparatus is gently pulled back against the resistance of the septum, until it is in the right atrium and no further resistance is felt. The blade should never be jerked, and strict fluoroscopic guidance should be assured. The blade is retracted by pulling back on the locking device. The process

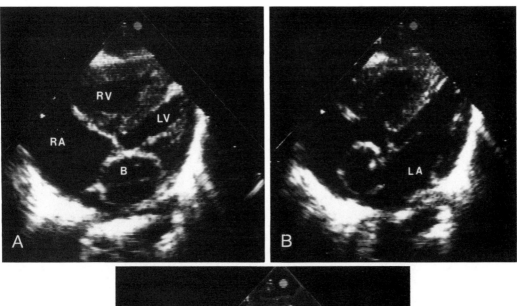

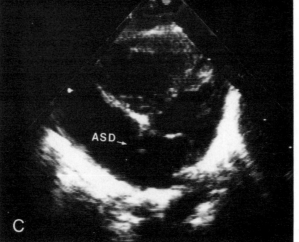

Figure 17.2. Two-dimensional echocardiograms of balloon atrial septostomy procedure, using long-axis subxyphoid view. **A,** Balloon is fully inflated in the left atrium, with the shaft pointing leftward, prior to pullback; **B,** balloon position in the right atrium following septostomy with its shaft assuming a more anterosuperior-posteroinferior direction; **C,** catheter is withdrawn, and flailed fragments of atrial septum with a new defect are visualized. *ASD* = atrial septal defect; *B* = balloon; *LA* = left atrium; *LV* = left ventricle; *RA* = right atrium; *RV* = right ventricle.

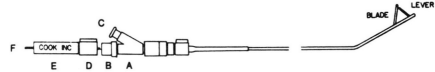

Figure 17.3. Blade septostomy catheter and assembly components. *A* = Y-connector; *B* = gasket to prevent leakage; *C* = sidearm for fluid infusion and pressure measurement; *D* = locking device for wire holder; *E* = blade control wire holder; *F* = control wire. (From Park SC, Neches WH, Mullins CE, et al. Blade atrial septostomy. *Circulation 66*:260, 1982; by permission of the American Heart Association, Inc.)

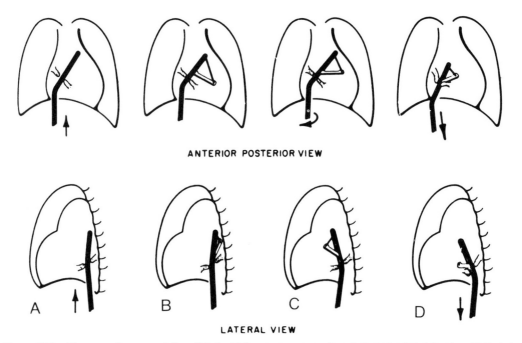

Figure 17.4. Diagrammatic representation of blade atrial septostomy procedure. **A,** Catheter tip in left atrium; **B,** blade is extruded; **C,** blade is rotated to face anteriorly, inferiorly, and leftward; **D,** catheter is pulled back across atrial septum. (From Park SC, Neches WH, Mullins CE, et al. Blade atrial septostomy. *Circulation 66*:260, 1982; by permission of the American Heart Association, Inc.)

should then be repeated one or more times after rotating the catheter slightly. Balloon septostomy may then be performed to enlarge the incision.

In the context of current trends in neonatal surgery, this procedure is primarily limited to children outside the neonatal age group with left or right atrioventricular valve atresia in whom BAS is unlikely to be successful.

PERCUTANEOUS BALLOON PULMONIC VALVULOPLASTY

Pulmonary valve stenosis in neonates is of "critical" severity if right ventricular systolic pressure is at systemic level or greater and/or if there is cyanosis due to right-to-left atrial level shunting. The clinical presentation varies from profoundly cya-

notic newborns to asymptomatic older neonates who may have mild desaturation and a precordial thrill. Pulmonary valve stenosis may be an isolated anomaly or associated with complex defects, such as single ventricle, double-outlet right ventricle, transposition of the great arteries, or tetralogy of Fallot.

Since the original description of the static balloon technique by Kan et al.,[53] several large series have demonstrated its short- and intermediate-term efficacy.[54-57] Application of balloon valvuloplasty to neonates with critical pulmonic stenosis had, until recently, been confined to single case reports[58] or occasional patients within a large series. This section will describe the methodology and recent experiences with this technique in neonates.

Technique

The sicker neonates require intravenous infusion of prostaglandin E_1 to maintain ductal patency and provide pulmonary blood flow, and many are best stabilized by tracheal intubation and assisted ventilation. Standard sedation is given. All neonates should have arterial pressure monitoring, either by umbilical or radial artery cannulation in the intensive care unit, or femoral artery cannulation in the catheterization laboratory. Crossing the pulmonary valve with an umbilical venous catheter is difficult, so the femoral venous approach is preferred. Once all catheters have been placed, the infant receives heparin intravenously, 100 U/kg.

The most important hemodynamic data include right ventricular and systemic arterial systolic pressures. A right ventriculogram is performed before a catheter and wire are passed across the pulmonary valve, and the valve anulus diameter is measured at the leaflet hinge points (Fig. 17.5). Measuring devices to correct for magnification include external grids, radiopaque calibrated catheters, or the known diameter of the catheter used for ventriculography. An echocardiographic estimate of anulus size is a helpful adjunct.

Negotiating the pulmonary valve orifice can be difficult and associated with bradycardia and hypotension. Large catheter loops, which may stretch a cardiac chamber, should be avoided, and supplemental oxygen and atropine may be required. Newborns receiving prostaglandin E_1 are usually more tolerant of the additional obstruction of the outflow tract by the catheter.[59] If the patient does not tolerate a catheter across the valve orifice, the catheter should be removed, without obtaining

a pulmonary artery pressure, and leaving only the guidewire in place. The orifice may be traversed with a 4- or 5-F, end-hole, balloon-directed catheter[60] or a 3- or 4-F angulated multipurpose catheter.[61] Floppy, high-torque wires (down to 0.014 cm) may be initially necessary, followed by wire and catheter exchanges up to the appropriate size. Despite these maneuvers, in two reports,[61,62] 3 of 16 neonates could not undergo this procedure due to inability to cross the valve. The final exchange wire should be the largest that will fit the balloon dilation catheter, 0.035 cm for most 8- to 10-mm balloon catheters down to 0.014 cm for the smallest coronary artery dilation balloon catheters.[60] This wire should be anchored distally in the pulmonary artery or descending aorta if the ductus arteriosus is patent. Several authors[60–62] advocate gradational valve dilation, starting with coronary artery balloons whose inflated diameter may be only 2 or 3 mm, and increasing the balloon size until the final diameter (usually 6, 8, or 10 mm) is 120 to 140% the anulus diameter. Use of oversized balloons has been shown to be safe and is associated with better relief of obstruction.[54,63,64] The balloon length should be as short as possible (usually 2 cm) to avoid damage to the right ventricular outflow tract. The safety of these balloon dimensions is based on work done in a neonatal lamb model.[65]

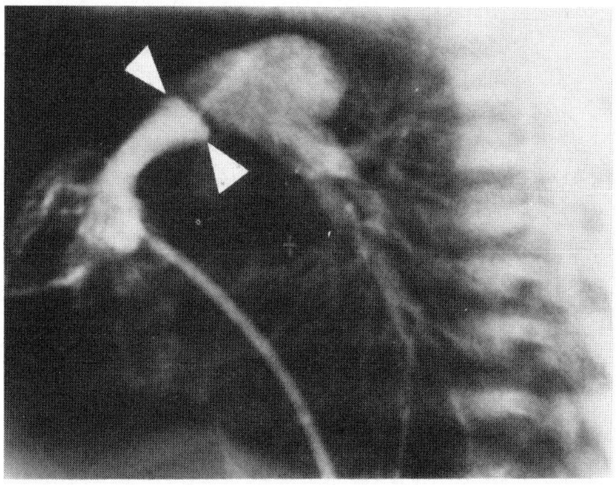

Smaller balloon catheters may be placed into the vein through a sheath, but most require direct entry over the guidewire. This requires twisting in the direction opposite of that in which the balloon is wrapped (so as not to unravel it), with constant negative pressure applied to the balloon inflation port in order to minimize the balloon profile. Dilute contrast (33%) is used to inflate the balloon. Unlike older children, it is not necessary to monitor inflation pressure with a manometer, as it does not require much force to dilate these valves. The balloon is centered across the anulus and inflated and deflated over 10 to 15 sec. Many valves never result in a distinct waist in the balloon, because the valves are so pliable (Fig. 17.6). Right ventricular pressure may be measured after inflations by exchanging the dilation catheter for a pigtail catheter with a Y-arm adaptor, so that the guidewire may remain in place. A right ventriculogram is performed following the final dilation.

Figure 17.5. Lateral projection of right ventriculogram in a neonate with critical pulmonic stenosis. The anulus diameter is measured between leaflet hinge points, indicated by arrowheads.

Results

In the neonate with critical pulmonic stenosis and right-to-left atrial level shunting and left-to-right

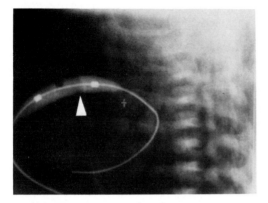

Figure 17.6. Lateral projection of an inflated valvuloplasty balloon across the pulmonary valve in a neonate with critical pulmonic stenosis. Only a minimal waist is seen (arrowhead).

ductal shunting, the transvalvular pressure gradient may underestimate the degree of obstruction. Nevertheless, large pressure gradient reductions have been achieved. In 18 consecutive patients, we were able to cross the pulmonary valve in 17. The peak systolic pressure gradient was reduced from 90 ± 21 to 14 ± 8 mm Hg, using a balloon to anulus ratio of 1.25 ± 0.16. The right ventricular pressure dropped from 115 ± 17 to 62 ± 27 mm Hg immediately following dilation, with a stable aortic pressure (75 ± 11 to 77 ± 17 mm Hg). Other reports have described similar results,[60–62] with improved arterial oxygen saturation.[60]

Intermediate-term follow-up has demonstrated maintenance of gradient reduction (mean peak systolic ejection gradient of 22 mm Hg[62]) after 11 months. Inadequate balloon size has been the most frequent explanation for the few infants who required repeat valvuloplasty.[61,62] Dysplasia of the valve has been offered as a reason for dilation failure in some older children,[66–68] but this has been a concern in neonates only rarely.[68] This may be due to selection bias, to greater responsiveness by the dysplastic valve to valvuloplasty at the younger age, or to a tendency for dysplastic valves to require attention at an older age.

Balloon pulmonary valvuloplasty has been used to improve pulmonary blood flow and reduce cyanosis in tetralogy of Fallot, in transposition of the great arteries (d- or l-) with a ventricular septal defect, in tricuspid atresia, and in single ventricle patients.[69–71] Most patients responded to valvuloplasty with better arterial oxygen saturations, increased pulmonary:systemic flow ratios, and, eventually, decreased hematocrits. Although most

of these patients were outside the neonatal period, theoretically, application to neonates in need of a palliative procedure for cyanosis is possible. This would avoid complications of systemic arterial to pulmonary artery shunts, such as pulmonary artery distortion. In a patient with severe tetralogy of Fallot and aortopulmonary collaterals, valve dilation may also allow subsequent transcatheter embolization. Severe subvalvular pulmonic stenosis is usually present, as well, limiting application of this technique.

Complications from pulmonary balloon valvuloplasty, even in sick neonates, are uncommon. Transient hypotension and bradycardia may be anticipated, and excessive blood loss requiring transfusion is not unusual. Conduction defects have been reported but are either transient or apparently clinically unimportant. During follow-up, pulmonary valve regurgitation is often evident by Doppler interrogation but is usually inaudible. Intimal dissection of the iliac vein without long-term disability[61] and femoral vein thrombosis at later catheterization[62] have been described.

Pulmonary balloon valvuloplasty for severe valvular stenosis in the neonate is an accepted therapeutic modality. The technical difficulty of accessing the pulmonary valve orifice, especially if the right ventricle is hypoplastic, occasionally limits its application. The greatest hazard of this technique is related to the generally increased risk of a potentially prolonged cardiac catheterization in a neonate.

PERCUTANEOUS BALLOON AORTIC VALVULOPLASTY

Neonates with critical aortic stenosis commonly present with signs of severe congestive heart failure or shock. Associated anomalies are common and include varying degrees of left ventricular hypoplasia and dysfunction, endocardial fibroelastosis, mitral valve hypoplasia or regurgitation, subaortic stenosis, coarctation, and patent ductus arteriosus. Even those neonates dependent on right-to-left ductal flow for systemic output may have only mild tachypnea, mild or differential cyanosis, or an unimpressive murmur, escaping diagnosis until the duct begins to close. This usually occurs in the first few days but can occur later within the first month. The diagnosis is established with Doppler echocardiography, which demonstrates valve morphology and gradient, the size of the aortic anulus, and the appearance of other left heart structures and associated anomalies.

Initial management is directed at reversing the state of shock and correcting metabolic abnormalities using ventilation, inotropic support, and prostaglandin E_1. Because not all patients will improve with medical management, definitive relief of the valvular obstruction should be undertaken without undue delay. Aortic valvotomy can be performed surgically or using balloon dilation. Surgical valvotomy, the traditional therapy, has been associated with a high mortality and relatively high incidence of aortic regurgitation and restenosis.[71–80] Balloon aortic valvuloplasty was first reported in 1983 in a child with congenital aortic stenosis[81] and has subsequently been performed in large numbers of older patients with both congenital and acquired stenosis.[82–84] Following initial reports of its use in neonates,[85,86] a retrospective study comparing surgical and percutaneous balloon valvuloplasty suggested the results of balloon dilation are at least as good as those obtained with surgical valvotomy.[87] This section will focus on the techniques and results of percutaneous balloon aortic valvuloplasty in neonates with critical aortic stenosis.

Technique

The purpose of the catheterization in these patients, who have had complete Doppler echocardiograms, is to perform the balloon valvuloplasty. Thus, while complete right and left heart hemodynamics can usually be obtained easily and quickly, wasting time or taking undue risks to obtain this information is counterproductive in these sick neonates. The catheterization can be performed with routine sedation, although most patients are intubated and paralyzed. A 5-F sheath and 5-F Berman catheter are placed in the femoral or umbilical vein. Umbilical artery access can usually be obtained in the first week of life. Catheter manipulation from the umbilical artery, because of the complex catheter course, is more difficult than from the femoral artery, but its use avoids the risk of damage to the femoral arteries. We, therefore, first try the umbilical artery approach and, if not successful within 30 minutes, use the femoral artery. A 3- or 4-F pigtail catheter is placed in the artery.

The patient is heparinized (100 U/kg) when access has been obtained. Right heart oxygen saturations and pressures are measured, and the venous catheter is advanced across the patent foramen ovale to the left ventricle. The transvalvular gradient is measured using the left ventricular and aortic catheters. A left ventriculogram is performed with the venous catheter to assess left ventricular volume and function, mitral regurgitation, the subvalvular area, the valve morphology, and to measure the valve anulus (Fig. 17.7). A predilation aortogram for aortic regurgitation and arch anatomy can be performed using the arterial catheter, but it may be prudent to forego this

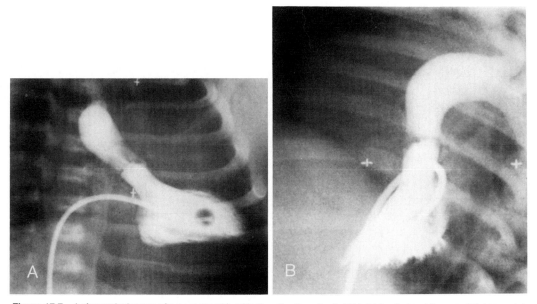

Figure 17.7. Left ventriculogram of a neonate with critical aortic stenosis. **A,** Mild right anterior oblique and **B,** long axial oblique projections.

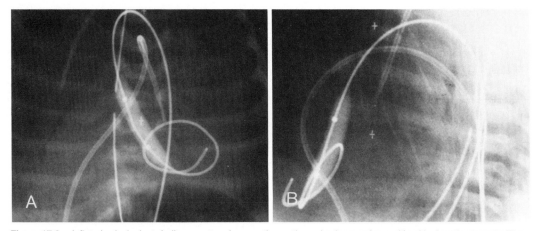

Figure 17.8. Inflated valvuloplasty balloon centered across the aortic anulus in a newborn with critical aortic stenosis. The guidewire is looped in the left ventricle, and a venous catheter is across the ductus arteriosus in the descending aorta. **A,** Anteroposterior and **B,** lateral projections.

injection in critically ill neonates with impaired renal function who have no aortic regurgitation by physical examination or Doppler.

The most difficult part of the procedure is crossing the aortic valve retrograde from the aorta. The easiest technique, in our experience, is to probe for the valve orifice with the soft end of a straight guidewire, 0.018 inch or smaller. This probing need not be entirely random because the commissure between the left and non-coronary cusps is almost always open in congenitally stenotic valves. Thus, at the same time one is probing with the wire, the pigtail catheter is manipulated to direct the wire posteriorly and to the left. This is easier if approximately half of the pigtail has been cut off. The probing must be done gently to avoid perforating a cusp or damaging the coronary arteries. If there is any difficulty in getting the pigtail or balloon catheter to follow the wire across the valve, even if the wire went easily, it should raise the question of cusp perforation.

The initial balloon diameter is chosen to be 75–90% of the anulus diameter. Animal and clinical studies[82,88–90] demonstrate balloon:anulus ratios > 1.0 are more likely to be associated with damage to the outflow tract and increased aortic regurgitation. The balloon should have the smallest shaft size available and should not exceed 2 cm in length. The pigtail catheter is exchanged for the dilation catheter over a guidewire. We do not usually flush the balloon prior to dilation in neonates because a distorted balloon may not cross the critically narrowed valve. The balloon is centered across the valve, inflated and deflated

rapidly, and pulled back to the descending aorta (Fig. 17.8). A waist at the valve during inflation is unusual in neonates, and a tight waist suggests the balloon is through a cusp. Videotapes are reviewed to measure balloon size and check balloon position. A postdilation gradient is measured using a pigtail and Y-arm adaptor to avoid losing wire position. If the left ventricular pressure and transvalvular gradient are unchanged and there is little aortic regurgitation, one can consider using a larger balloon. At the end of the procedure, an aortogram is performed to look for aortic regurgitation.

Results

Determining the immediate results of balloon dilation is difficult in these patients. Due to poor ventricular function and the patent foramen and ductus, the transvalvular gradient is not a reliable indicator of obstruction, and the output across the aortic valve and valve area cannot be calculated. Thus, although we look for a drop in transvalvular gradient and have found successful dilations are statistically associated with a drop in left ventricular end-diastolic pressure, the outcome is defined ultimately by the patient's postdilation course. The goal of the initial procedure should be to relieve the obstruction sufficiently to allow for clinical improvement. If, in addition to achieving this, the patient has at most mild aortic regurgitation and intact femoral pulses, the procedure is a success. Failure of the patient to improve could be due to an inadequate valvuloplasty or to other problems such as a hypoplastic left ventricle, ventricular dysfunction, mitral regurgitation, development of coarctation as the patent ductus arteriosus closes, or continued patency of the ductus. Left ventricular function and mitral regurgitation usually improve following successful dilation, but this may take weeks. The transvalvular gradient commonly increases in the postdilation period and is probably related to increased cardiac output across the valve. The fact that a patient may need to be redilated within weeks or months, a procedure that can be performed with minimal mortality and morbidity, should not be considered a sign of failure.

We have dilated 27 consecutive neonates with critical valvular aortic stenosis regardless of clinical condition, valve morphology, left ventricular size or function, or degree of mitral regurgitation. They ranged in age from 1 to 30 days and in weight from 2.2 to 5 kg. Unicommissural valves were present in 17 and bicommissural in 10. The left ventricular volume was greater than 80% of predicted normal in 16, 60–80% of normal in 7, and less than 60% of normal in 4. Using a balloon to anulus ratio of 0.90 ± 0.14, the peak systolic ejection gradient was reduced from 58 ± 27 to 27 ± 19, and the left ventricular end-diastolic pressure was also reduced significantly. New aortic regurgitation developed in 11, was mild in 8, and severe in 3 who died. If failure is defined as death ($N = 9$) or need for stage I palliation (Norwood procedure) for hypoplastic left heart syndrome ($N = 2$), there were 11 failures, and 9 occurred in the 11 patients with left ventricular volumes ≤80% of normal. Complications have included postprocedure sepsis in 1 patient, and cusp perforation and dilation in another; both patients died. Transient loss of pulse occurs in approximately 60% of neonates dilated from the femoral artery but is permanent in less than 10%. Transient left bundle branch block and ventricular arrhythmias are seen in 10–20%.

The mortality rate following surgical or transcatheter valvotomy in neonates is commonly 30–50%, but rates as low as 9% and as high as 86% have been reported. This variation is likely to be multifactorial reflecting factors such as changes in pre- and post-intervention care, changes in technique, expertise of the operator, and perhaps most importantly, patient selection. Some neonates with critical aortic stenosis have such severe left ventricular hypoplasia and/or endocardial fibroelastosis that survival with two ventricles even following a "perfect" valvuloplasty is unlikely. Few series in the literature have addressed this issue or

clearly defined the population of patients treated. For example, combining results in neonates and infants can be misleading. We have balloon-dilated 34 infants (1 to 12 months of age) with no mortality and results not significantly different than in older patients—results clearly different from the neonatal results. Carefully defining the patient population is important not only to allow comparison of results using different techniques but also in trying to improve management of groups with high mortality. Although our results demonstrate a high mortality in patients with small left ventricles undergoing balloon valvuloplasty, alternative forms of therapy in this group, stage 1 palliation of hypoplastic left heart syndrome or transplant, also have a high mortality. Presently, we perform balloon valvuloplasty in patients with relatively small left ventricles and then proceed to alternative therapy if the patient fails to improve.

PERCUTANEOUS BALLOON ANGIOPLASTY OF COARCTATION

Percutaneous balloon angioplasty of coarctation was first described in 1982[91] and has since been used in large numbers of older patients with native (unoperated)[92–94] and postoperative recoarctation.[95–97] We do not recommend dilating postoperative lesions in the first 4–6 weeks following surgery, and, therefore, dilation of recurrent coarctations in the first month of life is not really a consideration. Balloon angioplasty of native coarctations has been performed in a relatively small number of neonates, and follow-up is incomplete. Although the immediate results appear similar to results in older patients, the incidence of restenosis appears higher, and the incidence and natural history of aneurysms are unknown.

Technique

Using routine sedation, the femoral vein and artery are entered percutaneously, and the patient is heparinized. Coarctations can be dilated using the venous catheter and an antegrade approach, but the femoral artery approach is preferred. Right and left heart hemodynamics are measured. If the neonate has a patent ductus with right-to-left flow, the pressure gradient will not reflect the degree of obstruction. An aortogram is performed with the side-holes at or just proximal to the coarctation. The first biplane angiogram may be either anteroposterior and lateral or right anterior oblique and long axial oblique. More than one angiogram may be required to profile the lesion. The diameter of the narrowest area of coarctation and of the normal aorta proximally and distally are measured.

The initial balloon is chosen to be approximately 2 to 3 times the narrowest area but not greater than 1.5 times the normal aorta proximally or distally. The balloon dilation catheter should have the smallest shaft available and a 2-cm long balloon. Compared with older patients, high inflation pressures are rarely needed in neonates, and a waist is commonly not seen during inflation in neonates. The balloon is centered across the coarctation, inflated rapidly until fully expanded or to maximal inflation pressure, and deflated. Videotapes are reviewed to check balloon size (balloon size varies with inflation pressures) and position. The balloon catheter is exchanged for a pigtail, and a pressure pullback can be performed using a Y-arm adaptor without losing wire position. It is important not to lose wire position until the procedure is complete due to the danger of perforation when trying to recross the dilated area. An angiogram is performed following dilation to measure the diameter of the narrowing and to look for tears, aneurysms, or dissections.

Results

The controversy over whether to manage native coarctation surgically or with balloon angioplasty continues for all age groups. Currently, comparing results of surgery and balloon angioplasty in neonates is not really possible because so few neonates have been dilated. The major problem with surgery in neonates is the 10–30% incidence of recoarctation. The limited experience with balloon angioplasty of native coarctation suggests a gradient reduction is unrelated to age.[94] The major concerns with balloon angioplasty are the incidence and natural history of aneurysms and the incidence of restenosis. Angioplasty relieves obstruction by producing intimal and medial tears,[98] and this same mechanism, perhaps in combination with cystic medial necrosis or other factors, can lead to aneurysm formation. The incidence of aneurysms, which is reported to be 5–6%, may be lower in patients with discrete as opposed to long segment coarctation.[92–94] Though no large series have been reported, the incidence of restenosis following balloon angioplasty in neonates appears to be higher than in older patients.[99,100] In our experience with six neonates, balloon dilation resulted in excellent short-term relief of obstruction, but all eventually restenosed and underwent

surgery. This was a highly select group of very sick neonates, most of whom had complex congenital heart disease. The primary indication for dilation was to immediately improve hemodynamics in patients who were not responding to medical management, and we tended to use relatively small balloons. Whether this high incidence of restenosis will be found in all neonates remains to be seen.

Only careful, long-term follow-up of neonates undergoing balloon angioplasty will provide the information necessary to decide between surgery and balloon dilation. At present, we do not recommend routine dilation of neonatal coarctation but continue to use the procedure to achieve immediate hemodynamic improvement in sick neonates who are high surgical risks.

MISCELLANEOUS INTERVENTIONS

The last few years have seen a dramatic increase in the types of transcatheter interventions available to treat congenital heart disease. With the exception of the interventions already discussed, most have not been used widely in neonates, either because they are not appropriate or required in the neonatal period or because the hardware currently available is too large to be used routinely in neonates. An example of the latter are the double umbrellas used to close PDAs, ASDs, and VSDs, which currently require 8- or 11-F sheaths for delivery.[101–104] Despite these limitations, several of these interventions will be discussed briefly.

Gianturco coils have now been used in large numbers of patients with congenital heart disease to close aortopulmonary collaterals, systemic to pulmonary shunts, arteriovenous malformations (including pulmonary and hepatic), venous collaterals, and coronary artery fistulae.[105] A major advantage of coils is that they can be delivered through catheters as small as 3-F, and therefore, their use in neonates is technically feasible. Of a total of 191 vessels embolized in 112 patients, we have coil embolized 4 aortopulmonary collaterals and 2 hepatic arteriovenous malformations in 5 neonates, the smallest weighing 1.8 kg. There were no complications in these neonates.

Balloon angioplasty of branch pulmonary artery stenoses has rarely been performed in neonates. Many of the patients in whom the procedure is indicated have complex congenital heart disease with pulmonary atresia. These patients cannot be dilated until surgery establishes a source of pulmonary blood flow, preferably a right-ventricular to pulmonary artery connection, through which catheters can be passed to the pulmonary arteries. Second, most neonates with isolated branch pulmonary artery stenoses, a group who could technically be dilated, are either undiagnosed or asymptomatic in the neonatal period. Rothman et al.[106] reported results of balloon angioplasty of branch pulmonary stenoses in 135 patients. The patients ranged in age from 1 month to 38.5 years, but only seven patients were younger than 1 year. Over this age range, the success rate, defined in terms of vessel enlargement, was approximately 60% and did not correlate with age. Whether development or maturation of the pulmonary vasculature distal to the obstruction would be altered by successful dilation at an earlier age remains to be determined.

Endomyocardial biopsy is recognized as a safe and effective means of diagnosing a range of myocardial diseases in adolescent and adult patients[107] and can also be performed safely in neonates and infants.[108–110] Of 280 right and 45 left ventricular biopsies in 110 patients between 5 days and 18 years of age, we have performed right ventricular biopsies in 7 neonates weighing 2.5 to 4 kg. The indications were dilated cardiomyopathy in 4, suspected myocarditis in 2, and hypertrophic cardiomyopathy in 1. The right ventricular biopsies were performed from the femoral vein ($N = 3$) using a 5- or 6-F long sheath and 5- (Cook or Fehling-Inrad) or 5.5-F (Cordis) biopsy forceps. No complications were encountered in these neonates. Based on the relative safety of the procedure in neonates, indications for endomyocardial biopsy at our institution are the same as for older patients.

REFERENCES

1. Gutgesell HP, Garson A, McNamara DG. Prognosis for the newborn with transposition of the great arteries. *Am J Cardiol* 44:96–100, 1979.
2. Onoki H, Sato T, Kano I, Mochizuki K. Dye dilution curves after the artificial atrial septostomy in three infants with the transposition of the great arteries. *Tohoku J Exp Med* 100:39–46, 1970.
3. Watson H. Atrial septostomy. *Am Heart J* 75:143–144, 1968.
4. Singh SP, Astley R, Burrows FG. Balloon septostomy for transposition of the great arteries. *Br Heart J* 31:722–726, 1969.
5. McNamara DG. Twenty-five years of progress in the medical treatment of pediatric and congenital heart disease. *J Am Coll Cardiol* 1:264–273, 1983.
6. Gale GE, Levin SE, Pocock WA, Barlow JB.

Balloon atrial septostomy in transposition of the great arteries. *S Afr Med J* 45:975–979, 1971.
7. Tynan M. Survival of infants with transposition of the great arteries after balloon atrial septostomy. *Lancet* 1:621–623, 1971.
8. Baker F, Baker L, Zoltum R, Zuberbuhler JR. Effectiveness of the Rashkind procedure in transposition of the great arteries in infants. *Circulation* 43 (Suppl I):1–6, 1971.
9. Rashkind WJ, Miller WW. Creation of an atrial septal defect without thoracotomy. *JAMA* 196:173–174, 1966.
10. Bierman FZ, Williams RG. Subxiphoid two-dimensional imaging of the interatrial septum in infants and neonates with congenital heart disease. *Circulation* 60:80–90, 1979.
11. Leanage R, Agnetti A, Graham G, Taylor J, Macartney FJ. Factors influencing survival after balloon atrial septostomy for complete transposition of great arteries. *Br Heart J* 45:559–572, 1981.
12. Powell TG, Dewey M, West CR, Arnold R. Fate of infants with transposition of the great arteries in relation to balloon atrial septostomy. *Br Heart J* 51:371–376, 1984.
13. Tynan M. Haemodynamic effects of balloon atrial septostomy in infants with transposition of the great arteries. *Br Heart J* 34:791–794, 1972.
14. Tynan M, Carr I, Graham G, Carter RE. Subvalvar pulmonary obstruction complicating the postoperative course of balloon atrial septostomy in transposition of the great arteries. *Circulation* 39 (Suppl): 223–228, 1969.
15. Rashkind WJ. Atrial septostomy in congenital heart disease [Review]. *Adv Pediatr* 16:211–232, 1969.
16. Gutgesell HP, McNamara DG. Transposition of the great arteries. Results of treatment with early palliation and late intracardiac repair. *Circulation* 51:32–38, 1975.
17. Hawker RE, Krovetz LJ, Rowe RD. An analysis of prognostic factors in the outcome of balloon atrial septostomy for transposition of the great arteries. *Johns Hop Med J* 134:95–106, 1974.
18. Horst RL van der, Winship WS, Gotsman MS. Balloon atrial septostomy in complete transposition of the great vessels. *S Afr Med J* 44:916–919, 1970.
19. Korns ME, Garabedian HA, Lauer RM. Anatomic limitations of balloon atrial septostomy. *Hum Pathol* 3:345–349, 1972.
20. Aziz KU, Paul MH, Idriss FS, Wilson AD, Muster AJ. Clinical manifestations of dynamic left ventricular outflow tract stenosis in infants with d-transposition of the great arteries with intact ventricular septum. *Am J Cardiol* 44:290–297, 1979.
21. Tonkin IL, Sansa M, Elliott LP, Bargeron LM Jr. Recognition of developing left ventricular outflow

tract obstruction in complete transposition of the great arteries. *Radiology 134*:53–59, 1980.

22. Waldhausen JA, Boruchow I, Miller WW, Rashkind WJ. Transposition of the great arteries with ventricular septal defect. Palliation by atrial septostomy and pulmonary artery banding. *Circulation 39* (Suppl):215–221, 1969.

23. Parsons CG, Astley R, Burrows FG, Singh SP. Transposition of the great arteries. A study of 65 infants followed for 1 to 4 years after balloon septostomy. *Br Heart J 33*:725–731, 1971.

24. Rashkind W. Balloon atrioseptostomy. *Adv Cardiol 11*:2–10, 1974.

25. Mok Q, Darvell F, Mattos S, et al. Survival after balloon atrial septostomy for complete transposition of great arteries. *Arch Dis Child 62*:549–553, 1987.

26. deLeon VH, Hougen TJ, Norwood WI, Lang P, Marx GR, Castenada A. Results of the Senning operation for transposition of the great arteries with intact ventricular septum in neonates. *Circulation 70*:121–125, 1984.

27. Mullins CE, el Said GM, Neches WH, et al. Balloon atrial septostomy for total anomalous pulmonary venous return. *Br Heart J 35*:752–757, 1973.

28. Serratto M, Bucheleres HG, Bicoff P, Miller RA, Hastreiter AR. Palliative balloon atrial septostomy for total anomalous pulmonary venous connection in infancy. *J Pediatr 73*:734–739, 1968.

29. Neches WH, Mullins CE, McNamara DG. Balloon atrial septostomy in congenital heart disease in infancy. *Am J Dis Child 125*:371–375, 1973.

30. Lenox CC, Zuberbuhler JR. Balloon septostomy in tricuspid atresia after infancy. *Am J Cardiol 25*:723–726, 1970.

31. Sato T, Onoki H, Kano I, Horiuchi T, Ishitoya T. Balloon atrial septostomy in an infant with tricuspid atresia. *Tohoku J Exp Med 101*:281–288, 1970.

32. Trusler GA, Yamamoto N, Williams WG, Izukawa T, Rowe RD, Mustard WT. Surgical treatment of pulmonary atresia with intact ventricular septum. *Br Heart J 38*:957–960, 1976.

33. Starc TJ, Gersony WM. Progressive obstruction of the foramen ovale in patients with left atrioventricular valve stenosis. *J Am Coll Cardiol 7*:1099–1103, 1986.

34. Baker EJ, Allan LD, Tynan MJ, Jones OD, Joseph MC, Deverall PB. Balloon atrial septostomy in the neonatal intensive care unit. *Br Heart J 51*:377–378, 1984.

35. Hurwitz RA, Girod DA. Pecutaneous balloon atrial septostomy in infants with transposition of the great arteries. *Am Heart J 91*:618–622, 1976.

36. Kaye HH, Tynan M. Balloon atrial septostomy via the umbilical vein. *Br Heart J 36*:1040–1042, 1974.

37. Newfeld EA, Purcel C, Paul MH, Cole RB, Muster AJ. Transumbilical balloon atrial septostomy in 16 infants with transposition of the great arteries. *Pediatrics 54*:495–497, 1974.

38. Roguin N, Sujov P, Montag J, Zeltzer M, Riss E. Transumbilical balloon atrial septostomy for transposition of the great arteries in infants under the age of 60 hours. *Am Heart J 107*:174–176, 1984.

39. Lau KC, Mok CK, Lo RN, Leung MP, Leung CY. Balloon atrial septostomy under two-dimensional echocardiographic control. *Pediatr Cardiol 8*:35–37, 1987.

40. Allan LD, Leanage R, Wainwright R, Joseph MC, Tynan M. Balloon atrial septostomy under two dimensional echocardiographic control. *Br Heart J 47*:41–43, 1982.

41. Ozkutlu S, Ozme S, Saraclar M, Baysal K. Balloon atrial septostomy using echocardiographic monitoring. *Jpn Heart J 29*:415–419, 1988.

42. Tyrrell MJ, Moes CA. Congenital levoposition of the right atrial appendage. Its relevance to balloon septostomy. *Am J Dis Child 121*:508–510, 1971.

43. Moore JW, Bricker JT, Mullins CE, Ott DA. Infusion of blood from pericardial sac into femoral vein: A technique for survival until operative closure of a cardiac perforation during balloon septostomy. *Am J Cardiol 56*:494–495, 1985.

44. Blanchard WB, Knauf DG, Victorica BE. Interatrial groove tear: An unusual complication of balloon atrial septostomy. *Pediatr Cardiol 4*:149–150, 1983.

45. Sondheimer HM, Kavey RW, Blackman MS. Fatal over-distension of an atrioseptostomy catheter. *Pediatr Cardiol 2*:255–257, 1982.

46. Venables AW. Balloon atrial septostomy in complete transposition of great arteries in infancy. *Br Heart J 32*:61–65, 1970.

47. Hohn AR, Webb HM. Balloon deflation failure: A hazard of "medical" atrial septostomy. *Am Heart J 83*:389–391, 1972.

48. Ellison RC, Plauth WH Jr, Gazzaniga AB, Fyler DC. Inability to deflate catheter balloon: A complication of balloon atrial septostomy. *J Pediatr 76*:604–606, 1970.

49. Ehmke DE, Durnin RE, Lauer RM. Intra-abdominal hemorrhage complicating a balloon atrial septostomy for transposition of the great arteries. *Pediatrics 45*:289–291, 1970.

50. Matthews RA, Park SC, Neches WH, Fricker FJ, Lenox CC, Zuberbuhler JR. Iliac venous thrombosis in infants and children after cardiac catheterization. *Cathet Cardiovasc Diagn 5*:67–74, 1979.

51. Park SC, Zuberbuhler JR, Neches WH, Lenox CC, Zoltun RA. A new atrial septostomy technique. *Cathet Cardiovasc Diagn 1*:195–201, 1975.

52. Park SC, Neches WH, Mullins CE, et al. Blade atrial septostomy. *Circulation 66*:258–266, 1982.

53. Kan JS, White RI Jr, Mitchell SE, Gardner TJ. Percutaneous balloon valvuloplasty: A new method for treating congenital pulmonary valve stenosis. *N Engl J Med 307*:540–542, 1982.

54. Rao PS, Fawzy ME, Solymar L, Mardini MK. Long-term changes of balloon pulmonary valvuloplasty of valvar pulmonic stenosis. *Am Heart J* 115:1291–1296, 1988.

55. Mullins CE, Ludomirsky A, O'Laughlin MP, et al. Balloon valvuloplasty for pulmonary valve stenosis—two-year follow-up: Hemodynamic and Doppler evaluation. *Cathet Cardiovasc Diagn* 14:76–81, 1988.

56. Kan JS, White RI Jr, Mitchell SE, Anderson JH, Gardner TJ. Percutaneous transluminal balloon valvuloplasty for pulmonary valve stenosis. *Circulation* 69:554–560, 1984.

57. Sullivan ID, Robinson PJ, Macartney FJ, et al. Percutaneous balloon valvuloplasty for pulmonary valve stenosis in infants and children. *Br Heart J* 54:435–441, 1985.

58. Tynan M, Jones O, Joseph MC, Deverall PB, Yates AK. Relief of pulmonary valve stenosis in first week of life by percutaneous balloon valvuloplasty. *Lancet* 1:273, 1984.

59. Rao PS. Balloon valvuloplasty and angioplasty in infants and children. *J Pediatr* 114:907–914, 1989.

60. Khan MAA, Al-Yousef S, Huhta JC, Bricker JT, Mullins CE, Sawyer W. Critical pulmonary valve stenosis in patients less than 1 year of age: Treatment with percutaneous gradational balloon pulmonary valvuloplasty. *Am Heart J* 117:1008–1014, 1989.

61. Zeevi B, Keane JF, Fellows KE, Lock JE. Balloon dilatation of critical pulmonary stenosis in the first week of life. *J Am Coll Cardiol* 11:821–824, 1988.

62. Rey C, Marache P, Francart C, Dupuis C. Percutaneous transluminal balloon valvuloplasty of congenital pulmonary valve stenosis, with a special report on infants and neonates. *J Am Coll Cardiol* 11:815–820, 1988.

63. Radke W, Keane JF, Fellows KE, Lang P, Lock JE. Percutaneous balloon valvuloplasty of congenital pulmonary stenosis using oversized balloon. *J Am Coll Cardiol* 8:909–915, 1986.

64. Rao PS, Thaper MK, Kutayli F. Causes of restenosis after balloon valvuloplasty for valvular pulmonary stenosis. *Am J Cardiol* 62:979–982, 1988.

65. Ring JC, Kulik TJ, Burke BA, Lock JE. Morphologic changes induced by dilatation of the pulmonary valve annulus with overlarge balloons in normal newborn lambs. *Am J Cardiol* 55:210–214, 1985.

66. DiSessa TG, Alpert BS, Chase NA, Birnbaum SE, Watson DC. Balloon valvuloplasty in children with dysplastic pulmonary valves. *Am J Cardiol* 60:405–407, 1987.

67. Museive NN, Robertson MA, Benson LN, et al. The dysplastic pulmonary valve: Echocardiographic features and results of balloon dilatation. *Br Heart J* 57:364–370, 1987.

68. Marantz PM, Huhta JC, Mullins CE, et al. Results of balloon valvuloplasty in typical and dysplastic pulmonary valve stenosis; Doppler echocardiographic follow-up. *J Am Coll Cardiol* 12:476–479, 1988.

69. McCredie RM, Swinburn MJ, Lee CL, Warner G. Balloon dilatation pulmonary valvuloplasty in pulmonary stenosis. *Aust N Z J Med* 16:20–23, 1986.

70. Rao PS, Brais M. Balloon pulmonary valvuloplasty for congenital cyanotic heart defects. *Am Heart J* 115:1105–1113, 1988.

71. Boucek MM, Webster HE, Orsmond GS, Ruttenberg HD. Balloon pulmonary valvotomy: Palliation for cyanotic heart disease. *Am Heart J* 115:318–322, 1988.

72. Keane JF, Bernhard WF, Nadas AS. Aortic stenosis surgery in infancy. *Circulation* 69:554, 1984.

73. Kugler JD, Campball E, Vargo TA, McNamara DG, Hallman GL, Cooley DA. Results of aortic valvulotomy in infants with isolated aortic valve stenosis. *J Thorac Cardiovasc Surg* 78:553–558, 1979.

74. Messina LM, Turley K, Stanger P, Hoffman JIE, Ebert PA. Successful aortic valvotomy for severe congenital valvular aortic stenosis in the newborn infant. *J Thorac Cardiovasc Surg* 88:92–96, 1984.

75. Pelech AN, Dyck JD, Trusler GA, et al. Critical aortic stenosis: Survival and management. *J Thorac Cardiovasc Surg* 94:510–517, 1987.

76. Sink JD, Smallhorn JF, Macartney FJ, Taylor JFN, Stark J, de Leval MR. Management of critical aortic stenosis in infancy. *J Thorac Cardiovasc Surg* 87:82–86, 1984.

77. Brown JW, Stevens LS, Holly S, et al. Surgical spectrum of aortic stenosis in children: Thirty-year experience with 257 children. *Ann Thorac Surg* 45:393–403, 1988.

78. Dobell ARC, Bloss RS, Gibbons JE, Collins GF. Congenital valvular aortic stenosis: Surgical management and long term results. *J Thorac Cardiovasc Surg* 81:916–920, 1981.

79. Fulton DR, Hougen TJ, Keane JF, Rosenthal AR, Norwood WI, Bernhard WF. Repeat aortic valvotomy in children. *Am Heart J* 106:60–63, 1983.

80. Sandor GGS, Olley PM, Trusler GA, Williams WG, Rowe RD, Morch JE. Long term follow-up of patients after valvotomy for congenital valvular aortic stenosis in children: A clinical and actuarial follow-up. *J Thorac Cardiovasc Surg* 80:171–176, 1980.

81. Lababidi Z. Aortic balloon valvuloplasty. *Am Heart J* 106:751, 1983.

82. Scholler GF, Keane JF, Perry SB, Sanders SP, Lock JE. Balloon dilation of aortic stenosis: Results and influence of technical and morphological features on outcome. *Circulation* 78:351–360, 1988.

83. Rocchini AP, Beekman RH, Schachar GB, Benson L, Schwartz D, Kan JS. Balloon aortic valvuloplasty: Results of the valvuloplasty and angioplasty

of congenital anomalies registry. *Am J Cardiol* 65:784–789, 1990.

84. Cribier A, Savin T, Berland J, et al. Percutaneous transluminal balloon valvuloplasty of adult aortic stenosis: Report of 92 cases. *J Am Coll Cardiol* 9:381–386, 1987.

85. Lababidi Z, Weinhaus L. Successful balloon valvuloplasty for neonatal critical aortic stenosis. *Am Heart J 112*:913–916, 1986.

86. Wren C, Sullivan I, Bull C, Deanfield J, Percutaneous balloon dilatation of aortic valve stenosis in neonates and infants. *Br Heart J 58*:608–612, 1987.

87. Zeevi B, Keane JF, Castenada AR, Perry SB, Lock JE. Neonatal critical valvar aortic stenosis. A comparison of surgical and balloon dilatation therapy. *Ciculation* 80:831–839, 1989.

88. Helgason H, Keane JF, Fellows KE, Kulik TJ, Lock JE. Balloon dilation of the aortic valve: Studies in normal lambs and in children with aortic stenosis. *J Am Coll Cardiol* 9:816–822, 1987.

89. Waller BF, Girod DA, Dillon JC. Transverse aortic wall tears in infants after balloon angioplasty for aortic valve stenosis: Relation of aortic wall damage to diameter of inflated angioplasty balloon and aortic lumen in 7 necropsy cases. *J Am Coll Cardiol* 4:1235–1241, 1984.

90. Phillips RR, Gerlis LM, Wilson N, Walker DR. Aortic valve damage caused by operative balloon dilatation of critical aortic valve stenosis. *Br Heart J* 97:168–170, 1987.

91. Singer MI, Rowen M, Dorsey TJ. Transluminal aortic balloon angioplasty for coarctation of the aorta in the newborn. *Am Heart J 103*:131–132, 1982.

92. Morrow WR, Vick GW, Nihill MR, Mullins CE, Hedrick T, McNamara DG. Balloon dilation of unoperated coarctation of the aorta: Short- and intermediate-term results. *J Am Coll Cardiol 11*:133, 1988.

93. Beekman RH, Rocchini AP, Dick M. Percutaneous balloon angioplasty for native coarctation of the aorta. *J Am Coll Cardiol 10*:1078, 1987.

94. Tynan M, Finley JP, Fontes V, Hess J, Kan J. Balloon angioplasty for the treatment of native coarctation: Results of the valvuloplasty and angioplasty of congenital anomalies registry. *Am J Cardiol 65*:790–792, 1990.

95. Saul JP, Keane JF, Fellows KE, Lock JE. Balloon dilation angioplasty of postoperative aortic obstructions. *Am J Cardiol 59*:943–948, 1987.

96. Hellenbrand WE, Allen HD, Golinko RJ, Hagler DJ, Lutin W, Kan J. Balloon angioplasty for aortic recoarctation: Results of the valvuloplasty and angioplasty of congenital anomalies registry. *Am J Cardiol 65*:793–797, 1990.

97. Perry SB, Zeevi B, Keane JF, Lock JE. Interventional catheterization of left heart lesions, including aortic and mitral valve stenosis and coarctation of the aorta. *Cardiol Clin 7*:341–349, 1989.

98. Lock JE, Niemi T, Burke B, Einzig S, Castaneda-Zuniga W. Transcutaneous angioplasty of experimental aortic coarctation. *Circulation 66*:1280–1286, 1982.

99. Finley JP, Beaulieu RG, Nanton MA, Roy DL. Balloon catheter dilation of coarctation of the aorta in young infants. *Br Heart J 50*:411–415, 1983.

100. Rao PS. Balloon angioplasty for coarctation of the aorta in infancy. *J Pediatr 110*:713, 1987.

101. Rashkind WJ, Mullins CE, Hellenbrand WE, Tait MA. Nonsurgical closure of patent ductus arteriosus: Clinical application of the Rashkind PDA occluder system. *Ciculation 75*:583–592, 1987.

102. Lock JE, Rome JJ, Davis R, et al. Transcatheter closure of atrial septal defects: Experimental studies. *Circulation* [In press]

103. Lock JE, Block PC, McKay RG, Baim DS, Keane JF. Transcatheter closure of ventricular septal defects. *Circulation 78*:361–368, 1988.

104. Goldstein SAN, Perry SB, Keane JF, Rome J, Lock JE. Transcatheter closure of congenital ventricular septal defects. (Abstr) *J Am Coll Cardiol 15*:240A, 1990.

105. Perry SB, Radke W, Fellows KE, Keane JF, Lock JE. Coil embolization to occlude aortopulmonary collateral vessels and shunts in patients with congenital heart disease. *J Am Coll Cardiol 13*:100–108, 1989.

106. Rothman A, Perry SB, Keane JF, Lock JE. Early results and follow-up of balloon angioplasty for branch pulmonary artery stenosis. *J Am Coll Cardiol 15*:1109–1117, 1990.

107. Mason J. Endomyocardial biopsy: The balance of success and failure. *Circulation 71*:185–188, 1985.

108. Lurie PR. Revision of pediatric endomyocardial biopsy technique. *Am J Cardiol 60*:368–370, 1987.

109. Rios B, Nihill MR, Mullins CE. Left ventricular endomyocardial biopsy in children with the transseptal long sheath technique. *Cathet Cardiovasc Diagn 10*:417–423, 1984.

110. Bhargava H, Donner RM, Sanchez G, et al. Endomyocardial biopsy after heart transplantation in children. *J Heart Transplant 6*:298–302, 1987.

18

Transcatheter Closure of Abnormal Shunt Pathways

WILLIAM E. HELLENBRAND and JOHN T. FAHEY

Cardiac catheterization in infants, children, and adults is the most definitive diagnostic modality for understanding and defining congenital heart disease and has been performed for many years in patients. This procedure enables pediatric cardiologists to delineate the natural history of congenital heart defects, define pathologic anatomy, evaluate altered hemodynamics and physiology, and provide detailed diagnostic information for making surgical decisions. With the advent of newer forms of cardiac imaging such as two-dimensional echocardiography, Doppler ultrasound, and transesophageal echocardiography (TEE) along with computerized tomographic and magnetic resonance imaging scanning techniques, it has become apparent that cardiac catheterization is probably not indicated in all cases of congenital heart disease. With the report of balloon pulmonary valvuloplasty in 1982,[1] a new and exciting era for the pediatric cardiac catheterization laboratory has evolved, providing a different and important role for cardiac catheterization in the management of congenital heart disease.

Although therapeutic catheterization for congenital heart disease began with Dr. Rashkind's report of balloon atrial septostomy in 1966,[2] it is only since 1982 that the goals and indications for cardiac catheterization have dramatically changed, and therapeutic procedures presently account for as much as one-third of all catheterization procedures performed on patients with congenital heart disease in many pediatric cardiology centers. Balloon dilation procedures have been developed to relieve obstruction in both stenotic valves and blood vessels in pre-and post-operative patients[3–10] and are detailed in separate chapters. Newer techniques have been developed for children and adults to close abnormal shunt pathways such as

patent ductus arteriosus (PDA),[11–13] atrial septal defects (ASD),[14–17] ventricular septal defects (VSD),[18] pulmonary arteriovenous malformations,[19] and congenital or surgically created systemic-pulmonary collaterals.[20] The purpose of this chapter is to review the techniques and results of these new nonsurgical transcatheter approaches to closure of these abnormal shunt pathways.

CLOSURE OF THE PATENT DUCTUS ARTERIOSUS
Historical Perspective

Persistent PDA is a very common form of congenital heart disease,[21] which can present in infancy with congestive heart failure, can be an incidental finding in children and young adults, and can cause congestive heart failure and pulmonary vascular obstructive disease in the adult population. In 1971, the first report of nonsurgical closure of PDA was reported by Dr. Porstmann in 62 patients.[22] This technique required the simultaneous use of both the femoral artery and vein to allow the introduction of the occluding plug into the PDA. A large catheter was introduced into the femoral artery by either arteriotomy or percutaneous technique. The artery had to be dilated with an 18-F (6 mm) dilator to allow insertion of the ductal occluding device. A catheter was then passed from the femoral artery to the aorta and across the PDA into the pulmonary artery. A catheter was then advanced through the right heart into the inferior vena cava and out the contralateral femoral vein (Fig. 18.1). A long guidewire was passed through this catheter so that both ends of the guidewire extend outside the body. An Ivalon plug was prepared to conform to the shape of the ductus and was then inserted on the arterial end of

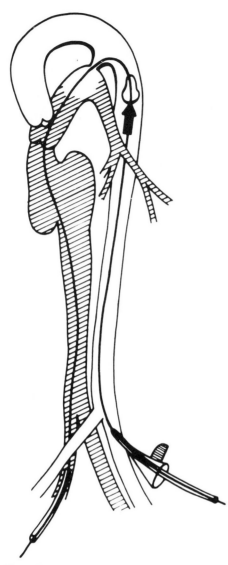

Figure 18.1. Diagrammatic representation of closure of a patent ductus arteriosus by Porstmann's technique. The Ivalon ductal plug is seen in the descending aorta as it is moved into position along a transductal wire loop extending from the left femoral artery to the right femoral vein. (Reproduced with permission from Radiology Clinics of North America 9:204;1971.)

was reported. There have been subsequent reports using this technique with some modifications with equally good results.[23]

Successful nonsurgical closure by this technique required that the ductus be conical in shape and that the diameter of the femoral artery used be greater than the narrowest diameter of the PDA in order to be able to introduce the proper-sized occluder into the femoral artery. Only 5 of the original 62 patients were less than 10 years of age, as this retrogade approach required a large femoral artery. Accordingly, this technique has not been widely accepted as it is not applicable to the majority of patients who undergo closure of this defect in the first five years of life. However, this technique served to demonstrate the feasibility of transcatheter nonsurgical closure of the PDA, avoiding the need for an extended hospital stay, general anesthesia, a lateral thoracotomy, and a prolonged convalescence.

Present Closure System

Following several years of experimentation in animals, the latest closure system currently in use has been designed as a double umbrella system that is applicable to all patients from small infants to adults. It does not require the use of a large catheter in the femoral artery and is a procedure that can be performed by cardiologists who are uniquely skilled in interventional procedures. The umbrella currently in use for closure of a PDA has been under investigation for the past six years and has been used in over 500 patients in five pediatric cardiac centers.

Technical Considerations: The PDA Umbrella

The umbrella is designed as two spring assemblies resembling two opposing discs (USCI Angiographic Systems, Tewksbury, MA) (Fig. 18.2A, B). There are two different sized devices measuring either 12 or 17 mm in diameter. In the 17-mm device, each spring assembly consists of four arms individually wound from surgical steel wire fashioned in such a manner as to create opposing spring tension between the two discs. The individual arms of each disc are attached centrally and are equally spaced 90° apart. The arms have been designed so that when they are extruded from the delivery catheter, they will spring open perpendicular to the delivery system. Each arm ends as a smooth round eye so there are no sharp or jagged points where the arms come into contact with the

the wire and introduced into the femoral artery. The plug was advanced over the wire with a catheter pushing the device ahead of it and was wedged into the aortic end of the PDA. The arterial catheter was then removed, and the wire pulled out via the femoral vein. In the initial report, the PDA was successfully closed in 56 of 62 patients. There was no mortality although some morbidity related to femoral artery complications

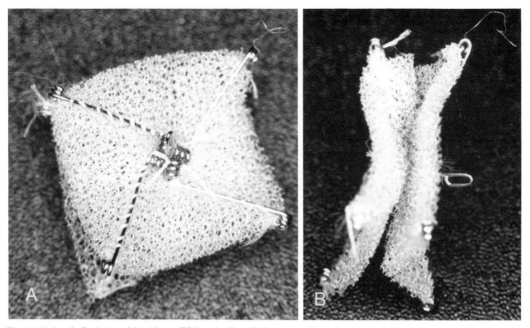

Figure 18.2. **A,** End view of the 17-mm PDA umbrella with the polyurethane foam sewn to the four arms. Each arm ends as smooth round eye. **B,** Profile view of the device with both discs parallel to each other. The elliptical loop that attaches the device to the delivery catheter is seen in profile.

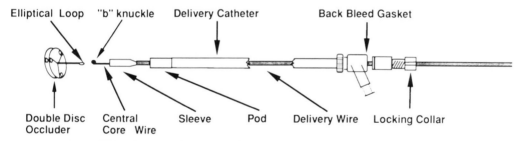

Figure 18.3.   Diagrammatic representation of the double disc PDA umbrella delivery system.

wall of the blood vessel. This is to prevent any damage or perforation as the device is placed in the PDA. Platinum is placed on each arm to facilitate fluoroscopic visualization of the device. An elliptical loop is located at the central hub of the proximal disc to allow attachment to the delivery catheter system. The 12-mm device is built in a similar fashion with three arms instead of four, spaced 120° apart, each made from a slightly lighter grade of stainless steel.

Each disc is covered with a piece of medical grade open pore polyurethane foam contoured to correspond to the diameter of the umbrella and sewn securely with very fine suture material to the spring assembly along each arm and through each distal eye.

Technical Considerations: The Delivery System

The delivery system is illustrated in Figure 18.3. It is designed as a coaxial system with a central core wire within a larger spring guide delivery wire that in turn is enclosed in a larger delivery catheter. At the distal end of the fine central core wire is a small polished b-shaped knuckle that will fit perfectly into the elliptical loop of the umbrella, attaching the umbrella to the delivery system. The distal end of the coiled delivery wire ends as a small sleeve through which the central core wire extends. At the proximal end of the system, the central core wire and the coiled delivery wire are both attached to the central wire control clamp that permits the

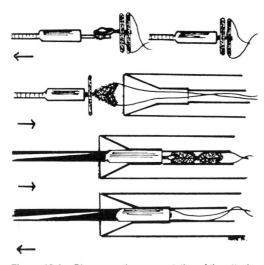

Figure 18.4. Diagrammatic representation of the attachment and loading sequence for the PDA umbrella. The four step process: (1) connection of the umbrella to the central wire and locking the knuckle/loop in the sleeve; (2) with traction on the suture, the distal arms are folded and advanced into the loader with the proximal arms following; (3) the folded disc is advanced to the narrowest part of the loader and the catheter advanced into the loader; (4) the folded double disc is withdrawn into the delivery catheter. (Reproduced with permission from *Circulation 75*:586, 1987.)

inner wire to be retracted into or pushed out of the sleeve at the end of the delivery wire. The entire central core/delivery wire system is contained within an 8-F delivery catheter. At the end of the delivery catheter there is a thin-walled stainless steel tubular pod, that is 8-F for the 12-mm device and 11-F for the 17-mm device. There is a locking collar on the delivery wire to control the movement of the delivery wire out the end of the delivery catheter. Figure 18.4 illustrates the attachment and loading sequence of the umbrella device. To attach the umbrella to the catheter, the elliptical loop at the center of the proximal disc is placed over the b-shaped knuckle at the end of the central core wire. The central wire is then withdrawn into the delivery wire, drawing the joined knuckle and elliptical loop into the sleeve at the end of the delivery wire. This is locked in the sleeve using the central wire control clamp. The precisely machined internal diameter of the sleeve holds the loop and the knuckle together until the central wire is advanced out of the sleeve. To help load the device into the catheter, each umbrella has a suture that passes through each eye of the distal disc and then through a central lumen of a specially designed plastic loader. Traction is applied to the suture on the opposite end of the loader, and the distal set of arms is folded to fit into the funnel within the

loader. As the device is pulled farther into the loader, the proximal arms fold backward. The two discs that have now been folded in opposite directions are then pulled into the narrow part of the loader and compressed so they can fit into the delivery pod at the end of the delivery catheter. The catheter can now be advanced into the narrow part of the loader, and the delivery wire is withdrawn into the pod drawing the folded device into the delivery pod. The locknut device is tightened to prevent the device from advancing out of the pod, the suture is cut, the catheter is flushed, and the umbrella is now ready to be placed in the PDA.

Placement of the PDA Umbrella Device

The umbrella device has been developed to allow percutaneous introduction of the system from either the femoral artery or vein. The most common approach has been from the venous system and will be described.

The patients are premedicated using standard medications for cardiac catheterization. General anesthesia need not be used for the entire procedure; however, most patients receive intravenous ketamine during the implantation. All patients are fully heparinized, and prophylactic antibiotics are used. Although both groins are prepped, usually only one groin will be used. The right femoral vein is cannulated with a short 8-F sheath, and the right femoral artery is entered using either 4-, 5-, or 6-F sheath, depending on the patient's size. Following a complete right and left heart catheterization, a descending aortogram is performed using a retrograde aortic catheter with calibrated markings to facilitate measurement of the ductus. Angiograms are obtained in the posteroanterior and lateral projections to demonstrate the location, size, and configuration of the ductus. In patients with a PDA up to 4 mm in diameter, a 12-mm diameter device is used. With a patent ductus greater than 4 or less than 8 mm in diameter, a 17-mm device is used. With the present umbrella devices, one should not attempt to close a PDA equal to or greater than 8 mm in diameter at its narrowest end. Following the decision to close the ductus in the catheterization laboratory, an end-hole catheter is advanced across the PDA from the venous system, and an exchange J-wire is passed through this catheter into the descending aorta below the level of the diaphragm. The catheter and short sheath are removed, and the 11-F long sheath and dilator (8-F for the 12-mm device) is advanced over the exchange wire through the right heart, across the PDA, and into the descending aorta (Mullin's modification.)[11] The wire and dilator are removed and the umbrella delivery system is advanced in the sheath until the delivery pod on the end of the catheter reaches the level of the tricuspid valve. At this point, it is extremely difficult to advance the catheter farther, and the sheath now is used as an extension of the pod. The locknut is loosened, and the delivery wire is advanced slowly delivering the umbrella out of the pod into the sheath (Fig. 18.5A). The delivery wire continues to be advanced until the umbrella is at the end of the sheath. The entire delivery system, including the sheath and the catheter, can now be withdrawn from the descending aorta until the end of the sheath is at the aortic end of the ductus (Fig. 18.5B). The delivery wire is then advanced carefully until the distal set of arms is extruded from the sheath and the distal disc springs open completely in the aorta (Fig. 18.5C). The entire delivery system (sheath, catheter, delivery wire, and device) is slowly withdrawn into the ductus with slight backward tension on the delivery wire so that the proximal arms will not open until the proper position for the distal arms is attained (Fig. 18.5D). This can be identified by any or all of three methods: (1) resistance to further withdrawal as the narrowest part of the ductus is reached, (2) flexing of the distal ribs within the ductus, or (3) distal arm position in relation to the trachea previously seen by aortography. This part of the procedure is complicated by positional changes of the ductus as the device is pulled into it. When the distal arms are in proper position, the central delivery wire is held in place, and the sheath is then retracted allowing the proximal arms to spring open in the pulmonary side of the ductus, thereby securing the umbrella in the ductus (Fig. 18.5E). It is important not to place any tension on the system at this time to prevent unexpected dislodgement of the device prior to release.

At this point, a repeat descending aortogram may be performed to confirm the proper position of the device before separation from the delivery system. If the device is not in proper position or it has pulled through into the pulmonary artery, the entire device can be withdrawn into the sheath and removed allowing a second approach with a new umbrella. If the umbrella is in the proper position, the release mechanism in the central wire control clamp is engaged allowing the sleeve to slide off the knuckle of the central control wire releasing the umbrella (Fig. 18.5F). The delivery system is then withdrawn into the sheath and removed.

Twenty minutes following the release of the umbrella, a repeat descending aortogram is performed to confirm complete closure. If there is a residual jet present, we place a balloon catheter into the pulmonary artery and try to press the foam on the proximal arm against the vessel wall to effect complete closure. Some investigators suggest soaking the umbrella in tropical thrombin just prior to implantation to ensure complete closure. Initially patients were kept overnight following this procedure; however, closure of the PDA is now performed as an outpatient procedure when possible. The patients are followed with echo-Doppler and chest x-ray immediately after the procedure and at one month and one year following implantation according to the current protocol.

Closing of the PDA from the femoral artery is an alternative approach. The only difference is that frequently the delivery pod can be delivered directly through the sheath into the pulmonary artery. This permits the sheath to be withdrawn into the aorta thus obviating use of the sheath as an extension of the pod.

Clinical Results

At Yale-New Haven Hospital, 75 patients have undergone attempted transcatheter closure of a patent ductus arteriosus (Table 18.1). The indications for catheter closure are the same as for surgery and relate to the clinical presence of a PDA. The age of the patients has ranged from 3 months to 70 years with 16 patients less than 1 year of age. There were 8 patients older than 18, 3 of whom were greater than 50 years of age. Two patients had previously undergone surgical closure of their PDA and had residual patency of the ductus arteriosus. There were 21 patients less than 10 kg, and 8 were less than 6 kg. The diameter of the PDA at its narrowest point ranged from less than 1 mm to 11 mm in diameter. Closure procedures in

Table 18.1.
Clinical Profile for PDA Closure ($N = 75$)

Age (3 months–70 years)	< 1 yr	16
	1–5 yr	36
	5–18 yr	15
	> 18 yr	8
Weight (4.3–88 kg)	< 6 kg	8
	6–10 kg	13
	10–20 kg	36
	> 20 kg	18
PDA (0.5–12.5 mm)	< 2.5 mm	25
(narrowest dimension)	2.5–4.4 mm	42
	> 4.5 mm	8

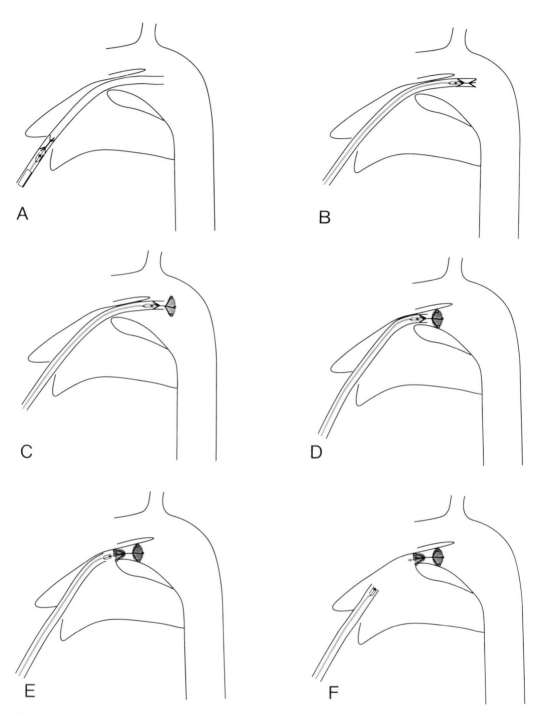

Figure 18.5.   A, Diagrammatic representation of the Mullins transseptal sheath across the PDA with the umbrella device extending from the delivery catheter into the sheath. **B,** The umbrella is at the end of the sheath, and the sheath has been withdrawn to the aortic end of the ductus. **C,** The distal disc has been extruded from the sheath and is fully open in the descending aorta. **D,** The sheath and umbrella are within the ductus with the distal disc wedged into the ductus. **E,** Both discs are open in the ductus with the umbrella still attached to the delivery system. **F,** Detached umbrella is now within the ductus and the delivery system is withdrawn into the sheath. (Reproduced with permission from *Cardiology Clinics 7*:354, 1989.)

patients with a ductal diameter of less than 2 mm were sometimes complicated by the inability either to enter the PDA from the pulmonary artery with the guidewire or to pass the delivery system across the PDA over the guidewire. In the former group, the ductus was first crossed with a small catheter from the aortic end of the PDA, and a 400-mm wire was passed through the catheter into the main pulmonary artery where it was retrieved with a basket retrieval catheter (Meditech multipurpose basket or forceps) and extracted out the femoral vein. The long sheath was then delivered across the PDA over the wire. In the latter group of patients, the PDA was dilated with small angioplasty catheters to facilitate placement of the delivery system across the PDA.

The PDA umbrella has been successfully implanted in the ductus in 67 of 75 patients (89%) at Yale-New Haven Hospital (Table 18.2). Most of the failures to implant occurred in the early part of the protocol, and the last 45 patients have had successful implantation. Of the 8 unsuccessful implantations, only 1 would not be attempted at the present time because the ductus was too large. The other 7 would most likely be successful at the current time and represent our learning curve. Despite proper placement of the device, there has been a 10% incidence of residual left-to-right shunt through the device on long-term follow-up. Of the 7 patients with residual leaks, 4 have both clinical (continuous murmur) and echo-Doppler evidence of a PDA, and the other 3 have only echocardiographic documentation. The patients with clinical evidence of a residual left-to-right shunt will undergo placement of a second umbrella in the near future.[12,13] We have delayed this

Table 18.2.
Clinical Results for PDA Closure (*N* = 75)

Successful implantation	67/75 (89%)	
	1983–1986	22/29 (76%)
	1987–1990	45/46 (98%)
Implantation	60/67[a] (90%)	
Complete closure	1983–1986	20/22 (91%)
	1987–1990	40/45 (89%)
Implantation	7/67[a] (10%)	
Residual L-R shunt	1983–1986	2/22 (9%)
	1987–1990	5/45 (11%)
Umbrella	8/75 (11%)	
embolization	1983–1986	7/29 (24%)
	1987–1990	1/46 (2%)

PDA = patent ductus arteriosus; L-R = left to right.
[a]number of patients who had successful implantation

procedure as late closure has been documented in several patients.

In our adult series of 8 patients over 18 years of age, 7 have had successful implantation of the umbrella device with complete closure.

CASE STUDIES

A 4.7 kg, three-month-old female with congestive heart failure presented with a classical PDA and was brought to the catheterization laboratory on the day after admission. A PDA whose narrowest diameter measured 3 to 4 mm was identified, and a transcatheter closure was performed successfully with a 12-mm umbrella (Fig. 18.6*A*, *B*). The patient was discharged the next day asymptomatic, with no cardiac murmurs, on no cardiac medications, and has been followed for two years with no clinical or echo-Doppler evidence of a residual shunt and normal growth and development.

A 26-year-old asymptomatic female was found to have a PDA and was referred for catheter closure. The ductus, which was 12 mm in diameter at its aortic end and 4 to 5 mm in diameter at the pulmonary end, was identified (Fig. 18.7*A*). A 17-mm device was successfully placed straddling the narrow end of the ductus, and repeat angiography demonstrated complete closure (Fig.18.7*B*). This patient has no clinical or echo-Doppler evidence of a PDA at long-term follow-up.

A 70-year-old woman who had been followed for a murmur for many years presented with congestive heart failure and underwent cardiac catheterization where pulmonary hypertension with a large left-to-right shunt at the great vessel level was found. A 7-mm PDA was identified (Fig. 18.8*A*), and successful transcatheter closure was performed using a 17-mm device (Fig. 18.8*B*). The pulmonary artery peak systolic pressure, which was initially 70 mm Hg, fell to 35 mm Hg 20 min after implantation of the device. The symptoms of congestive heart failure have disappeared, and the patient is currently doing well.

COMPLICATIONS

The only significant complication has been related to embolization of the device into the pulmonary artery. This event always occurred immediately after release, and there have been no late embolizations. In our experience, there have been a total of 8 embolized umbrellas, all to the pulmonary artery (Table 18.2). Three of these umbrellas have been retrieved during the catheterization procedure. A retrieval catheter (Meditech multipurpose basket or

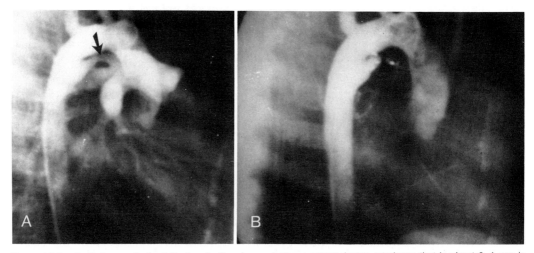

Figure 18.6. **A,** Aortogram in the lateral projection demonstrates a patent ductus arteriosus that is about 3–4 mm in diameter in a 3-month-old infant. **B,** Repeat aortogram 15 min after insertion of the PDA umbrella demonstrates complete closure of the PDA. (Reproduced with permission from *Cardiology Clinics* 6:434, 1988.)

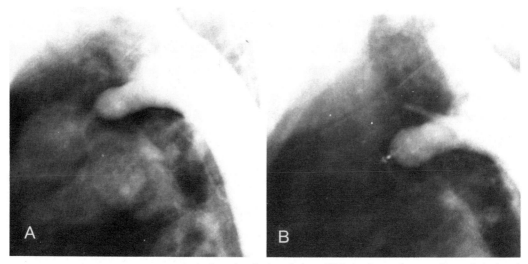

Figure 18.7. **A,** Descending aortogram in the lateral projection shows a PDA that is very large at the aortic end and narrows considerably at the pulmonary end before it enters the pulmonary artery. **B,** Following proper implantation of the 17-mm umbrella, a repeat angiogram demonstrates complete closure of the PDA with the device in the proper position.

forceps) was employed to grasp the device in the pulmonary artery, withdraw the device into a large sheath in the pulmonary artery, and then remove the umbrella. The opened device should not be pulled through the RV as it will become entangled with the tricuspid valve apparatus. In 2 of these 3 patients, a second device was placed successfully in the PDA. In 3 patients, the embolized umbrella was removed at surgery at the same time the ductus was ligated. Two devices were left in the distal part of the left pulmonary artery with no long-term

effects. In one of these patients, a second device was properly placed in the PDA. Embolization of the device has not occurred in the last 45 procedures.

Transcatheter closure of the PDA thus provides a reasonable alternative to surgical closure in both the pediatric and adult population. Successful implantation can now be achieved in greater than 95% of cases, and new modifications of the device will decrease the incidence of residual left-to-right shunts. The complication rate is now extremely low, with subsequent operative repair available if the ductus cannot be successfully occluded.

CLOSURE OF ATRIAL SEPTAL DEFECTS

Historical Perspective

Atrial septal defect is another common form of congenital heart disease,[21] presenting in children and young adults usually as an incidental finding or as mild congestive heart failure. In adults, arrhythmias, congestive heart failure, and pulmonary vascular obstructive disease can occur. The first approach to transcatheter closure of this abnormality was described by King and Mills in 1975.[14] A double umbrella closure system (Fig. 18.9) was placed across the atrial defect via a large delivery catheter (23-F) to close the atrial communication. The first (or left atrial) umbrella was opened in the left atrium and pulled against the left side of the atrial septum. The right atrial umbrella was then advanced through the delivery catheter, opened in the right atrium, and advanced to the right side of the atrial septum where it is locked to the left atrial umbrella closing the atrial defect. This procedure was used successfully in several patients. However, this approach has not been adopted by other pediatric cardiology centers, and no further reports have appeared in the literature.

More recently, a different approach was attempted.[12,24] A single umbrella was designed that

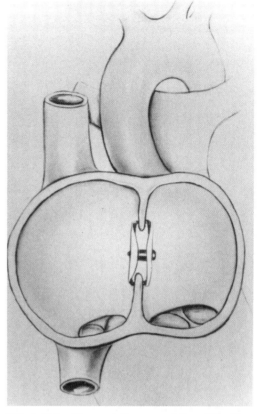

Figure 18.9. Diagrammatic representation of the King ASD umbrella with both the left and right discs locked together on either side of the ASD. (Reproduced with permission, *Surgery* 75:386, 1975.)

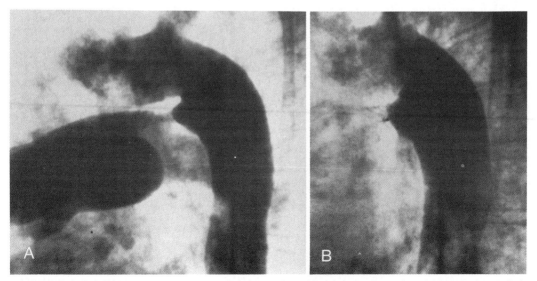

Figure 18.8. **A,** Aortogram in a 70-year-old woman demonstrating a PDA and a markedly dilated pulmonary artery. **B,** A repeat aortogram 20 min after placement and release of the umbrella demonstrates complete occlusion of the PDA. (Reproduced with permission from *Cardiology Clinics* 6:434, 1988.)

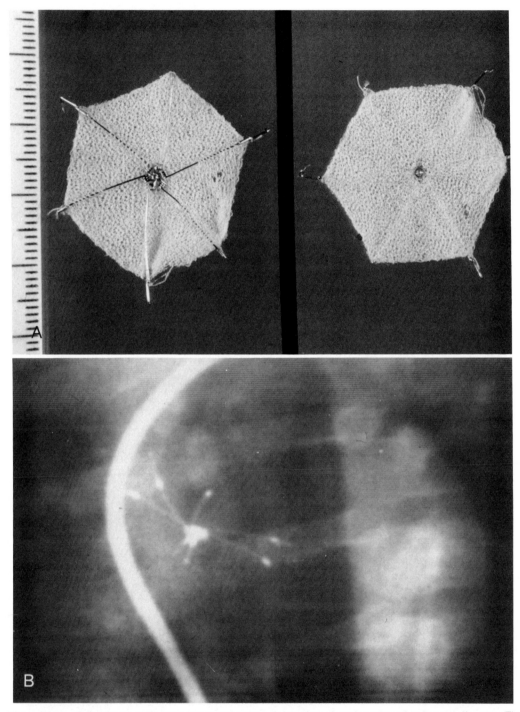

Figure 18.10.   A, The 25-mm ASD single disc closure device. Polyurethane foam is contoured and sewn to the arms. The barbed hooks can be seen at the end of every other arm. **B,** The ASD device is well seated on the atrial septum following implantation. (Reproduced with permission from *Cardiology Clinics 6*:435, 1988.)

consisted of a stainless steel frame with six arms covered with a disc of polyurethane foam (Fig. 18.10*A*). Every other arm had a barbed hook at the end to attach to the atrial septum. This device was delivered to the left atrium via a 16-F sheath and opened in the middle of the left atrium and withdrawn against the atrial septum with the hooks embedded into the septum surrounding the defect (Fig.18.10*B*). This procedure was tried in a number of patients with limited success. This device was abandoned because the success rate was low, and, because of the hooks, this device could not be withdrawn if placed in the wrong position. Accordingly, a new device was suggested by Dr. James Lock similar to the PDA umbrella and is presently in clinical investigation.[17]

Technical Considerations: The Present ASD Umbrella and Delivery System

The ASD closure device presently being tested is designed as two spring assemblies resembling two opposing umbrellas (USCI Angiographic Systems, Tewksbury, MA) (Fig. 18.11*A, B*). Each spring assembly consists of four arms that are wound in such a way that when opened they create an opposing spring tension between the two umbrellas. The individual arms are spaced 90° apart and are attached to a central spring area. In addition, each arm has a second spring in the middle, so that when the occlusion device is extruded from the delivery catheter, it will spring open with the free ends of the arms of the opposing umbrellas tending to overlap one another, past perpendicular. When the device is appropriately placed, with each umbrella on opposite sides of the interatrial

septum, the septal tissue will prevent overlap of the arms. This will assure secure attachment of the device to the limbus of the defect. There are no barbed hooks on the arms, and the device is held in place only by the opposing tensions of the umbrellas. Each spring assembly is covered with a square disc of medical grade Dacron fabric virtually identical to the Dacron fabric used in surgical repair. The atrial septal defect umbrella currently under investigation comes in five different diameters (17, 23, 28, 33, and 40 mm). The delivery system is virtually identical to the one used for the PDA umbrella, except there is only one size, designed as an 8-F catheter and an 11-F delivery pod of varying lengths. The assembly fits through an 11-F sheath. The ASD device is loaded into the delivery catheter in a similar fashion to the PDA umbrella.

Technical Considerations: Implantation Technique

The initial portion of the catheterization procedure involves right and left heart catheterization performed via the right femoral artery and vein. Intracardiac pressures and shunt measurements are performed in standard fashion.

Angiocardiography is performed with the venous catheter positioned in the right upper pulmonary vein or the left atrium, with the frontal image intensifier positioned in hepatoclavicular orientation (four-chamber, 35° LAO and 35° cranial angulation), in order to profile the interatrial septum. This facilitates identification of the location and dimensions of the atrial communication. A precalibrated NIH marking catheter (USCI Angiographic Systems, Tewksbury, MA), with

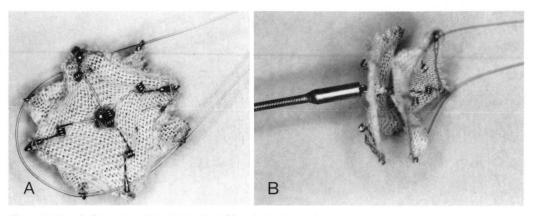

Figure 18.11. **A,** Front view of the double disc ASD umbrella device demonstrating the four arms of one disc attached centrally and a second spring approximately in the middle of each arm. Dacron fabric is sewn to the disc. **B,** Side view of ASD device showing the two discs slightly pulled apart from each other.

radiopaque markers spaced 1 cm apart, is located in the descending thoracic aorta at the level of the left atrial cavity. These markets enable measurement of the size of the atrial defect with accurate correction for magnification.

Thereafter the venous catheter is exchanged for a vascular sizing balloon catheter (USCI Angiographic Systems, Tewksbury, MA), which is placed over a flexible guidewire into the left atrial cavity. The balloon is inflated in the left atrium to a size that exceeds the size of the atrial defect. The balloon is retracted against the left atrial aspect of the atrial septum, and gentle traction is applied to the catheter as the balloon is gradually deflated

(Fig. 18.12*A*, *B*). When the balloon "pops through" the defect, the balloon dimension is measured fluoroscopically and echocardiographically. This measurement represents what is called the "stretched diameter" of the atrial defect. A device twice the size of the "stretched diameter" of the atrial defect is selected to be implanted.

A special long 11-F sheath is then advanced over a flexible guidewire into the left atrial cavity. The delivery catheter is advanced through the sheath, and the distal arms of the occluder are extruded from the delivery pod into the sheath and then opened in the left atrial cavity. The entire occluder system is withdrawn until the distal arms

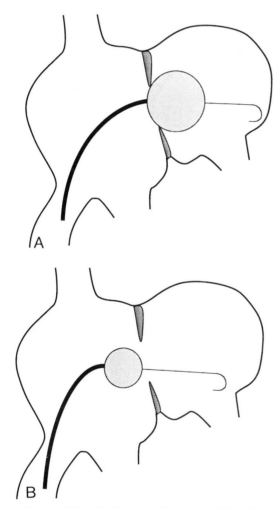

Figure 18.12. **A,** Diagrammatic representation of a secundum atrial septal defect with a sizing balloon inflated larger than the atrial defect in the left atrium and withdrawn against the septum. **B,** The balloon has been partially deflated to allow it to come across the defect, to measure the "stretched diameter."

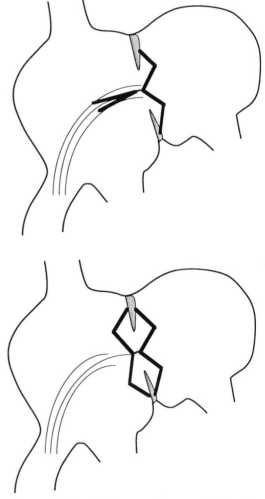

Figure 18.13. **A,** Diagrammatic representation of a secundum atrial septal defect with a long sheath in the left atrium and the distal (left atrial) arms of the occluder opened and pulled against the left side of the atrial septum. **B,** The sheath has been withdrawn into the right atrium and the proximal (right atrial) arms have opened and are seated on the right side of the atrial septum.

begin to engage the left side of the interatrial septum (Fig. 18.13*A*). The sheath is then withdrawn over the proximal arms of the occluder allowing the proximal arms to spring open and engage the right side of the interatrial septum (Fig. 18.13*B*). Appropriate positioning of the device is ascertained fluoroscopically by determining that none of the spring arms of one umbrella overlap the arms of the opposite umbrella disc. Once proper positioning of the device is confirmed, the device is released from the delivery catheter. If proper position is not attained, this device can be withdrawn into the sheath and removed and a second device implanted.

Transesophageal echocardiography (TEE) is now routinely used at our institution during the catheterization procedure to aid in determining the position and size of the defect, to determine whether there are multiple atrial defects, and to facilitate the proper placement of the closure device. The pediatric patients are placed under general anesthesia and intubated, and an 11-mm TEE probe (Hewlett-Packard, Andover, MA) is passed into the esophagus for imaging of the interatrial septum.

Comprehensive TEE examinations are performed, using a sequence of transducer positions and tomographic sections, as has been described by workers at the Mayo Clinic.[25] Transducer positioning is selected to provide optimum imaging of the interatrial septum, which is best examined in short-axis and four-chamber imaging planes. Imaging is continuous and performed simultaneously with fluoroscopy during the closure procedure. The TEE probe remains in the esophagus a maximum of 30 min in the smaller patients to prevent damage to the surrounding structures.

Clinical Results

Twelve patients have undergone attempted transcatheter closure of their ASD using this technique at our hospital (Table 18.3). The indications for closure are the clinical presence of an atrial-level shunt with echocardiographic confirmation of a secundum ASD. The patients ranged in age from 13 months to 45 years and in weight from 11.6 to 77 kg. The diagnosis was isolated secundum atrial septal defect in 8, residual atrial septal defect following an arterial switch procedure for transposition of the great arteries in 2 patients, and following a Fontan procedure in one patient. One patient had severe pulmonary stenosis along with a secundum ASD and underwent balloon valvuloplasty and closure of the atrial defect. In 10 patients, the shunt at the atrial level was left to right with a $Q_p:Q_s$ ratio ranging from 1.5 to 2.8. Two patients had right-to-left flow leading to hypoxemia, one following an arterial switch for transposition of the great arteries and one following

Table 18.3.
Clinical Data for ASD Closure

				Atrial Septal Defect Size						
Pt #	Diagnosis	Age (yrs)	Wt (kg)	Precordial Echo (mm)	TEE (mm)	Angiography (mm)	Balloon Sizing (mm)	Occluder Size (mm)	$Q_p:Q_s$	Clinical Result
1	ASD	12	29.0	10		10	15	28	2.0	implanted/closed
2	ASD	9	50.0	8		4	12	28	1.5	implanted/closed
3	d-TGA, S/P arterial switch	1	11.6	9		10	14	28	1.6	not implanted
4	d-TGA, S/P arterial switch	4	15.5	8		8	10	23	0.9	implanted/closed
5	ASD	2	12.5	12		12	17	33	2.8	implanted/closed
6	ASD	4	19.3	10	10	10	12	23	1.9	implanted/small residual L-R shunt
7	ASD	8	37.0	10	12	12	17	33	2.0	implanted/closed
8	ASD	45	77.0	15	18	18	24	40	2.1	implanted/closed
9	PS, ASD	4	13.7	8		10	13	28	1.8	implanted/closed
10	mitral atresia, S/P Fontan	3	14.6	4		6,4		17,17	0.6	implanted/closed
11	ASD	10	42.0	12	12	12	14	28	1.8	implanted/closed
12	ASD	16	66	10	13	13	17	33	2.5	implanted/closed

ASD = atrial septal defect; d-TGA = d-transposition of the great arteries; PS = pulmonic stenosis.

a Fontan procedure. Defect diameter ranged from 4 to 18 mm as measured from both transthoracic and transesophageal echocardiography. The stretched diameter measured during catheterization ranged from 10 to 24 mm and averaged 37% larger than measured by echocardiography.

The device was implanted in 11 of the 12 patients, and the atrial defect was completely closed in 10 patients. In one patient there was a tiny residual left-to-right shunt seen by color flow Doppler with no clinical evidence of a residual ASD. Unsuccessful implantation occurred in the youngest patient, age 13 months, and will be reattempted when he is older.

In two patients, proper placement of the device could not be attained during an initial procedure. Repeat attempts were made with the use of TEE, and successful implantation with complete closure was accomplished. Presently, all procedures are performed with both fluoroscopic and TEE monitoring.

CASE STUDIES

An 11-year-old weighing 42 kg presented with a classical physical examination for an ASD and was asymptomatic. The $Q_p:Q_s$ ratio was 2.0:1 with normal pulmonary artery pressure. The ASD measured 12 mm both by angiography and TEE (Fig. 18.14*A–C*) and had a stretched diameter of 14 mm (Fig. 18.15*A, B*). A 28-mm device was inserted without difficulty under simultaneous fluoroscopic and TEE monitoring. During implantation, TEE provided visualization of the defect and its margins and was used to ascertain that the multiple arms of the device were properly aligned and well seated on both sides of the atrial septum (Fig. 18.16*A–C*). Following release of the device, color flow mapping confirmed closure, and no further angiography was necessary. In the hepato-clavicular view, the TEE probe did not interfere with fluoroscopy (Fig. 18.16*A*). The patient was discharged home the next day, and long-term follow-up has demonstrated continued proper position of the umbrella with no residual shunt.

A three-year-old weighing 14.6 kg underwent a Fontan procedure for mitral atresia and single ventricle. Following the surgery, he was noted to be severely cyanotic with an arterial saturation of 75%. Cardiac catheterization 10 days after surgery demonstrated a significant right-to-left shunt with two separate defects between the intra-atrial tunnel and the pulmonary venous atrium, each measuring 4–5 mm in diameter (Fig. 18.17*A*). Two separate 17-mm devices were placed in each defect (Fig. 18.17*B*), and the shunt was eliminated. The patient was discharged two days after the procedure with an arterial saturation of 95%.

A 45-year-old woman weighing 77 kg presented with a history of atrial flutter and mild exertional intolerance. Cardiac catheterization demonstrated a $Q_p:Q_s$ of 2:1 with an ASD that measured 18 mm by echocardiography and had a stretched diameter of 24 mm. A 40-mm device was inserted, and TEE demonstrated proper position of the device (Fig. 18.18) with only minimal residual shunting. Follow-up with repeat echocardiography has demonstrated closure of the defect. Her symptoms have improved, and her atrial flutter is well controlled.

COMPLICATIONS

The only significant complication that has occurred has been embolization of the device to the right ventricle in one patient following release of the umbrella. This was retrieved with a basket retrieval catheter and pulled out the femoral vein. This procedure was done initially without TEE, and the device had not been positioned properly. Subsequently, with the aid of TEE, an umbrella was placed with complete closure of the defect.

In the only unsuccessful procedure in the 13-month-old, the opened device was pulled through the defect still attached to the delivery system. The device became lodged in the iliac vein as the venous system was too small to remove the umbrella, and a surgical procedure was required to remove the device.

There have been no complications related to the use of TEE.

OTHER CONCLUSIONS

Atrial septal defects up to 20 mm in diameter can now be effectively closed using the transcatheter method. This technique may be applied to pediatric and adult patients with simple ostium secundum defects and will avoid the need for open-heart surgery. This technique will be especially useful in patients with right-to-left atrial shunts following open-heart surgery and in adults with paradoxical emboli associated with small atrial defects or a patent foramen ovale.[26] The technique may also be useful to close created ASDs following some Fontan procedures.

CLOSURE OF VENTRICULAR SEPTAL DEFECTS

With the success of transcatheter closure of both the PDA and the ASD, it became possible to apply these same principles to close defects in the

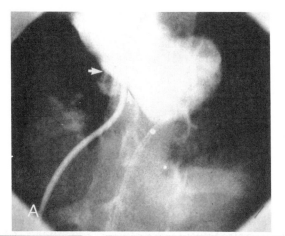

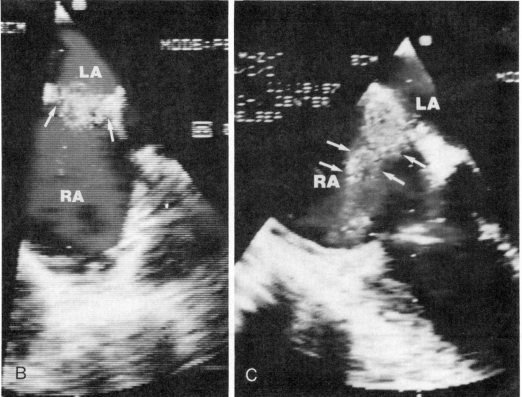

Figure 18.14.   A, A four-chamber angiographic projection of a left atrial angiogram with the atrial septal defect (straight arrows) well delineated in the middle of the atrial septum. A marker catheter is in the descending aorta. **B,** Short-axis transesophageal scan of atrial septum, showing atrial septal defect (arrows) with shunt flow (area between arrows) from the LA to the RA. **C,** Four-chamber transesophageal scan demonstrating the atrial septal defect. Shunt flow from LA to RA is seen as a jet across the defect (between the straight arrows). LA = left atrium; RA = right atrium.

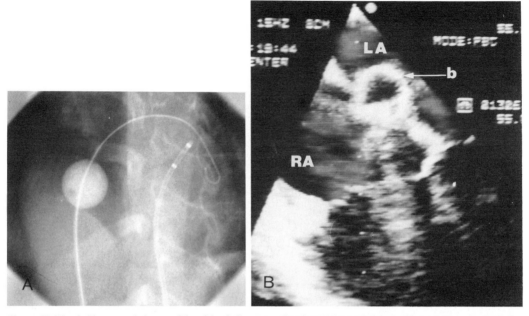

Figure 18.15. **A,** Fluoroscopic image of the sizing balloon crossing the atrial septal defect with a marker catheter in the descending aorta. **B,** Four-chamber transesophageal scan of interatrial septum. Sizing balloon (*b*) is pulled through the atrial defect to obtain the "stretched diameter" of the defect. LA = left atrium; RA = right atrium; b = balloon.

ventricular septum. The initial approach involved the use of the PDA umbrella to close both postinfarction and certain congenital ventricular septal defects.[18] Since the right side of the septum is heavily trabeculated, it was felt to be too difficult to cross a muscular defect from the right side. Accordingly a double catheter approach was designed (Fig. 18.19). A balloon end-hole catheter was passed in a retrograde manner from the femoral artery to the left ventricle and manipulated across the VSD, sometimes with the help of a wire, and then placed in either the pulmonary artery or the right atrium. A 400-cm exchange wire was then passed through the catheter and retrieved either from the internal jugular vein for defects in the apical or midmuscular septum or from the femoral vein for defects in the membranous septum. After withdrawal of the wire out the venous system, a long sheath was introduced and advanced through the VSD under fluoroscopic guidance. The ductal umbrella was placed in the defect using a similar approach as for PDA closure. The distal arms were opened in the left ventricle and pulled against the left side of the ventricular septum. The proximal arms were then released on the right side of the septum. As seen in Figure 18.20, this approach met with some success and demonstrated it was possible to close a VSD in the catheterization

laboratory. However, the PDA device was not large enough to safely close most postinfarction defects (some of which are multiple), and larger devices were needed.

The newer ASD umbrella provides a larger range of device sizes and potentially could close the defects more effectively because of the double spring assembly. Accordingly, a new protocol has been devised for closure of VSDs with the ASD umbrella. The approach is virtually identical to that described by Lock et al.[18] for VSD closure except that the left ventricle is now approached via the atrial transseptal route. Preliminary results for congenital defects have demonstrated the ability to close surgically inaccessible apical or muscular ventricular septal defects in patients with either isolated defects or as part of a combined catheterization and surgical approach to multiple defects.[27] In Figure 18.21*A*, a left ventricular angiogram demonstrates an anterior muscular ventricular defect in a 17-month-old weighing 8.7 kg with a significant left-to-right shunt. The defect was measured both angiographically and with a sizing balloon and found to have a diameter of 12 mm. A 28-mm ASD septal umbrella was placed across the defect, and repeat angiography demonstrated complete closure (Fig. 18.21*B*). This promising technique is presently undergoing a multicenter trial similar to the ASD trial protocol.

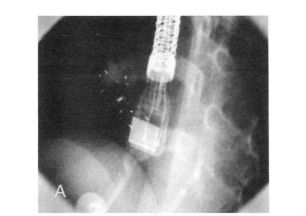

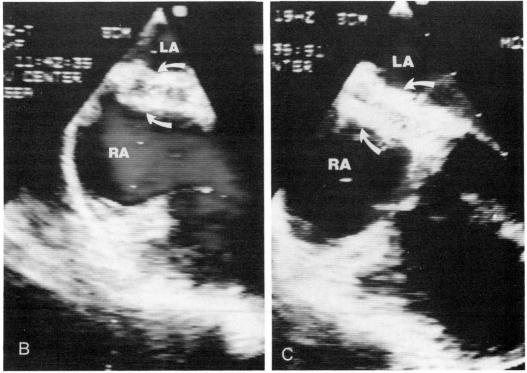

Figure 18.16.   A, Fluoroscopic image of the fully opened umbrella properly aligned along the atrial septum completely covering the atrial septal defect. The transesophageal probe can be seen in the esophagus. **B,** Short-axis transesophageal scan of atrial septum shows the atrial defect to be completely occluded by the two opposing umbrellas (curved arrows). **C,** Four-chamber transesophageal scan of the interatrial septum shows the atrial defect to be completely occluded by the two opposing umbrellas (curved arrows).

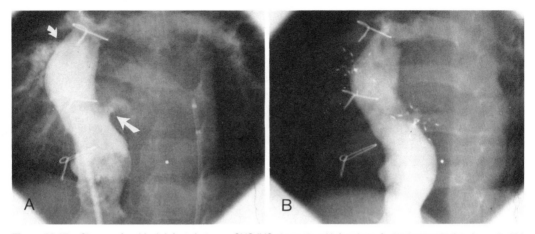

Figure 18.17.   Closure of residual defects between SVC-IVC channel and left atrium. **A,** Angiogram in the channel within the right atrium connecting the IVC to the SVC in a patient following a total caval pulmonary anastomosis for mitral atresia. Two separate residual defects (white arrows) are well seen allowing flow from this venous channel into the new left atrium. **B,** Repeat angiogram following insertion of two 17-mm ASD devices demonstrates closure of both defects.

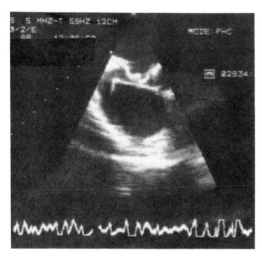

Figure 18.18.   TEE in a 45-year-old patient with a 40-mm ASD device properly straddling an atrial defect.

EMBOLOTHERAPY

Nonsurgical transcatheter closure of blood vessels that are abnormal or detrimental to the patient has been demonstrated to be an effective form of therapy that does not require a prolonged hospitalization or convalescence. There are several devices currently available for embolization and closure such as detachable balloons,[19,28,29] foam,[30,31] and Gianturco coils.[20,32] These have been used for a variety of indications including closure of pulmonary arteriovenous malformations (both congenital and acquired), systemic to pulmonary collaterals, and surgically created systemic to pulmonary

shunts. With the addition of the PDA and ASD closure devices to the available armamentarium, even larger vessels can be closed successfully, and any vessel that can be reached by a vascular catheter can be effectively embolized. Application of these new procedures has avoided the need for further surgery following complex open-heart surgery and has allowed for closure of collateral vessels prior to definitive repair.

Pulmonary Arteriovenous Malformations (PAVM)

These malformations can be congenital and part of a syndrome such as hereditary hemorrhagic telangiectasia[19] or acquired fistulae in the right lower lobe of the lung many years following a superior vena cava–right pulmonary artery anastomosis (Glenn shunt).[33] The PAVM represents a direct communication between the pulmonary artery and the pulmonary vein without an intervening capillary bed. This allows desaturated blood in the pulmonary artery to enter the pulmonary vein leading to systemic desaturation and varying degrees of hypoxemia and cyanosis. In addition, the filter function of the lung is compromised and allows for direct transfer from the venous to the systemic circulation of bland and septic emboli. These thin-walled PAVMs may rupture into a bronchus and lead to hemoptysis.

These malformations have been embolized with both coils and detachable balloons (Fig. 18.22*A*,*B*). Coils are made of stainless steel wires covered with synthetic Dacron strands that coil up to a prespecified diameter. The sizes vary from 2 to

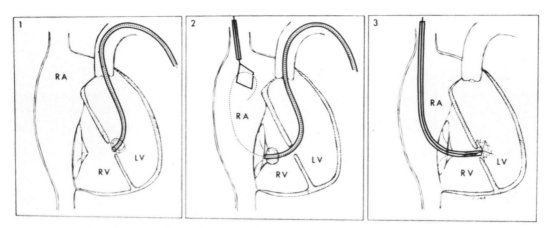

Figure 18.19. Method for transcatheter closure of ventricular septal defects. (1) An end-hole balloon catheter is passed retrograde into the LV and allowed to seat itself on the defect. (2) It is passed across the defect and a long exchange wire is passed through the catheter and retrieved on the right side of the heart and withdrawn out the jugular vein. (3) The long sheath is then passed over the wire from the jugular vein across the VSD allowing placement of the double disc device. (Reproduced with permission from *Circulation 78*:362 1988.)

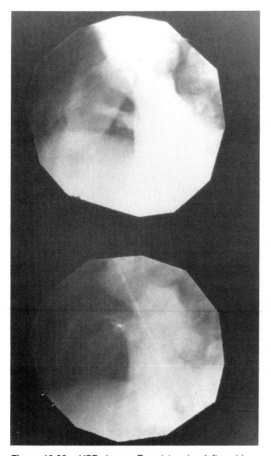

Figure 18.20. VSD closure. Top picture is a left ventricular angiogram demonstrating a moderate ventricular septal defect in the low membranous septum. Lower picture is a repeat angiogram following implantation of a 17-mm PDA device across the ventricular septal defect demonstrating complete absence of a left-to-right communication. (Reproduced with permission from *Circulation 78*:364 1988.)

20 mm in diameter and from 1 to 5 cm in length. A coil with a diameter slightly larger than the vessel to be occluded is chosen, and frequently multiple coils are placed in the same vessel. These coils are delivered to the vessel via an end-hole catheter that is advanced to the site where the coil is to be placed.

Detachable balloons come in two different sizes. The 1-mm balloon is used for vessels up to 4 mm in diameter, and the 2-mm balloon can close vessels up to 8 to 9 mm in diameter. The small balloon is delivered through a 4.9-F catheter and the larger balloon through an 8.8-F catheter. The balloon is delivered to the vessel to be occluded and inflated within the vessel. If not in the proper position, it can be deflated and the position changed. When proper placement is attained, the balloon is easily detached from the delivery system.

Figure 18.23 shows an angiogram in a young patient with a congenital PAVM consisting of a single artery and a draining vein. A detachable balloon was placed in the feeding artery proximal to the malformation, and repeat angiography prior to release of the balloon demonstrates complete elimination of flow through the fistula.

In patients with fistula formation following a Glenn shunt, the feeding vessels frequently are multiple and can be very large (Fig. 18.24A). These patients have presented with both cyanosis and hemoptysis. Frequently we have used a combination of both coils and balloons to try and close the multiple vessels in these patients (Fig. 18.24B, C). If the vessel is larger than 9 mm, large coils are placed in the vessel first, and then a balloon is placed inside the coils and inflated to prevent embolization of the balloon.

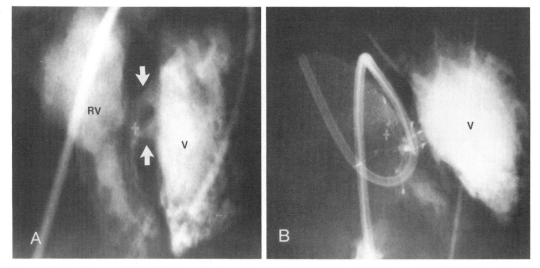

Figure 18.21. Closure of VSD. **A,** Left ventricular angiogram demonstrating an anterior muscular VSD with two sites of entry on the left ventricular side of the septum and one exit site into the right ventricle (white arrows). **B,** Repeat left ventricular angiogram following placement of a 28-mm septal occlusion device shows complete closure of the VSD. (Reproduced with the permission of Dr. James Lock.) LV = left ventricle; RV = right ventricle.

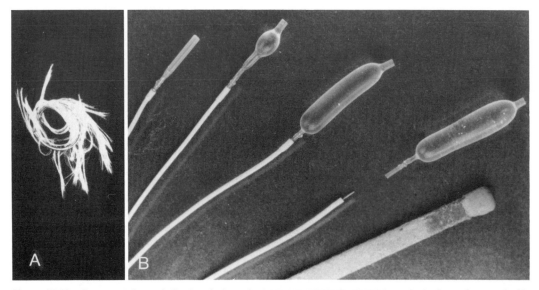

Figure 18.22. Representative embolization devices. **A,** A 10-mm coil made of stainless steel wire and covered with synthetic fibers. **B,** A 2-mm detachable balloon attached to a delivery catheter. The balloon is inflated slowly and when fully expanded is released from the delivery system.

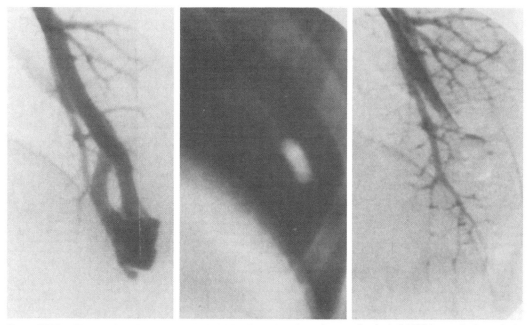

Figure 18.23. Closure of a pulmonary arteriovenous malformation. **A,** Angiogram of a single PAVM demonstrating a single artery and draining vein. A single balloon is inflated distally in the artery and repeat angiography demonstrates distal occlusion with preservation of proximal arterial branches. (Reproduced with permission from *Radiology 169*:664, 1988.)

Systemic to Pulmonary Connections

These communications result from congenital systemic-pulmonary collaterals in patients with cyanotic congenital heart disease or from surgically created shunts between the systemic circulation and the pulmonary artery to maintain pulmonary blood flow. These vessels need to be closed at the time of definitive surgical correction, and frequently they are either very difficult to approach at the time of surgery or significantly lengthen the procedure. Therefore, transcatheter embolization is usually performed to close these vessels in the perioperative period.

In Figure 18.25*A*, an angiogram was performed in a patient following complete repair of tetralogy of Fallot. A persistently patent Blalock-Taussig shunt was found. Several coils were placed in the subclavian artery leading to the left pulmonary artery, and a follow-up angiogram (Fig. 18.25*B*) demonstrated complete occlusion of the shunt, avoiding the need for repeat surgery.

Similarly, a hypertensive systemic pulmonary collateral was identified in a patient with pulmonary atresia and a ventricular septal defect (Fig. 18.26*A*, *B*). This vessel was completely occluded by several coils prior to surgery, eliminating the need for surgical ligation.

Hemoptysis is a well-described complication in patients with systemic collaterals, especially in older adolescents and adults with complex cyanotic heart disease who are not surgically correctable. This occurs when a large bronchial collateral ruptures into a bronchus and may severely compromise pulmonary function in a patient who is already hypoxemic. Transcatheter embolization of the bronchial arteries in these patients may be performed and avoid the need for emergency lobectomy.[31]

Embolization of Miscellaneous Vessels

There are a number of other situations in congenital heart disease that may have previously required surgery for closure of certain blood vessels (or could not be treated at all) that can now be definitively treated with a transcatheter approach.

In cyanotic patients with a Glenn shunt, all the flow from the superior vena cava is drained directly to the right pulmonary artery to increase both pulmonary blood flow and systemic oxygenation. If there is any collateral vessel that allows egress of blood from the head and neck back to the heart, bypassing the superior vena cava, the Glenn shunt is less effective. Figure 18.27*A* is an angiogram of the left innominate vein in a patient with tricuspid

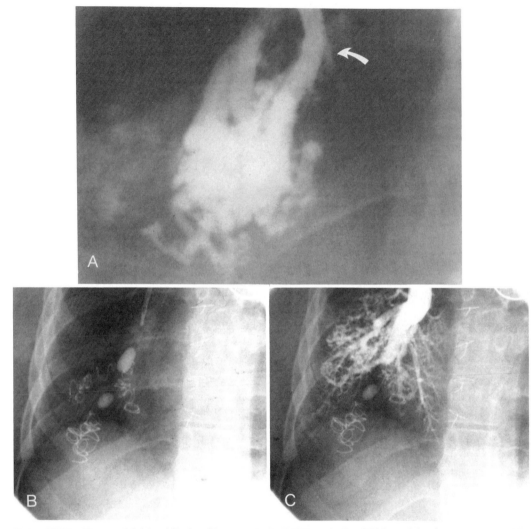

Figure 18.24. Closure of fistulae following Glenn shunt. **A,** Angiogram in the right lower lobe demonstrates multiple fistulous connections to the pulmonary veins. There is a large proximal arterial feeder (white arrow) and two large draining veins. **B,** Fluoroscopic image of multiple coils and several detachable balloons in the distal and proximal portions of the arteries leading to the fistulae. **C,** Repeat angiography in the right lower lobe demonstrates virtual closure of the feeding vessels to the fistulae.

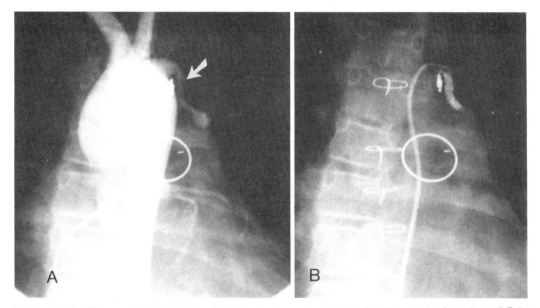

Figure 18.25. Closure of Blalock-Taussig shunt. **A,** Aortogram in a patient following repair of tetralogy of Fallot demonstrating a persistently patent left Blalock-Taussig shunt. **B,** Two coils were placed in the shunt, and repeat angiography confirms complete closure.

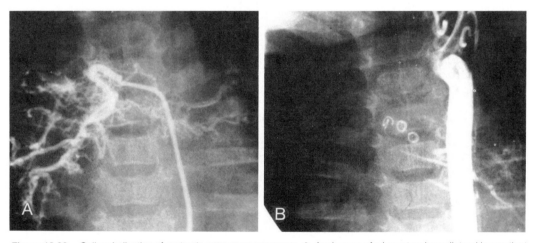

Figure 18.26. Coil embolization of systemic-pulmonary collaterals. **A,** Angiogram of a hypertensive collateral in a patient with pulmonary atresia and VSD prior to definitive surgical correction of the congenital defects. There are no obvious areas of narrowing within this vessel originating from the descending aorta. **B,** Repeat angiography in the descending aorta following placement of three coils in the proximal part of the collateral shows complete closure of the vessel.

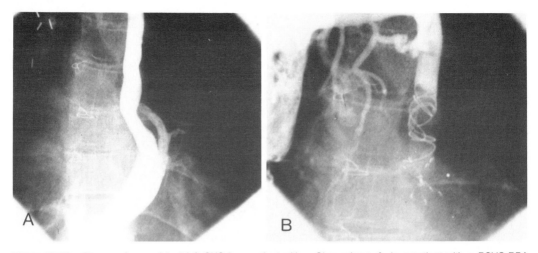

Figure 18.27. Closure of a persistent left SVC in a patient with a Glenn shunt. **A,** in a patient with a RSVC-RPA anastomosis Angiogram demonstrates a persistent left SVC draining to the coronary sinus. **B,** Following placement of a 17-mm PDA umbrella in the mid-portion of the LSVC and several large coils proximal to the device, a repeat angiogram demonstrates complete closure of the vessel.

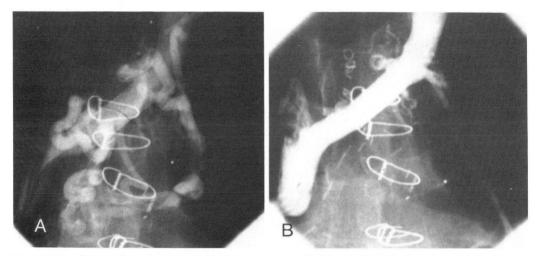

Figure 18.28. Closure of innominate vein to left atrial collaterals. **A,** Contrast injection in the innominate vein in a patient following a Fontan procedure demonstrates several collaterals draining venous blood directly to the left atrium. **B,** Following placement of multiple coils in these collaterals, angiography demonstrates closure of these anomalous vessels.

atresia and a Glenn shunt. There is a persistent left superior vena cava draining blood to the coronary sinus bypassing the right pulmonary artery. A large PDA umbrella was placed in this vessel proximal to the coronary veins to occlude this vessel (Fig. 18.27B). Proximal to the PDA occluder, several large coils were placed to ensure complete closure. Coils alone would have embolized to the heart, and the ductal occluder prevented their migration to the heart. The combination of these two devices for embolization allowed for safe and effective closure leading to improved flow in the Glenn shunt and improved oxygenation.

Figure 18.28A shows an angiogram in the innominate vein in a patient with single ventricle and a Fontan procedure who has moderate cyanosis. There were multiple collaterals connecting the left innominate vein directly to the left atrium, causing the patient to have a right-to-left shunt with hypoxemia. Multiple coils were placed in several of these vessels to eliminate this right-to-left shunt, and follow-up angiography shows virtual elimination of flow through the collaterals (Fig. 18.28B). There was significant improvement in the level of oxygen in the arterial blood.

A young adult presented with a very rare form

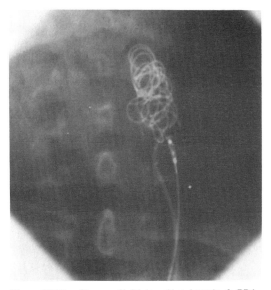

Figure 18.29. Closure of left internal jugular vein. **A,** PDA closure device and multiple coils in the left internal jugular vein effectively closing this vessel.

of severe tinnitus and was found to have a markedly enlarged left internal jugular vein. When this vessel was temporarily occluded with a large balloon catheter all the symptoms disappeared. This syndrome[34] had been previously treated with ligation of the affected jugular vein. Instead of undergoing surgery, a large ductal device was placed in the jugular vein and multiple coils were place cephalad to the device (Fig. 18.29). The internal jugular vein was effectively closed, and her tinnitus resolved.

With the availability of many different type and size devices for occlusion, most abnormal vessels can be effectively embolized and closed without the need for surgery.

SUMMARY

Ongoing clinical trials are proving transcatheter closure of abnormal shunt pathways to be safe, successful, and markedly cost-effective. The most experience has been attained with closure of the PDA. These studies are completed, and the device should soon be available for general use. At our institution, transcatheter closure of PDA is the treatment of choice for children and adults. The experience with transcatheter closure of atrial septal defects is more limited, but, thus far, the results are equally as encouraging. We feel that, eventually, the majority of secundum ASDs will be approachable using this technique. Attempts at transcatheter closure of carefully selected VSDs, both congenital

and acquired, are just beginning, and much more experience must be gained before conclusions regarding its general applicability can be made.

Although the indications for transcatheter closure of these shunt pathways are currently the same as for surgical closure, transcatheter therapy may extend beyond this group of patients. For example, patients who are not considered surgical candidates due to other medical problems such as chronic lung or renal disease may be good candidates for transcatheter therapy. In addition, patients with repeated cerebrovascular accidents or transient ischemic attacks and who are found to have a patent foramen ovale by contrast echocardiography may not be considered candidates for open-heart surgery and yet may benefit from transcatheter closure of the foramen ovale. As more experience is gained, the indications for transcatheter interventions will extend even further.

REFERENCES

1. Kan JS, White RI, Mitchell SE, et al. Percutaneous balloon valvuloplasty: A new method for treating congenital pulmonary valve stenosis. *NEJM 307*: 540–542, 1982.
2. Rashkind WJ, Miller WW. Creation of an atrial septal defect without thoracotomy: A palliative approach to complete transposition of the great vessels. *JAMA 196*:991–992, 1966.
3. Stanger P, Cassidy SC, Girod DA, Kan JS, Lababidi Z, Shapiro SR. Balloon pulmonary valvuloplasty: Results of the valvuloplasty and angioplasty of congenital anomalies registry. *Am J Cardiol 65*:775–783, 1990.
4. Rao PS. Balloon pulmonary valvuloplasty: A review. *Clinical Cardiology 12*:55–74, 1989.
5. Sholler GF, Keane JF, Perry SB, Sanders SP, Lock JE. Ballon dilation of congenital aortic valve stenosis: Results and influence of technical and morphological features on outcome. *Circulation 78*:351–360, 1988.
6. Rocchini AP, Beekman RH, Shachar GB, Benson L, Schwartz D, Kan JS. Balloon aortic valvuloplasty: Results of the valvuloplasty and angioplasty of congenital anomalies registry. *Am J Cardiol 65*:784–789, 1990.
7. Tynan M, Finley JP, Fontes V, Hess J, Kan JS. Balloon angioplasty for treatment of native coarctation: results of valvuloplasty and angioplasty of congenital anomalies registry. *Am J Cardiol 65*:790–792, 1990.
8. Beekman RH, Rocchini AP, Dick M, Snider AR, Crowley DC, Serwer GA, Spicer RL, Rosenthal A. Percutaneous balloon angioplasty for native coarctation of the aorta. *J Am Col Cardiol 10*:1078–1084, 1987.

9. Hellenbrand WE, Allen HD, Golinko RJ, Hagler DJ, Lutin WA, Kan J. Balloon angioplasty for aortic recoarctation; Results of the valvuloplasty and angioplasty of congenital anomalies registry. *Am J Cardiol* 65:793–797, 1990.

10. Kan JS, Marvin WJ, Bass JL, Muster AJ, Murphy J. Balloon angioplasty—Branch pulmonary artery stenosis: Results from the valvuloplasty and angioplasty of congenital anomalies registry. *Am J Cardiol* 65:798–801, 1990.

11. Rashkind WJ, Mullins CE, Hellenbrand WE, Tait MA. Nonsurgical closure of patent ductus arteriosus: Clinical application of the Rashkind PDA occluder system. *Circulation* 75:583–592, 1987.

12. Hellenbrand WE, Mullins CE. Catheter closure of congenital cardiac defects. *Cardiology Clinics* 7(2): 351–368, 1989.

13. Musewe NN, Benson LN, Smallhorn JF, Freedom RM. Two-dimensional echocardiographic and color flow Doppler evaluation of ductal occlusion with the Rashkind prosthesis. *Circulation* 80:1706–1710, 1989.

14. King TD, Mills NL. Secundum atrial septal defect: Nonoperative closure during cardiac catheterization. *JAMA* 235:2506–2509, 1976.

15. Lock JE, Rome JJ, Davis R, Van Praagh S, Perry SB, Van Praagh R, Keane JF. Transcatheter closure of atrial septal defects: Experimental studies. *Circulation* 79:1091–1099, 1989.

16. Lock JE, Hellenbrand WE, Latson L, Mullins CE, Benson L, Rome JJ. Clamshell umbrella closure of atrial septal defects: Initial experience (Abstr). *Circulation* 80:II-592, 1989.

17. Rome JJ, Keane JF, Perry SB, Spevak PJ, Lock JE. Double umbrella closure of atrial defects: Initial clinical applications. *Circulation* 82:751–758, 1990.

18. Lock JE, Block PC, McKay RG, Baim DS, Keane JF. Transcatheter closure of ventricular septal defects. *Circulation* 78:361–368, 1988.

19. White RI, Lynch-Nyhan A, Terry P, Buescher PC, Farmlett EJ, Charnas L. Pulmonary arteriovenous malformations: Techniques and long term outcome of embolotherapy. *Interventional Radiology* 169: 663–669, 1988.

20. Perry SB, Radtke W, Fellows KE, Keane JF, Lock JE. Coil embolization to occlude aortopulmonary collateral vessels and shunts in patients with congenital heart disease. *JACC* 13:100–108, 1989.

21. Anderson RH, Macartney FJ, Shinebourne EA, Tynan M. *Paediatric Cardiology*, London, Churchill Livingstone, 1987.

22. Portsmann W, Wierny L, Warnke H, Gerstberger G, Romaniuk PA. Catheter closure of patent ductus arteriosus: 62 cases treated without thoracotomy. *Radiology Clinics of North America 9*:203–218, 1971.

23. Sato K, Fujino M, Kozuka T, et al. Transfemoral plug closure of patent ductus arteriosus: Experiences with 61 consecutive patients treated without thoracotomy. *Circulation* 51:337–341, 1975.

24. Beekman RH, Rocchini AP, Snider R, Rosenthal A. Transcatheter atrial septal defect closure: Preliminary experience with the Rashkind occluder device. *J Interven Cardio* 2:1–7, 1989.

25. Seward JB, Khandheria BK, Oh JK, Abel MD, Hughes RW, Edwards WD, Nichols BA, Freeman WK, Tajik AJ. Transesophageal echocardiography : Technique, anatomic correlations, implementations and clinical applications. *Mayo Clinic Proceedings* 63:649–680, 1988.

26. Scott WW, Siegelman SS, Harrington DP, White RI. Diagnosis and pathophysiology of paradoxical embolism. *Radiology 121*:59–62, 1976.

27. Goldstein SA, Perry SB, Keane JF, Rome J, Lock JE. Transcatheter closure of congenital ventricular septal defects (Abstr). *JACC 15*:240A, 1990.

28. Barth KH, White RI, Kaufman SL, Terry RB, Roland JM. Embolotherapy of pulmonary arteriovenous malformations with detachable balloons. *Radiology 142*:599–606, 1982.

29. Grinnell VS, Mehringer CM, Hieshima GB, Stanley P, Lurie PR. Transaortic occlusion of collateral arteries to the lung by detachable valved balloons in a patient with tetralogy of Fallot. *Circulation* 65:1276–1278, 1982.

30. Zuberbuhler JR, Ankner E, Zoltun R, Burkholder J, Bahnson H. Tissue adhesive closure of aortic-pulmonary connections. *Am Heart J* 88:41–46, 1974.

31. Kaufman SL, Kan JS, Mitchell SE, Flaherty JT, White RI. Embolization of systemic to pulmonary artery collaterals in the management of hemoptysis in pulmonary atresia. *Am J Cardiol* 58:1130–1132, 1986.

32. Gianturco C, Anderson JH, Wallace S. Mechanical devices for arterial occlusion. *Am J Roentgenol 124*:428–435, 1975.

33. Glenn WWL, Hellenbrand WE, Henisz A. Superior vena cava-right pulmonary artery anastomosis: Present status. In: *Obstructive Lesions of the Right Heart*, Eds: Tucker, B. L; Lindesmith, GG; Takahashi, Masato, Baltimore, University Park Press, 1984, pp. 121–134.

34. Buckwalter JA, Sasaki CT, Virapongse C, Kier EL, Bauman N. Pulsatile tinnitus arising from jugular megabulb deformity: A treatment rationale. *Laryngoscope 93*:1534–1539, 1983.

19

Impact of Interventional Catheter-Directed Techniques on Congenital Heart Repair—A Surgical Perspective

ROSS M. UNGERLEIDER and FRANK HANLEY

Increasing enthusiasm for interventional catheter-directed therapy for a variety of congenital heart defects has resulted in a subtle but definite change in the role of the cardiac catheterization laboratory in the management of infants and children with congenital heart defects. Echocardiography with color flow mapping techniques has, in many instances, replaced the need for cardiac catheterization in establishing the diagnosis of congenital heart defects. Nevertheless, the volume of patients being evaluated in cardiac catheterization facilities remains high due to the variety of therapeutic maneuvers that can be performed in this environment. Surgeons who specialize in the treatment of congenital heart defects have not only learned the techniques that enable safe neonatal cardiac surgery with one-stage reconstruction for a variety of complex congenital heart defects,[1] but they have also learned to incorporate the variety of options provided by their cardiology colleagues to expand the choices available for optimal treatment of these defects. These developments have blurred the traditional distinction between the catheterization laboratory and the operating room and have spawned the emergence of a new collaboration between the interventional cardiologist and the surgeon. This has resulted in great clinical benefit to certain groups of infants and children with complex congenital heart disease.

This chapter is not intended to provide a detailed explanation of how interventional techniques are performed in the treatment of congenital heart disorders. Those techniques are more fully described by our cardiology counterparts in other sections of this book. Instead, we hope to provide a surgical perspective on how interventional catheter-directed technology can enhance the "surgical" approach to congenital heart lesions and on how a committed surgical team can enhance the efforts in the interventional catheterization laboratory.

HISTORICAL PERSPECTIVE

The use of cardiac catheterization as more than a diagnostic procedure dates back to the time that surgeons were first beginning to perform open cardiac corrections using extracorporeal circulation. In 1954, attempts at pulmonary valvotomy were reported using catheter-guided techniques.[2] Nevertheless, catheter-directed therapy was not widely accepted and utilized until the experience of Rashkind and Miller[3,4] produced a clinically successful method of performing an atrial septostomy to enhance atrial level mixing for patients with transposition of the great arteries. These techniques have maintained themselves into the current therapeutic armamentarium, although the manner with which balloon septostomy is performed has been greatly simplified by the ability to perform balloon septostomy in the intensive care unit under echocardiographic guidance.[5,6] In this sense, it is ironic that the first interventional catheter technique to gain wide acceptance has now been, in many cases, removed from the catheterization laboratory and placed in the environment of intensive care as an accepted first maneuver to stabilize patients with transposition. The cardiac catheterization laboratories are now the environment for a variety of other procedures that have a great impact on the field of congenital heart surgery. Figure 19.1 demonstrates the dramatic increase in cardiac catheterization procedures being performed for therapeutic indications at one large children's hospital.[7] This increase in therapeutic catheterization is the reason a chapter such as this has relevance, because these data clearly indicate that cardiologists now possess the ability to treat diseases that were previously only approached by surgeons. It is the prudent congenital heart surgeon who accepts this change in the structure of care for these patients. Some of these techniques have been pioneered and encouraged by surgeons who have attempted catheter balloon angioplasty of otherwise inaccessible areas during the course of an operation to repair a specific defect.[8–10]

The impact of interventional techniques on surgical approaches to congenital heart disease has resulted in several changes. In some cases, certain straightforward lesions can now be corrected in the catheterization laboratory, as a result, the surgeon no longer treats these patients. In other instances, interventional techniques provide a therapeutic option, for patients who are felt to be unsuitable candidates for surgery. This enables preliminary

treatment to be provided without subjecting these infants or young children to the anesthetic and physiologic risks of operative intervention. Interventional techniques can also be employed to change the approach to some defects and can simplify the operations to such an extent that a long, arduous, and potentially risky procedure can be reduced to a shorter and potentially more successful endeavor. This collaboration has led to altered surgical indications, changes in the actual conduct of operations, and creation of new surgical procedures. Finally, the advent of interventional techniques inevitably produces new problems that the surgeon must learn to repair. Oftentimes, these are due to complications of the catheter-directed therapy, and surgeons must be willing and supportive participants in this aspect of the care for these patients.

INTERVENTIONAL TECHNIQUES AS A "TREATMENT OF CHOICE"

Catheter-directed therapy for certain congenital heart defects is now considered the first treatment option, and in these instances, surgical therapy is only rarely necessary. Table 19.1 lists several examples of interventional techniques that have replaced surgical procedures.

Atrial septostomy and septectomy. Atrial septostomy is routinely performed to enhance sys-

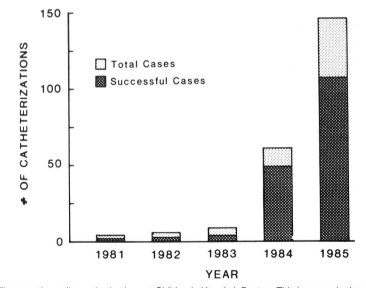

Figure 19.1. Therapeutic cardiac catherizations at Children's Hospital, Boston. This increase in therapeutic catheterizations occurred with total case volumes ranging from 650 (in 1983) to 825 (in 1985), representing an increased incidence of procedures from 1.5 to 18%. (Locke JE, Keane JF, Fellows KE. The use of catheter intervention procedures for congenital heart disease (Editorial). *JACC* 7:1420–1423, 1986 (with permission.)

Table 19.1.
Interventional Techniques That Have
Replaced **Surgical Procedures**

Atrial Septostomy
Atrial Septectomy
Pulmonary Valvotomy
Angioplasty for Recurrent Aortic Coarctation
Angioplasty for Peripheral Pulmonary Stenosis
Angioplasty for Systemic Venous Baffle Obstruction
Embolization of Systemic-Pulmonary Collaterals
Removal of Embolized Foreign Bodies
Ventricular Biopsy

temic and pulmonary venous mixing in patients with transposition of the great arteries and related lesions. As discussed elsewhere in this book, atrial septostomy is also a valuable adjunct for initial palliation in patients with left-sided outflow obstruction necessitating unrestrictive left-to-right atrial shunting (such as in patients with mitral atresia or hypoplastic left heart syndrome) as well as for patients with a need for unrestrictive right-to-left atrial level shunting (such as in tricuspid or pulmonary atresia). Although the Blalock-Hanlon atrial septectomy was initially designed to provide for unrestrictive atrial level shunting, the safe application of Rashkind's balloon technique[3–7,11–13] has largely eliminated surgical septectomy as a consideration for these patients. The safety with which a balloon septostomy can be performed and its role in decompressing the left atrium in patients with transposition have placed balloon septostomy high on the list of recommended therapeutic maneuvers for the initial stabilization of these patients. The fact that balloon septostomy can be safely performed under echocardiographic guidance,[5,6] has made it even more desirable as an initial stabilization maneuver, since it can be so readily performed in the intensive care unit after initial evaluation of the patient.

The use of surgical septectomy is reserved for patients outside the neonatal age group in whom balloon septostomy has been found to be less effective due to thickening of the intraatrial septum. The introduction of blade septectomy[14] provides an alternative to surgical septectomy that is extremely effective and safe. These procedures employ a specially designed catheter to incise a flap of atrial tissue, allowing unrestrictive mixing between the right and left atria. As in surgical septectomy, the communication provided by this technique must be large enough to enable un-

restrictive blood flow. Results with this procedure in experienced hands have been excellent, and although restenosis of the atrial communication can occur, it appears to be no less common than the restenosis rate occurring after surgical septectomy.[15] The combination of balloon septostomy and blade atrial septectomy has all but eliminated the Blalock-Hanlon procedure from surgical textbooks, and it is probably accurate to say that surgeons in the 1990s will no longer utilize the Blalock-Hanlon procedure. Occasionally, when blade septectomy is unsuccessful surgeons may find it convenient to perform a direct atrial septectomy under inflow occlusion or during a short run on cardiopulmonary bypass. This may or may not be combined with a more complete operative procedure, depending on the nature of the patient's congenital heart defect.

Pulmonary valvular stenosis. Infants and children with pulmonary valvular stenosis are now almost exclusively treated with catheter-guided techniques. In most instances, balloon pulmonary valvotomy is now considered to be the "treatment of choice"[7,12,16,17,92] for patients with isolated pulmonary stenosis. For this reason, very few pulmonary valvotomies are performed by surgeons as an initial isolated procedure. This marks a significant evolution in the surgical treatment of this disease over the past decade, since open pulmonary valvotomy was formerly a common surgical procedure. The initial success in terms of reduction in the gradient across the stenotic valve from balloon pulmonary valvotomy can range as high as 90%,[11,16] and there appears to be no significant restenosis over periods of short-term follow-up.[18–20] In this sense, balloon pulmonary valvotomy is possibly a curative procedure. The mechanism by which pulmonary valvotomy works has been evaluated,[21,22] and it is important for the clinician to clearly appreciate that while the procedure usually results in splitting the valvular commissures, valvotomy may also produce a tear in the cusp of a valve leaflet or avulsion of the leaflet from the anulus (Fig. 19.2). Our own experience performing intraoperative balloon valvotomy on stenotic pulmonary valves has confirmed that although commissural splitting occurs in most instances, valves that are particularly dysplastic without well-formed commissures are more likely to split through the substance of the leaflet material itself and can be deformed in such a manner that they are no longer securely anchored by the anulus. Although this does not seem to pose any acute hemodynamic problem with respect to pulmonary

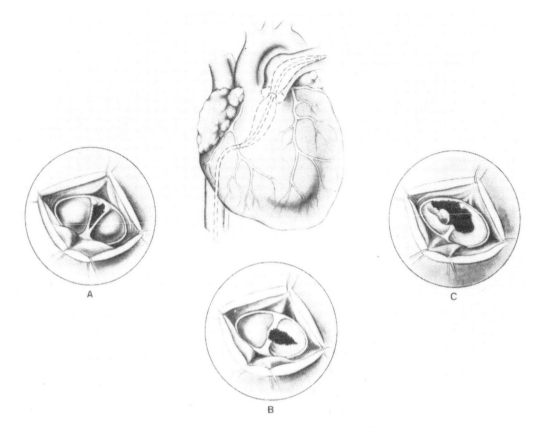

Figure 19.2.   Operative inspection of pulmonary valves after pulmonary valvotomy demonstrates that balloon angioplasty opens stenotic valves by (**A**) commissural splitting, (**B**) cusp tearing, or (**C**) cusp avulsion. (Walls JT, Lababidi Z, Curtis JJ, Silver D. Assessment of percutaneous balloon pulmonary and aortic valvuloplasty. *J Thorac Cardiovasc Surg 88*:352–356, 1984, with permission.)

regurgitation, these anatomic considerations take on greater importance in the treatment of valvular stenosis of the aortic valve. It has also been observed that cusp avulsion is more likely to occur when pulmonary stenosis occurs at both the valvular and infundibular level,[21] and it is recommended by some that this combination should be considered a potential indication for surgical rather than catheter valvotomy.

Older infants and children with pulmonary stenosis can usually be well treated by balloon valvotomy alone. In the neonatal age group[23] the clinical presentation is more complex and requires a more flexible management plan.[92] It is preferable that these neonates initially be treated with a prostaglandin E_1 infusion to provide blood flow through the ductus arteriosus at the time of valvotomy. The most difficult features to performing valvotomy in these patients include obtaining femoral venous access to enable placement of

adequate-sized balloon catheters and advancing a guidewire across what is frequently only a pinhole opening in these valves. Nevertheless, in a reported series of seven patients from the Children's Hospital of Boston[12,23] the procedure was successful in six. These patients were then able to be weaned off of their prostaglandin infusion within a few days after valvotomy. This treatment is not dissimilar from that recommended by Foker[25] for the one-stage surgical treatment of patients with pulmonary atresia and intact ventricular septum whereby a surgical right ventricular outflow patch is placed and a prostaglandin infusion is maintained. This avoids placement of an aorta to pulmonary shunt. The surgical approach to neonates with critical pulmonary stenosis can be dictated by the abilities of the cardiologist at a given institution and may depend in part on the size of the right ventricular chamber.[92] Pulmonary valvotomy is an option if a guidewire can be placed across the stenotic pulmonary valve with maintenance of the pulmonary blood flow by prostaglandin for a few days around the time of valvotomy. If a valvotomy cannot be performed in the cardiac catheterization laboratory or if pulmonary atresia makes such a procedure impossible, then the appropriate surgical approach is open valvotomy or the placement of a right ventricular outflow tract patch. The decision to construct a systemic to pulmonary shunt or to continue maintenance of prostaglandin can then be made based on the adequacy of antegrade flow into the pulmonary artery system.

Peripheral pulmonary stenosis. It is not uncommon for patients with valvular pulmonary stenosis, tetralogy of Fallot, or other complex congenital heart defects to have areas of stenosis in the branch pulmonary arteries. In some instances, these areas of stenosis correspond to areas of dynamic ductal tissue[26] that further constrict after birth. In other instances, peripheral pulmonary stenosis may result from previously placed shunts or other surgical procedures. Finally, the peripheral stenosis may be due to an intrinsic abnormality of the branch pulmonary artery itself. Regardless, these areas of stenosis can result in increased right ventricular pressure and can also worsen pulmonary insufficiency in patients with incompetent pulmonary valves (such as after pulmonary valvotomy or transannular patching to repair tetralogy of Fallot). Treatment options for these patients are directed at enlarging these areas of stenosis, with patch angioplasty being the most frequent surgical consideration. Unfortunately, surgical exposure of the stenosis is oftentimes extremely difficult. The effect of balloon angioplasty on peripheral pulmonary stenosis has been evaluated[27] and appears to result in tearing of the intima with stretching of the vessel lumen that is subsequently fixed by scar tissue to produce a larger lumen size. Although dilation of peripheral pulmonary stenosis is less successful than dilation of pulmonary valvular stenosis, the success rate is still quite reasonable (60–65%), and considering the difficult nature of surgically repairing these problems, balloon dilation of peripheral pulmonary stenosis remains the first appropriate therapeutic option in the majority of these patients.[11,20]

Coarctation of the aorta (recurrent). Although treatment of native coarctation by balloon angioplasty remains controversial and will be considered in a later section of this chapter, it is becoming fairly clear that balloon angioplasty dilation of restenotic areas after coarctation repair has become a desirable option for this problem.

This position has been influenced by the difficulty in providing adequate surgical treatment to these patients as well as by the increasing success obtained by angioplasty techniques.[28–30] Although several surgical approaches are still available for the treatment of recurrent coarctation and may be recommended in certain unique instances,[31] restenosis after aortic arch repair is not uncommon and can be easily treated by balloon angioplasty. Nevertheless, balloon angioplasty produces an intimal tear, and late aneurysms of the aorta can form even when the vessel is surrounded by scar tissue. This is especially true for patients after recurrent stenosis following repair of an interrupted aortic arch.[12,85] These late aneurysms often require surgical intervention.

Embolization of collaterals. Several congenital heart defects present with systemic to pulmonary artery collateral vessels, usually arising from the descending aorta. These are often inaccessible to ligation through a median sternotomy although techniques for exposing these vessels have been described. The experience with embolization of these collateral vessels using gel foam, Gianturco coils, or detachable balloons has been excellent[20,32] and has provided excellent long-term results in over 80% of patients,[11] including young infants.[33] The ability of cardiologists to place catheters selectively into the orifices of small collateral vessels and then to occlude them by embolization of foreign material has greatly simplified the surgical approach to these patients and has largely eliminated ligation of collaterals as a surgical concern in the treatment of this aspect of congenital heart disease. This technology has now been extended to the embolization of previously created systemic to pulmonary artery shunts.[34–36] In many instances this has provided a successful therapeutic option to surgery for the elimination of persistent or recurrent flow through these artificially created shunts.

Other indications. There are several other instances where interventional techniques have replaced surgery as a first option in the treatment of congenital heart defects. Although atrial level repairs for transposition of the great arteries are now being infrequently performed as an elective procedure, patients who received intraatrial baffle procedures (Mustard, Senning) occasionally present with obstruction of the SVC from the intraatrial baffle. Surgical correction of this problem is difficult, and balloon angioplasty of these baffles can often be used as a first option.[37] Although success is variable, several of these patients can be adequately treated by interventional catheter techniques and thus be spared the necessity of undergoing a difficult and risky surgical procedure.[16] Catheter techniques are also employed exclusively for ventricular biopsy in the evaluation of patients with cardiomyopathy and in the follow-up assessment of patients after cardiac transplantation. These catheter-guided biopsies can even be performed in infants[12] and have eliminated the need for surgical assistance with these biopsy procedures. Catheter-guided removal of embolized foreign material such as sheared catheter tips is also extremely successful[11,38,39] and makes surgical intervention for these problems an infrequent occurrence.

INTERVENTIONAL TECHNIQUES AS A LEGITIMATE THERAPEUTIC OPTION

The successful application of the techniques mentioned previously has allowed extention of interventional therapy to other lesions. Future experience with these techniques will dictate their appropriate place in patient management. Table 19.2 provides a list of such controversial indications.

Aortic stenosis. Balloon aortic valvotomy was first reported in 1984,[40] and experience with this technique has shown clear success in a number of instances.[41–43] Although balloon valvotomy of stenotic aortic valves can relieve valvular gradients, the inherent risks of valve destruction leading to early valve replacement make individualization of the application of this therapy mandatory. The morphology of the stenotic aortic valve is an important consideration, and evaluation of the valve and its mobility is essential in planning the therapeutic strategy.[43] Furthermore, careful attention to the details of the aortic valvotomy procedure are crucial in preventing significant aortic regurgitation.[44]

Critical aortic stenosis in neonates is a particularly serious problem, especially because it is often

Table 19.2.
Lesions for Which Interventional Techniques Are Under Investigation

Aortic Stenosis
Native Aortic Coarctation
Patent Ductus Arteriosus
Atrial Septal Defect
Ventricular Septal Defect

associated with other significant cardiac defects such as endocardial fibroelastosis or hypoplasia of the left ventricle or its outflow tract. The mortality for surgical valvotomy in these patients ranges from 9% to 85%,[45] due in large part to the nature of the underlying defects. Balloon valvotomy for these patients can be successful although the mortality may still approach 50% (5 of 12 neonates in one series).[45] Follow-up of these patients suggests that balloon dilation in neonates may not be much better than surgical valvotomy.[12] Nevertheless, the dysplastic nature of the valve in neonatal aortic valvular stenosis may lend itself nicely to balloon angioplasty, and this technique should certainly be considered as a therapeutic option, especially in critically ill infants.[46–50] It is particularly helpful if these infants are first stabilized by infusion of prostaglandin E_1,[51] and after this stabilization, the decision between balloon valvotomy and surgical valvotomy can be made. This decision is often influenced by the nature of coexisting defects. Echocardiography is important in the selection of patients appropriate for catheter valvotomy[43,52] as data from the echocardiogram helps predict the likelihood of post dilation aortic insufficiency and may identify those patients who might receive little relief by balloon techniques. The use of balloon valvotomy to treat *subvalvular stenosis* is more controversial, and although it can be successful in certain selected instances, most cases of subvalvular stenosis are best treated surgically.[20,53]

Coarctation of the aorta. Despite the current enthusiasm for balloon dilation of native aortic coarctation,[5,12,54–59] careful consideration must be given to whether or not this technique has clinical merit.[60] Balloon dilation of a native aorta results in an intimal tear.[61–65] Whether or not these intimal tears will eventually result in aneurysm formation is unknown.[64] Such aneurysms have been reported after dilation of native coarctations by some authors[22,57,66,67] but have not been seen in other series.[55,68–70] Late aneurysm formation has been reported with longer follow-up studies. Furthermore, the surgical approach to native aortic coarctation has been excellent over recent years. Renewed enthusiasm for removal of the area of coarctation, which represents a region of pathology, and primary end-to-end anastomosis of the proximal and distal segments may lead to superb long-term results. The fact that surgical repair of aortic coarctation in neonates can be accomplished with a low mortality, and because the long-term impact of balloon dilation is unknown, one must be cautious in recommending primary angioplasty techniques in the treatment of native coarctation. Balloon dilation, however, is an important consideration for treating the occasional exceptional patient in whom surgical intervention seems ill-advised.

Patent ductus arteriosus. The use of the Rashkind double umbrella to occlude a patent ductus arteriosus beyond the neonatal period[20] is now routine at some institutions, but for the most part, occlusion of the ductus arteriosus by a catheter-introduced device should still be considered experimental. This is largely due to the fact that surgical ligation of a ductus arteriosus carries a negligible morbidity and mortality with an almost guaranteed likelihood of success. Nevertheless, as experience with interventional techniques improves, it can be expected that closure of a ductus arteriosus beyond the neonatal period may become a safe and acceptable procedure to be performed in the cardiac catheterization suite.

A recent review of the experience at the Children's Hospital in Boston[43] suggests that this technique can be applied safely in the majority of instances with minimal complications. However, it should be cautioned that this is in the hands of experienced technicians. Even in this series, there were some initial problems with embolization of the device to the distal pulmonary arteries as well as with incomplete closure of the ductus, necessitating surgical ligation in some instances and producing a persistent risk of bacterial endarteritis in others.

The fact that a ductus arteriosus can be obliterated with a catheter-introduced device should now enter into surgical decision making, especially for patients who are otherwise high-risk or inappropriate candidates for surgery. It is entirely likely that over the next few years catheter closure techniques will take on an increasing clinical role.[20] In addition to obliteration of the ductus arteriosus, there has been a report of dilation of a stenotic ductus to provide enhanced pulmonary blood flow in a patient with hypoplastic left heart syndrome.[71]

Other intracardiac communications. Closure of atrial septal defects and ventricular septal defects can now also be accomplished by catheter-introduced devices.[72–74] The location of secundum atrial septal defects away from critical cardiac structures makes them particularly amenable to closure by "clam-shell" devices. These can be safely introduced in the catheterization laboratory and appear to endothelialize over several months to produce permanent closure of the atrial septal communication. The ability to close atrial septal defects without surgery takes on unique relevance by enabling congenital heart surgeons to leave atrial septal defects during initial repair of complex lesions, knowing that these can subsequently be closed without requiring further operation. The indications for this will be discussed later in this chapter. Likewise, ventricular septal defects can also be closed by catheter-inserted devices. Selected cases of both residual ventricular septal defects[20] and muscular ventricular septal defects have been successfully closed. Although catheter-directed closure of intracardiac communications cannot currently be considered the treatment of choice at most centers, the feasibility of these techniques is improving and its application will likely become widespread.

Dilation of prosthetic valves. Prosthetic valves within conduits calcify, obstruct, and eventually require conduit replacement. In certain patients, the gradient across a conduit is produced primarily by valve stenosis as opposed to an intimal peel. In these cases, conduit replacement can be postponed by balloon dilation of the conduit valve. This often gives excellent short-term palliation[75] and can, in selected instances, be considered a superb management option. Nevertheless, this approach is by no means curative and will not obviate the need for eventual conduit replacement. It may, however, help to minimize the number of operations necessary, especially for patients who have received conduits in infancy and who might face multiple replacements. The increased use of pulmonary and aortic allografts as valve conduits may reduce the necessity for this type of procedure in the future.

INTERVENTIONAL TECHNIQUES THAT ALTER OR SIMPLIFY THE SURGICAL APPROACH TO CONGENITAL HEART REPAIR

Some congenital heart lesions cannot be totally corrected by interventional techniques, but the application of catheter-directed therapy can alter the surgical approach and, in some cases, simplify an otherwise formidable procedure. By understanding the application of interventional methods, a surgeon can plan an operation to take full advantage of this improved technology and produce overall surgical results that could not otherwise be achieved. These examples, of which several will be given subsequently, provide the most remarkable testimony to the synergistic impact of interventional techniques combined with creative surgical procedures to produce operative results that provide for optimal patient care.

Fontan procedures. With the application of the Fontan procedure to more complex forms of cardiac anatomy, there have recently been recommendations to proceed by stages that slowly prepare the patient physiologically for the hemodynamics after Fontan surgery. In many instances, surgeons have recommended the creation of a bidirectional Glenn shunt prior to completion of the Fontan procedure.[76] Others have recommended leaving an atrial septal defect surrounded by a purse-string and controlled by a subcutaneously placed snare that can be slowly pulled, closing the atrial septal defect over the ensuing weeks following the Fontan operation.[77] The justification for these approaches is that patients receiving a Fontan-type procedure often have high systemic venous pressures at the completion of the operation. Frequently, these high pressures are produced by transient elevations in pulmonary vascular resistance as a result of cardiopulmonary bypass. Unfortunately, these physiologic changes in a patient after a Fontan procedure may result in reduced cardiac output due to inadequate pulmonary blood flow. Staging toward a Fontan procedure by preliminary production of a Glenn shunt or by leaving an atrial septal communication enables maintenance of a forward cardiac output by allowing some of the systemic venous return to flow to the left-sided circulation without crossing the pulmonary vascular bed. Of course, this results in persistent cyanosis, and eventually the communication between systemic and pulmonary venous return will need to be obliterated.

Experience with closing atrial septal defects using "clam-shell" devices[72,74] allows for a staged Fontan procedure requiring only one operation. The surgeon, at the time of operation, simply creates a small atrial level communication that can be percutaneously closed several days to weeks after surgery when the pulmonary vascular resistance has returned toward normal. In this sense, the Fontan procedure is completed by interventional catheter techniques, and the need for a second operation is avoided. This approach has a number of advantages compared to the "purse-string" closure of the atrial communication. At the time of the closure in the catheterization laboratory careful hemodynamic measurements are made before and after temporary occlusion of the defect to assure that the permanent closure will be tolerated. Preliminary experience with this operative technique has been extremely promising and warrants future consideration. It can also be expected that patients with residual atrial septal shunts who present in the years following a Fontan procedure (often with increasing cyanosis) can be best served by catheter-guided closure of these communications, thus avoiding the need for another operative intervention and the consequent risk imposed by placing these patients once again on cardiopulmonary bypass.

Intraoperative angioplasty. In certain instances of peripheral pulmonary stenosis, especially in patients who have shunts and in whom catheter access to the peripheral pulmonary arteries may be limited by catheter techniques, balloon dilation of the peripheral pulmonary lesion can be performed by the surgeon through the opened pulmonary artery at the time of operative reconstruction. Results with these techniques have been very satisfying in several instances,[8,9] and the willingness of the surgeon to perform these maneuvers during the time of operative intervention expands the scope of what the surgeon can do. It also avoids the expense and ordeal of putting the patient through a separate invasive procedure when surgery will be required to repair the defect. Surgeons can also take advantage of the experience gained by the interventional cardiologist and use balloon dilation techniques to perform valvotomy on pulmonary and aortic valves as part of a more complex operative repair. An excellent example is dilation of an aortic valve by retrograde insertion of a catheter across the aortic arch at the time of aortic coarctation repair. The disadvantages of this latter procedure are similar to those of percutaneous aortic valvotomy, especially in the absence of fluoroscopic control to guide selection of balloons. Nevertheless, in selected patients, these techniques can have value.

Simplification of operations. Reconstruction for certain types of complex congenital heart lesions can be complicated by the presence of a number of bothersome secondary lesions including stenotic areas in the distal pulmonary arteries from previously placed shunts, excessive pulmonary blood flow from systemic to pulmonary artery collaterals, or the presence of small muscular ventricular septal defects (VSD) that increase pulmonary blood flow. Many of these problems can be dealt with in the catheterization laboratory prior to operative intervention. This combined approach shortens and simplifies the surgery for certain patients who have multiple complex defects.

The overall management approach to the patient with a complex lesion that includes peripheral pulmonary artery stenosis is a classic example of the collaboration between the cardiac surgeon and the interventional cardiologist. Tetralogy of Fallot accompanied by branch pulmonary artery stenoses illustrates this point. The details of the individual case will dictate the exact approach; however, several general considerations can be outlined. Preoperative balloon dilation of the peripheral pulmonary artery stenosis may allow closure of the VSD at the time of the right ventricular outflow tract (RVOT) reconstruction in certain cases that otherwise would require a second operation for VSD closure. Under other circumstances, balloon dilation after surgical RVOT reconstruction may subsequently make it possible to close the VSD surgically in certain cases where it might otherwise never be possible. Finally in cases with unacceptably high right ventricular pressure after surgical RVOT reconstruction and VSD closure, balloon dilation of peripheral pulmonary artery stenoses may avoid a technically demanding second operation. Numerous other combinations of "surgical" and "interventional" techniques are also possible and depend on the subtleties of the individual case.

The availability of catheter occlusive techniques has created increased flexibility for the cardiac surgeon. For example, the decision to place a systemic to pulmonary artery shunt at the time of pulmonary valvotomy for pulmonary atresia or critical pulmonary stenosis when a "borderline-size" right ventricle is present is made easier knowing that the shunt can be physiologically "removed" without the need for further surgery.

A further example is that of a patient with congenital aortic stenosis who presented after three previous operations that included two aortic valvotomies and then placement of a porcine valved conduit from the left ventricular apex to the descending aorta. At the time of presentation, the porcine valve had degenerated, leading to severe "aortic insufficiency." The patient was studied in the cardiac catheterization laboratory and underwent temporary balloon occlusion of the conduit on the day before scheduled surgery. This was followed by uneventful "orthotopic" anular enlargement and aortic valve replacement without the need to remove or even expose the conduit at surgery.

Catheter-directed techniques for closure of septal defects can particularly influence the surgeon's approach when a septal defect is part of a more complex lesion that will require an extensive surgical approach. In a number of cases, patients have presented with lesions such as transposition of the great arteries and multiple inaccessible VSDs. The approach to these problems has involved preoperative catheter-directed device closure of all inaccessible VSDs (i.e., muscular and apical) followed by total surgical correction of the lesion including closure of any remaining VSDs (usually perimembranous or conoventricular). This type of collaboration can change a prohibitively complex surgical procedure into a manageable one.

Other instances in which interventional techniques may be advantageous would be in management of residual VSDs and ASDs following surgical attempts at closure. Successful interventional closure of residual interatrial communications following atrial level repair of transposition of the great arteries and following Fontan-type operations has been performed. Finally, during neonatal and infant repair of lesions such as tetralogy of Fallot and total anomalous pulmonary venous return, it may be physiologically advantageous to leave a patent foramen ovale or a small atrial septal defect. The benefit of leaving the defect must always be weighed against the possibility that a significant left-to-right shunt that requires future closure may ultimately develop. The option of catheter-directed closure of these communications instead of further surgery can support the surgeon's decision to leave them open.

Unconventional palliation. Although the standard treatment for patients with univentricular anatomy who are cyanotic on the basis of pulmonary stenosis is the placement of a systemic to pulmonary artery shunt until such a time that the patient is a candidate for a Fontan procedure, experience with pulmonary valvotomy in this setting has demonstrated increased pulmonary blood flow and increased systemic oxygen saturation.[12] This eliminates an operative intervention in these patients and allows them to grow to an age and size appropriate for a more definitive Fontan-type procedure. Likewise, pulmonary valvotomy in certain patients with tetralogy of Fallot may provide excellent palliation[20,78] by similarly increasing pulmonary blood flow and reducing cyanosis and allowing these patients to receive correction of their tetralogy lesion at a later date. In both of these instances, careful controlled pulmonary valvotomy can provide an excellent alternative to classical shunt procedures and can be considered as an important part of the surgical decision making.

Although the use of pulmonary artery bands is becoming less commonplace, there are still occasions where patients with univentricular anatomy, who will be candidates for a Fontan procedure, will need to have their pulmonary vascular bed protected from excessive pulmonary blood flow. The use of pulmonary artery bands in these patients is a reasonable alternative to more extensive forms of palliation (e.g., stage one Norwood procedure). The recent development of expandable bands[79,80,90] provides the potential for balloon dilation of the band at a future date to further extend the duration of acceptable palliation.

The initial surgical approach to infants with pulmonary atresia, VSD, and diminutive pulmonary arteries can also be modified because of the potential for subsequent catheter interventional approaches. Instead of creating a systemic to pulmonary artery shunt, a homograft valved conduit is placed between the right ventricle and the pulmonary artery bifurcation, leaving the VSD open. This procedure, like the shunt, provides pulmonary blood flow and encourages pulmonary artery growth. However, it also provides simple access to the pulmonary artery bed so that an angioplasty catheter can be advanced through the conduit to selectively dilate areas of discrete stenosis, which commonly develop in this lesion. When the pulmonary arteries have enlarged and the discrete stenoses have been dilated percutaneously, the VSD can be surgically closed, thus completing a total repair.

Planning for operative procedures. Interventional techniques can also assist the surgeon in planning the proper surgical procedure. An example of this is balloon occlusion of an atrial septal defect in patients with questionable right ventricular anatomy in order to demonstrate tolerance to the absence of an intracardiac "pop-off" and maintenance of the cardiac output via antegrade flow across the pulmonary outflow tract.[81] If patients tolerate balloon occlusion of their atrial septal defect for a period of time in the catheterization laboratory, then the surgeon can close the atrial septal defect with confidence. Furthermore, increased experience with transcatheter occlusion of atrial septal defects may enable these patients to be treated without surgery.

COMPLICATIONS OF INTERVENTIONAL TECHNIQUES THAT REQUIRE SURGICAL REPAIR

It is important for surgeons to understand that the trade-off for acquiring experience in interventional techniques is the occasional production of a complication requiring surgical support. Although many patients will benefit from interventional techniques and be spared the need for surgery or will have the nature of their surgical procedure greatly modified, occasional patients will come to the operating room as a direct result of a failed intervention. Examples of this can include atrial tears after septostomies[82,83] or following blade septectomies.[14] Balloon angioplasty can result in vessel rupture[20] or in the formation of an aneurysm at the angioplasty site several years after the procedure. Some of these aneurysms may require surgical intervention. Balloon valvotomy, especially of the aortic valve, can result in avulsion of the aortic valve cusp producing severe aortic insufficiency requiring immediate operative repair of the valve (Fig. 19.3). A mitral or tricuspid valve can be damaged during balloon septostomy[84] and can occasionally present the surgeon with a complicated problem. Coils used for embolization of collaterals can be inadvertently embolized to the wrong vessel. Fortunately, these coils can also sometimes be removed by interventional techniques.[43] The loss of pulses and injury to peripheral vessels secondary to insertion of the large catheters used for interventional techniques is commonplace and sometimes requires involvement of a cooperative vascular surgeon. The use of heparin and thrombolytic agents to treat arterial thrombosis after catheterization can also delay surgical planning for these patients.

Devices used to close septal defects can dislodge, requiring surgical retrieval, which often requires cardiopulmonary bypass. Devices that have dislodged from their proper place in the heart have been surgically removed from the pulmonary arteries, from various points in the aorta, and from the chordae of the atrioventricular valves. In general, patients tolerate the surgical intervention quite well. The present practice has been to retrieve the device and to simultaneously perform the corrective procedure only if this can be easily accomplished. For example, if a "clam-shell" device dislodges from a secundum atrial septal defect and becomes tangled in the tricuspid valve apparatus, then surgical closure of the defect would be performed at the time of the device retrieval. On the other hand, if the device embolizes to the mid-abdominal aorta, only device retrieval would be accomplished. Further evaluation is then performed before a decision is made as to whether elective surgical closure of the defect or another attempt at device closure should be undertaken.

Occasionally, a device fails to close a patent

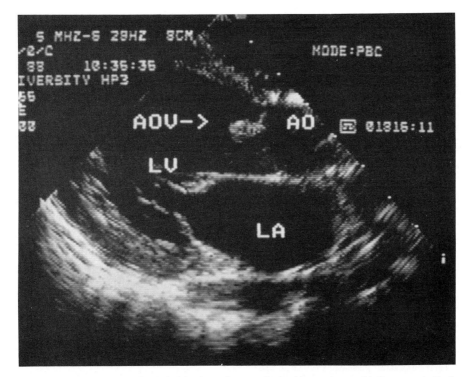

Figure 19.3. This is a long-axis two-dimensional echocardiogram obtained from a 4-year-old after attempted balloon aortic valvotomy for aortic stenosis. Valvotomy resulted in avulsion of an aortic valve leaflet from the anulus (AOV) resulting in severe aortic insufficiency. The patient was taken to the operating room where the aortic valve was repaired resulting in relief of the aortic insufficiency, and she now continues to grow and develop well two years following her surgery. Intraoperative color flow images demonstrating the severity of her aortic insufficiency and the successful outcome after repair are available in the literature.[91] (Key: AO = aorta; AOV = avulsed aortic valve leaflet; LV = left ventricle; LA = left atrium).

ductus arteriosus. If the device embolizes, then the approach outlined previously is taken. The device, however, may remain in place but not completely occlude the lumen, leaving a significant residual shunt. The approach to these patients is surgical ligation of the ductus on an elective basis. Surgically exposing the ductus arteriosus is greatly complicated by the presence of a "clam-shell" device within its lumen, as the risks of serious bleeding are increased significantly. The "arms" of the device have often penetrated the wall of the ductus and may have punctured the wall thickness to such a degree that the tips of the device are clearly visible externally. The surgical dissection is awkward and proceeds slowly in order to avoid hemorrhage. Care must be taken not to dislodge the device during this time. Simple ligation of the ductus includes entrapping the device securely.

It is also important for surgeons to recognize the circumstances in which percutaneous interventional techniques have not been successful. Neither surgical nor balloon angioplasty techniques for enlargement of pulmonary venous obstructions have been successful,[37,86] and future therapy for these patients must still be planned. It may be that interventional techniques will prove most useful if the introduction of stents into stenotic pulmonary veins can produce relief of obstruction. Experimental evidence suggests that this may be possible.[87-88] Balloon angioplasty is not successful in enlarging previous surgical systemic to pulmonary artery shunts. This may not be of considerable surgical importance since with the increasing trends toward neonatal repair,[1] the need for long-lived shunts may be relatively infrequent. Finally, balloon angioplasty is fairly unsuccessful in relieving right ventricular infundibular obstruction in postsurgical patients.[89] Most of these patients will need to have surgical intervention directed at the outflow obstruction.

THE FUTURE

The extraordinary advances made in interventional cardiology over the past decade and the consequent influence on the surgical approach to congenital heart defects make it imperative for surgeons to look toward the future utilization of this technology. With the advent of intravascular guided echo,[24] more precise diagnosis and a better understanding of the results of interventions can be expected. Improvements with device closure techniques should lead to more consistent application of interventional cardiology for the management of routine atrial septal defects, certain types of ventricular septal defects, and systemic to pulmonary artery connections. Finally, the recent application of valvuloplasty techniques to a human fetus suggests an entirely new arena for expansion of this technology. Concomitant advances in fetal cardiac surgery may provide interventional cardiologists with the opportunity of impacting on blood flow patterns in the developing fetus and thereby altering the natural history of congenital heart lesions.

Overall, it is important for the surgeon to recognize the efficacy of standard interventional techniques and to readily accept the advantages of these techniques when making surgical decisions. The enhanced care that is possible for patients with complex congenital heart lesions is in large part due not only to advances in surgical technique but also to the cooperative efforts now available in the interventional cardiac catheterization laboratory.

REFERENCES

1. Castaneda AR, Mayer JE Jr, Jonas RA, Lock JE, Wessel DL, Hickey PR. The neonate with critical congenital heart disease: Repair—A surgical challenge. *J Thorac Cardiovasc Surg* 98:869–875, 1989.
2. Rubio V, Limon Lason R. Treatment of pulmonary valvular stenosis and of tricuspid stenosis using a modified catheter. Program abstract, Second World Congress on Cardiology, Washington, D.C., pp. II-205, 1954.
3. Rashkind WJ, Miller WW. Creation of an atrial septal defect without thoracotomy—Palliative approach to complete transposition of the great arteries. *JAMA* 196:991, 1966.
4. Rashkind WJ, Miller WW. Transposition of the great arteries: Results of palliation by balloon atrioseptostomy in thirty-one infants. *Circulation* 38:453, 1968.
5. Allan LD, Leanage R, Wainwright R, et al. Balloon atrial septostomy under two dimensional echocardiographic control. *Br Heart J* 47:41, 1982.
6. Lin AE, DiSessa TG, Williams RG, et al. Balloon and blade atrial septostomy facilitated by two dimensional echocardiography. *Am J Cardiol* 57:273, 1986.
7. Lock JE, Keane JF, Fellows KE. The use of catheter intervention procedures for congenital heart disease (Editorial). *JACC* 7:1420–1423, 1986.
8. Walls JT, Lababidi Z, Curtis JJ. Operative balloon pulmonary valvuloplasty. *J Thorac Cardiovasc Surg* 93:792–793, 1987.
9. Pfeiffer RB Jr, String ST. Adjunctive use of the balloon dilatation catheter during vascular reconstructive procedures. *J Vascular Surg* 3:841–845, 1986.
10. Murphy JD, Sands BL, Norwood WI. Intraoperative balloon angioplasty of aortic coarctation in infants with hypoplastic left heart syndrome. *Am J Cardiol* 59:949–951, 1987.
11. Hoffer FA, Fellows KE, Wyly JB, Lock JE. Therapeutic catheter procedures in pediatrics. *Pediatric Clinics of North America* 32:1461–1476, 1985.
12. Zeevi B, Perry SB, Keane JF, Mandell VS, Lock JE. Interventional cardiac procedures in neonates and infants: State of the art. *Clinics in Perinatology* 15:633–658, 1988.
13. Rashkind WJ. Transcatheter treatment of congenital heart disease. *Circulation* 67:711–716, 1983.
14. Park SC, Neches WH, Mullins CE, et al. Blade atrial septostomy: Collaborative study. *Circulation* 66:258–266, 1982.
15. Perry SB, Lang P, Keane JF, Jonas RA, Sanders SP, Lock JE. Creation and maintenance of an adequate interatrial communication in left atrioventricular valve atresia or stenosis. *Am J Cardiol* 58:622–626, 1986.
16. Miller GAH. Balloon valvuloplasty and angioplasty in congenital heart disease. *Br Heart J* 54:285–289, 1985.
17. Lababidi Z, Wu J. Percutaneous balloon pulmonary valvuloplasty. *Am J Cardiol* 52:560–562, 1983.
18. Radtke W, Keane JF, Fellows KE, et al. Percutaneous balloon valvotomy of congenital pulmonary stenosis using oversized balloons. *J Am Coll Cardiol* 8:909, 1986.
19. Ring JC, Kulik TJ, Burke BA, et al. Morphologic changes induced by dilation of the pulmonary valve annulus with overlarge balloons in normal newborn lambs. *Am J Cardiol* 55:210, 1984.
20. Perry SB, Keane JF, Lock JE. Interventional catheterization in pediatric congenital and acquired heart disease. *Am J Cardiol* 61:109G–117G, 1988.
21. Walls JT, Lababidi Z, Curtis JJ, Silver D. Assessment of percutaneous balloon pulmonary and aortic valvuloplasty. *J Thorac Cardiovasc Surg* 88:352–356, 1984.
22. Walls JT, Lababidi Z, Curtis JJ. Morphologic effects of percutaneous balloon pulmonary valvuloplasty. *Southern Medical Journal* 80:475–478, 1987.
23. Zeevi B, Keane JF, Fellows KE, Lock JE. Balloon dilation of critical pulmonary stenosis in the first week of life. *JACC* 11:821–824, 1988.
24. Harrison JK, Sheikh KH, Davidson CJ, Kisslo KB, Leithe ME, Himmelstein SI, Kanter RJ, Bashore TM. Balloon angioplasty of coarctation of the aorta evaluated using intravascular ultrasound. *JACC* 15: 906–909, 1990.

25. Foker JE, Braulin EA, St. Cyr JA, et al. Management of pulmonary atresia with intact ventricular septum. *J Thorac Cardiovasc Surg 92*:706, 1986.

26. Momma K, Takao A, Imai Y, Kurosawa H. Obstruction of the central pulmonary artery after shunt operations in patients with pulmonary atresia. *Br Heart J 57*:534–542, 1987.

27. Edwards BS, Lucas RV Jr, Lock JE, Edwards JE. Morphologic changes in the pulmonary arteries after percutaneous balloon angioplasty for pulmonary arterial stenosis. *Circulation 71*:195–201, 1985.

28. Lock JE, Bass JL, Amplatz K, Fuhrman BP, Castaneda-Zuniga W. Balloon dilation angioplasty of aortic coarctations in infants and children. *Circulation 68*:109–116, 1983.

29. Lababidi ZA, Daskalopoulos DA, Stoeckle H Jr. Transluminal balloon coarctation angioplasty: Experience with 27 patients. *Am J Cardiol 54*:1288–1291, 1984.

30. Singer MI, Rowen M, Dorsey TJ. Transluminal aortic balloon angioplasty for coarctation of the aorta in the newborn. *Am Heart J 103*:131–132, 1982.

31. Ungerleider RM, Ebert PA. Midline approach to aortic coarctation in infants and children. *Ann Thorac Surg 44*:517–522, 1987.

32. Perry SB, Radtke W, Fellows KE, Keane JF, Lock JE. Coil embolization to occlude aortopulmonary collateral vessels and shunts in patients with congenital heart disease. *JACC 13*:100–108, 1989.

33. Fuhrman BP, Bass JL, Castaneda-Zuniga W, Amplatz K, Lock JE. Coil embolization of congenital thoracic vascular anomalies in infants and children. *Circulation 70*:285–289, 1984.

34. Culham JAG, Izukawa T, Burns JE, et al. Embolization of a Blalock-Taussig shunt in a child. *AJR 137*:413–415, 1981.

35. Fellows KE. Therapeutic catheter procedures in congenital heart disease: Current status and future possibilities. *Cardiovasc Intervent Radiol 7*:170–177, 1984.

36. Morag B, Rubinstein ZJ, Smolinsky A, et al. Percutaneous closure of a Blalock-Taussig shunt. *Cardiovasc Intervent Radiol 7*:218–220, 1984.

37. Lock JE, Bass JL, Castaneda-Zuniga W, Fuhrman BP, Rashkind WJ, Lucas RV Jr. Dilation angioplasty of congenital or operative narrowings of venous channels. *Circulation 70*:457–464, 1984.

38. Dworsky M, Kohaut E, Jander HP, et al. Neonatal embolism due to thrombosis of the ductus arteriosus. *Radiology 134*:645–646, 1980.

39. Smith PL. Umbilical catheter retrieval in the premature infant. *J Pediatr 93*:499–502, 1978.

40. Lababidi Z, Wu J, Walls JT. Percutaneous balloon aortic valvuloplasty. Results in 23 patients. *Am J Cardiol 53*:194–197, 1984.

41. Sanchez GR, Mehta AV, Ewing LL, Brickley SE, Anderson TM, Black IFS. Successful percutaneous balloon valvuloplasty of the aortic valve in an infant. *Pediatr Cardiol 6*:103–106, 1985.

42. Rao PS, Thapar MK, Wilson AD, Levy JM, Chopra PS. Intermediate-term follow-up results of balloon aortic valvuloplasty in infants and children with special reference to causes of restenosis. *Am J Cardiol 64*:1356–1360, 1989.

43. Rome JJ, Lock JE. New developments in pediatric interventional heart catheterization (Editorial). *G Ital Cardiol 18*:255–258, 1988.

44. Sholler GF, Keane JF, Perry SB, Sanders SP, Lock JE. Balloon dilation of congenital aortic valve stenosis. *Circulation 78*:351–360, 1988.

45. Zeevi B, Keane JF, Castaneda AR, Perry SB, Lock JE. Neonatal critical valvar aortic stenosis. A comparison of surgical and balloon dilation therapy. *Circulation 80*:831–839, 1989.

46. Brown JW, Robinson RJ, Waller BF. Transventricular balloon catheter aortic valvotomy in neonates. *Ann Thorac Surg 39*:376, 1985.

47. Lababidi Z, Weinhaus L. Successful balloon valvuloplasty for neonatal critical aortic stenosis. *Am Heart J 112*:913, 1986.

48. Phillips RR, Gerlis LM, Wilson N, et al. Aortic valve damage caused by operative balloon dilation of critical valve stenosis. *Br Heart J 57*:168, 1987.

49. Rupprath G. Newhaus KL. Percutaneous balloon valvuloplasty for aortic valve stenosis in infancy. *Ann J Cardiol 55*:1655, 1985.

50. Waller BF, Girod DA, Dillon JC. Transverse aortic wall tears in infants after balloon angioplasty for aortic valve stenosis. *J Am Coll Cardiol 4*:1235, 1984.

51. Jonas RA, Lang P, Mayer JE, et al. The importance of prostaglandin E_1 in resuscitation of the neonates with critical aortic stenosis. (Letter) *J Thorac Cardiovasc Surg 39*:314, 1985.

52. Sholler GF, Keane JF, Perry SB, Sanders SP, Lock JE. Balloon dilation of aortic stenosis: Influences of valve morphology and technique on outcome. *Circulation 76* (Suppl. IV):554, 1987.

53. Lababidi Z, Weinhaus L, Stoeckle H Jr, Walls JT. Transluminal balloon dilatation for discrete subaortic stenosis. *Am J Cardiol 59*:423–425, 1987.

54. Brodsky SJ, Percutaneous balloon angioplasty. *Am J Dis Child 138*:851, 1984.

55. Lababidi Z, Daskalopoulos DA, Stoeckle H Jr. Transluminal balloon coarctation angioplasty: Experience with 27 patients. *Am J Cardiol 54*:1288, 1984.

56. Lock JE, Bass JL, Amplatz K, et al. Balloon dilation angioplasty of coarctations in infants and children. *Circulation 68*:109, 1983.

57. Marvin WJ, Mahoney LT, Rose EF. Pathologic sequelae of balloon dilation angioplasty for unoperated coarctation of the aorta in infants and children (Abstr.) *JACC 7*:117A, 1986.

58. Morrow WR, Vick III GW, Nihill MR, et al. Balloon dilation of unoperated coarctation of the aorta: short and intermediate-term results. *JACC 11*:113, 1988.

59. Sperling DR, Dorsey TJ, Rowen M, et al. Percutaneous transluminal angioplasty of congenital coarctation of the aorta. *Am J Cardiol 51*:562, 1983.

60. Lock JE. Now that we can dilate, should we? *Am J Cardiol 54*:1360, 1984.

61. Sos T, Sniderman KW, Rettek-Sos B, et al. Percutaneous transluminal dilation of coarctation of thoracic aorta postmortem. *Lancet 2*:970, 1979.

62. Castaneda-Zuniga WR, Lock JE, Vlodaver Z, et al. Transluminal dilation of coarctation of the abdominal aorta. *Radiology 143*:693, 1982.

63. Finley JP, Beaulien RG, Nanton MA, et al. Balloon catheter dilatation of coarctation of the aorta in young infants. *Br Heart J 50*:411, 1983.

64. Lock JE, Niemi T, Burke B, et al. Transcutaneous angioplasty of experimental aortic coarctation. *Circulation 66*:1280, 1982.

65. Lock JE, Castaneda-Zuniga WR, Bass JL, et al. Balloon dilatation of excised aortic coarctation. *Radiology 143*:689, 1982.

66. Boxer RA, La Corte MA, Singh S, et al. Nuclear magnetic resonance imaging in evaluation and follow-up of children treated for coarctation of the aorta. *JACC 7*:1095, 1986.

67. Cooper RS, Ritter SB, Rothe WB, et al. Angioplasty for coarctation of the aorta: Long-term results. *Circulation 75*:600, 1987.

68. Allen HD, Marx GR, Ovitt TW, et al. Balloon dilation angioplasty for coarctation of the aorta. *Am J Cardiol 57*:828, 1986.

69. Rao RS. Ballon angioplasty for coarctation of the aorta in infancy. *J Pediatr 110*:713, 1987.

70. Rocchini AP, Beekman RH. Balloon angioplasty in the treatment of pulmonary valve stenosis and coarctation of the aorta. *Tex Heart Inst J 13*:377, 1986.

71. de Lezo JS, Lopez-Rubio F, Guzman J, et al. Percutaneous transluminal angioplasty of stenotic ductus arteriosus. *Catheterization and Cardiovasc Diag 11*:493–500, 1985.

72. Lock JE, Cockerham JT, Keane JF, Finley JP, Wakely PE Jr, Fellows KE. Transcather umbrella closure of congenital heart defects. *Circulation 75*:593–599, 1987.

73. Lock JE, Block PC, McKay RG, Baim DS, Keane JF. Transcatheter closure of ventricular septal defects. *Circulation 78*:361–368, 1988.

74. Lock JE, Rome JJ, Davis R, et al. Transcatheter closure of atrial septal defects. Experimental studies. *Circulation 79*:1091–1099, 1989.

75. Lloyd TR, Marvin WJ Jr, Mahoney LT, Lauer RM. Balloon dilation valvuloplasty of bioprosthetic valves in extracardiac conduits. *Am Heart J 114*:268–274, 1987.

76. Zellers TM, Driscoll DJ, Humes RA, Feldt RH, Puga FJ, Danielson GK. Glenn shunt: effect on pleural drainage after modified fontan operation. *J Thorac Cardiovasc Surg 98*:725–729, 1989.

77. Billingsley AM, Laks H, Boyce SW, George B, Santulli T, Williams RG. Definitive repair in patients with pulmonary atresia and intact ventricular septum. *J Thorac Cardiovasc Surg 97*:746–754, 1989.

78. Bouchek MM, Webster HE, Orsmond GS, et al. Balloon pulmonary valvotomy: Palliation for cyanotic heart disease. *Am Heart J 115*:318, 1988.

79. Vince DJ, Culham JAG. A prosthesis for banding the main pulmonary artery capable of serial dilation by balloon angioplasty. *J Thorac Cardiovasc Surg 97*:421–427, 1989.

80. Lock JE. Invited letter concerning: Enlargeable prosthesis for banding the main pulmonary artery. *J Thorac Cardiovasc Surg 97*:473, 1989.

81. Bass JL, Fuhrman BP, Lock JE. Balloon occlusion of atrial septal defect to assess right ventricular capability in hypoplastic right heart syndrome. *Circulation 68*:1081–1086, 1983.

82. Neches WH, Mullins CE, McNamara DG. Balloon atrial septostomy in congenital heart disease in infancy. *Am J Dis Child 125*:371, 1973.

83. Sondheimer HW, Webb Kavey RE, Blackman MS. Fatal overdistension of an antrioseptostomy catheter. *Pediatr Cardiol 2*:255, 1982.

84. Attia I, Weinhaus L, Walls JT, Lababidi Z. Rupture of tricuspid valve papillary muscle during balloon pulmonary valvuloplasty. *Am Heart J 114*:1233–1235, 1982.

85. Saul JP, Keane JF, Fellows KE, Lock JE. Balloon dilation angioplasty of postoperative aortic obstructions. *Am J Cardiol 59*:943–948, 1987.

86. Kirklin JW, Barratt-Boyes BG. *Cardiac Surgery*. New York, John Wiley and Sons, 1986, p. 1107.

87. O'Laughlin MP, Vick III GW, Mayer D, et al. Implantation of balloon expandable intravascular grafts by catheterization in pulmonary arteries and systemic veins (Abstr). *JACC 9*(Suppl):131A, 1987.

88. Sigwart U, Puel J, Mirkovitch S, et al. Intravascular stents to prevent occlusion and restenosis after transluminal angioplasty. *N Engl J Med 316*:701, 1987.

89. Zeevi B, Keane JF, Perry SB, Lock JE. Balloon dilation of postoperative right ventricular outflow obstructions. *JACC 14*:401–408, 1989.

90. Rocchini AP, Gundry SR, Beekman RH, et al. A reversible pulmonary artery band: Preliminary experience, *JACC 11*:172–176, 1988.

91. Ungerleider RM, Greeley WJ, Sheikh KH, Kern FH, Kisslo JA, Sabiston DC Jr. The use of intraoperative echo with Doppler color flow imaging to predict outcome after repair of congenital cardiac defects. *Ann Surg 210*:526–534, 1989.

92. Caspi J, Coles JG, Benson LN, et al. Management of neonatal critical pulmonic stenosis in the balloon valvotomy era. *Ann Thorac Surg 49*:273–278, 1990.

Index

Page numbers followed by "f" denote figures; those followed by "t" denote tables.